Culture, Health and Illness

To my daughter Zoe

Culture, Health and Illness

Fourth Edition

Cecil G. Helman MB ChB MRCGP Dip Soc Anthrop

Associate Professor, Department of Human Sciences, Brunel University;
Senior Lecturer, Department of Primary Care and Population Sciences,
Royal Free and University College Medical School, University College London;
Honorary Research Fellow, Department of Anthropology, University College London;
Former Visiting Fellow in Social Medicine and Health Policy, Harvard Medical School, USA

Marquisa LaVelle, PhD
Anthropology

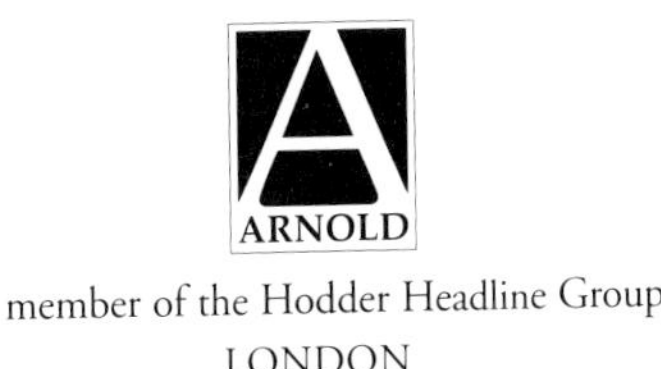

A member of the Hodder Headline Group
LONDON

First edition published in 1984 by John Wright and Sons Ltd
Paperback edition 1985
Second edition published in 1990 by Butterworth Heinemann
Third edition published in 1994 by Butterworth Heinemann
Reprinted 1995, 1996, 1997 (twice), 1998
Fourth edition published in 2000 by Butterworth Heinemann

This impression published in 2001 by
Arnold, a member of the Hodder Headline Group,
338 Euston Road, London NW1 3BH

http://www.arnoldpublishers.com

Co-published in the USA by
Oxford University Press Inc.,
198 Madison Avenue, New York, NY10016
Oxford is a registered trademark of Oxford University Press

British Library Cataloguing in Publication Data
A catalogue record for this book is available from the British Library

Library of Congress Cataloging-in-Publication Data
A catalog record for this book is available from the Library of Congress

ISBN 0 7506 4789 8

1 2 3 4 5 6 7 8 9 10

Printed and bound in Great Britain by The Bath Press

Contents

Preface to the fourth edition

Since the first edition of *Culture, Health and Illness* – a slim, red volume – appeared in 1984, both it and the subject of medical anthropology have come of age. Since that year, the book itself has almost doubled in size and in popularity. In its English language version, as well as in several translations, it has now been used in 37 different countries as a course textbook in universities, medical schools, and nursing colleges. In the USA alone, it has been used as a textbook in over 100 universities or medical schools in different parts of the country.

Also since 1984, medical anthropology has become an established academic subject in many different countries – Western and non-Western, rich and poor. It has also been recognized as an essential part of many international aid programmes and health promotion strategies. At a time of major global health problems – such as AIDS, tuberculosis, malaria, diarrhoeal diseases and malnutrition, as well as the social problems linked to poverty, urbanization and overpopulation – a global, cross-cultural perspective is increasingly necessary. It has now become vital to have some form of overview of the diversity of the world's population, their cultures, social structures, health beliefs and practices, and how this diversity can be addressed in terms of international health policy. This fact was officially recognized by the World Health Organization and UNESCO, when they jointly declared 1996 to be the Year of Culture and Health. The list of topics of interest to WHO and UNESCO, listed in their publication *World Health*, echoed many of the topics described in more detail throughout this book.

Like the three previous editions, this fourth edition emphasizes the role that medical anthropology can play in understanding health problems in a variety of cultural settings, and how to prevent and deal with them. However, the book now includes a large number of new topics, either absent from the first three editions or else insufficiently covered in them. These many additions to the fourth edition include new material and discussion of: the AIDS epidemic and its cultural dimensions; anthropological perspectives on the human lifecycle, especially childhood and old age; children's perception of illness and medical care; refugee health and the experience of collective stress; the problem of 'somatization' cross-culturally; the concept of 'psychosomatic' disorders; the new 'culture-bound syndromes' of the late twentieth century; narratives of illness and misfortune; the effect on self image of medical technology, transplants, *in vitro* fertilization and other innovations; the socio-cultural aspects of physical disability and impairment; the relationship of gender to alcohol abuse; the role of traditional healers (such as the Malaysian *bomohs*) in the treatment of drug addiction; the impact of 'globalization' on global diet, especially in developing countries; the relation of nutrition to cancer risk; the cultural dimensions of tuberculosis prevention; and many others. A large, new section on malaria and the problems of prevention in different cultural contexts has been included, as well as an entirely new chapter on new research methods in medical anthropology.

To help the reader explore the subject of medical anthropology even further, a list of relevant journals and websites has been included. Finally, to supplement the text, a number of illustrations have also been added.

In preparing this book, I would like to thank my family and friends for their support, and to acknowledge the help of many colleagues including Audrey Callum, Alizon Draper, Vari Drennan, Ronald Frankenberg, David Gellner, Arthur Kleinman, Gerald Mars, Hugh MacMillan, Isaac Mwanzo, Ian Robinson, Leslie Swartz, Christiane Woleczko, the Research Council on Complementary Medicine (UK), and also – of course – my loyal and supportive publisher, Dr Geoffrey Smaldon of Butterworth-Heinemann.

As with the first three editions, my hope is that in some way this edition will help readers to understand and deal with many of the health problems, some very major, that we now face in an increasingly diverse, yet interconnected, world.

1 Introduction: the scope of medical anthropology

Medical anthropology is about how people in different cultures and social groups explain the causes of ill health, the types of treatment they believe in, and to whom they turn if they do get ill. It is also the study of how these beliefs and practices relate to biological, psychological and social changes in the human organism, in both health and disease.

To put this subject in perspective, it is necessary to know something about the discipline of anthropology itself, of which medical anthropology is a comparatively new offshoot. Anthropology – from the Greek, meaning 'the study of man' – has been called 'the most scientific of the humanities and the most humane of the sciences'[1]. Its aim is nothing less than the holistic study of humankind – its origins, development, social and political organizations, religions, languages, art and artefacts.

Anthropology, as a field of study, has several branches. *Physical anthropology* – also known as human biology – is the study of the evolution of the human species, and is concerned with explaining the causes for the present diversity of human populations. In its investigation of human pre-history it utilizes the techniques of archaeology, palaeontology, genetics and serology, as well as the study of primate behaviour and ecology. *Material culture* deals with the art and artefacts of mankind, both in the present and the past. It includes studies of the arts, musical instruments, weapons, clothes, tools and agricultural implements of different populations, and all other aspects of the technology that human beings use to control, shape, exploit and enhance their social or natural environments. *Social* and *cultural anthropology* deal with the comparative study of present-day human societies and their cultural systems respectively, though there is a difference in emphasis between these two approaches.

In the UK, *social anthropology* is the dominant approach, and emphasizes the social dimensions of human life. Man is a social animal, organized into groups that regulate and perpetuate themselves, and it is man's experience as a member of society that shapes his view of the world. In this perspective culture is seen as one of the ways that man organizes and legitimizes his society, and provides the basis for its social, political and economic organization. In the USA, *cultural anthropology* focuses more on the systems of symbols, ideas and meanings that comprise a culture, and of which social organization is just an expression. In practice, the differences in emphasis of social and cultural anthropology provide valuable and complementary perspectives on two central issues – the ways that human groups organize themselves, and the ways that they view the world they inhabit. In other words, when studying a group of human beings it is necessary to study the features of both their society and their culture.

Keesing[2] has defined a *society* as 'a population marked by relative separation from surrounding populations and a distinctive culture'. The boundaries between societies are sometimes vague, but in general each has its own territorial and political identity. In studying any society, anthropologists investigate the ways that members of that society organize themselves into various groups, hierarchies and roles. This organization is revealed in its dominant ideology and religion, in its political and economic systems, in the types of bonds that kinship or close residence creates between people, and in the division of labour between different people from different backgrounds and different genders. The rules that underpin the organization of a society and the ways that it is symbolized and transmitted are all part of that society's culture.

The concept of culture

What then is *culture* – a word that will be used on many occasions throughout this book? Anthropologists have provided many definitions of it, perhaps the most famous being Tylor's[3] definition, in 1871: 'That complex whole which includes knowledge, belief, art, morals, law, custom and any other capabilities and habits acquired by man as a member of society'. Keesing[4], in his definition, stresses the ideational aspect of culture. That is, cultures comprise: 'Systems of shared ideas, systems of concepts and rules and meanings that underlie and are expressed in the ways that human beings live'.

From these definitions one can see that culture is a set of guidelines (both explicit and implicit) that individuals inherit as members of a particular society, and that tell them how to view the world, how to experience it emotionally, and how to behave in it in relation to other people, to supernatural forces or gods, and to the natural environment. It also provides them with a way of transmitting these guidelines to the next generation – by the use of symbols, language, art and ritual. To some extent, culture can be seen as an inherited 'lens' through which the individual perceives and understands the world that he inhabits and learns how to live within it. Growing up within any society is a form of enculturation, whereby the individual slowly acquires the cultural 'lens' of that society. Without such a shared perception of the world, both the cohesion and continuity of any human group would be impossible.

The American anthropologist Edward T. Hall[5] has proposed that in each human group there are actually three different *levels* of culture. These range from the explicit manifest culture ('tertiary level culture') visible to the outsider, such as social rituals, traditional dress, national cuisine and festive occasions, to much deeper levels known only to members of the cultural group themselves. While the tertiary level is basically the public 'facade presented to the world at large', below it lies a series of implicit assumptions, beliefs and rules which constitute that group's 'cultural grammar'. This deeper level includes 'secondary level culture', where these underlying rules and assumptions are known to the members of the group but rarely shared with outsiders, and 'primary level culture'. This is the deepest level of culture 'in which the rules are known to all, obeyed by all, but seldom if ever stated. Its rules are implicit, taken for granted, almost impossible for the average person to state as a system, and generally out of awareness'.

In Hall's view, while the manifest, tertiary level of culture is easiest to observe, change and manipulate, it is the deeper levels (primary and secondary) that are the most hidden, stable and resistant to change. This in turn has major implications for the applied social scientist, especially for those involved in aiding or educating populations from cultures different to their own.

One crucial aspect of any culture's 'lens' is the division of the world, and of the people within it, into different *categories*, each with their own name. For example, all cultures divide up their members into different social categories – such as men or women, children or adults, young people or old people, kinsfolk or strangers, upper class or lower class, able or disabled, normal or abnormal, mad or bad, healthy or ill. And all cultures have elaborate ways of moving people from one social category into another (such as from 'ill person' to 'healthy person'), and also of confining people – sometimes against their will – to the categories into which they have been put (such as 'mad', 'disabled' or 'elderly').

Anthropologists such as Leach[6] have pointed out that virtually all societies have more than one culture within their borders. For example, most societies have some form of social stratification into social classes, castes or ranks, and each stratum is marked by its own distinctive cultural attributes, including use of language, manners, styles of dress, dietary and housing patterns and so on. Rich and poor, powerful and powerless – each will have their own inherited cultural perspective. To some extent, both men and women can have their own distinctive 'cultures' within the same society, and are expected to conform to different norms and different expectations. In addition to such social strata, one can see that most modern complex societies, such as those in North America and Western Europe, now include within them religious and ethnic minorities, tourists, foreign students, recent immigrants, political refugees and migrant workers, each with their own distinctive culture. Many of these groups will undergo some degree of *acculturation* over time, whereby they incorporate some of the cultural attributes of the larger society, but others will not. In addition, an increasing number of the followers of different new religions, cults and lifestyles are beginning to appear in most Western societies, each with their own unique view of the world. A further subdivision of culture within complex societies is seen in the various professional *sub-cultures* that exist, such as the medical, nursing, legal or military professions. In each case these people form a group apart with their own concepts, rules and social organization. While each sub-culture is developed from the larger culture, and shares many of its concepts and values, it also has unique, distinctive features of its own. Students in these professions – especially in medicine and nursing – also undergo a form of enculturation, as they slowly acquire the 'culture' of their chosen career over many years. In doing so, they also acquire a very different perspective on life from those who are outside the profession. In the case of the medical profession, its sub-culture also reflects many of the social divisions and prejudices of the wider society (see Chapters 4 and 6), and this might interfere with both health care and doctor–patient communication, as illustrated later in this book. All this means that most complex societies are now a patchwork of different sub-cultures, with many different views of the world co-existing – sometimes uneasily – within the same territory.

The context of culture

Overall, therefore, cultural background has an important influence on many aspects of people's lives, including their beliefs, behaviour, perceptions, emotions, language, religion, rituals, family structure, diet, dress, body image, concepts of space and of time, and attitudes to illness, pain and other forms of misfortune – all of which may have important implications for health and health care. However, the culture into which you are born, or in which you live, is never the only such influence. It is only one of a number of influences on health-related beliefs and behaviours, which include:

- *individual* factors (such as age, gender, size, appearance, personality, intelligence, experience, physical and emotional state)
- *educational* factors (both formal and informal and including education into a religious, ethnic or professional sub-culture)
- *socio-economic* factors (such as social class, economic status, occupation or unemployment, and the networks of social support from other people)
- *environmental* factors (such as the weather, population density or pollution of the habitat, but also including the types of infrastructure available, such as housing, roads, bridges, public transport and health facilities).

In any particular case, moreover, all of these factors will play some role, but in different proportions. Thus in some situations – depending on the context – people will act more 'culturally' than in others. At other times their behaviour may be determined more by their personality, economic status, what they have been educated to believe or the characteristics of the environment in which they live.

Furthermore, the concept of culture itself has sometimes been misunderstood or even misused. For example, cultures are never homogeneous, and therefore one should always avoid using generalizations in explaining people's beliefs and behaviours. One cannot make broad generalizations about the members of any human group without taking into account the fact that differences among the group's members may be just as marked as those between the members of different cultural groups. Statements such as 'the members of group X do not do Y' (such as smoking, drinking or eating meat) may be true of some or even most members of the group, but not necessarily of all. One should therefore differentiate between the rules of a culture, which govern how one *should* think and behave, and how people actually behave in real life. Generalizations can also be dangerous, for they often lead to the development of stereotypes and then to cultural misunderstandings, prejudices and discrimination. Another reason not to generalize is that cultures are never static; they are usually influenced by other human groups around them, and in most parts of the world they are in a constant process of adaptation and change. Increasingly this is due to economic globalization and the growth of global communication systems such as radio, television and the Internet, as well as to jet travel and mass tourism. In the modern age, therefore, what is true of a particular group's culture one year may not be true of it the next.

Therefore, an important point in understanding the role of culture is that it must always be seen in its particular *context*. This context is made up of historical, economic, social, political and geographical elements, and means that the culture of any group of people, at any particular point in time, is always influenced by many other factors. It may therefore be impossible to isolate 'pure' cultural beliefs and behaviour from the social and economic context in which they occur. For example, people may act in a particular way (such as eating certain foods, living in a crowded house or not going to a doctor when ill) not because it is their culture to do so, but because they are simply too poor to do otherwise. They may have high levels of anxiety in their daily lives, not because their culture makes them anxious, but because they are suffering discrimination or persecution from other people. Therefore, in understanding health and illness it is important to avoid 'victim blaming' – that is, seeing the poor health of a population as the sole result of its culture, instead of looking also at their economic or social situation.

Economic factors are an important cause of ill health, since poverty may result in poor nutrition, overcrowded living conditions, inadequate clothing, physical and psychological violence, psychological stress, and drug and alcohol abuse. The unequal distribution of wealth and resources, both between countries and within each country itself, can lead to this situation. As an example of this, the Black Report[7] of 1982 showed how, in the UK, health could clearly be correlated with income, and people in the poorer social classes had more illness and a much higher mortality than their fellow citizens in the more affluent classes. In the developing world too, whatever the local culture, poor health is usually associated with a low income, since this influences the sort of food, water, clothing, sanitation, housing and medical care that people are able to afford[8]. For example, Unterhalter's[9] study of infant mortality rates among different ethnic communities in Johannesburg, South Africa, between 1910 and 1979 found very much higher rates among blacks and other non-white groups than among whites, and this clearly correlated with the economic and social inequalities imposed on them by the apartheid system. Preston-Whyte[10] has described how the legacy of this political system has made the control of AIDS in South Africa much more difficult today. This is because apartheid was a system that, in the rural areas, often separated men from their wives, sending them to work in the cities for many years. Here they lived in male-only hostels, and this helped institutionalize multiple-partner sex relationships for many of them. At the same time, back in the rural areas poor women sometimes had to depend on selling sex in order to earn money for their own survival and that of their children.

Thus culture should never be considered in a vacuum, but only as one component of a complex mix of influences on what people believe and how they live their lives.

A final misuse of the concept of culture – especially in medical care – is that its influence may be over-emphasized in interpreting how some people present their symptoms to health professionals. Symptoms or behaviour may be ascribed to the person's culture, when they are really due to an underlying physical or mental disorder[11]. Similarly, physical disorders may be confused with mental illness in certain cultural contexts. Thus Weiss[12] has described how, in India and elsewhere, some cases of cerebral malaria have been mistakenly diagnosed as mental illness.

Medical anthropology

Although *medical anthropology* is a branch of social and cultural anthropology, its roots also lie deep within medicine and other natural sciences, for it is concerned with a wide range of biological phenomena, especially in relation to health and disease. As a subject it therefore lies – sometimes uncomfortably – in the overlap between the social and natural sciences, and draws its insights from both sets of disciplines. In Foster and Anderson's[13] definition it is: 'A biocultural discipline concerned with both the biological and sociocultural aspects of human behaviour, and particularly with the ways in which the two interacted throughout human history to influence health and disease'.

Anthropologists studying the socio-cultural end of this spectrum have pointed out that, in all human societies, beliefs and practices relating to ill health are a central feature of the culture. Often these are linked to beliefs about the origin of a much wider range of misfortunes (including accidents, interpersonal conflicts, natural disasters, crop failures, theft and loss), of which ill health is just one form. In some societies the whole range of these misfortunes is blamed on supernatural forces, or on divine retribution, or on the malevolence of a witch or sorcerer. The values and customs associated with ill health are part of the wider culture, and cannot really be studied in isolation from it. One cannot really understand how people react to illness, death or other misfortunes without an understanding of the type of culture they have grown up in or acquired – that is, of the 'lens' through which they are perceiving and interpreting their world. In addition to the study of culture it is also necessary to examine the *social organization* of health and illness in that society (the health care system), which includes the ways in which people have become recognized as ill, the ways that they present this illness to other people, the attributes of those they present their illness to, and the ways that the illness is dealt with.

This group of 'healers' is found in different forms in every human society. Anthropologists are particularly interested in the characteristics of this special social group; their selection, training, concepts, values and internal organization. They also study the way these people fit into the social system as a whole – their rank in the social hierarchy, their economic or political power, and the division of labour between them and other members of the society. In some human groups the healers play roles beyond their healing functions – they may act as 'integrators' of the society, who regularly reassert the society's values (see Chapter 9), or as agents of social control, helping to label and punish socially deviant behaviour (see Chapter 10). Their focus may not be only on the ill individual, but rather on his 'ill' family, community, village or tribe. It is therefore important when studying how individuals in a particular society perceive and react to ill health, and the types of health care that they turn to, to know something about both the *cultural* and the *social* attributes of the society in which they live. This is one of the main tasks of medical anthropology.

At the biological end of the spectrum, medical anthropology draws on the techniques and findings of medical science and its various subfields – including microbiology, biochemistry, genetics, parasitology, pathology, nutrition and epidemiology. In many cases it is possible to link biological changes found by these techniques to social and cultural factors in a particular society. For example, a hereditary disease transmitted by a recessive gene may occur at a higher frequency in a particular population due to that group's cultural preference for endogamy – that is, for marrying only within one's own family or local kin group. To unravel this problem, one needs a number of perspectives:

- *clinical medicine*, to identify the clinical manifestation of the disease
- *pathology*, to confirm the disease on the cellular or biochemical level
- *genetics*, to identify and predict the hereditary basis of the disease and its linkage to a recessive gene
- *epidemiology*, to show its high incidence in a particular population in relation to 'pooling' of recessive genes and certain marriage customs
- social or cultural *anthropology*, to explain the marriage patterns of that society and to identify who may marry whom within it.

Medical anthropology tries to solve this type of clinical problem by utilizing not only anthropological findings but also those of the biological sciences – by being, in other words, a 'biocultural discipline'.

Medical anthropology and the human life cycle

One important aspect of medical anthropology is the study of the human life cycle, and of all the stages from birth to death. The term *age-grade* is used in anthropology for the category of persons who happen to fall within a particular culturally defined age range (such as child, adult or elder)[14]. Each of these age-grades is not just a universal biological stage of life; its beginning and end are also defined by the culture, as are the events expected within it. Furthermore, each age-grade also has profound social and psychological dimensions for those passing through it. In general, these define quite precisely how people within an age-grade should behave, and how other people should behave towards them. Just as every society has a profound split between the types of behaviour expected of males and of females (see Chapter 6), so are there major differences between what is expected of each of the age-grades.

Later in this book the two extremes of the human life cycle, birth and death, are discussed in more detail from the perspective of medical anthropology (Chapters 6 and 9). There is also more discussion of how, particularly in Western society, many of the normal milestones of the life cycle (such as puberty, menstruation, pregnancy, childbirth, menopause and even dying) seem gradually to have become medicalized – turned into pathological, rather than natural states.

In recent years, medical anthropology has paid considerable attention to the cultural characteristics of two particular stages of human growth and development: childhood and old age. To some extent, both children[15] and the elderly[16] can be said to have their own cultures, or rather sub-cultures; their own unique view of the world, and ways of behaving within it. Although each is always imbedded within the wider culture, they also have certain distinct characteristics of their own.

Childhood

Like old age, the definition of childhood is not something fixed and finite and based only on biological criteria. Cross-cultural studies indicate there are wide variations in how childhood is defined, its beginning and end, and the behaviour considered appropriate for children and for those around them. James and colleagues[17] point out that definitions of childhood are always, to some extent, 'socially constructed', and this is why they tend to vary quite widely between different human groups. For example, different societies set different ages at which children can be educated, take part in certain religious rituals, work outside the home, have sexual relations, control their own finances, make independent decisions (about their health, education or place of residence), have their own identity documents or passports, take legal responsibility for their actions and so on. In some traditional cultures children were even expected to marry, and a betrothal ceremony would take place arranged by their parents and close kin. Although such arranged child marriages are now increasingly uncommon, especially in urban areas, in the past they existed in parts of India, China, Japan, Africa and southern Europe[18]. Among the Hausa of Nigeria, for example, childhood effectively ended for a girl when, at the age of 10, she was betrothed to her future husband and was expected to take on 'the social responsibilities of a wife'[19]. In other cultural settings, children have been expected to become full combatants in war – especially in civil wars and insurrections[20] – or to work full-time outside the home, often for very low wages[20]. The notion of childhood being a unique, protected time – a notionally carefree existence, with its own mores, leisure pursuits, dress codes, diets, treats, toys, books, computer programmes, movies, videos and magazines – seems to be a feature of economically developed societies, where huge profits are being made from this conceptual 'separateness' of childhood. By contrast, in poorer societies children are in effect 'trainee adults', expected to perform almost all the usual adult tasks, such as child care, cooking, hunting, herding and earning money, as early as possible.

In the construction of childhood culture, both at home and at school, children are not just passive recipients of the process. They too develop their own lore and language[15], and contribute to the development of their own identity. As James and colleagues[21] put it: 'children are not formed by natural and social forces, but rather ... they inhabit a world of meaning created by themselves and through their interaction with adults'. Increasingly, medical anthropology is focusing on certain aspects of childhood culture that relate to health and illness – in particular, the needs and perceptions of the sick child, their beliefs about health and illness and their attitudes to medical treatment (see Chapter 5).

On the international level, the anthropological study of childhood is of growing importance because of the health implications of a number of contemporary social issues. These include the use of child labour[20], the sexual and physical abuse of children[20,22], the widespread prevalence of child prostitution[20], the increased use of children in warfare[20], and the increasing numbers of 'street children' in many poorer countries.

Later in this book there will be discussion of some of those areas where medical anthropology has already contributed to a fuller understanding of infant and child health. They include the issues of disability (Chapter 2), male and female circumcision (Chapter 2), nutrition and infant feeding practices (Chapter 3), perceptions of illness (Chapter 5), pregnancy and childbirth (Chapter 6), self-medication and substance abuse

(Chapter 8), family structure (Chapter 10) and immunizations, family planning and primary care (Chapter 13).

Old age

A relatively new branch of medical anthropology, *cross-cultural gerontology*, is the study of aging and social attitudes towards it across different cultures. It is of growing importance, since the number of aged people in the world is rapidly increasing. World-wide, the population aged 60 or over is expected to more than double from 500 million in 1990 to about 1.2 billion by the year 2035, and 72 per cent will be living in developing countries[23]. Most of this growth is expected to be in Africa, Asia and Latin America. Throughout the world, the 'oldest old' (aged 85 or older) are the most rapidly increasing age group among the older population[23]. At the same time, economic modernization, a falling birth rate, changing gender roles, and the mobility of populations has often meant the breakdown of the extended family structure, with more of the elderly than ever before being left to fend for themselves.

Anthropologists have pointed out that, in every culture, biological aging is not necessarily the same as social aging, or even as psychological aging. A particular chronological age defined as old in one culture may not be considered so in another. Similarly, behaviour defined by one group as inappropriate for the elderly, such as having sexual relations or wearing brightly-coloured clothes, may be considered quite normal in another. Also, self-perception and psychological aging are often independent of chronological age. Despite the body's physical decline, most older people retain within themselves a sense of what Kaufman[16] terms 'the ageless self'.

Cultures vary widely in the status that they give to the elderly. Unlike in Western industrial societies – where loss of productivity with age, and retirement, usually means a steep drop in social status – the respect accorded to the elderly is usually much higher in traditional, more rural societies. In non-literate societies particularly, the elders are the living repositories of oral history and ancient traditions; of cultural mores, beliefs, myths and ritual expertise. Under these circumstances, the unexpected death of a respected elder is almost equivalent to the effect of a library burning down in a more literate, developed society.

In general, modern Western industrial society, with its emphasis on youth, productivity, individualism, autonomy and self-control, is often quite intolerant of old people. As Loustaunau and Sobo[24] ironically put it: 'Aging is unpopular in the United States'. Increasingly, those societies that have entered the information age of computers, global telecommunications and artificial intelligence give an increased cultural importance to the brain (see Chapter 2). They especially value its cognitive functions; reasoning, memory, calculation, and the absorption and retention of large amounts of data. Such a cultural bias tends to devalue many of the elderly, especially if they suffer from some form of memory loss or cognitive impairment. This prejudice against the loss of cognitive skills is clearly seen in the presence of Alzheimer's or other forms of dementia (even if quite mild). In an age where the computer (with its advanced skills of memory, logic and calculation) has become the respected 'second self'[25] of much of the population, many of the normal signs of aging have become pathologized.

As Desjarlais and colleagues[23] point out, this attitude is in contrast to many other cultures, where dementia is not seen as such a major public health problem. Instead it is regarded as an expected, or at least understandable, part of aging. In many non-Western societies, such as China, a certain amount of 'childishness' in the very old is seen as a condition to be tolerated and not as something abnormal and requiring medical treatment. Although Chinese families are generally very caring and supportive of the elderly, Desjarlais and colleagues point out that the increasing life expectancy (resulting in increased mental and physical disabilities) and the paucity of resources (such as homes for the elderly) is now creating considerable emotional and financial hardship for many families there. They quoted another study from India that also suggests that senile dementia is less frequent or less severe there, either due to lower longevity or because there is greater tolerance for the demented aged there than in the West. It is important, though, not to over-romanticize the care of the elderly in non-industrialized societies. Although the elderly are generally well cared for by their relatives, they are sometimes abandoned or abused. In some societies demented old women can be in danger of being accused of being a witch and even put to death[23] – probably a similar situation to that which prevailed in the 'witch-crazed' hysteria of sixteenth and seventeenth century England.

An aging population also poses a growing challenge to the medical model, with its current emphasis on the dramatic 'quick-fix' types of treatment (see Chapter 4). In a world where an increasing number of the population will be suffering from chronic diseases (both physical and mental) this will require a major shift in the medical paradigm, with a move away from acute, more dramatic treatment towards longer-term, more holistic management – a shift from 'cure' to 'care'.

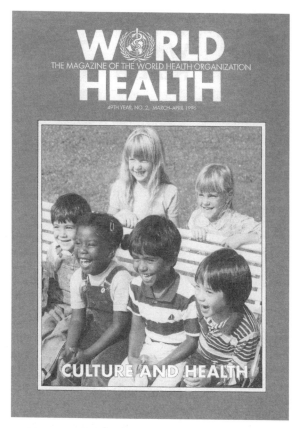

Figure 1.1 Cover of the journal *World Health*, in which the WHO and UNESCO declare 1996 to be the year of 'Culture and Health'. (Source: WHO, Front cover, *World Health*, No. 2, March–April 1996).

Clinically applied medical anthropology

Within medical anthropology, some researchers have concentrated on its theoretical aspects while others (especially those involved in clinical practice, health education programmes or international medical aid) have focused more on its applied aspects in health care and preventive medicine.

Interest in this field of *clinically applied medical anthropology* has grown steadily in the past few years. Medical anthropologists have become involved in a variety of projects, in many parts of the world, aimed at improving health and health care. They have worked both in the non-industrialized world and within the cities and suburbs of Europe and North America.

A number have become 'clinical anthropologists'[26], closely involved in patient care within a hospital or clinic setting, often as members of a multidisciplinary health care team. Here their role has been either that of teacher – raising their colleagues' awareness of the importance of cultural factors in health and illness – or of a health professional or therapist in their own right, with their own specific area of expertise.

Some have widened their focus beyond clinical care to include the more 'macro' influences on health. *Critical medical anthropology* focuses on the political and economic inequality between and within many of the societies in today's world, and especially on the close relationship between poverty and disease[27,28]. Other anthropologists have worked for international aid agencies, such as the World Health Organization or UNICEF, on health problems in various parts of the non-industrialized world. Here they have helped in the planning and evaluation of different forms of health care and health education, or acted as advocates for particular patients or their communities. As well as monitoring the responses of various communities to health care programmes, they have also studied the aid agencies themselves, observing how their organization and sub-culture can either help or hinder the success of the programmes[29]. In both the industrialized world and elsewhere, medical anthropologists have been especially involved in the areas of primary health care, family planning, maternal and child health, infant feeding, nutrition, mental illness, immunizations, the control of drug abuse and alcoholism, and the prevention of AIDS, malaria and tuberculosis.

The importance of cultural factors to many different aspects of international health was officially recognized in 1996 by the World Health Organization and UNESCO, who declared it the Year of Culture and Health. In their joint declaration, the Directors General of both organizations proposed 'further avenues for cooperation so that health and culture can be developed in a mutually supportive manner which will benefit all peoples in all countries'[30].

Case study: Oral rehydration therapy in Pakistan

A study by the Mulls[33] in rural Pakistan showed widespread ignorance or rejection of ORT by mothers despite the fact that the use of ORT has been promoted on a national level by the Ministry of Health since 1983, and packets of oral rehydration solution (ORS) are available free of charge through government health outlets; also, more than 18 million packets of ORS are produced annually by Pakistan's own pharmaceutical industry. The researchers found that many of the mothers were ignorant of how the ORS should be used, and some of them saw the diarrhoea (which was very common in that area) as a natural and expected part of teething and growing up and not as an illness. Some believed it was dangerous to try to stop the diarrhoea, lest the trapped 'heat' within it spread to the brain and caused a fever. Others explained infant diarrhoea as due to certain folk illnesses (see Chapter 5) such as *nazar* (evil eye), *jinns* (malevolent spirits) or *sutt* (a sunken or fallen fontanelle said to cause difficulty in infant sucking), which should be treated with traditional remedies or by traditional healers without recourse to ORT. Some of these mothers did not connect the fallen fontanelle with severe dehydration, and tried to raise it by applying sticky substances to the top of the infant's head or pushing up on the hard palate with a finger. Many mothers in the group saw diarrhoea as a 'hot' illness (see Chapter 3) which required a 'cold' form of treatment, such as a change in maternal diet or giving certain foods and herbs to the infant, in order to restore the sick infant to a normal temperature. They classified most Western medicines, such as antibiotics and even vitamins, as also 'hot', and therefore inappropriate for a diarrhoeal child. A few even rejected ORS (which contains salt) because they thought that salt 'was bad for diarrhoea'.

To illustrate how medical anthropology may be useful in dealing with a particular health problem in a particular part of the world, take the example of diarrhoeal diseases. According to the WHO[31], the high incidence of these diseases poses a major health problem world-wide, especially in the non-industrialized world. There they are usually associated with poverty and the resultant malnutrition, poor sanitation, contaminated drinking water and vulnerability to infection. They kill about 5–7 million people every year. A long-term solution to this problem is not in the hands of health professionals or social scientists, since it will involve major and comprehensive economic, social and political changes, both within those countries and in their relation to the rest of the world.

In terms of an immediate treatment, however, oral rehydration therapy (ORT) provides a safe, inexpensive and simple way to prevent and treat the life-threatening dehydration associated with the diarrhoea, in both infants and children. Despite this, mothers in many parts of the world are reluctant to use this relatively simple form of treatment, even when it is free and easily available to them. Anthropological research, as illustrated in the case history opposite has found that this is partly due to indigenous beliefs about the causes and dangers of diarrhoeal disease and how they should best be treated[32].

As this and other case studies illustrate, therefore, health care programmes should always be designed not only to address medical concerns, but also to involve community participation. They need to take into account the specific needs and circumstances of different communities, their social, cultural and economic backgrounds, and what the people living in them actually believe about their own ill health and how it should be treated.

Research methods in anthropology

In studying societies and cultural groups around the world – including their health beliefs and practices – anthropologists have used two main approaches to research, both unique to anthropology. The *ethnographic* approach involves the study of small-scale societies or relatively small groups of people in order to understand how they view the world and organize their daily lives. The aim is to discover, in so far as this is possible, the 'actor's perspective'; that is, to see how the world looks from the perspective of a member of that society. To discover this, the anthropologists often carry out fieldwork, using the 'participant observation' technique. Here they live with and observe a group of people over a period of time (usually one or more years at least), and learn to see the world through their eyes while at the same time retaining the objective perspective of the social scientist. Although the work of anthropologists is 'concerned with meanings rather than measurements'[34], it often involves quantitative studies as well – such as counting the population, measuring their diet or income, or listing the inhabitants of various households. Ethnography then leads on to a second stage, the *comparative* approach, which seeks to distil the key features of each society and culture and compare these with other societies and cultures in order to draw conclusions about the universal nature of human beings and their social groupings.

In its earlier years, anthropology was mainly concerned with studies of small-scale tribal societies within or at the borders of the colonial empires. Modern anthropology, however, is just as concerned with doing ethnographies in complex Western societies. The 'tribe' of a modern anthropologist might easily be a sect in New York, a suburb in London, a group of surgeons in Los Angeles or patients attending a clinic in Melbourne. In all these cases, both the ethnographic and comparative approaches are used – as well as some of the interviewing and measurement techniques of sociology or psychology.

As detailed in Chapter 14, the range of research techniques available to anthropology has steadily increased. As well as long-term 'participant observation', techniques now often include the use of open-ended questionnaires, videos or tape recordings, computer analyses, aerial photography, the compilation of family histories and analysis of genealogies, the collection of individual narratives, and the examination of written or printed material such as diaries, letters, family photographs, newspaper articles, maps, census reports and local historical records.

More recently, to meet the increasing needs of international aid programmes, a number of 'rapid ethnographic assessment' techniques have been developed[35]. These usually involve a short, intensive period of research by a team of anthropologists and their assistants, and can last anything from several weeks to several months. They tend to focus on a particular problem (such as a high rate of diarrhoeal diseases) in a particular community or region. Used in conjunction with longer-term fieldwork, the data from these studies can be very useful in the planning and evaluation of international aid programmes.

Many of these new research methods now available to medical anthropology are described in more detail in Chapter 14.

In its general approach, this book arises mainly from the growing field of clinically applied medical anthropology, which has been briefly described above. Many examples of its application, especially in relation to contemporary health issues of global concern, are described in each of its chapters. Overall, the aim of the book is to demonstrate the clinical significance of cultural and social factors in illness and in health, in preventive medicine and health education, and in the actual delivery of health care.

Recommended reading

Medical anthropology

Anderson, R. (1996). *Magic, Science and Health*. Harcourt Brace.

Foster, G. M. and Anderson, B. G. (1978). *Medical Anthropology*. Wiley.

Hahn, R. A. (1995). *Sickness and Healing: An Anthropological Perspective*. Yale University Press.

Johnson, T. M. and Sargent, C. F. (eds) (1991). *Medical Anthropology*. Praeger.

Kleinman, A. (1980). *Patients and Healers in the Context of Culture*. University of California Press.

Landy, D. (ed.) (1977). *Culture, Disease, and Healing*. Macmillan.

Social and cultural anthropology

Keesing, R. M. and Strathern, A. (1997). *Cultural Anthropology: A Contemporary Perspective*. Harcourt Brace.

Leach, E. (1982). *Social Anthropology*. Fontana.

Peacock, J. L. (1986). *The Anthropological Lens*. Cambridge University Press.

Research techniques in anthropology

Pelto, P. J. and Pelto, G. H. (1978). *Anthropological Research: The Structure of Inquiry*. Cambridge University Press.

Journals

AM: Rivista della Societa Italiana di Antropologia Medica (Italy)
Anthropology and Medicine (UK)
Journal of Cross-Cultural Gerontology (USA)
Culture, Medicine and Psychiatry (USA)
Curare: Zeitschrift fur Ethnomedizin und Transkulturelle Psychiatrie (Germany)
Ethnicity and Health (UK)
Kallawaya: Órgano del Instituto Antropológico de Investigaciones en Medicina Tradicional (Argentina)
Medical Anthropology (USA)
Medical Anthropology Quarterly (USA)
Nieuwsbrief Medische Antropologie (Holland and Belgium)
Transcultural Psychiatry (Canada)
Social Science and Medicine (UK/USA)
Sociology of Health and Illness (UK)

Web sites

Medical Anthropology Quarterly(USA)
http://www.ameranthassn.org/smapubs.htm
Royal Anthropological Institute (UK)
http:/www.lucy.ukc.ac.uk/rai
Society for Applied Anthropology (USA)
http://www.telepath.com/sfaa
Society for Medical Anthropology (USA)
http://www.people.memphis.edu/~sma
Traditional Chinese Medicine
http://www.mic.ki.se/China.html
Traditional Indian Medicine
http://www.mic.ki.se/India.html
Traditional Islamic Medicine
http://www.mic.ki.se/Arab.html
World Health Organization
http://www.who.org

2 Cultural definitions of anatomy and physiology

To the members of all societies, the human body is more than just a physical organism fluctuating between health and illness. It is also the focus of a set of beliefs about its social and psychological significance, its structure and function. The term *body image* has been used to describe all the ways that an individual conceptualizes and experiences his or her body, whether consciously or not. In Fisher's[1] definition, this includes 'his collective attitudes, feelings and fantasies about his body', as well as 'the manner in which a person has learnt to organize and integrate his body experiences'. The culture in which we grow up teaches us how to perceive and interpret the many changes that can occur over time in our own bodies and in the bodies of other people. We learn how to differentiate a young body from an aged one, a sick body from a healthy one, a fit body from a disabled one; how to define a fever or a pain, a feeling of clumsiness or of anxiety; how to perceive some parts of the body as public, and others as private; and how to view some bodily functions as socially acceptable and others as morally unclean.

The body image, then, is something acquired by every individual as part of growing up in a particular family, culture or society – although there are, of course, individual variations in body image within any of these groups.

In general, concepts of body image can be divided into four main areas:

1. Beliefs about the optimal shape and size of the body, including the clothing and decoration of its surface
2. Beliefs about the boundaries of the body
3. Beliefs about the body's inner structure
4. Beliefs about how the body functions.

All four are influenced by social and cultural background as well as by individual factors, and can have important effects on the health of the individual.

The shape, size, clothing and surface of the body

In every society, the human body has a *social* as well as a physical reality. That is, the shape, size and adornments of the body are a way of *communicating* information about its owner's position in society, including information about age, gender, social status, occupation and membership of certain groups, both religious and secular. Included in this form of communication are bodily gestures and postures, which frequently differ between cultures, and between different groups within a culture. The body language of, for example, doctors, priests, policemen and salespeople is very different from one another, and conveys different types of messages. Clothing is also of particular importance in signalling social rank and occupation; in the Western world mink coats, jewels and designer clothes are usually worn as displays of wealth, in contrast to the ill-fitting and mass-produced clothes of the poor. Similarly, the white coat of the Western doctor or the starched cap of the nurse do not only have a practical aspect (cleanliness and the prevention of infection) but also a *social* function, indicating their membership of a prestigious, powerful occupational group, with its own specific rights and privileges (see Chapter 9). A change in social position is often signalled by a change in clothing; the black dress and shawl adopted by widows in a Greek village is a public indicator of their transition from married woman to solitary mourner. Similarly, new graduates at a Western university wear, at least temporarily, a uniform of academic gown and mortarboard. Thus many aspects of the body's adornments, especially clothing, have both a social function (signalling information about an individual's current position in society) and the more obvious utilitarian function of protecting the body from the environment.

Artificial changes in the shape, size and surface of the body, which are widespread throughout the world, can also have a social function. This applies also to the more extreme forms of bodily mutilation, which will be mentioned below. Inherent in most of these are culturally defined notions of 'beauty' – usually of women – and of the optimal size and shape of the body. Polhemus[2] has listed some of the more extreme forms of body alteration practised now and in the past among non-industrialized peoples. These include:

- artificial deformation of infants' skulls in parts of Peru
- filing and carving of teeth in pre-Columbian Mexico and Ecuador
- scarification of the chest and limbs in New Guinea and parts of Central Africa
- binding of women's feet in Imperial China
- artificial fattening of girls in some parts of West Africa
- tattooing of the body in Tahiti and among some Native Americans
- insertion of large ornaments into the lips and earlobes in the Brazilian Amazon, East Africa and Melanesia
- the wearing of nose- and ear-rings among the people of Timbuktu, Mali.

The most widespread form of bodily mutilation is male circumcision. It has been common in some communities for almost 5000 years, and today is practised by about one-sixth of the world's population[3]. The most controversial[4] is probably female circumcision in its various forms. It usually involves the removal of all or part of the external genitalia, and is carried out on girls ranging in age from 1 month to puberty. An estimated 80 million girls and women living today have undergone circumcision, especially in sub-Saharan Africa, the Arab world, Malaysia and Indonesia, and some immigrant groups in Western countries[5]. In many of these regions, and especially in rural areas, women who are not circumcised may be stigmatized and find it difficult to get married. In 1982 the World Health Organization urged health professionals not to carry out female circumcision under any circumstances.

The health risks of such bodily mutilations are obvious. Female circumcision, for example, carries with it the dangers of infection, haemorrhage, damage to adjacent organs, scar tissue formation and long-term difficulties with micturition, menstruation, sexual intercourse and childbirth[5,6]. However, some forms of bodily mutilation may bring health benefits to the population, even if indirectly. Early male circumcision was once believed to be one of the factors protecting women from developing cancer of the cervix, but this is now disputed[7]. However, it may protect against some infections in the penile area, as well as phimosis (tight foreskin). In addition, as has been found among the Mende of Sierra Leone, the use of ritual scarring by a community may make them accept the 'ritual scars' of vaccination more enthusiastically than other groups without these customs[8]. Both scarification and tattooing (which carry with them the dangers of local infection, hepatitis B and AIDS) are now less commonly seen in the West, except among sailors and servicemen, though recently the popularity of tattooing has begun to increase again among adolescents.

Various forms of self-mutilation or alteration are used in Western societies, especially by women, to conform to culturally defined standards of beauty. These include the widespread use of orthodontics, plastic surgery, breast implants, ear piercing, bodybuilding regimens and hair implants, and the use of false teeth, eyelashes and fingernails. Also included here are the various forms of dieting used by women (like the millions who regularly attend Weight Watchers™ and other self-help groups) in order to reduce their weight to 'attractive' dimensions. It has been hypothesized that anorexia nervosa, often accompanied by loss of periods, is an extreme, pathological form of dissatisfaction with body image in a society which values and rewards female slimness[9]. Thus it can only be understood within the context of certain wider cultural values and influences, especially the 'ideal' body shape of the times[10]. Rintala and Mutajoki[11], for example, have analysed the size, shape and proportions of the mannequins displaying women's clothing in the windows of fashion stores. They show how these have become progressively thinner over the past 80 years until they are now virtually anorexic in appearance. As women need at least 17 per cent of their weight as fat in order to begin menstruating and 22 per cent in order to have regular cycles, they calculate that 'a woman with the shape of a modern mannequin would probably not menstruate', as she would be so underweight. Orbach[12] has suggested further that anorexia is not only a cultural phenomenon, but may even represent a symbolic 'hunger strike' by some women against their oppression in Western society. By contrast, in parts of West Africa wealthy men frequently sent their daughters to 'fatting-houses' where they were fed on fatty foods, with minimal exercise, so as to be plump and pale – a culturally defined shape believed to indicate both wealth and fertility[13]. Similarly, among the Enga people of the New Guinea Highlands a 'sleek, fat body' was regarded as the most important physical asset of a young woman, and 'a thin girl is considered unlikely to make a good marriage'[14]. Men, too, often value a plump body shape, as a sign of health and affluence. Among the Massa people of Northern Cameroon, for example, de Garine[15] has described how male 'fattening sessions' are common, and social attitudes to obesity are much more positive than in the Western world. Among this group, and in many of the surrounding peoples, neither fatness nor obesity are frowned upon, or considered 'conducive to psychological unrest and a passport to death'. By contrast, slim people are seen as weak and tired and their body shape as ugly and ridiculous.

In the Western world, however, obesity is seen as a major health problem, and also carries with it a significant social stigma. Ritenbaugh[16] points out that medical descriptions of the causes of obesity – over-eating and under-exercising – are often just a modern, medicalized version of the traditional moral disapproval of gluttony and sloth (Chapter 5), as well as of a lack of self-control.

Not only is body shape altered to fit in with culturally prescribed patterns, but special clothes are also worn that make this possible. These include women's corsets and other constrictive underwear, and high-heeled or platform shoes, all of which may have a negative effect on health. Cosmetics and deodorants, which may cause skin allergies or contact dermatitis, are also part of the Western mode of communication, where personal body odour is considered to be offensive – a belief not shared by many other cultures.

While the body is protected by its clothes, some areas of the body surface are sometimes considered to be more vulnerable than others. For example, in the author's study[17] of English lay beliefs about chills, colds and fevers, the body image included certain areas of skin (the top of the head, the back of the neck, and the feet) considered more vulnerable than other parts to penetration by environmental cold, damp or draughts. You 'caught cold' if you went out into the rain without a hat on (or after a haircut), or stepped in a puddle or on a cold floor. At the same time, fevers were believed to result from the penetration of germs or bugs or viruses through other breaks in the body's surface – such as the anus, urethra, throat, nostrils or ears.

As well as these cultural influences, medical or surgical treatments may also have a profound impact on body image. This applies particularly to operations such as amputations, mastectomies and plastic surgery, and to treatments such as radiotherapy and chemotherapy that may result in hair loss or other physical changes. Similarly, some women may, after a hysterectomy, experience a sense of the loss of their female identity – at least for a while.

Individual and social bodies

As the section above illustrates, each human being has, in a symbolic sense, two bodies; an *individual* body-self (both physical and psychological) which is acquired at birth, and a *social* body that is needed in order to live within a particular society and cultural group[18].

The social body is an essential part of the body image, for it provides each person with a framework for perceiving and interpreting physical and psychological experiences[18]. It is also the means whereby the physical functioning of individuals is influenced and controlled by the society in which they live. This larger society, or 'body-politic', exerts a powerful control over all aspects of the individual body – its shape, size, clothing, diet and postures, its behaviour in sickness and in health, and its reproductive, work and leisure activities[19].

Douglas[18] points out that there is a two-way relationship between bodily and social imagery, with each influencing the other. Not only does society shape and control the bodies within it, but the body also provides us with a collection of 'natural symbols' with which to understand society itself and how it is organized – from the 'head' of government and the 'heart' of a community', to the 'left' and 'right' sides of the political spectrum. Gordon[20] notes that this close relationship between bodily and social imagery means that different types of society produce very different images of the body. For example, Western society sees itself as made up of autonomous, individual citizens, and it assumes that the body, too, is made up of individual organs, which can be removed and replaced by spare-part surgery without threatening the survival of the whole. As described below, this Western body image is very different from that found elsewhere – for example, in Japan.

In practice, however, the body image derived from society is not really external to or separate from the individual body-self, nor from its physical reality. Csordas[21] points out that body and culture (like body and mind) are not really separate from one another. To a large extent, individuals *embody* the culture that they live in. Their sensations, perceptions, feelings and other bodily experiences are all culturally patterned. So is the body's awareness of other bodies within that society, and the ways that it relates towards them. Bodily sensations and perceptions (the 'somatic modes of attention') are the means by which people are aware of other bodies, and are able to create and maintain the networks of relationships with them. Thus they are 'culturally elaborated ways of attending to and with one's body in surroundings that include the embodied presence of others'. In a general sense, therefore, the body *is* culture – an expression of its basic themes. A full understanding of any human body gives, at the same time, a fuller understanding of the culture embodied within it.

The boundaries of the body

Symbolic skins

In every human group the boundaries of individuals' sense of self are not necessarily the same as the boundaries of their body, and their sense of personal identity extends far beyond the borders of their skin. They are surrounded by a series of what I would term *symbolic skins* – some of them invisible, others not. Hall[22], for example, has identified four invisible, concentric circles of space and distance that surround the bodies of middle-class Americans. They are:

1. *Intimate* distance (0 to 18 inches) [0–45 cm] – this can only be entered by those who have an intimate physical relationship with the individual
2. *Personal* distance (18 inches to 4 feet) [45–120 cm] – this involves less intimate contact and relationships, but is still within the zone of personal space; it is 'a small protective sphere or bubble that an organism maintains between itself and others'
3. *Social* distance (4 to 12 feet) [1.2–3.6 m] – this is the distance at which impersonal business transactions and casual social interactions take place
4. *Public* distance (12 feet to 25 feet or more) [3.6–7.5 m or more] – this is the distance at which no social or personal interaction is taking place.

Hall stresses that the size and shape of these invisible 'bubbles' varies widely between different social and cultural groups within the USA, as well as in different parts of the world – for example, between Americans, British, French, Germans and Arabs. In each case, penetration by a stranger (including a health professional) of one of these unseen skins, especially the inner two, may be experienced by the individual in that culture as rude, invasive or very threatening.

Other 'symbolic skins' that help define people's sense of self may include their clothing, the walls of their rooms (or houses), their cars, the outer limits of their suburbs, cities or villages, their membership of an ethnic group or social class, or even the borders of their nation state (whose symbolic 'orifices' are airports, harbours and border posts). In those cultures where the group is considered to be more important than the individual, these skins usually include other people (members of the same family, clan, ethnic group, village or workplace), and sometimes even livestock, a dwelling or a piece of ancestral land. This collective sense of self, enclosed within a symbolic boundary far beyond the human body, is common in many parts of the world. For example, Tamura and Lau[23] note how, in Japan, the group is generally considered to be more central than the individual, and is thus intimately involved in the individual's sense of self – unlike the 'skin-encapsulated ego' common in the West. This in turn has implications when trying to define the moment of an individual's death, as discussed below. In many other societies, too, individuals do not necessarily 'own' their body in the way they would expect to in the West. Jadhav[24] describes how, in parts of northern India, the folk concept of *ārdha-angāni* ('half-body') can be found. Here, the left half of a married woman's body is believed to belong to her husband and his kinsfolk; in this cultural setting women may 'embody' any marital conflict by developing pain, paralysis or other symptoms of that side of their bodies.

The boundaries of an individual's body image are not static, however. They may alter with emotional state, disease or disability, surgery (amputations, mastectomies, breast augmentations, spare-part surgery) and medical treatments (radiotherapy, *in vitro* fertilization), as well as in physiological states such as pregnancy, obesity and weight loss. They also vary with age. In adolescence, an increasing body awareness is linked to the individual's need to develop the series of symbolic skins characteristic of their own culture or social group. These are acquired, one by one, as part of the transition from childhood to adult status. Often these new 'skins' are experienced as potentially fragile and easily disrupted by other people, especially adults. To most adolescents, an important boundary (or symbolic skin) of their sense of self is that of their peer group, and thus exclusion from it can be very traumatic for them.

In many traditional societies, the individual's status is physically 'written' onto the surface of their body. Tattooing, scarification, circumcision and piercing of ears, lips or other parts of the body are all permanent and visible forms of cultural skin. As well as status, they usually signal permanent membership of a particular community. Among groups such as the New Zealand Maori, for example, complex full-body tattoos were especially common. For the Maori warriors they were even a type of spiritual armour that protected them, as well as an expression of deeper cultural and religious beliefs[25]. Thus to the anthropologist Claude Levi-Strauss[26], the purpose of these tattoos was 'not only to imprint a drawing onto the flesh but also to stamp onto the mind all the traditions and philosophy of the group'. In Western society, by contrast, tattoos are voluntary, but in recent years have become increasingly common. This phenomenon may represent – especially among younger people – a craving for a more permanent, fixed identity in an age of unpredictability and constant flux.

Changes in body image are common in certain severe, crippling diseases. For example, Kaufman[27] has described the impact of a stroke on American patients as 'an assault on the taken-for-granted body – the "natural", "right" sense of self'. Faced with its crippling effects, and the fact that it cannot be cured, the neat equation between body and self often breaks down. The healthy self – determined to get better as soon as possible – finds itself in conflict with its permanently damaged body. Because contemporary US culture assumes that 'the individual can acquire the ability, through training and perseverance, to reverse disease outcomes and, in fact, to overcome nature'[27], the stroke victims' inability to master or cure their disability may be interpreted by them (and by others) as a sign of moral weakness, personal failure or loss of control.

The inner structure of the body

To most people the inner structure of the body is a matter of mystery and speculation. Without the benefit of anatomical dissections, charts of the skeletal and organ structures or X-ray photographs, beliefs about how the body is constructed are usually based on inherited folklore, books and magazines, personal experience and theorizing. The importance of this 'inside-the-body' image is that it influences people's perception and presentation of bodily complaints. It also influences their responses to medical treatment. For example, a 20-year-old London woman was told, on the basis of her symptoms, that she was suffering from 'heartburn', and an antacid mixture was prescribed. A week later, with the same symptoms, she saw another doctor and admitted she had not taken any antacid. Asked why she hadn't followed the first doctor's advice she replied, 'Of course I didn't take his mixture. How could he know I had heartburn if he didn't even listen to my heart?'

Several studies have been done on people's conceptions of what lies inside the body. Boyle[28] studied 234 patients, with the aid of multiple choice questionnaires, to discover their knowledge of bodily structure and function, and then compared the answers with those of a sample of 35 doctors. He found a wide discrepancy between the two sets of answers, especially on

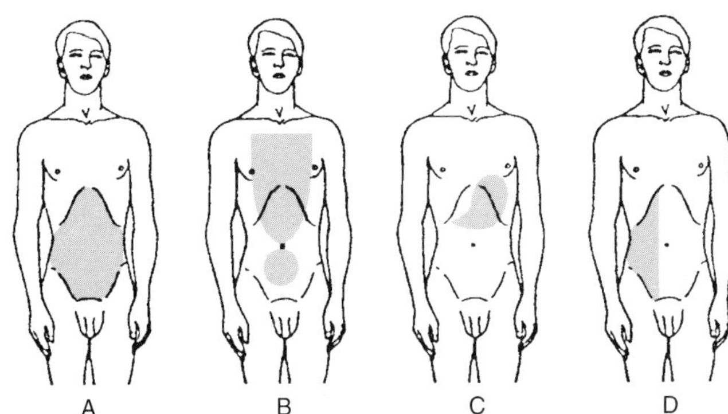

Distribution of positions of the stomach. A, 67 patients (58.8%), no doctors. B, 22 patients (19.3%), no doctors. C, 23 patients (20.2%), 35 doctors (100%) χ^2 43.21; D.F. 1; P<0.0005 (doctors > patients). D, 2 patients (1.8%), no doctors

Figure 2.1 The position of the stomach: from a British study of doctors' versus patients' understanding of common anatomical terms[28] (Source: Boyle, C. M. (1970) Difference between patients' and doctors' interpretation of some common medical terms. *Br. Med. J.*, **ii**, 286–9, Fig. 4).

the location of internal organs. For example: 14.9 per cent of the patients placed the heart as occupying most of the thoracic cavity; 58.8 per cent located the stomach as occupying the entire abdomen, from waist to groin; 48.7 per cent located the kidneys low down in the groin; and 45.5 per cent saw the liver as lying in the lower abdomen, just above the pelvis. In another study of 81 men and women in hospital awaiting major abdominal surgery Pearson and Dudley[29] found that, out of a total of 729 responses dealing with organ location, only 28 per cent were correct; 14 per cent were only vague answers, and 58 per cent were incorrect. Fifteen per cent equated the stomach with the abdominal cavity, 14 per cent marked in two livers on opposite sides of the body, and 18 per cent said the gallbladder was concerned with urine, or located it in the lower pelvic area, or both. Such bodily perceptions obviously influence how patients interpret, and present, certain bodily symptoms. For example, a vague discomfort anywhere in the chest may be interpreted as 'heart trouble', whether the doctor confirms this or not. A patient complaining of a pain in the stomach may be referring to virtually anywhere in the abdominal cavity.

Conceptions of what lies inside the body are also not static. They can vary with certain physical and psychological states, and seem to vary with age. A study by Tait and Ascher[30] examined these conceptions in 107 hospitalized psychiatric patients, 105 candidates for admission to a Naval Academy, 55 military men hospitalized in medical or surgical wards and 22 sixth-grade pupils in New York. Many of the drawings the psychotics produced 'exhibited disorderly arrangement, confusion, vagueness and pronounced and bizarre distortions of shape, relative size and position of [bodily] parts'. In the children's drawings the sexual organs were omitted, while the skeletomuscular system was prominently drawn. In medical and surgical patients there was a tendency to emphasize the organ or system involved in the illness for which they were hospitalized, such as the lung, the kidneys, or the skeletomuscular system. One patient with neurodermatitis drew the skin surface of the body, with only the faintest indication of ribs as the inside of the body.

Illness may also involve reifying a diseased organ or bodily part – thinking of it as though it were an 'it'; something partly alien to the body and only partially under its control[31]. In this way unpleasant or worrying bodily experiences can be denied, or separated from the type of body-image now idealized in the modern world; a body which is healthy, happy, independent and in full control of all its functions[32]. This is particularly the case in severe diseases, such as cancer, where both the disease and the affected body part are often seen as somehow separate or alien to the patient's body (see Chapter 5). In one study of psychosomatic disorders, for example, patients put the blame for their embarrassing symptoms (such as unexpected vomiting or diarrhoea) on a part of their body that was weak, unreliable and only partly under their control, such as an 'irritable colon', a 'nervous stomach' or a 'weak chest'[32].

The effect of body image is also seen in the presentation of non-organic, i.e. psychogenic, signs and symptoms. Waddell and colleagues[33] studied the distribution of physical signs for

Case study: Body image in a patient in Boston, USA

Kleinman and colleagues[35] described a case which illustrates the clinical significance of patients' beliefs about their bodies and how these can affect their behaviour and the reactions of clinicians. A 60-year-old white woman was admitted to a medical ward in Massachusetts General Hospital, Boston, suffering from pulmonary oedema secondary to atherosclerotic cardiovascular disease and chronic congestive heart failure. As she began to recover, her behaviour became increasingly bizarre; she forced herself to vomit and urinated frequently in her bed. A psychiatrist was called in for an opinion. On close questioning he discovered that, from her point of view at least, her behaviour made sense. She had been told by the doctors that she had 'water in the lungs'. She was the wife and daughter of plumbers, and her concept of the structure of the body had the chest connected by 'pipes' to the mouth and urethra. She was therefore trying to remove as much of the 'water in the lungs' as possible by vomiting and urinating frequently. She compared the latter to the effect of the 'water pills' that she had been prescribed, and which she had been told would get rid of the water in her chest by making her urinate. Once the actual 'plumbing' of the human body had been explained to her, using diagrams, her bizarre behaviour immediately ended.

which no organic cause could be found in 350 British and American patients with low back pain. The distribution of these signs (such as numbness, weakness or tremor) did not match accepted neuroanatomical distribution. Instead, it corresponded to lay divisions of the body into regions such as knee, groin or waist. In another study by Walters[34], hysterical pain or psychogenic regional pain was found to occur in distributions which matched patients' body images – especially their beliefs about parts of the body supplied by a particular nerve, rather than their actual anatomical innervation. Examples of this are the 'glove' or 'stocking' distribution of hysterical pain, numbness or paralysis.

The functioning of the body

While beliefs about the body's structure can have clinical importance, those about how it functions are probably more significant in how they affect people's behaviour. Beliefs about function usually deal with one or more of the following inter-related aspects of the body:

1. Its inner workings.
2. The effect on these of diet, environment and other outside influences.
3. The nature (and disposal) of the by-products of the body's functioning, such as faeces, urine and menstrual blood.

From the wide range of lay theories of physiology that have been studied, a few have been selected for closer examination.

Balance and imbalance

In all of these theories, the healthy working of the body is thought to depend on the harmonious *balance* between two or more elements or forces within the body. To a variable extent this balance is dependent on external forces such as diet, environment or supernatural agents, as well as on internal influences such as inherited weakness or state of mind. The most widespread of these theories is the *humoral* theory, which has its roots in ancient China and India but was elaborated into a system of medicine by Hippocrates, who was born in 460 BC. In the Hippocratic theory, the body contained four liquids or humours; blood, phlegm, yellow bile and black bile. Health resulted from these four humours being in optimal proportions to one another; ill health from an excess or deficiency of one of them. Diet and environment could affect this balance, as could the season of the year. Treatment for imbalance/disease consisted of restoring the optimal proportion of the humours by removing excess (bleeding, purging, vomiting, starvation) or replacing the deficiency (by special diets, medicines, etc.). It also included a theory of personality types, based on the predominance of one of the humours, the four types being: sanguine (excess blood), phlegmatic (excess phlegm), choleric (excess yellow bile) and melancholic (excess black bile). Hippocratic medicine was restored and further elaborated by Galen (130–200 AD), a Greek physician living in Rome. In the centuries that followed, Galen's work gradually diffused throughout the Roman world and into the Islamic world. In the ninth century, under the Abbasid Dynasty of Baghdad, large portions of his work were translated into Arabic. Foster[36] has described how, during the Moorish occupation of the Iberian Peninsula, much of this humoral medicine was taken over by Spanish and Portuguese physicians and later carried by their descendants to South and Central America and the Philippines. However, some anthropologists believe that certain indigenous humoral and 'hot–cold' beliefs preceded the European conquest of Latin America[37], although others dispute this claim[36]. In any case, humoral medicine remains the basis of lay beliefs about health and illness in much of Latin America, is also prominent in the Islamic world, and is a component of the Ayurvedic medical tradition in India.

In Latin American folk medicine, the humoral theory – often called the 'hot–cold theory of disease' – postulates that health can only be maintained (or lost) by the effect of heat or cold on the body[36]. As Logan[38] points out, 'hot' and 'cold' here do not pertain to actual temperature but to a symbolic power contained in most substances, including food, herbs and medicines. In addition, all mental states, illnesses, natural and supernatural forces are grouped in a binary fashion into 'hot' or 'cold' categories. To maintain health, the body's internal 'temperature' balance must be maintained between the opposing powers of 'hot' and cold, especially by avoiding prolonged exposure to either quality. In illness, health is restored by re-establishing the internal temperature balance by exposing oneself to, or ingesting, items of an opposite quality to that believed to be responsible for illness. Certain illnesses seen as 'hot' are believed to result from over-exposure to sun or fire, or from ingesting hot foods or beverages. Both pregnancy and menstruation are considered to be hot states and, like other hot conditions, are treated by the ingestion of cold foods and medicines or by cold treatments such as sponging with cool water. Such beliefs can have dangerous effects on women's health. For example, postpartum or menstruating women from some parts of Latin America may avoid certain fruits and vegetables, which they classify as 'cold' and liable to clot their hot menstrual blood. The avoidance of such foods in women who already have a diet deficient in vitamins may eliminate even more of these vitamins from their diet. In one US study[39], a group of postpartum Puerto Rican women believed that if the lochia was 'clotted' by cold foods, it would be re-absorbed to cause nervousness or even insanity. As a preventive measure, they drank tonics containing 'hot' foods such as chocolate, garlic and cinnamon.

Humoral medicine is still one component of the pluralistic medical system in Morocco, as described by Greenwood[40], but most of the emphasis is now placed on two of the humours; blood and phlegm. As in Latin America, this theory of health and illness relates the inner workings of the body to outside influences such as diet and environment. There are 'hot' and 'cold' foods and environmental factors, the imbalance of which in the body can cause hot or cold illnesses that are treated by foods of the opposite quality. Food is commonly used as a treatment, as most foods are considered hot and most illnesses cold. Excess blood is seen as a feature of 'hot' illnesses, and excess phlegm in the body as a feature of 'cold' ones. Most hot illnesses are caused by overexposure to sun, heat or hot winds, or by eating excess foods in summer. The heat then enters the blood, which rises to the head, causing flushing, fever and other symptoms. Treatment in this Moroccan humoral model is removal of the excess hot blood by cooling the body's surface, eating cold foods and also using cupping and leeching at the neck to draw off some of the blood.

In the ancient Indian Ayurvedic system, there are similar highly complex concepts of the physiology of the body that equate health with balance. As described by Obeyesekere[41], there are five *bhūtas* or basic elements in the universe; ether, wind, water, earth and fire. These are the basic constituents of all life, and also make up the three *dōsas* or humours (wind, bile and phlegm) and the seven *dhātus* or components of the body. Food which contains the five elements is 'cooked' by fires in the body and converted into bodily refuse and a refined portion, which is successively transformed into the seven basic components of the body: food juice, blood, flesh, fat, bone, marrow and semen. The five elements also go to make up the three humours in the body; the wind element becomes wind or flatulence, fire appears as bile and water as phlegm. The harmonious working of the body results from an optimal balance of these three humours, and illness results from relative excess or deficiency of one or more of the humours. As in Latin America, there are 'cooling' and 'heat-producing foods' that are used to reduce excess of a humour; hot foods can cause excess bile, and thus illness must be treated by a diet of cold food and other medication. Ayurveda also includes a theory of temperament and its relationship to ill health. For example, a patient whose temperament results from an excess of bile is believed to be especially vulnerable to illness caused by an excess of this humour, and thus should avoid heat-producing food which may increase even further the amount of bile in the body.

Like Ayurveda, traditional Chinese medicine also saw health as a harmonious balance, in this case between two contrasting cosmic principles: *yin*, described as dark, moist, watery and female; and *yang*, hot, dry, fiery and male. The organs of the body were either predominantly *yin* (such as the heart, lungs, spleen, kidneys and liver) or *yang* (such as the intestines, stomach and gallbladder). Illness was believed to result from an imbalance, usually an excess of one principle within an organ, which might then have to be removed by acupuncture or moxibustion[42].

The humoral concept has largely disappeared from the UK and other European societies, but concepts of restoring health by counteracting one element in the body with another still persist. In English folk beliefs about colds and chills, which are thought of as being due to the penetration of environmental cold or damp into the body, a common treatment was to counteract cold by heat. Heat was administered in the form of warm drinks, warm foods (which help generate the body's own heat) and rest in a warm bed. The aphorism 'feed a cold, starve a fever' sums up this approach. To prevent colds and chills a variety of patent tonics were used, such as cod liver oil and malt extract, to generate heat inside the body. As one elderly patient put it, if you went outdoors after taking a tonic 'you felt warm inside', for the tonic was an internal protection against excess cold[17].

Humoral medicine has, of course, also disappeared from modern scientific medicine. Nevertheless, modern physiology does include numerous examples of diseases that are caused by a deficiency or excess of certain substances in the body, such as hormones, enzymes, electrolytes, vitamins, trace elements and blood cells, which can be corrected by replacing the deficient substance or counteracting the excess. The concept of the negative feedback loop in endocrinology, whereby the rise of one hormone in the bloodstream results in a decline in another, might also be seen as a balance/imbalance view of ill health, though it also includes notions simultaneously of deficiency/excess.

Symbolic anatomies

In traditional systems of healing, such as traditional Chinese medicine, Tibetan medicine or Ayurveda, practitioners are working not only with concepts of balance but also with their own models of the body's structure and function. Usually these are part of much wider cosmologies, linking the individual body to greater forces in the universe. Often they deal with the flow, blockage, concentration or imbalance of mystical forces (usually translated into our Western idiom as 'energy'). Being part of much larger cosmologies, these traditional 'maps' of the human body bear little relation to the illustrations in a Western

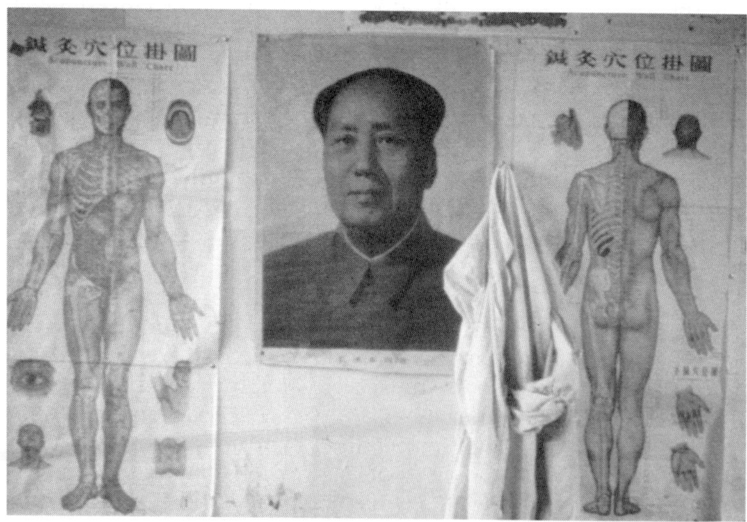

Figure 2.2 Acupuncture charts on the walls of a clinic in Qinghai, China. The charts show the various acupuncture points on the body, and the meridians or channels along which flows its vital energy or *chi* (Source: Catherine Platt/Panos Pictures).

anatomy textbook. In traditional Chinese acupuncture, for example, the body is criss-crossed by a series of meridians, or invisible channels, along which flow *chi* – the vital energy or life force of the human body. Any interruptions or imbalances in its flow may be linked to disease, both physical or mental. Treatment is by needling some of the 309 acupuncture points along the meridians in order to restore the flow of *chi* and the harmonious balance between *yin* and *yang*[42]. In the Tantric tradition of both Hinduism and Buddhism, the *chakras* (or 'wheels') are concentrations and receptors of energy along the central axis of the body. Thus in the Hindu version the body is traversed by a number of channels (or *nadis*) along which flow a vital force, or *prana*. The central one of these channels, rising from the anus up to the crown of the head, is the *sushumna*. Along it lie the seven *chakras*, each located at a key point for the body's functioning[43]. In Tibetan Buddhism, usually only five or six chakras are described[44]. In both traditions, healing – by means of certain rituals, yoga practices, herbs, acupuncture or moxibustion – aims to restore, strengthen or rebalance the flows of vital energy within and beyond the body, especially in relation to the *chakras*.

To the scientific medical mind, these 'maps' of the body are merely symbolic – mystical metaphors that bear no relation to physical reality. To the practitioners of these ancient forms of healing, however, they represent true models of how the body functions in both health and disease, and are rooted in religious traditions many thousands of years old.

The 'plumbing' model of the body

In the Western industrialized world, many contemporary concepts of the body's structure and function seem to be borrowed partly from the worlds of science and technology. Familiarity with drainage systems in the home, electricity, machines and the internal combustion engine all provide the models in terms of which people conceptualize and explain the structure and workings of the body. A common version of this might be termed the 'plumbing' model, as illustrated in the case study above. Here the body is conceived of as a series of hollow cavities or chambers, connected with one another and with the body's orifices by a series of pipes or tubes. The major cavities are usually the chest and the stomach, which almost completely fill the thoracic and abdominal spaces respectively.

This type of subdivision of the body into large volumes with a single name was demonstrated in Boyle's[28] study, mentioned above, where 58.8 per cent of the sample saw the stomach as occupying all of the abdominal cavity. Lay vocabulary of ill health also reflects this conception; for example, 'I've got a cold on my chest' or 'my chest's full of phlegm'. The cavities are connected to each other and to the orifices by pipes such as the intestines, the bowel, the windpipe and the blood vessels. Central to this model is the belief that health is maintained by the uninterrupted *flow* of various substances – including blood, air, food, faeces, urine and menstrual blood – between cavities, or between a cavity and the body's exterior via one of the orifices. Disease, then, is seen as the result of blockage of an internal tube or pipe.

The implications of this model in clinical practice were well demonstrated in the example quoted from Kleinman *et al.*[35]. A further example, in the UK, is the widespread folk concept of the dangers of constipation – that is, of a 'blockage in the bowels'. In this model, more common in the older generation, the retained faeces were thought to diffuse into the bloodstream and somehow contaminate it with impurities and 'toxins' – and this then affected both the complexion and one's general health. Self-prescribed laxatives are still widely used in order to achieve a 'good clear out' and so preserve good health and a good complexion. The notion of a 'good clear out' is also applied to menstrual and postpartum blood, and will be described more fully below.

The plumbing model does not necessarily cover all aspects of the body's physiology and anatomy, but mostly deals with the respiratory, cardiovascular, gastrointestinal and genitourinary systems. It is not a coherent or internally consistent system, but rather a series of metaphors used to explain the body's functioning. Often different physiological systems are lumped together if they occur in the same area (e.g. the chest). A man with nasal catarrh and cough, for example, described his self-treatment as: 'I gargled with salt water to get the catarrh out – and I always swallow a bit of it to loosen the cough'[17].

The model can also be used to express emotional states, especially lay notions of 'stress' or 'pressure' (see Chapter 11), in images borrowed from the Age of Steam – 'I blew my top', 'I need to let off steam', 'I almost burst a boiler'.

The body as a machine

The conceptualization of the body as an internal combustion engine or as a battery-driven machine has become more common in Western society. These machine and engine metaphors are increasingly encountered by health professionals, who may in turn reinforce them, especially by the use of such explanatory phrases as 'your heart isn't pumping so well', 'you've had a nervous breakdown', 'the current isn't flowing so well along your nerves' or 'you need a rest – your batteries need recharging'. Central to the body as a machine concept is the idea of a renewable fuel or battery power needed to provide energy for the smooth working of the body. 'Fuel' here includes various foodstuffs or beverages, such as tea or coffee, and the large number of self-prescribed vitamins, tonics and other patent remedies. Some people may conceive of alcohol, tobacco or psychotropic drugs as forms of essential fuel without which they could not function in everyday life.

The machine model includes the idea that individual parts of the body, like the parts of a motor car, may fail or stop working, and may sometimes need to be replaced. Modern spare-part surgery (see below), with its widespread usage of organ transplants and artificial organs and body parts, as well as the use of electronic aids such as pacemakers and transistor hearing-aids, all help to reinforce the image of the body as a repairable machine, with treatment consisting of 'new parts for old'[45]. This, in turn, may result in unrealistic expectations of medical treatment. Certain diagnostic procedures such as electrocardiographs or electroencephalograms, which measure the body's 'electrical currents' or waves, as well as the use of foetal monitors in obstetrics (see Chapter 6), may all reinforce the machine metaphor in the minds of both patients and health professionals.

Allied with this image of the body as a machine is that of the mind as a computer. The increasing use of computers has influenced the ways many people in the industrialized world think about themselves. We now live in a new psychological culture, in what Turkle[46] calls a 'computational culture', with new metaphors for the mind as mainly a processor and storehouse of information. In this model, thoughts, ideas, creativity, memory and personality are all seen as forms of 'software' or programs hidden inside the 'hardware' of the brain and the skull. Thus mental illness or deviant behaviour can now be conceived of as faulty wiring or programming of the individual brain, to be cured by merely reprogramming or rewiring – a new and simplified image of human thought and behaviour that has important social implications. At the same time, just as the mind is seen as a computer, so can the computer be seen as a sort of external mind – a second brain outside the skull, an advanced organ of memory, logic and calculation; what Turkle[46] terms a 'second self'. In the modern information age, loss of a computer or of its electronic memory can seem to some individuals almost as traumatic as a brain injury or a stroke.

The body in space and time

The concept of symbolic skins, outlined above, means that the body's existence is always shaped and altered by cultural notions of *space*. These usually extend the body's boundaries far beyond its natural, physical border of skin. In spatial terms, these symbolic skins – some of them invisible, others not – may enlarge the body (and the sense of self that it contains) by an enormous distance. Some writers, such as McLuhan[47], have even argued that the media (radio, television) can now extend the body's special senses (listening, looking) to virtually every part of the world. With their help one can now 'hear' or 'see' events on the other side of the globe at the very moment that they occur. The phenomenal growth of the Internet in recent years has also added to this process.

Other cultural concepts of the body, described earlier, deal more with ideas of internal space. They include the arrangement of the bodily organs and systems or, in the case of *ārdha-angāni,* the penetration of social categories to within the borders of skin. The recent growth of medical technology (see Chapter 4) has also altered the spatial reality of the human body. X-rays, scans and MRIs have now made it 'transparent' both to medical science and to patients themselves. In a symbolic way, this may be slowly weakening or dissolving people's sense of their own skin as the first, most intimate and fixed border of the self[48]. Similarly, life support systems and monitoring machines, as well as the development of the new reproductive technologies (see Chapter 6), all help to extend the body's boundaries even further. In the case of dialysis machines, for example, it is as if certain organs – in this case the kidneys – have now become external to the body itself[48].

The human body exists in *time*, as well as in space. This is partly due to cultural concepts of the development and changes of the body as it travels from birth towards death. Much of the Western medical model of 'normal' physical and mental development is based on a rigid, linear image of time, divided into a series of clearly defined milestones of development. Failure to achieve these milestones at exactly the right time (according to the textbook) is often regarded as a sign of abnormality; of being in some way undeveloped or even retarded.

Hall[49] has described the two concepts of time most common in Western countries. These are:

1. *Monochronic* time, which is linear, clock time. Here time is seen as a line or ribbon stretching from past to future, and divided into segments known as years, months or days. Every phenomenon is assumed to have a beginning and an end, and in between the two one can only do 'one thing at a time'. Monochronic time is a form of external social organization imposed on people, and is essential for the smooth functioning of industrial society. It is particularly strong in organizations and bureaucracies. In these settings, time is almost tangible; it can be spent, wasted, invested, bought or saved. Time can be converted into money, just as money can be converted into time. This type of time implies, however, a complete dominance over the body and its processes by clocks, calendars, diaries and schedules.
2. *Polychronic* time, which, by contrast, is much more human time, where personal relationships and interactions take precedence over the rigid schedules of the calendar and the clock. Time is not experienced as a line, but as a point at which relationships or events converge. Polychronic people are not so dominated by clock time; instead, they 'are oriented towards people, human relationships, and the family, which is the core of their existence'. In Hall's view, monochronic time in the USA is more public, 'male' time, while polychronic is more private, 'female' time – the time of the home, leisure and family life.

Both forms of time, but especially monochronic time, imply different types of cultural pressure that impact upon the human body in modern society. An example of this is the damaging physiological effect of driving in heavy traffic during 'rush hours', to and from work, each day of the week. Some of the other effects of clock time, on heart disease for example, are discussed further in Chapter 11. In the case of the contraceptive pill, too, a rigid 28-day cycle of clock time is imposed onto the woman's physiology, and for some women this may possibly have emotional, or physical consequences. Throughout the Western world, moreover, monochronic time is a widespread feature of almost all medical institutions, including hospitals, clinics, doctors' offices and medical bureaucracies. In these health care settings, the overuse of rigid schedules such as hospital visiting times or appointment systems may be seen by some ill people as inhuman and impersonal. They and their families may see it as a way avoiding human contact, of not dealing with their illness and the emotional reality of their situation.

The 'disabled' body

One of the key cultural categories, found in virtually all societies, is the division between the 'able' and the 'disabled' body. Despite this division, anthropologists have pointed out how these definitions vary widely between different social and cultural groups, as do the meanings they ascribe to these particular labels.

Some attempts have been made to standardize the classification of disabilities internationally, such as the World Health Organization's *International Classification of Impairments, Disabilities, and Handicaps*[50] of 1980. From an anthropological perspective, however, it is the social dimensions of how people (whether disabled or not) interpret and respond to these cultural categories that is of the greatest interest. This phenomenon is of growing importance, since it was estimated in the 1980s that there were about 500 million severely disabled people in the world[51]. Since then this number has greatly increased, due partly to various wars and civil conflicts, and to the large numbers of landmine victims in Cambodia, Mozambique, Afghanistan and elsewhere.

'Disability' versus' impairment'

The sociologist Michael Oliver[52], in a radical critique of the subject, makes a useful distinction between *impairment* and *disability*. The former describes a body lacking part or all of a limb, or having a defective limb or some other bodily mechanism, while the latter refers to the many social and other disadvantages imposed by society on people with physical impairments. He criticizes the medical model of disability, which focuses solely on the individual and their physical condition instead of on the society in which disability occurs. His model emphasizes how the very concept of disability is socially constructed, and how this category helps create a large number of people who are dependent, marginal and supposedly unproductive economically. Society's narrow definitions of physical normality lead it to ignore and marginalize those who do not fit within that definition. Thus it does not provide the facilities (such as ramps for wheelchairs) for those who are physically different from the majority of the population. This radical model represents, therefore, a shift in focus from individual to social pathology. Disability is not seen as an individual problem, but as one of society. In some ways, therefore, this perspective resembles the 'socially labelling' model of psychiatric disorders described in Chapter 10. Furthermore, Oliver argues that, because disability is largely 'socially constructed', it follows that not all impaired people need necessarily be 'disabled': this state is not necessarily an inherent aspect of the individual, but is determined rather by the meanings that society ascribes to it and the state of dependency that it often imposes.

Disability and stigma

In many societies, anthropologists have described how people with different physical shapes, sizes and bodily functions are often subject to considerable *stigma*, as well as to prejudice and discrimination[53,54]. Even though the disabled body is not necessarily a sick body, these people often encounter a variety of social disadvantages – especially in finding a marriage partner. In Uganda, for example, Sentumbwe[55] describes how blind girls usually have much reduced marriage opportunities. It is widely assumed that, although they are able to have sexual ('lover') relationships, they will normally not be acceptable as a potential wife, since 'the management of a home requires sight and complete physical functioning'. Many men therefore see them merely as sexual objects, and try to exploit the situation. Despite this, Sentumbwe points out that many blind women in Uganda *do* get married, raise children, have employment and contribute towards the economic and social life of the community. He anticipates a time when, through public education, 'the sighted might come to see the blind as persons with a visual impairment rather than as people who are blind and therefore socially and physically handicapped'. Devlieger[56] also describes how, among women of the Songye people of former Zaire, a major disability of the limbs which may inhibit daily domestic tasks can make getting married very difficult; however, this does not apply to men with similar disabilities. Similarly, anthropologists[54] have described the social difficulties of physically impaired young people in Dakar, Senegal, and how marrying off a disabled daughter means accepting a lower 'bridewealth' for her than would be paid for a 'normal' woman, but obtaining a wife for a disabled son requires the payment of a much larger than normal bridewealth – a sum that can take many years to accumulate.

The degree of stigma and the economic effect of physical impairment can depend on a number of factors. These include the type of impairment, the socio-economic position of the person and their family *vis-á-vis* the wider society, the types of rehabilitation or treatment available, and the level of technology and social organization of the society itself. In an age of computers, information technology, telecommunications and the Internet, for example, many types of physical impairment are no longer a barrier to a full working and social life. In other cultures, stigma can be avoided or lessened in different ways. In Botswana, Ingstad[57] has described how the parents of a physically impaired child are able to avoid the stigmatizing label of *mopakwane* – a disability believed to be caused by the parents having broken the taboo against having sexual relations while the baby is very young. They do this either by claiming that it is something that 'just happened' (that is, without any social cause), or that the child is *mpho ya modimo*, a 'gift from God'. Actually naming the child in this way can in some ways protect it from stigma in its future life.

Positive aspects of disability

It should be emphasized, however, that the stigmatization of *all* physical impairment is not universal. In many cultures different forms of impairment are seen in a more positive light, and disabled people play a full role in community life. For example, Levinson and Gaccione[58] list several cultures where people with certain types of physical impairment are highly valued and believed to have special powers or abilities. In rural Korea, in a cultural tradition that goes back 1000 years, some blind men have been *pongsa* – a special group of diviners who act as fortune tellers, select sites for buildings and graves, pray for rain and place curses. They are believed to have a special type of sight, the 'eyesight of mind'. Among the Tiv people of Nigeria, too, blind people are often believed to develop this special type of sight, and are respected accordingly. Reynolds-Whyte and Ingstad[54] also note how, in many cultures, blind people are more likely to become learned religious men, storytellers or singers – such as the *Surdasi*, the blind singers of India. They also mention how, particularly in some very poor countries in Africa and Asia, physical disability can sometimes be turned to economic advantage. In these contexts, beggars often 'use their impairment as a tool to work for their families', and can sometimes earn more than the physically able.

Theories of causation of disability

As with other human problems, physical impairments are often blamed on a variety of causes – originating either in individual behaviour or in the natural, social or supernatural worlds (see Chapter 5). Supernatural theories are particularly common, even among the disabled themselves. In one study of 104 blind people in rural Ethiopia[59], for example, 45 per cent of them blamed their blindness on a febrile illness and 15 per cent on accidents, but 33 per cent blamed supernatural forces such as 'curses' or divine punishment. In that same study, almost all the fully and partially sighted people in the community thought that blindness prevented education and that educational opportunities should not be given to the blind. In many other non-industrialized societies, too, considerable attention is paid to the *cause* of the impairment. Often a physical abnormality is seen as the result and expression of some abnormality in that person's relationships to their social or supernatural environment. Among the Songye people, for example, Devlieger[56] describes how physical impairment is often seen as 'a symptom of something more important'. It can be the result of sorcery (often resulting from social or familial conflict) or the breaking of taboos (such as those against sex during pregnancy), or from a lack of respect given to a dead ancestor. For example, a person with a club foot may be seen as having been born 'with the spirit of the ancestor', since this could mean that that the ancestor was not well buried and his coffin was too small so that his legs were compressed. If no other social cause can be found, the condition may simply be ascribed to the act of God (*Efile Mukulu*).

In general, but without over-romanticizing the picture, the ethnographic evidence suggests that in many small scale societies the physically impaired are treated with more care – as a more normal, accepted part of everyday life – than in many Western, industrialized societies. But even within these Third World communities, attitudes towards disabled people are usually not uniform. Often those with different types of impairment are labelled differently and then treated in a different way. Devlieger[56], for example, has described how, among the Songye, physically unusual or 'abnormal' children are divided into three categories: 'bad' (*malwa*) children include albino, dwarf and hydrocephalic children; 'faulty' (*bilema*) children include those with deformed upper or lower limbs (such as from polio or birth injuries) or congenital abnormalities (such as club foot); while 'ceremonial' (*mishinga*) children include twins, or children born with the hands or feet first or with the cord around their neck. Those in the last category are given special attention and a higher social status, and are believed to have special powers of healing. The 'bad' children, by contrast, are treated as marginal, inferior beings that are not fully human. There is believed to be something supernatural about them, since their origin is believed to be associated with sorcery, and thus they were recently in contact 'with the anti-world of sorcerers'. Although given basic care, they are expected to die fairly soon, since 'they come into this world to stay for a short time and afterwards return to their own world'. The third, probably more common group, includes *mwana wa kilema* ('a child with a fault'). These children do not only have distorted bodies, but their condition is believed to arise from distorted relationships within their family or community. Little effort is made to improve their physical functioning, but they are not necessarily treated in a negative way. Instead, 'the person with a disability is seen not as an abnormal, a marginal or a deviant figure, but as a liminal one' (for discussion of such 'liminal' identity, see Chapter 9). Furthermore, they are often valued as confidants for their wisdom, and for their unique perspective on the world.

Finally, many of the supernatural explanations for the disabled body attach to congenital conditions rather than to those acquired later in life, where 'personhood has already been established'[54]. Despite this, an acquired physical impairment can have almost as dramatic psychological and social effects on the individual concerned. Two classic monographs on this theme are those of the Dutch journalist Renate Rubinstein[60] and of Oliver Sacks[61], the neurologist and writer. Rubinstein describes her emotions of powerlessness when she developed multiple sclerosis, her new dependence on doctors and technology, and the feeling of being 'not quite human anymore' – at least in a social sense. Sacks, too, gives a poignant and graphic account of his experience of a severe leg injury, of the many shifts in body image and the sense of self that this involved, and how incomprehensible much of his experiences were to the doctors and nurses involved in his care.

Overall, then, the category of the disabled body is not fixed. It is a complex and variable one, and its definition depends on social, cultural, economic and historical context. In industrial societies particularly there is a concerted attempt to shift this definition from disability, with all the disadvantages this label implies, towards the more neutral definition of physical impairment.

'New bodies' of the twentieth century

Over several decades now a number of 'new bodies' – or new ways of conceptualizing the human body – have appeared in the Western, industrialized world. Each of them is the result of advances in both medical treatment and diagnostic technology. Their effect has been to alter radically the ways that the modern body, including its boundaries and interior, is conceived of, not only by doctors but also by much of the lay public. Five of these new conceptualizations are described below.

The composite body

As a result of the success of spare-part surgery, it has become possible to replace diseased or damaged organs or body parts either by implanting an artificial organ or by transplanting an organ from another person. Artificial body parts, made of metal, plastic, nylon or rubber, now include hips, knees, arteries, larynx, limbs, teeth, heart valves, corneas and oesophagus. Transplanted organs include hearts, kidneys, corneas, cartilage, bone, hair, liver, lungs, pancreas and parathyroid. Many thousands of people, especially the aged, now have bodies that are partly artificial or are composites of parts of other bodies. Despite their obvious medical and psychological advantages, these spare parts may be subtly altering the contemporary body image and the sense of what is self and what is non-self[45]. They also create new links of 'kinship' between the donors and recipients of these organs, whether living or dead, and between the recipients of artificial organs and those who have manufactured or implanted them.

The 'cyborg'

Cyborgs are advanced fusions of human beings and machines. Modern medical technology has enabled many people to be kept alive or to function better by attaching the body to a machine, large or small, for most of the time. These now include dialysis machines (for kidney failure), life support systems (such as heart–lung machines and 'iron lungs'), incubators (for premature infants), artificial hearts, and smaller machines such as transistor hearing aids and heart pacemakers. By creating bodies which are partly machine, medical technology has profoundly influenced the contemporary body image – a fact reflected in the imagery of popular culture[48]. For many people, it has further reinforced the body-as-a-machine metaphor described above.

The brain

For several decades medical research and practice has increasingly focused on the study of the brain and the monitoring of its functions. This has followed advances in neurophysiology and in diagnostic technologies such as the electroencephalograph (EEG). In symbolic terms, however, it seems to have resulted in a contemporary shift in body image – locating the true site of 'personhood' and the self (as well as of the personality and the unconscious) within the brain itself rather than in the body as a whole. As such it echoes older cultural models, such as *phrenology* in the nineteenth century, which emphasized the head and brain as the most important part of human anatomy. This shift is illustrated by changing medical definitions of death. Since the late 1960s death has increasingly been defined as 'brain death'; that is, the end of cerebral functions rather than the cessation of other bodily functions such as heartbeat or respiration[62]. In many Western countries it is now possible for comatose patients to be declared legally dead on the basis of an EEG, and their organs 'harvested' for transplantation to other people, even if their heart is still beating and they are still breathing with the aid of a life support system[63]. Increasing focus on the brain is reflected in a huge increase in brain research, in the declaration by the US Congress of the 1990s as 'The Decade of the Brain'[64], and in the growth of the 'brain banks' – collections of brain and neural tissue for research – in the USA and elsewhere. For example, the National Neurological Research Specimen Bank at Veterans Administration Wadsworth Hospital, University of California, Los Angeles, holds more than 2000 brains and collects 150 more each year[65], while in Russia the Moscow Brain Institute still has 30 000 slices of Lenin's brain for study, as well as those of other prominent people[66].

Nudeshima[67], however, points out that in Japan there is considerable cultural resistance to the Western approach to brain death, followed by organ harvesting. For this reason, many Japanese who needed a transplant have had to travel abroad to get one. This is because 'the traditional Japanese notion of person had a communal, not an individual, basis'; the death of an individual's brain was not necessarily equated with the actual death of that individual. Death was seen as a long process rather than as a single event, and was only recognized as being final after a series of rituals conducted by the family and community (see Chapter 9) and which sometimes lasted several years. Despite the Organ Transplant Law of 1997, which for the first time recognized brain death as the end of life, and the distribution of 23 million organ donor cards throughout Japan, a year later not a single transplant operation had been performed[68].

The medical body

The essential reductionism of modern medicine coupled with advances in diagnostic technology (see Chapter 5) has led to a focus on progressively smaller areas of the body. Medical diagnosis routinely deals with abnormalities at the biochemical, cellular and even molecular levels. This is reflected in the illustrations in medical textbooks over the past century or two. Gradually they have shifted from gross anatomy to micro-anatomy; from depictions of the body itself to those of individual organs, and finally of cells or even of molecular structures within those cells. Arguably, the 'body' in which modern medicine is now most interested is that of the cell itself. Much of the medical discourse on AIDS, for example, focuses mainly on this cellular level, especially in relation to the immune system. Also, since 1895 the development of X-rays and, more recently, ultrasound, CT, and MRI scans has made the human body more 'transparent', with its structure and interior easily visible[69]. Many thousands of patients have been shown scans or X-rays of their own bodies, in hospitals, doctors' offices and antenatal clinics. Together with medicine's reductionist view of the body, which the public increasingly learns about via the media, magazines or Internet or during consultations with a doctor, this has undoubtedly influenced in subtle ways how people perceive their own bodies.

The external womb

Advances in the medical treatment of infertility (the new reproductive technologies), such as *in vitro* fertilization (IVF) or surrogate motherhood (see Chapter 6), have influenced the view many women have of their own bodies and reproductive functions[70]. For example, whereas ovulation, fertilization and pregnancy used to take place within the same woman's body, it is now possible for one or more of these to take place outside her body or even in the bodies of other women. A baby's gestation, birth and development may now involve three different women; the genetic mother, the carrying mother, and the nurturing mother[71] – one supplying the ovum, another carrying the foetus during pregnancy, and a third caring for the baby once it has been born. Although welcome to infertile women, these advances in reproductive technology, like spare-part surgery, have influenced both body image and assumptions about body boundaries. If one woman's child can be carried in the womb of another (an external womb, as it were), then traditional notions of what is body, self and non-self will all have been radically altered. For the ovum donor, moreover, the ova themselves can become an external body part – one that will soon blend into the body of another woman[72].

The body during pregnancy

All cultures share beliefs about the *vulnerability* of the mother and foetus during pregnancy; to a variable extent, this extends after birth, usually throughout the early postpartum or lactation period. Cultural concepts of the physiology of pregnancy are often evoked after the child is born, in order to explain *post hoc* any unwanted outcomes of pregnancy such as a deformed, ailing or retarded child. In most cultures it is believed that the mother's behaviour – her diet, physical activity, state of mind, moral behaviour, use of drink, drugs or tobacco – can directly affect the physiology of reproduction and cause damage to the unborn child. Anthropologists have argued that not all the taboos and restrictions surrounding pregnant women can be explained as protecting the mother and foetus from physical damage; the pregnant woman is also in a state of *social* vulnerability and ambiguity. She is in a state of transition between two social roles; those of wife and mother[73]. In this marginal state, as in other states of social transition (see Chapter 9), the person involved is seen as somehow in an ambiguous and 'abnormal' state, dangerous both to herself and to others. The rituals and taboos surrounding pregnancy therefore serve both to mark this transition and to protect mother and foetus during this dangerous period.

Several studies have been carried out by Snow *et al.*[39,74,75], at public antenatal clinics in Michigan, USA, into lay beliefs about the physiology and dangers of pregnancy. In many cases these beliefs were markedly different from those of the clinicians involved in their care. In one study of 31 pregnant women[74], 77 per cent of them believed that the foetus could be 'marked' – that is, permanently disfigured or even killed – by strong emotional states on the part of the mother, divine punishment for behavioural lapses, the 'power of nature' or the evil intentions of others. The Mexican-American women in the sample believed that too much sleep or rest during pregnancy would harm the baby by causing it to 'stick to the uterus', making delivery difficult or impossible. They also feared the effect on the child if they saw a lunar eclipse, believing that if a pregnant woman goes out unprotected at this time her child may be born dead, or with a cleft palate or part of the body missing. Wearing a key suspended around the waist was thought to be adequate protection at this time. Many in the study also believed that excessive emotion in the mother – fear, hate, jealousy, anger, sorrow, pity – could all be dangerous to the unborn child. If the pregnant woman saw something that frightened her, like a cat or a fish, the child might be born resembling that object. One woman frightened by a fish during her pregnancy gave birth to a child that 'has two holes in the roof of her mouth and can swim like a fish'. Fetal damage could also result from behavioural lapses on the part of the mother; making fun of a cripple or retarded person during pregnancy could result in God afflicting the infant with a similar disability. Finally, the malevolence of another person could cause foetal damage and even death. Similar lay beliefs are found throughout the world, with local variations.

Beliefs about the effects on the foetus of maternal diet were also investigated in the Michigan study[39]. Ninety per cent of a sample of 40 women thought that pregnant women should change their diets in some way, while 38 per cent believed that food cravings could 'mark' the child permanently if these cravings were not satisfied. In most cases the baby was believed to be marked by unsatisfied food cravings. One woman thought that if a pregnant woman craved chicken but did not get it, the baby could be born 'looking like a chicken'. Other beliefs related to the effect of particular types of food on the foetus; for example, a baby might be born with red spots if the mother ate too many cherries or strawberries during pregnancy, or have a 'chocolate mark' if she ate (or even sat upon) any chocolate. Snow points out that some of these dietary beliefs may be dangerous in pregnancy, as they may provide the rationale for undesirable eating habits by the women. Another factor among some Latin American women is the use of 'hot' or 'cold' foods in pregnancy, irrespective of their nutritional properties, in order to maintain their internal 'balance'. Similar beliefs are found among women from the Indian subcontinent. Homans[73] quotes a British-born Asian woman as saying, 'my mother said not to have "hot" things, not to sit in front of the heater and not to have Coca Cola ... The body acquires too much heat and this can lead to miscarriage'.

Beliefs about the state of the uterus during pregnancy can also affect a pregnant woman's health. In the Michigan study[75], a widely held belief was that the uterus was a hollow organ that was 'tightly closed' during pregnancy to prevent the loss of the foetus. One woman believed that pregnant women could not contract venereal disease (and therefore did not need to take precautions against it) during pregnancy as 'the uterus is closed and germs cannot enter'.

Beliefs about the physiology and dangers of pregnancy have social, psychological and physical aspects. They set pregnant women apart as a special category of person surrounded by what their culture tells them are protective taboos and customs, and these help to explain retrospectively any physical damage or deformity in newborn children. Both aspects, as illustrated above, may have damaging effects on the pregnant woman and her unborn child.

Beliefs about blood

To illustrate further some of the clinical implications of cultural conceptions of physiology, a number of beliefs about the nature and function of human *blood* are described below. The human experience of blood – as a vital liquid circulating within the body, and which appears at the surface at times of injury, illness, menstruation or childbirth – provides the basis for lay theories about a variety of illnesses. In general these illnesses are ascribed to changes in its *volume* ('high blood', due to too much blood), *consistency* ('thin blood' causing anaemia), *temperature* ('hot illnesses' caused by 'heat in the blood' in Morocco), *quality* ('impurities' in the blood, from constipation) or *polluting power* (menstrual blood causing 'weakness' in males). It should also be remembered that lay concepts of blood deal with much more than its perceived physiological actions; blood is a potent image for a number of things, social, physical and psychological. It is what Turner[76] calls 'a multi-vocal symbol', that is, it signifies a number of elements at the same time. Among the cluster of meanings associated with blood cross-culturally are: an *index* of emotional state (blushing or pallor); personality type (hot-blooded, cold-blooded); illness (flushed, or feverish); kinship ('blood is thicker than water'); social relationships ('bad blood between us'); physical injury (bleeding, bruises); gender (menstruation); danger (menstrual and postpartum blood); and diet ('thin blood' from a bad diet). The clinician should thus be aware of the possible hidden symbolism in any lay conceptualizations of blood.

Case study: Beliefs about blood in South Wales, UK

Skultans[77] studied the beliefs about menstruation among women in a mining village in South Wales. She found two types of belief about menstrual blood. The first was that menstrual blood is 'bad blood', and menstruation the process by which the system is purged of badness or excess. The emphasis was on losing as much blood as possible, as this was the method whereby 'the system rights itself'. The women said they felt huge, bloated, slow and sluggish 'if they do not have a period or if they do not lose much'. One woman felt 'really great' after a heavy period, and most insisted on the value of having a monthly 'good clearance'. Skultans found that this group had relatively undisturbed and stable married lives, and regarded the menstrual process as 'essential to producing and maintaining a healthy equilibrium' by regular purging of badness. These women also saw menstruation as a state of increased vulnerability, and particularly feared anything which might stop the flow; this would obviously give them a pessimistic attitude towards the menopause, while at the same time they might not worry about menorrhagia or an exceptionally heavy bleed, regarding it instead as 'a good clearance'. The second group of women believed that menstruation was damaging to their overall health, and were fearful of 'losing their life's blood'. They wished to cease menstruating as early as possible and, unlike the first group, were much more positive about the menopause and its attendant symptoms. Skultans found that this group, who viewed periods as 'a nuisance', seemed to be associated with irregular or disturbed conjugal relationships.

Case study: Beliefs about menstruation among the Zulu of South Africa

Ngubane[78] described beliefs about menstrual blood among the Zulu people of South Africa. Menstruating women are believed to have a contagious pollution, which is dangerous both to other humans and to the natural world. Men's virility may be weakened by this blood, especially if they have intercourse with a menstruating woman. A menstruating woman should also avoid sick people or their medicines during her period, and crops may be ruined or cattle fall ill if she walks among them. In other African societies, women may be confined each month to an isolated 'menstrual hut' to protect the community from their dangerous pollution. Similar beliefs about the 'uncleanness' and polluting powers of menstrual blood are found, especially among men, in cultures and religious groups in many parts of the world[79].

Case study: Beliefs about menstruation in Michigan, USA

Snow and Johnson[39,75] examined the views of low-income women in a public clinic in Michigan. Many of them saw menstruation as a method of ridding the body of impurities that might otherwise cause illness or poison the system. They saw the uterus as a hollow organ that is tightly closed between periods while it slowly fills with 'tainted blood', and then opens up to allow the blood to escape during the period. As a result they reasoned that one could only get pregnant just before, during or just after the period, 'while the uterus is still open'. While the uterus was open, the women believed themselves to be particularly vulnerable to illness, caused by the entry of external forces such as cold air or water, germs or witchcraft. One woman in the group speculated that one should not attend a funeral during menstruation lest the germs that caused the deceased's death enter the open uterus and cause disease. A recurrent fear among the women studied was of stopped or impeded menstrual flow, or of the flow of blood in the postpartum or post-abortion period. Latin American women in particular feared that certain 'cold' foods (or cold water or air) might clot the 'hot' blood, and interrupt the flow. The stopped flow might then 'back up' in the body and cause a stroke, cancer, sterility or 'quick TB'. 'Cold' foodstuffs included fresh fruits, especially citrus, tomatoes and green vegetables. As one Mexican-American woman put it '*Le da mucha friadad a la matriz*' ('Such things make the womb very cold')[39]. The researchers point out that avoidance of such foods during vaginal bleeding associated with menstruation, post-abortion or postpartum states can eliminate much-needed vitamins from a diet which, for many low-income women, is already deficient in vitamins. The fear of impeded menstruation may also lead some women to avoid some methods of contraception (oral contraceptives, intrauterine contraceptive devices) that may cause changes in menstruation.

Case study: 'High blood' in the Southern United States

Snow[80] has described a common lay belief among low-income patients in the Southern USA, both black and white, called 'high blood'. The central belief is that the blood goes up or down in volume depending on what one eats or drinks, and this can cause either 'high blood' or 'low blood'. 'Low blood' is believed to result from eating too many acid or astringent foods, such as lemon juice, vinegar, pickles, olives, sauerkraut and Epsom salts, and causes lassitude, fatigue and weakness; it is thought to occur particularly in pregnant women and should be treated by ingesting certain red foods or drink – beets, grape juice, red wine, liver and red meat. 'High blood', by contrast, results from eating too much rich food, especially red meat. Home remedies include taking lemon juice, vinegar, sour oranges, Epsom salts and the brine from pickles or olives. The clinical implications of this belief are not only the effects on health of this type of diet (for example, one with a very high salt content), but also the effect on compliance with a doctor's instructions by one who confuses 'high blood' with high blood pressure. Patients who interpret a diagnosis of high blood pressure as 'high blood' may increase the amount of salt in their diet and reduce the intake of red meat in a diet that may already be deficient in protein.

Case study: 'Sleeping blood' in the Cape Verde Islands

Like and Ellison[81] described the case of a 48-year-old woman from the Cape Verde Islands who was admitted to a neurology ward in a hospital in the USA. She was suffering from paralysis, numbness, pain and tremor of her right arm. It was discovered that 2 years previously she had suffered bilateral Colles' fractures of her wrists, and after that her neurological symptoms gradually appeared. No physical cause for her illness could be found, until it was realized that she believed herself to be suffering from a Cape Verdean folk illness, 'sleeping blood' (*sangue dormido*). In this lay model, traumatic injuries (in this case, her wrist fractures) may cause a person's normal 'living blood' (*sangue vivo*) to leak out into the skin, turn black (i.e. form a haematoma) and become 'sleeping blood'. It is feared that deeper deposits of blood develop between the muscles and the bones and, if not removed, their volume may expand over time and obstruct the circulation distal to the traumatized area. In addition, the internal 'living blood' may dam up and cause various disorders such as pain, tremor, paralysis, convulsions, stroke, blindness, heart attack, infection, miscarriage and mental illness. The patient explained her neurological disabilities as due to the blockage resulting from the 'sleeping blood'. She was eventually treated by withdrawing 12 ml of blood from her right wrist (the *sangue dormido*) on two occasions, and by the application of cold packs, after which her tremor, paralysis and pain completely disappeared.

Case study: Blood as a non-regenerative liquid

Foster and Anderson[82] pointed out that the belief that blood is a non-regenerative liquid which, when lost through injury or disease, cannot be replaced, leaving the victim permanently weakened, is common in many parts of the world. In parts of Latin America people are most reluctant to part with their precious blood, and this may be one of the reasons why blood banks are less successful in getting donations of blood than in the USA and in Europe.

Case study: 'Dirty' or 'lost' blood among the Mende of Sierra Leone

Bledsoe and Goubaud[83] described how, among the Mende people of Sierra Leone, blood is seen as a vital liquid that it is almost impossible to replace if lost. Debilitating sicknesses, injuries and infestation with small organisms and worms (*fulu-haisia*) are all said to make blood 'dirty', or to drain it. Blood can also be 'lost' by having blood samples taken at hospital, or by donating blood; thus 'the Mende view with great fear the attempts of hospital workers to induce them to give blood'. Attempts are made to replace, build or purify the blood by the use of certain foods (especially palm oil and greens such as spinach or potato leaves) and certain medicines (especially those that are red in colour). *All* red medicines are considered desirable, whatever they contain, provided they are red, brown or even orange in colour – for example, Fanta, Guiness Stout or Vimto are also taken during illness. Because palm oil is the favourite remedy for dirty or inadequate blood, young children may be fed only soft rice (which develops the body) and palm oil (which makes it produce blood) until well into their second year.

Recommended reading

de Garine, I. and Pollock, N. J. (eds). (1995). *Social Aspects of Obesity*. Gordon and Breach.

Foster, G. M. (1994). *Hippocrates' Latin American Legacy: Humoral Medicine in the New World*. Gordon and Breach.

Helman, C. (1992). *The Body of Frankenstein's Monster: Essays in Myth and Medicine*. W. W. Norton.

Ingstad, B. and Reynolds-Whyte, S. (eds) (1995). *Disability and Culture*. University of California Press.

Polbemus, T. (ed.) (1978). *Social Aspects of the Human Body*. Penguin.

Sacks, O. (1991). *A Leg to Stand On*. Picador.

Scheper-Hughes, N. and Lock, M. M. (1987). The mindful body: a proglomenon to future work in medical anthropology. *Med. Anthropol. Q.* (new series), **1(1)**, 6–41.

3 Diet and nutrition

Food is more than just a source of nutrition. In all human societies it plays many roles and is deeply embedded in the social, religious and economic aspects of everyday life. For people in these societies it also carries with it a range of symbolic meanings, both expressing and creating the relationships between man and man, between man and his deities, and man and the natural environment. Food, therefore, is an essential part of the way that any society organizes itself, and of the way it views the world that it inhabits.

The anthropologist Claude Levi-Strauss[1] has argued that, just as there is no human society which does not have a spoken language, so also is there no human group which does not in some way process some of its food supply through cooking. In fact, the constant transformation of raw into cooked food is one of the defining features of all human societies, a key criterion of *culture* as opposed to *nature*.

Anthropologists have further pointed out how cultural groups differ markedly from one another in many of their beliefs and practices related to food. For example, there are wide variations throughout the world as to what substances are regarded as food and what are not. Foodstuffs that are eaten in one society or group may be rigorously forbidden in another. There are also variations between cultures as to how food is cultivated, harvested, prepared, served and eaten. Each culture usually has a set of implicit rules that determine who prepares and serves the food and to whom; which individuals or groups eat together; where and on what occasions the consumption of food takes place; the order of dishes within a meal; and the actual manner of eating the food. All of these stages in food consumption are closely patterned by culture, and are part of the accepted way of life of that community.

In most parts of the world the actual preparation of food is usually the task of *women*[2], but in many societies they are also closely involved in its production – milking animals, caring for poultry and livestock, and planting, tending and harvesting a wide variety of crops. In many rural parts of the Third World women also play a leading role in the retail marketing of food – such as the famous 'market women' of West Africa, the Caribbean and parts of Latin America.

Cultural classifications of food

Because of the central role of food in daily life, especially in social relationships, dietary beliefs and practices are notoriously difficult to change, even if they interfere with adequate nutrition. Many well-meaning nutritionists, nurses and doctors have discovered this fact in dealing with cultures other than their own. Before these beliefs and practices can be modified or improved, it is important to understand the way that each culture views its food and the way that it *classifies* it into different categories. In general, five types of food classification systems can be identified, though in practice they overlap, and several of them usually co-exist within the same society. They are:

1. Food *versus* non-food
2. Sacred *versus* profane foods
3. Parallel food classifications

4. Food used as medicine, and medicine as food
5. Social foods (which signal relationships, status, occupation, gender or group identity).

Their clinical significance is that they may severely restrict the types of foodstuffs available to people, and that diet may be based on cultural rather than nutritional criteria.

Food *versus* non-food

Each culture defines which substances are edible and which are not, although this definition often leaves out substances that *do* have a nutritional value. In the UK, for example, snakes, squirrels, otters, dogs, cats and mice are all edible, but are rarely classified as food. In France snails and frogs' legs are food, but usually not so in the UK. In parts of the Far East dogs and cats are commonly eaten, but this does not occur in the Western world. Irrespective of cultural background, however, virtually no human groups in the world define human flesh as food.

In some cases, the definition of substances as non-food may be due to their historical associations; for example, Jelliffe[3] suggested that the spleen is rarely eaten in Britain because, in the ancient Galenic humoral system, it was the prime seat of the melancholic humour. Definitions of what is considered edible and what is not tend to be flexible, however, especially under conditions of famine, economic deprivation and foreign travel. In addition, there is a spectrum among the substances defined as food ranging between those that are regarded as nutritious, and are eaten during meals, and those eaten between meals as snacks. In some cases the manufacturers of certain of these snacks, such as sweets, candies, chocolates and cakes, have sought to promote their products as a nutritious food, something that 'fills the energy gap' between proper mealtimes.

Whatever the origins of these definitions, classifying a substance as non-food on cultural grounds may leave out useful nutriments from the diet, and this seems to be a universal phenomenon. 'No group', as Foster and Anderson[4] put it, 'even under conditions of extreme starvation, utilizes all available nutritional substances as food'.

Sacred *versus* profane foods

The term 'sacred' foods is used here to refer to those foodstuffs the use of which is validated by *religious* beliefs, while foodstuffs expressly forbidden by the religion can be termed 'profane'. This latter group is usually the subject of strict taboos that not only prohibit ingestion of the food but also forbid physical contact with it. In most cases, this profane food is also seen as unclean and dangerous to health. The sacred/profane dichotomy applies to much more than food, since it is usually part of a wider moral framework including dress, behaviour, speech and certain ritual actions – such as regular prayers, or ritual bathing and other rites of purification. The priestly castes and officiators within these groups are more likely to be subject to these strict rules, which maintain their purity and holiness, than the average worshipper. On certain occasions or fasts, all – or certain – foodstuffs are considered profane, and must be avoided. Examples of this are the Jewish *Yom Kippur* (a 25-hour fast) and the Muslim fast of *Ramadhan* where, for the ninth month of the lunar year, food and drink are avoided between dawn and sunset by all Muslims above the 'age of responsibility' (15 years for boys, 12 for girls) unless they are ill, menstruating, pregnant or lactating. Regular food abstentions are also a feature of Hinduism and, according to Hunt[5], many observant Hindus spend 2 or 3 days a week 'fasting' – that is, eating only 'pure' foods such as milk, fruit, nuts and starchy root vegetables like cassava and potatoes.

Strict taboos against certain types of food are characteristic of a number of religious faiths.

Hinduism

Orthodox Hindus are forbidden to kill or eat any animal, particularly the cow. Milk and its products may be eaten, since they do not involve taking the animal's life. Fish and eggs are infrequently eaten.

Islam

Neither pork nor any pig products may be eaten. The only meat permitted is that from cloven-hooved animals that chew the cud, and it must be *halal* – or ritually slaughtered. Only fish that have fins and scales may be eaten, and shellfish, shark and eels are therefore forbidden.

Judaism

As with Islam, all pig products are forbidden, and also fish without fins or scales, birds of prey and carrion. Only animals that chew the cud, have cloven hooves, and have been ritually slaughtered are *kosher* and may be eaten. Meat and milk dishes are never mixed within the same meal.

Sikhism

Beef is strictly forbidden, but pork is allowed though it is rarely eaten. The meat must also be slaughtered in a special ritual way known as *jhatka*.

Rastafarianism

Many Rastafarians are vegetarian, although some follow dietary restrictions similar to Judaism[6]. As with many other religious groups, alcohol is strictly prohibited.

A more secular example of food taboos is found in the contemporary *whole food* movement in the UK and USA. Here the sacred/profane dichotomy is between 'whole foods' on the one hand and 'junk foods' on the other; but also between natural and artificial, between the purity of the past and the pollution of the present. Junk foods are associated with ideas of uncleanliness and danger, especially from their additives, dyes, preservatives and other pollutants. In the ideology of the movement these additives are often associated with the supposed evils of modernity, and of the urban, industrial way of life. Similarly, the modern movement of *vegetarianism* – which Twigg[7] sees as offering 'a this-worldly form of salvation in terms of the body' – sees meat and its various products as dangerous and profane. They associate a vegetarian diet with purity, lightness, wholeness and spirituality while, by contrast, meat and blood are associated with aggressiveness, base sexual instincts, an 'animal nature' and a disharmonious world.

As will be illustrated below, all these forms of food taboos may exclude much-needed nutriments from the diet by classifying some foodstuffs as profane and therefore forbidden. They may also result in some forms of medication being rejected on religious grounds – for example, insulin made from beef or pork is unacceptable to many Hindus and Muslims.

Parallel food classifications

The division of all foodstuffs into two main groups, usually called 'hot' and 'cold', is a feature of many cultural groups in the Islamic world, the Indian subcontinent, Latin America and China. In all these cultures, this binary system of classification includes much more than food; medicines, illnesses, mental and physical states, natural and supernatural forces, are all grouped into either hot or cold categories. The theory of physiology on which this is based, and which equates health with *balance* between these two categories, has been fully described in Chapter 2.

In many cases this view of health and illness represents a survival of the humoral theory of physiology, especially in Latin America and North Africa. In China and India, while hot/cold dichotomies are also found, they have a different genealogy – from the YinYang and Ayurvedic systems respectively. The notions of hot and cold do not refer to actual temperature, but rather to certain symbolic values associated with each category of foodstuffs. Because health is defined as a balance between these categories, ill health is treated by adding hot or cold foods or medicines to the diet in order to restore the balance. For example, among some Latin American groups living in the USA, a 'cold' disease like arthritis may be treated by hot foods or medications, while in Morocco, 'hot' illnesses like sunstroke are treated by cold substances. In most cases these parallel food classifications are not based on a logically consistent principle, nor are foodstuffs that are classified as hot in one culture or region necessarily seen as hot in another.

Local historical and cultural factors, as well as personal idiosyncrasies, may play a part in assigning foods to these two categories. For example, in his study in Morocco, Greenwood[8] found significant disagreements among his informants as to which foods were 'hot' and which were 'cold', though they all agreed on the tastes, physiological effects and therapeutic value expected of the two categories. In some cases the choice of category was based mainly on personal experience. For example, one man noted that goat's meat tasted sour and caused indigestion and joint stiffness (cold conditions) and that goats could not tolerate being outside in the winter; however, cattle could, and therefore goat's meat was cold while beef was hot.

Table 3.1 Hot–cold classification of foods among New York Puerto Ricans

Hot (caliente)	*Cool (fresco)*	*Cold (frio)*
Alcoholic beverages	Barley water	Avocado
Chili peppers	Bottled milk	Bananas
Chocolate	Chicken	Coconut
Coffee	Fruits	Lima beans
Cornmeal	Honey	Sugar cane
Evaporated milk	Raisins	White beans
Garlic	Salt-cod	
Kidney beans	Watercress	
Onions		
Peas		
Tobacco		

Source: Harwood, 19719.

Parallel food classifications sometimes include intermediate categories such as cool, warm or neutral, so that there is a spectrum between hot and cold rather than a clear division. Harwood[9] described an example of this form of classification among a group of Puerto Ricans in New York City. While diseases were grouped into hot and cold categories, foodstuffs and medications were divided into hot (*caliente*), cool (*fresco*) or cold (*frio*). Arthritis, colds, menstrual periods and joint pains were all cold diseases, while constipation, diarrhoea, rashes, tenesmus and ulcers were all hot. The hot medicines included aspirin, castor oil, penicillin, cod liver oil, iron and vitamins, while cold medicines were bicarbonate of soda, mannitol, nightshade and milk of magnesia.

The three categories of foods are shown in Table 3.1, though this division is not necessarily typical of all Puerto Ricans, whether in New York or elsewhere. Harwood notes how the classification he described is not based on relative temperatures – iced beer, for example, is still considered hot because it is an alcoholic beverage.

Cold illnesses are sometimes blamed on eating too many cold foods, which cause a stomach chill or *frialdad del estomago*. Similarly, a person with a cold may refuse to drink fruit juices recommended by a physician as they are also classified as cold.

During pregnancy a woman in this group would avoid hot foods or medications (including iron and vitamin supplements) lest her child be born with a hot illness, such as a rash. After delivery and during menstruation cold foods are avoided lest they clot the blood and impede the flow, causing it to go backwards into the body and cause nervousness or insanity.

Table 3.2 Hot–cold classification of foods among Indians in the UK

Hot	*Cold*
Wheat	Rice
Potato	Plantains
Buffalo milk	Cow's milk
Fish	Buttermilk
Chicken	Greengram
Horse gram	Peas
Groundnut	Beans
Drumstick	Onions
Bitter gourd	Green tomatoes
Carrots	Pumpkin
Radish	Spinach
Fenugreek	Ripe mango
Garlic	Bananas
Green mango	Guava
Paw-paw	Lemons
Dates	

Source: Hunt, 1976[5].

Hunt[5] has described the hot–cold classification system among some Asian immigrants (from India, Pakistan and Bangladesh) living in Britain, including both Hindus and Muslims. The Indian classification of foodstuffs into hot and cold is shown in Table 3.2. As with the Puerto Rican example, illnesses were treated by restoring the balance of hot and cold forces within the body; a febrile illness, for instance, is treated with cold foods such as rice, greengram and buttermilk.

In another study, by Tann and Wheeler[10], a group of London Chinese mothers believed that their diet should be modified according to the general health of the infant receiving their breast milk. If the baby had a cold illness, they avoided cold foods that might turn the breast milk cold and thus aggravate the illness. In some cases this led to a considerable restriction in the sources of nutrition available to the mother. In this case, as in others, parallel food classifications are usually used by patients as a form of self-medication, which in some circumstances may prove damaging to their health.

Food as medicine, medicine as food

This category system usually overlaps with parallel food classifications when the two coexist in the same society, as in the cases of Morocco, India and Puerto Rico quoted above. However, in other societies special diets may also be seen as a form of 'medicine' for certain illnesses or psychological states. Some examples of this have been quoted in the previous chapter, such as 'feed a cold, starve a fever' in the case of common viral or bacterial infections, or the use of certain foods or vitamins (a form of concentrated food) to prevent colds and chills. In the case of special physiological states (such as pregnancy, lactation and menstruation) certain foods are sometimes avoided, or else prescribed to aid in the physiological process. The effect of hot and cold foods on these states has already been described in the case of women from Latin America. In a study[11] of 40 women attending a public clinic in Michigan, 11 believed the foetus could be 'marked' if the mother's food cravings were not satisfied, 12 thought that the diet should be altered in the postpartum period and four believed it should be changed during lactation. Twelve women in the sample admitted to having eaten starch, clay or dirt during pregnancy – as one pregnant woman put it, it was a good idea to eat earth since it acts as 'a scrub brush through the organs'. One woman believed that, during lactation, the supply of breast milk could be increased by drinking red raspberry tea and avoiding acid foods and cabbage. In many of these cases, cultural prescriptions about the appropriate food and drink to 'treat' or advance a physiological process may have negative effects on the patients' health.

The American folk illness 'high blood' (and its opposite, 'low blood'), described in Chapter 2, is a further example of food as medicine. 'High blood' is treated by taking lemon juice, vinegar, sour oranges, pickles, olives or sauerkraut, while the treatment of 'low blood' involves an increased consumption of beets, grape juice, red wine, liver and red meat. Where a patient confuses the diagnosis of high blood pressure with 'high blood', much needed sources of protein may be cut from the diet and replaced with foods with a high salt content – which may be dangerous in a case of hypertension.

Etkin and Ross[12] studied the use of plants, both as medicine and as food, among the Hausa people of Northern Nigeria. They found that many of the plants were used as folk medicines and as food. For example, cashew nuts were chewed for treatment of intestinal worms, diarrhoea and dyspepsia, but were also added to soups and used as a condiment in vegetable foods. By analysing both the nutritional and pharmacological properties of many of these substances, they concluded that many plants taken as medicine may in fact also have nutritional value, while some of the plants used mainly as food also have a medicinal effect. Therefore, only by examining all the many uses of plants can an estimation of their overall nutritional value be made. They also suggest that agricultural development programmes that attempt to reduce crop diversity in order to maximize calorie and protein availablity may reduce the range of nutrients available to food-producing populations, as well as the plants available both as medicines and as dietary constituents.

More recently, and especially in the USA, there has been increasing interest in 'nutriceuticals' – foods or nutritional supplements that are believed to prevent or treat a variety of physical and mental disorders. When included in the diet, these 'functional foods' are said to give a variety of health benefits beyond basic nutrition.

Medicines, whether medically or self-prescribed, may also come to be regarded as a form of food or nutriment without which the patient might weaken or die. Examples of this are certain cardiac or hypotensive drugs, insulin therapy, and thyroid and other hormone replacement therapy. When these drugs are regularly taken at mealtimes, they may become incorporated into the meal as a symbolic form of food. Other substances such as vitamins and tonics, alcohol, tobacco and psychotropic drugs, if taken regularly, might also come to play this role (see Chapter 8).

In the industrialized world, recent food scares have led many people to regard some types of foodstuffs as a potential 'poison'. For example, there has been widespread anxiety about contamination of food by micro-organisms (such as the virus of bovine spongiform encephalopathy, or BSE, in some British beef), the carcinogenic effects of food additives, and the possible health effects of genetically-modified crops. This new classification – 'food as poison' – has led more people to vegetarianism (see above), to eat organically-grown or whole foods, and to reject pre-packaged and processed convenience foods.

Social foods

Social foods are those that are consumed in the presence of other people, and which have a *symbolic* as well as nutritional value for all those concerned. A snack eaten in private is not a social food, but the constituents of a family meal or religious feast usually are. In every human society, food is a way of creating and expressing the *relationships* between people. These relationships may be between individuals, between the members of social, religious or ethnic groups, or between any of these and the supernatural world. Food used in this way has many of the properties of the ritual symbols described later in this book (Chapter 9). In particular, when food is consumed in the formalized atmosphere of a communal meal it carries with it many associations, telling the participants much about their relationship with one another and with the outside world. Most meals have a ritual aspect, in addition to their purely practical role in providing nutrition for a number of people at the same time. Like all ritual occasions, they are tightly controlled by the norms of a particular culture or group. These norms, or rules, determine who prepares and serves the food, who eats together, and who clears up afterwards. They also determine the times and setting of meals, the order of dishes within a meal, the cutlery or crockery used, and the precise way in which the food may be consumed (table manners). The food itself is subject to cultural patterning, which determines its appropriate size, shape, consistency, colour, smell and taste. Both the formal occasion of a meal and the types of food served within it can therefore be viewed as a complicated *language*, which can be decoded to reveal much about the relationships and values of those sharing in the food. Each meal is a restatement and recreation of these values and relationships.

Different types of meal convey different messages to those taking part in them. Farb and Armelagos[13] point out that, in North America, cocktails without a meal are for acquaintances or people of lower social status, meals preceded by alcoholic drinks are for close friends and honoured guests, and a cold lunch is 'at the threshold of intimacy' but not quite there. Social intimacy is symbolized by invitation to a complete meal, with a sequence of courses contrasted by hot and cold; the buffet, the 'cookout' and the barbecue extend friendship to a greater extent than an invitation to morning coffee, but less so than an invitation to a complete sit-down meal.

Meals can also be used to symbolize social *status*, often by serving rare and expensive dishes – what Jelliffe[3] calls 'prestige foods'. According to him, these are usually protein (and often animal), are difficult to obtain or prepare (as they are rare, expensive or imported), and are often linked historically with a dominant social group (such as venison, which was the preserve of the upper classes in Europe during the Middle Ages). Among the prestige foods that can be identified are venison and game birds in Northern Europe, the T-bone steak in America, caviar in much of the Western world, the camel hump among Bedouin Arabs, and the pig in New Guinea. Status can also be acquired by giving enormous feasts, where large amounts of food are conspicuously eaten or wasted. A well-known example of this, from the anthropological literature, is the *potlach* feast of the Indians of north-western USA and Canada. Here, different families competed with one another to throw huge, lavish feasts, each one greater than the next, and where large amounts of food were wasted. The aim was to humiliate rival families by throwing a feast that could not be matched by them.

In other societies, the display and sharing of food is also used to obtain prestige, but without the wastage characteristic of the *potlach*. In the Trobriand Islands off Papua New Guinea, for example, a farmer who has produced much food during a season is regarded as having shown great skill and prowess in farming, and to have been especially favoured by supernatural powers. He is now able to demonstrate his success and increase in status by displaying large piles of food he has grown at any of the tribal group ceremonies (such as harvest or mourning rituals), and to distribute this food to relatives and friends that he wishes to honour. Belshaw[14] pointed out that this does not result in a gluttonous feast, since the food, when distributed, is cooked and eaten in the home of the recipient.

In other social systems, such as the Hindu caste system in India, social rank is usually marked by the types of food prepared and eaten by each caste. The highest prestige is given to raw foods, which are considered suitable for the priestly Brahmins and other upper castes. Cooked food is less valued unless it contains *ghee*, a form of butter from which the water has been removed. Inferior cooked foods include pickles, cheap curries and barley cakes, all of which lacks *ghee*. Food may not be accepted from, or prepared by, the members of lower castes, although food can travel downwards in the caste system as payment for goods or services. In this society, food functions both as a form of currency and as an indicator of social position.

In many parts of the world, light-coloured foods such as white bread or white rice have a higher status than dark-coloured foods. In Europe, it was the peasants who ate rough, brown bread while the aristocracy ate white bread or cakes, and the same pattern existed elsewhere. In the Third World, as Trowell and Burkitt[15] note, westernization has led to the increased status of white bread and rice and other refined foods. Cereals are increasingly refined to produce low-fibre white wheat flour and polished white rice, resulting in a decreased intake of dietary fibre. Some of the Western diseases that possibly result from this change will be mentioned below.

As well as signalling status, food can be used as a badge of *group identity* – whether the group is based on regional, familial, ethnic or religious criteria. Each country has its national dish, and often regions within those countries are known by their local cuisine. Food produced and eaten locally is closely identified with the sense of continuity and cohesion of the community, and its dietary practices are often carried to other countries when members of the community emigrate. In their new countries, the immigrants may continue to eat their traditional diet – with its familiar taste, smells and mode of preparation – or merely revert to it only on special occasions. For example, Jerome[16] studied the changes in diet and the pattern of meals in African-Americans who had migrated from rural areas in the South to large cities in the North. The traditional Southern pattern consisted of two meals: breakfast, which comprised fried meats of various kinds, rice, grits, biscuits, gravy, fried sweet Irish potatoes, coffee and milk; and the 'heavy boiled dinner', which took place in the mid-afternoon and comprised boiled vegetables or dry legumes seasoned with a variety of meat items. The main dish was accompanied by cornbread, potatoes, a sweet beverage or milk, and an occasional dessert or fruit. In the Northern, urban environment, under the influence of occupational schedules, the pattern changed. The heavy boiled dinner was now served at 4–6 pm and renamed 'supper' whilst the large breakfast usually persisted for about 18 months after migration, with lunch consisting of leftovers from it. Eventually a new pattern was established with three meals: breakfast, comprising eggs, or bacon or sausage with eggs, hot biscuits, 'light' bread and coffee; lunch of sandwiches, soup, crackers, raw fruits and a fruit drink; and dinner, either 'heavy boiled' or fried food. The traditional large breakfasts were reserved for weekends, 'off-days' and holidays.

As Jerome's study illustrates, the internal structure and content of meals can be remarkably uniform within a social or cultural group. A similar study, of working-class British meals, was carried out by Douglas and Nicod[17]. They found that meals, unlike snacks, were highly structured events, with certain combinations of foods served in the appropriate sequence. Breakfast, where the dishes were served in any order, was usually not regarded as a meal. At meals, careful combinations were made between salty and sweet, moist and dry, and hot and cold foods. When food was very hot it had to be accompanied by a cold drink, while a dessert taken with a hot beverage had to be cold, dry and solid (cake or biscuits). Douglas and Nicod were able to decipher the underlying recurrent grammar of these meals, and point out that improvement in their nutritional qualities had to take this structure into account rather than trying to impose the opinions of the middle-class dietician.

Because of their central role in defining and recreating group identity and cohesion, communal meals or feasts mark many of the important occasions in the life of the group. Examples of

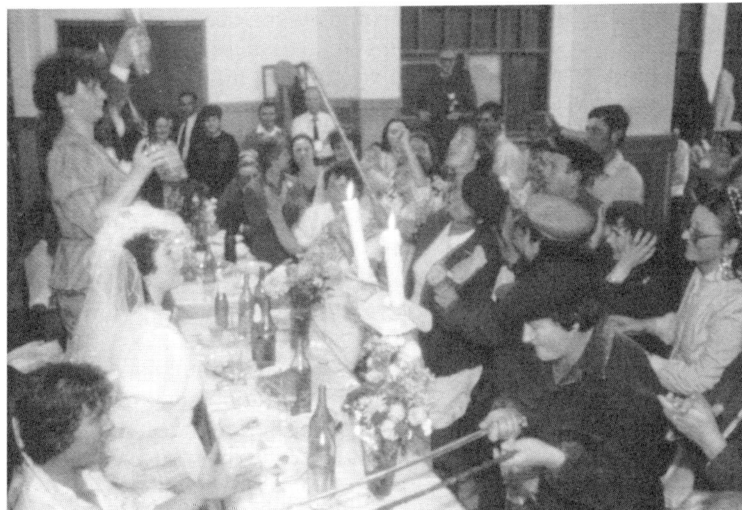

Figure 3.1 In all cultures, special meals and drinks mark important landmarks in the human life cycle, and other festive occasions. A wedding celebration in St Gheorghe, Romania. (Source: Caroline Penn/Panos Pictures.)

this are feasts associated with weddings, christenings, circumcisions, wakes, *barmitzvahs* and religious festivals and services. Foods consumed during religious occasions are more likely to have a symbolic rather than a nutritional significance – for example, the Communion wafer or Host, or the Passover *matzoh*. Consuming these foods confirms and re-establishes the relationship between man and his deity, as well as between man and man. More secular group festivals, where the group's history and experiences are celebrated, also utilize special foods – for example, the turkey eaten at the American Thanksgiving. Farb and Armelagos[18] note how the pumpkin, originally a commonly used vegetable, has gradually assumed more symbolic and less nutritional significance as a decoration at Halloween or Thanksgiving. They estimate that every autumn nearly three million pumpkins are sold in Massachusetts, and that 90 per cent of them will never be eaten – instead being carved into 'jack-o-lanterns', or used to decorate front porches, window sills and dining tables.

A further example of a social food with ritual significance is the British wedding cake. Charsley[19] suggests that the wedding cake – comprising three tiers, each covered with smooth white icing and surrounded by elaborate ornaments and decorations (silver or gold horseshoes, slippers or flowers) – is symbolic of the bride herself, in her long white dress and veil. Furthermore, the joint cutting of the 'virginal white' cake by the new bride and groom has a sexual significance, symbolic of the couple now 'becoming one flesh'.

These many examples of social foods illustrate the multiple roles that food plays in human society: creating and sustaining social relationships; signalling social status, occupation and gender roles; marking important life changes, anniversaries and festivals; and reasserting religious, ethnic or regional identities. Because of their many social roles, dietary beliefs and practices are sometimes difficult to discard, even when they are dangerous to health.

Culture and malnutrition

The five systems of food classification described above illustrate how food may be eaten for cultural as well as nutritional reasons. From a clinical perspective, these cultural influences may affect nutrition in two ways:

1. They may exclude much-needed nutriments from the diet by defining them as non-food, profane, alien or lower-class food, or food on the wrong side of a hot/cold dichotomy
2. They may encourage the consumption of certain foods or drinks, by defining them as food, sacred, 'medicine', or as a sign of social, religious or ethnic identity, which are actually injurious to health.

When both of these influences co-exist there is likely to be an increased risk of *malnutrition* – manifesting either as *under*nutrition (a deficiency of vitamins, proteins, energy sources or trace elements) or as *over*nutrition (especially obesity and its consequences). Other cultural factors can also have an indirect effect on nutrition, such as beliefs about the structure and functioning of the body, its optimal size and shape, and the role of diet in health and disease. Also, the rules of food use and distribution within a family may contribute towards malnutrition – for example, by giving larger portions of food to male members of the family than to females.

However, it should always be remembered that cultural influences alone *do not* account for the vast majority of malnutrition world-wide, although they may be one of the factors contributing towards it. To be fully understood, malnutrition should always be placed in its wider social, political, economic and environmental context. For example, various forms of *deprivation* – that is, the lack of available food or of the means to obtain what food there is – accounts for most cases of undernutrition, especially in the developing world. Such deprivation may result from a number of factors, especially:

- poverty, due to the unequal distribution of resources within a society or between societies
- natural disasters, such as floods, tidal waves, tornadoes and drought
- wars (especially civil wars) and other forms of violent social upheaval
- crop failures, due to locusts and other insects or parasites.

Another factor, fully described by Keesing[20], is the international *political economy* of food production and consumption. He notes how in many parts of the Third World, both under colonialism and afterwards, people were encouraged and sometimes forced to grow commodities for export (such as tobacco, sugar cane, coffee or cotton) rather than staple foods for internal consumption. In large areas of the developing world, more and more land was devoted to producing these 'cash crops' for export. In the 1970s, for example, cash crops occupied an estimated 55 per cent of the cropland in the Philippines, 80 per cent in Mauritius and 50 per cent of all cultivated land in Senegal. Many developing countries are therefore at the mercy of fluctuations in the world market for their cash crops, and are also increasingly reliant on imported food for subsistence. Furthermore, advertising from firms in the industrialized countries has promoted the use of less nutritious and more expensive artificial foods, such as soft drinks, canned foods and infant formula feeds (see below). In many countries an over-emphasis on the production of raw materials, such as coal, copper, tin, gold or oil, or even on the tourist industry, may play a similar role to cash crops: increasing dependence on international markets, and reducing the land and population available for food production.

Recently, more attention has been paid to the phenomenon of *globalization* and its effect on global diet[21,22]. This process involves the diffusion of Western modes of food production, marketing and consumption to many parts of the world, especially to poorer countries. One effect of this is to concentrate power over these processes into fewer and fewer hands, especially in the Western corporate sector. This in turn implies a shift in power from the producer of food – the farmer peasant, or agricultural worker – to the distributor of that food (often a multinational corporation or 'agribusiness')[21]. Overall, the effects of this process on nutrition include the rapid change of centuries-old traditional diets, the introduction of a variety of nutritionally inadequate fast foods ('burgerization'[21]), and a shift towards high fat, high salt, and high calorie diets as part of this 'nutrition transition'[22] (see below).

In many cases of malnutrition, therefore, the causes lie outside the control of individuals, their families and their communities. Thus cultural factors, as well as personal factors such as ignorance or idiosyncrasy, are only one part (though they may be an important part) of the complex mix of influences on the individual that determine whether his or her diet is nutritionally adequate or not.

Case study: Malnutrition among children in Farimabougou, Mali

Dettwyler[23] described some of the 'intricate web of interacting factors' that contribute to child malnutrition in Farimabougou, near Bamako, Mali. Based on a sample of 136 children, her study indicates that relative poverty alone cannot completely explain variations in diet and nutritional status within the community. Other studies in Mali also indicate that 'rising income is not correlated with an increase in quantity or an improvement in the nutritional quality of the diet'. In each case of severe malnutrition, therefore, 'a variety of biological, social, and cultural factors' – *in addition* to low incomes – has contributed to the child's poor growth, a situation that she terms 'socio-cultural malnutrition'. These factors include:

- differences in maternal age, experience, competence and attitudes to child-rearing
- the support networks available to mothers and the breakdown of the extended family unit under the influence of the wage economy
- maternal illness, such as malaria or measles
- marital problems, family conflicts and the difficult position of women in a polygamous society
- decisions on how household resources are to be allocated
- traditional infant feeding practices, such as weaning as soon as the mother gets pregnant again, or letting children themselves decide whether and how much they want to eat.

In one case, a 16-year-old unmarried mother with twins, living as a low-status foster child in another family's compound, was given little help by them with either infant feeding or child-care; nor was she supported by the father of her children. She resented the twins because 'they were a burden to her', and with two small children 'she had little chance of marrying'. As a result of these and other factors, the children were neglected and failed to thrive. In another case, a father spent most of his income on his moped and on clothes for himself and his wife, leaving little over to pay for the children's food.

Dettwyler thus pointed out that, although in some circumstances one factor – such as drought, famine or war – may be responsible for malnutrition, 'the vast majority of malnutrition in Third World populations does not have one primary cause'. Since 'all poor people are not the same', she warns against simplistic solutions of the problem. Poverty, however, does play a crucial role in the 'web of causation' of childhood malnutrition in Mali. Apart from having less money to spend on food for the children, a contaminated environment (due to the complete lack of sewage and garbage disposal) and inadequate primary health care both contribute to frequent childhood diarrhoea and other causes of poor health. Furthermore, in a situation of deprivation, ill, malnourished or stressed parents are less able to deal with the demands of childcare and to ensure adequate nutrition of their children.

To illustrate further the contributory role of culture in malnutrition, three topics are discussed below, with examples.

Immigrants and ethnic minorities in the UK: some nutritional problems

Most immigrant groups bring with them their own dietary culture – their traditional beliefs and practices relating to food. Not only does this ensure a sense of cultural continuity with their countries of origin, but it also plays many symbolic, religious and social roles in their daily lives. Food habits are one of the important indicators of acculturation, together with dress, behaviour and family structure, and are often among the last cultural traits to go if immigrants seek to discard their original cultures. In addition to dietary habits, other factors beyond the control of the immigrants themselves may affect their health and nutrition. These include discrimination or rejection by the host community; unemployment; physical violence or racial harassment[24]; substandard or overcrowded living conditions; low incomes; little leisure time; long working hours; social isolation; and the stressful effects of culture change itself (see Chapter 11).

Stroud[25] has reviewed the commonest nutritional problems of southern Asian (India, Pakistan and Bangladesh) and West Indian immigrants in the UK. These include osteomalacia and rickets among Asians, various forms of anaemia among both Asians and West Indians, and over-nutrition (obesity) in some West Indian infants. Another study, by Ward and colleagues[26], also identified rickets among some of the children of West Indian Rastafarians. It should be noted that many of these studies apply mainly to the first generation of immigrants, rather than to their descendants who were born and raised in the UK.

Rickets

Considerable research has been done on Asian rickets in the UK, which has occurred at a much higher rate than among the white population. It is especially common among those aged 9 months to 3 years, 8–14 years, and among pregnant and lactating Asian women[27,28]. Several factors have been blamed for this high incidence, including:

- a deficiency of vitamin D in the Asian vegetarian diet
- the phytase content of Asian diets (in chapattis), which binds with calcium and prevents its absorption
- skin pigmentation (skin pigments absorb ultraviolet light, with consequent reduction in vitamin D production)
- genetic factors
- a lack of exposure to ultraviolet light due to poor inner-city housing, confinement of women indoors, and types of female dress which cover large areas of skin surface.[29,30]

While the lack of dietary vitamin D is not the sole cause of rickets (one should include, for example, the fear of racial attacks, which may keep some Asian women indoors[24]), it is still an important cause of the condition. Hunt[5] points out that the Asian diet supplies about 1.5 mg of vitamin D daily, compared with 2.9 mg daily in the rest of the UK population, who derive most of their vitamin D from margarine and fish – both of which are hardly used by Asians. Hindus reject fish for religious reasons, while some Muslims believe that margarine contains pig fat. The lack of dietary vitamin D is especially important in girls during their growth spurt at puberty and in pregnant women – in both cases, social seclusion and dress also play a part. Rickets in infancy has also been blamed on the Asian practice of weaning babies directly onto cow's milk, without using vitamin drops or vitamin D enriched baby foods. Stroud[25] points out that cow's milk and human milk contain 20–40 iu/litre of vitamin D, while the recommended allowance for infants is 400 iu/day; therefore, a baby fed entirely on human or non-proprietary cow's milk will have much less than the recommended daily allowance. Vitamin D supplements have been suggested for both infants and pregnant Asian women. According to the *Lancet*[29], doctors should 'regard all pregnant Asian women as potentially osteomalacic and ensure that they receive adequate supplementary vitamin D (400 iu daily) throughout pregnancy and lactation', though some obstetricians are not convinced of the value of these supplements[31]. Furthermore, Mares and her colleagues[32] have argued recently against this over-emphasis on the role of Asian diet in causing rickets. They suggest that only about a quarter of British Asians – mainly Hindus, but usually not Muslims or Sikhs – are, to a lesser or greater extent, vegetarian; that many Asians do in fact eat large amounts of dairy products; and that the positive role of vegetarian diets in protecting against heart disease and many other disorders should be emphasized.

Nutritional rickets has also been described among some West Indian infants whose parents belong to the Rastafarian religion. Ward and colleagues[26] have described four cases of children aged between 11 and 20 months who were found to have clinical rickets. Their parents were strict Rastafarians, and ate a vegetarian diet that also excluded fish. They were breast-fed until the second half of the first year of life, when they were weaned on an essentially vegetarian diet known as *1-tal*. None had received vitamin supplements during infancy, nor had they completed a full course of immunizations. Like many Asians, they had low incomes and lived in depressed inner-city areas where opportunities for outdoor play are few and exposure to sunlight is likely to be limited.

Anaemia

Stroud[25] also reported higher rates of iron-deficiency anaemia among both Asian and West Indian infants and children. Part of this may be due to prolonged breast-feeding or to weaning directly on to cow's milk, since both types of milk are deficient in iron, containing 0.3 mg/l and 1.0 mg/l respectively. According to Hunt[5], the diet of adult Asians is devoid of easily assimilated iron from animal sources; although iron is added to chapatti flour, only about 3 per cent of it is absorbed when eaten as part of an Asian diet. In some cases the anaemia may result from hookworm (ankylostoma) infestations, because of the demands such infestations may make on body proteins; however, according to Stroud this is rare in the UK in all communities. Hunt also points out that megaloblastic anaemias – due to folic acid or vitamin B12 deficiency – are more common among Asians in Britain, especially Hindus. Asian cooking habits may destroy much of the folic acid, for example by boiling pulses for about an hour, or by the prolonged gentle heating of finely cut up foods. In addition, the habit of boiling the milk, tea leaves and water together for 5 minutes when making tea is thought to destroy much of the vitamin B12, which is especially important in Hindus, whose vegetarian diet lacks other sources of vitamin B12.

Overnutrition

A final problem among immigrants in the UK is that of overnutrition, a condition that is by no means confined to immigrant or ethnic minority communities, nor to the UK. In Stroud's opinion, West Indian children in Britain may be in more danger from obesity than from undernutrition. Since many of their families come from communities where malnutrition was common, 'many of the West Indian mothers seem to have a very deep-seated desire to see their children as big, fat babies, and are not satisfied with their average growth along the fiftieth centile'. Some of the issues relating to the world-wide growth in childhood obesity are discussed below.

Case study: Beliefs about food and diabetes among British Bangladeshis, London, England

Greenhalgh and colleagues[33] studied beliefs about diabetes mellitus, including diet, among 40 Bangladeshi immigrants in London. While some of these beliefs overlapped with the medical model, others were very different. The whole group recognized the importance of diet in diabetes control, and believed that one of the main causes of diabetes was too much sugar. They also blamed heredity, 'germs' and stress. In terms of foodstuffs, however, they divided them into two symbolic categories in terms of their perceived 'strength' (nourishing power), and 'digestibility'. Strong foods were perceived as energy-giving, and included white sugar, lamb, beef, *ghee* (derived from butter), solid fat and spices. Such foods were considered crucial to maintain or restore health, and also essential for certain festive occasions. They were considered dangerous, however, for the old or the debilitated (including diabetics), for whom weak foods (such as boiled rice or cereals) were more appropriate. Raw foods, and those baked or grilled, were considered indigestible, as were all vegetables that grow under the ground. They were considered unsuitable for the elderly, the very young or those who were very ill. Thus the recommendation that diabetics should bake or grill their foods rather than fry them would not accord with their food beliefs. By contrast, molasses – a dark form of raw sugar, liquid at room temperature – was considered safe for diabetics to eat, and very different from lighter coloured white sugar, butter, *ghee* and solid fat, which was forbidden. The whole sample believed that the onset and control of diabetes depended on the *balance* between food entering the body and emissions from the body, such as semen, sweat, urine and menstrual blood. An excess of any of these emissions was believed to cause illness and weakness, as in diabetes. In the Bangladeshi community, because communal feasts, festivals and social occasions are common (and usually involve the consumption of sweets and rich foods), a calculated compromise between social obligations and dietary compliance had to be made by both diabetics and their families. Finally, the value of physical exercise and weight-reduction had little cultural meaning for the sample. In general, larger body size (but not obesity) was viewed as an indicator of more health, while thinness was a sign of less health.

Infant feeding practices: cross-cultural comparisons

The care and feeding of infants is a central concern in every human group. There are widespread differences, however, in the techniques of infant feeding, whether breast, bottle or artificial feeds are used, and in the age and technique of weaning. Despite medical advice that, for a variety of physiological and emotional reasons, 'breast is best', breast-feeding has declined in most countries in the world this century. This is particularly the case in urban, industrialized societies or in non-Western societies undergoing modernization and urbanization. In most cases, moving from the countryside into the city results in a decline in breast-feeding. For example, the 1984 *World Fertility Survey*[34], based on data from 42 developing countries, found that rural women in those countries breast-fed an average of 2–6 months longer than their urban counterparts. As Farb and Armelagos[35] put it, 'mothers in many parts of the world often consider breast-feeding to be a vulgar peasant custom, to be abandoned as soon as the bottle can be afforded'. This decline in human lactation has been described as the greatest nutritional crisis in today's world[20]. Several reasons have been advanced for the shift from breast to bottle, including urbanization, the breakdown of the extended family and the increased employment of women outside the home[36]. A further factor in some non-industrialized countries, especially in Africa, are the huge advertising campaigns in favour of bottle-

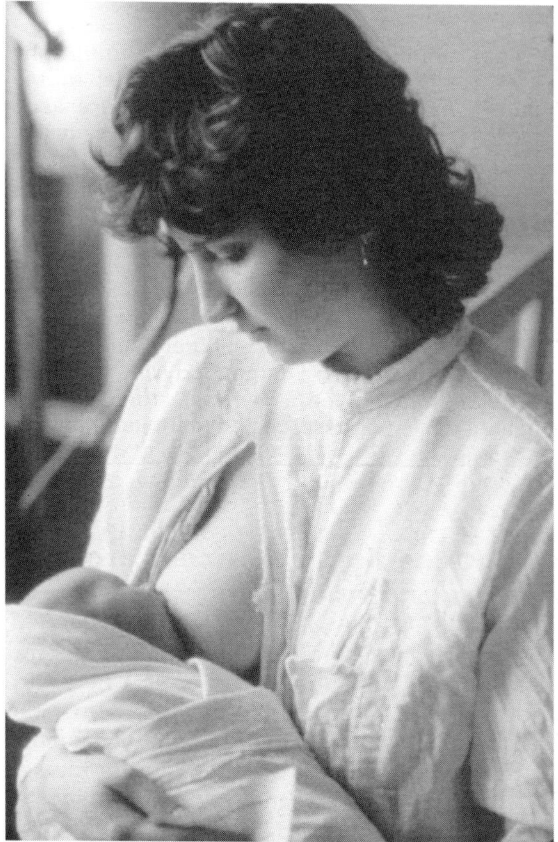

Figure 3.2 Despite medical advice that – for a variety of emotional and physical reasons – 'breast is best', many women are unable or else unwilling to breast-feed their infants (Source: © Jeremy Hartley/Panos Pictures).

feeding, promoted by the Western manufacturers of artificial infant foods. These campaigns have been heavily criticized for depriving babies of the nutritional and immunological advantages of breast milk, and for increasing the dangers of malnutrition and the risk of diarrhoeal diseases. In many areas mothers may not have the facilities to prepare infant feeds with properly boiled water and sterilized bottles, thus increasing their babies' risk of infection.

A reverse trend is appearing in many industrialized countries, as the past few years have seen a gradual return to breast-feeding among many mothers in the upper socio-economic classes. At the same time, many women in the developing world who are HIV positive are now being advised *not* to breast-feed. This is because an estimated half of all mother-to-child HIV transmissions in developing countries occurs during breast-feeding[37].

In any particular country or community, therefore, there is always a range of factors – social, cultural, personal and economic – that influence whether and for how long women breast-feed their infants, how they explain a failure to breast-feed to themselves and to others, and when and how they wean their infants. This is illustrated by an example from Egypt, as well as by four case studies from different communities in the UK.

Case study: Beliefs about breast-feeding and weaning in a poor urban neighbourhood in Cairo, Egypt

Harrison and colleagues[38], in a study of 20 mothers in Boulaq El Dakrour, Cairo, found a range of beliefs about whether a woman could breast-feed or not. All the women aimed to breast-feed their babies well into the second year of life, but did not assume that ability to breast-feed was automatic. Successful breast-feeding was believed to require patience, time, a sense of responsibility, good luck, a healthy mental state and specific changes in diet and behaviour. They cited many reasons why some women could breast-feed and others not. Some believed that adequate breast milk is a 'gift from God', and that only 'a lucky mother can breast-feed'. Others saw maternal emotional state as very important, since they believed that unhappiness turns the maternal body and its breast milk 'hot', and that this 'sadness milk' or 'grief milk' could cause diarrhoea in the infant. Thus, some mothers going through a stressful time would express much of their milk manually and discard it. By contrast, several would increase their breast-feeding if the baby was ill. The child itself was believed to influence the amount of milk that was available; certain children were seen as more 'blessed', a characteristic that ensures a plentiful supply of breast milk. Nursing another woman's baby of the same age as one's own was also common in this community, as elsewhere in Egypt. This act had considerable symbolic significance, creating a quasi-kinship relationship between the women and babies involved and resulting in a lifetime prohibition against marriage between children breast-fed by the same woman. There was also a range of beliefs about when to wean the infant. Many based their decision on the infant's developmental milestones, such as when it had all its teeth, or was able to walk or eat adult food. Others cited maternal illness, pregnancy, employment outside the home, medical advice and the use of oral contraceptives as reasons to stop breast-feeding. Seasonal and religious factors also had an influence on when to wean; some mothers preferred summer to winter, some stopped breast-feeding because they had decided to fast during *Ramadhan*, while others avoided *Muharam* (the first month of the Islamic calendar), which was thought to be an unsuitable time for weaning.

Case study: Infant feeding practices in Glasgow, UK

Goel and colleagues[39] studied the infant feeding practices of 172 families from various communities in Glasgow. These included 206 Asian, 99 African, 99 Chinese and 102 Scottish children. It was found that, after arrival in Britain, most immigrant mothers did not want to breast-feed their babies. Those immigrant children born outside Britain were more likely to have been breast-fed than those born within Britain; 83.7 per cent of Asian, 79.2 per cent of African and 80.9 per cent of Chinese children born abroad had been breast-fed. Ninety-nine per cent of the Scots children had been exclusively bottle-fed. The commonest reasons given by the immigrant mothers for not breast-feeding were embarrassment, inconvenience and insufficient breast milk. Two-thirds of the breast-fed Asian children were fed for at least 6 months and only 5 per cent of the African babies were breast-fed for more than 1 year, but Chinese mothers often breast-fed for 1–3 years, and many of their children were not given solid foods till they were 1 year or over. Asian children born in the UK usually had solids by 6 months (but were given these at 1 year if they had been born abroad). Both African and Scottish children were given solids at 6 months. The authors suggest that all Asian children be given vitamin D supplements, since 12.5 per cent of the Asian children in the sample were found to have rickets.

Case study: Breast-feeding versus bottle-feeding in London, UK

Jones and Belsey[40] surveyed 265 mothers of 12-week-old infants in the London Borough of Lambeth. Sixty-two per cent of the mothers had attempted to breast-feed (compared to 16 per cent in Dublin, 39 per cent in Newcastle and 52 per cent in Gloucestershire). The different communities showed different rates of breast-feeding; British 58 per cent, African 86 per cent, West Indian 84 per cent, Asian 77 per cent, European 59 per cent and Irish 64 per cent. The ethnic background of the mothers was an important influence here, since in many communities breast-feeding was the accepted norm. Several reasons were given for not breast-feeding, especially because they 'disliked the thought of breast-feeding'; 54 per cent of bottle-feeders said this, while 44 per cent thought bottle-feeding was more convenient since it required less privacy than breast-feeding. Only 13 per cent of the bottle-feeders thought the method they had chosen was the healthiest for the baby, compared with 85 per cent of the breast-feeders. Social, as well as ethnic factors were important in the choice of feeding technique, though the two were related; mothers were more likely to continue breast-feeding after 6 weeks if they had friends who had breast-fed. African and West Indian mothers more often had friends who breast-fed successfully than mothers in other ethnic groups, as did women in the upper socio-economic classes. Little evidence was found that either antenatal or postnatal medical advice affected the type of feeding chosen by mothers.

Case study: Feeding patterns in Chinese children, London, UK

Tann and Wheeler[41] assessed feeding patterns and growth rates of 20 London Chinese children, aged between 1 and 24 months, over a period of 6 months. All the families had originated from the New Territories, a rural area of Hong Kong. With one exception, all the children were bottle-fed, and soft canned food and rusks of the British type were introduced at between 1 and 6 months. Subsequent to this, at 6–10 months, most mothers introduced *congee*, a traditional Chinese weaning food prepared by boiling rice in large quantities of watery meat broth. Soft boiled rice was introduced at about 10 months, and then gradually the full range of Chinese foods was introduced. The mothers had chosen not to breast-feed mainly because of the 'inconvenience', although in Hong Kong nearly 60 per cent of mothers wholly or partially breast-feed their children. Most of the sample believed that milk quality was affected

continued

by the quality of the food eaten by the mother after delivery; in Hong Kong, Chinese mothers were usually confined at home for 30 days after delivery, during which nutritious (i.e. meaty) food was served to them by female relatives. In London they could not afford such a luxurious post-confinement period, as they had to get on with work or household chores. As a result, they believed they were not sufficiently well nourished to produce good milk for the babies. Meat served in hospital after delivery was not considered nourishing enough, since it should have been cooked in a traditional way with special spices, herbs and wines. The authors found that despite this, all the Chinese children in the sample were well nourished. The role of 'hot–cold' foods in the mother's diet has been mentioned previously.

Case study: Feeding patterns in infants in Sheffield, UK

Taitz[42] studied 261 normal full-term infants born in Sheffield, at birth and at 6 weeks old. Only 21 of the babies were breast-fed. It was found that the majority of the artificially fed infants were substantially overweight at 6 weeks, in relation to their expected weight at that age. For example, 40.4 per cent of the males and 37.3 per cent of the females were above the 90th percentile for their age on the Tanner centile charts. Taitz ascribes this overnutrition to encouragement by doctors, welfare clinics, health visitors and grandmothers, and to 'the popular notion of the "bonny" baby with bloated cheeks and limbs, protuberant belly, and the various signs of the "Michelin Tyre Man" syndrome'. In addition, 'the apparently low resistance of present-day mothers to the crying infant and the tendency to provide instant gratification in a caloric form may also play its part'. Taitz points out the danger of overnutrition in infancy, since it may result in obesity in later childhood and adulthood.

The four case studies from the UK indicate the range of infant feeding practices among different communities in the country, and the effects this may have on the babies' health. However, as noted above, the effects of cultural factors on maternal diet (and therefore on the infant's health) are also relevant. For example, both foetal and neonatal rickets among Asian babies have been reported in Britain as a result of maternal vitamin D deficiency[29]. The reasons for choosing one type or amount of infant feeding over another are many. Some of these reasons have been described above, but they include cultural conceptions of what a healthy, bonny baby should look like, the type of lifestyle the mother should follow after delivery, and whether public breast-feeding is acceptable or not. It should also be remembered that in some parts of the world lactation is seen as an effective contraceptive, and this may influence the choice of type of infant feeding. In some of these societies this is backed up by taboos that prohibit sexual intercourse until the infant is weaned. Where breast-feeding is optional, and other forms of contraceptive are available, cultural beliefs and fashions, as well as economic factors, will determine whether most mothers choose this form of infant feeding or not.

The 'nutrition transition': globalization, dietary changes and disease

An area of growing importance to nutritionists is the globalization of the human diet. In particular, they have studied the impact of social and economic change on nutrition and health – especially in those communities throughout the world that are undergoing urbanization, industrialization and westernization. As incomes rise in these societies, and their populations become more urbanized, they enter the different stages of what has been called the *nutrition transition*[21,22]. Both economic growth and the enormously rapid increase in urbanization world-wide (see Chapter 13) have had major effects on global dietary habits. Compared to rural diets, urban diets – especially in developing countries – are usually characterized by the consumption of more polished grains (rice and wheat, instead of corn or millet), more fats and animal products, more refined sugar, more processed foods, and more food consumed away from home[22]. Analysing data from 1962–1994, Drewnowski and Popkin[22] have shown how the global availability of cheap vegetable oils and fats has led to a greatly increased consumption of fat, and to a lesser extent sugar, among low income countries. One of the first stages of the nutrition transition is usually a major increase in the domestic production and imports of oilseeds and vegetable oils (including soyabean, sunflower, rapeseed, palm and peanut oils), rather than increased imports of meat and milk. Between 1991 and 1997, for example, global production of vegetable fats and oils rose from 60 million to 71 million metric tonnes. As a result, vegetable oils now contribute more energy to the human food supply than do meat or animal fats. Previously, high-fat diets were a privilege of the richer countries, but this is no longer the case. Throughout Asia, for example, despite the fact there is now a greater diversity of foodstuffs available, the diets of both rich and poor countries show a decline in the proportion of energy derived from complex carbohydrates and a corresponding increase in the energy derived from fats. In Japan, for example, in the years 1946–1987, the fat content of the diet almost tripled from 9 per cent to 25 per cent of the total energy. The overall impact of this nutrition transition is seen especially in child health, with a significant rise in obesity world-wide. In many parts of the world now, such as Latin America, the Caribbean and even the USA, 'the poor are more likely to be obese than the rich'. Drewnowski and Popkin predict that a diet that contains about 30 per cent of energy from fat may well become the global norm, and this will have major health implications in the future.

Lang[21] has criticized the economic basis of globalization and its impact on global nutrition, especially in poorer countries. He points out that while there is nothing new in the exchange of foods, diets, recipes and products between different parts of the world – a process that began with the birth of agriculture – modern globalization is significantly different. What is new is the pace and scale of change, and the systematic way in which control over global food production and distribution can now be exercised. For the first time, also, such control is concentrated in relatively few (and mainly Western) hands. The growth of a global food market has shifted power away from the local producers of food and towards the multinational corporations who closely control its processing, distribution and sale. Farmers who produce food are encouraged to increase the size of their lands or herds, and to compete not only with other farmers locally but also globally. The implications of this, and the growth of cash crops in many poorer countries, have been discussed above. Globalization also makes possible the world-wide diffusion of new types of foods from the West, such as genetically modified products or branded processed foods. The world-wide growth of US-style fast food chains – a process Lang terms 'burgerization' – is contributing to the disappearance of local cuisines and dietary traditions, and may have important impacts on health. At the same time, however, most northern countries have imported food habits from the poorer south – such as Mexican food in the USA, south Asian curries in Britain, and north African couscous in France. Overall, therefore, all these trends mean that we live in an age of rapid nutrition transition; global diet is in a constant state of flux, and the health implications of this are only now beginning to emerge.

The 'diseases of Western civilization': dietary changes and disease

Burkitt[43] has examined many of the diseases that have become common in the Western world itself, particularly in Europe and the USA, in the past century. These same diseases are rare or unknown in traditional, non-Western societies, but they increase in frequency under the influence of culture change – that is, where Western customs and lifestyles are adopted. These 'new' diseases include: appendicitis, diverticular disease, benign colonic tumours, cancer of the large bowel, ulcerative colitis, varicose veins, deep vein thrombosis, pulmonary embolism, haemorrhoids, coronary heart disease, gallstones, hiatus hernia, obesity and diabetes.

Burkitt sees obesity as the 'commonest form of malnutrition in the West', and it is also associated with some of the other 'Western diseases'. He estimates that over 40 per cent of people in the UK are overweight, and the problem is just as serious in the USA. He relates the dramatic increase in frequency of the various diseases to dietary changes in the past century. Between the years 1860 and 1960, fat consumption increased by less than 50 per cent while sugar consumption doubled. Over the past 100 years, the quantity of fibre consumed in the diet has markedly dropped. In 1860 the fibre content of white flour was 0.2–0.5 per cent and the amount of fibre supplied daily in bread was between 1.1 and 2.8 g. With bread consumption halved and the fibre content of white flour reduced to 0.1–0.01 per cent, the daily fibre intake from bread is about 10 per cent of the pre-1860 level. In addition, porridge oats, with a high fibre content, has gone out of fashion and been replaced by low-fibre packaged cereals. In non-Western societies who become westernized, traditional diets are usually changed by the addition of sugar, the substitution of white bread for high-fibre cereals and, often, an increase in meat consumption. Burkitt points out, however, that in none of the 'Western diseases' is fibre deficiency a *sole* causative factor, but that it might be one important aetiological factor – although its precise link to these diseases and the actual types of fibre (such as fruit and vegetables) that protect against them remain unclear [44].

Burkitt's study thus suggests how changes in technology and dietary culture may possibly be related to the increased incidence of certain diseases. However, a recent study[45] in the USA has cast doubt on whether a high-fibre diet could actually reduce the risk of colorectal cancer and adenomas in women, and therefore much further research into the precise role of fibre in certain diseases still needs to be carried out.

Diet and cancer

The study of a culture's dietary patterns and preferences is not only important in the search for malnutrition, or for any one of the 'Western diseases' listed by Burkitt and others. A number of studies suggest that, in some cases, different types of diet may be linked to certain forms of cancer. It has been suggested that one-third or more of all cancers may be related to dietary and nutritional factors[46]. Lowenfels and Anderson[47], in reviewing the evidence for this hypothesis, found that differences in food intake patterns can be positively correlated with differences in the incidence of various cancers in world populations. This is especially the case in colonic and gastric cancer. In addition to the food consumed, such variables as total caloric intake, nutritional excess or deficit, the exposure to carcinogens and the consumption of alcohol also increase the risk of cancer. Many of these dietary factors, as noted earlier, may be affected by cultural beliefs and practices. In another review of the subject, Newberne[48] also cites the evidence linking dietary patterns to a number of cancers, including cancers of the stomach, colon, oesophagus and breast (which has been linked to an increased intake of fat in the diet). He points out that, in the USA, food habits have gradually changed in the past 40 years, a period in which cancer has increased in some populations. A further study by Kolonel and colleagues[49] examined the incidence rate of stomach cancer in four populations: Japanese in Japan; Japanese in Hawaii; Caucasians in Hawaii; and the general population of American whites. The highest rates were in Japanese in Japan, followed by the Hawaii Japanese, with the white groups at a much lower level. There was a positive association of high rates of the cancer with consumption, early in life, of the traditional Japanese foods of rice, pickled vegetables and dried/salted fish. It was postulated that stomach cancer might be caused by endogenous nitrosamines formed from dietary precursors – the nitrates, nitrites and secondary amines that are at high levels in the Japanese diet[50]. Other studies indicate that in India and other parts of Asia, the high incidence of cancers of the oral cavity (lips, tongue, pharynx, floor of mouth and the salivary glands) may be related to chewing mixtures of tobacco, betel nuts and other substances[51]. In India a chewing mixture called *pan* (containing betel leaf, betel nut, tobacco, lime and aromatic substances), and in parts of Afghanistan and the former Soviet Central Asia a mixture known as *nass* (containing betel, tobacco leaf and lime treated with certain oils) have both been implicated in causing these cancers[51]. A diet rich in fats (especially saturated fats) and in calories has been blamed for increasing the risk of colon, breast and other cancers[48]. Certain food contaminants, especially the *aflatoxins* (found in mouldy peanuts or grains), have been linked to high rates of liver cancer in parts of Asia and Africa[46]. By contrast, certain types of diet may actually *protect* against some forms of cancer. A high intake of fresh fruits and vegetables (see below) has been found to reduce the incidence of cancers of the oral cavity, oesophagus, stomach and lung, while a low-fat, high-fibre diet may protect against cancers of the breast and colon[46]. A recent study in Shanghai, China, found that a diet rich in certain vegetables, garlic and fruits (especially oranges and tangerines) was protective against laryngeal cancer, but the risk of laryngeal cancer was increased by eating salt-preserved meat and fish, as well as by other factors[52]. Relating specific dietary components to the causation of specific cancers still remains problematic, however. A recent survey of the subject by oncologists[53] agreed that 'although diet is likely to be a very important factor in carcinogenesis, there are not yet sufficient data to allow classification of specific nutritional factors among the established carcinogens'. Nevertheless, there was evidence that some nutrients and food groups may be involved in either increasing or decreasing cancer risk. Overall, they concluded that:

> It is important that although no causal relation has been definitely established between any nutritional factor and any of the indicated cancers, a clear pattern of protection appears to characterize a high intake of fruits and vegetables, whereas a less clear pattern of increased risk appears to characterize positive energy balance and excessive intake[53].

A recent comprehensive review of the subject by the World Cancer Research Fund and the American Institute for Cancer Research[54] concluded that 30–40 per cent of cancer cases throughout the world, or 3–4 million cases a year, could be prevented by dietary means. This particularly applies to cancers of the mouth, pharynx, stomach, colon, rectum, liver and breast. As with several other studies, their recommendations included:

1. The basic diet should be adequate and varied, and based mainly on foods of plant origin, including vegetables, fruits, and pulses (legumes), as well as minimally processed starchy staple foods
2. The diet should always include a high intake of fruits and vegetables, which should provide 7 per cent or more of total energy
3. Total fats and oils in the diet should provide nor more than 15–20 per cent of total energy, thus fatty foods (especially of animal origin) should be avoided
4. If eaten at all, red meat should provide less than 10 per cent of the total energy
5. Dietary salt from all sources should amount to less than 6 g/day (0.25 oz) for adults, so herbs and spices rather than salt should be used to season food
6. A variety of starchy or protein-rich foods of plant origin should provide 45–60 per cent of energy, and these include cereals (grains), pulses, roots, tubers, and plantains
7. Intake of refined sugar should be limited, and should provide less than 10 per cent of total energy
8. Perishable food, if not consumed promptly, should be frozen or chilled, and stored in ways that minimize fungal contamination
9. Meat and fish should be cooked at relatively low temperatures and not charred or grilled, and cured and smoked meats should be avoided
10. In the presence of an adequate, balanced diet, dietary supplements (such as vitamins) are 'probably unnecessary, and possibly unhelpful' for reducing cancer risk.

In addition to these dietary changes, they also recommended adequate physical exercise, avoiding being overweight, and drastically reducing alcohol intake and tobacco smoking.

As the examples in this chapter indicate, a large number of diseases can be linked to dietary beliefs and practices, though these cultural factors are mainly relevant where enough food is available for nutrition in the first place. Attempts to modify or improve diets should therefore take into account the important cultural roles that food plays in all societies and cultural groups.

Recommended reading

Dettwyler, K. A. (1992). The biocultural approach in nutritional anthropology: case studies of malnutrition in Mali. *Med. Anthropol.*, **15**, 17–39.

Drenowski, A. and Popkin, B. M. (1997). The nutrition transition: new trends in the global diet. *Nutr. Rev.*, **55**, 31–43.

Farb, P. and Armelagos, G. (1980). *Consuming Passions: The Anthropology of Eating*. Houghton Muffin.

Lang, T. (1999). Diet, health and globalization: five key questions. *Proc. Nutr. Soc.*, **58**, 335–43.

Snow, L. F. and Johnson, S. M. (1978). Folklore, food, female reproductive cycle. *Ecol. Food Nutr.*, **7**, 41–9.

World Cancer Research Fund/American Institute for Cancer Research (1997). *Food, Nutrition and the Prevention of Cancer: A Global Perspective*. WCRF/AICR.

4 Caring and curing: the sectors of health care

In most societies people suffering from physical discomfort or emotional distress have a number of ways of helping themselves or of seeking help from other people. They may, for example, decide to rest or take a home remedy, ask advice from a friend, relative or neighbour, consult a local priest, folk healer or 'wise person', or consult a doctor, provided that one is available. They may follow all of these steps, or perhaps only one or two of them, and may follow them in any order. The larger and more complex the society in which the person is living, the more of these therapeutic options are likely to be available, provided the individual can afford to pay for them. Modern urbanized societies, whether Western or non-Western, are more likely, therefore, to exhibit *health care pluralism.* Within these societies there are many people or individuals, each offering the patient their own particular way of explaining, diagnosing and treating ill health. Though these therapeutic modes co-exist, they are often based on entirely different premises and may even originate in different cultures, such as Western medicine in China, or Chinese acupuncture in the modern Western world. To the ill person, however, the origin of these treatments is less important than their efficacy in relieving suffering.

Health care pluralism: social and cultural aspects

Anthropologists have pointed out that any society's *health care system* cannot be studied in isolation from other aspects of that society, especially its social, religious, political and economic organization. It is interwoven with these, and is based on the same assumptions, values and view of the world. Landy[1] points out that a system of health care has two inter-related aspects: a *cultural* aspect, which includes certain basic concepts, theories, normative practices and shared modes of perception; and a *social* aspect, including its organization into certain specified roles (such as patient and doctor) and rules governing relationships between these roles in specialized settings (such as a hospital or a doctor's office). In most societies one form of health care, such as scientific medicine in the West, is elevated above the other forms, and both its cultural and social aspects are upheld by law. Besides this official health care system, which includes the medical and nursing professions, there are usually smaller, alternative systems such as homeopathy, herbalism and spiritual healing in many Western countries, which might be termed *health care sub-cultures.* Each has its own way of explaining and treating ill health, and the healers in each group are organized into professional associations, with rules of entry, codes of conduct and ways of relating to patients. Medical sub-cultures may be indigenous to the society or they may be imported from elsewhere; in many cases immigrants to a society often bring their traditional folk healers along with them, to deal with their ill health in a culturally familiar way. In the UK, examples of these healers are the Muslim *hakims* or Hindu *vaids*, sometimes consulted by immigrants from the Indian subcontinent. In looking at health care pluralism, wherever it occurs, it is important to examine both the cultural and social aspects of the types of health care available to the individual patient.

In this chapter the pluralistic health care systems of complex, industrialized societies will be examined, in order to illustrate:

1. The range of therapeutic options available in these societies
2. How and why choices are made between the various options.

Health care pluralism in the UK will also be discussed, and the implications of this for the delivery of health care.

The three sectors of health care

Kleinman[2] has suggested that, in looking at any complex society, one can identify three overlapping and interconnected sectors of health care; the *popular* sector, the *folk* sector and the *professional* sector. Each sector has its own ways of explaining and treating ill health, defining who is the healer and who is the patient, and specifying how healer and patient should interact in their therapeutic encounter.

The popular sector

This is the lay, non-professional, non-specialist domain of society, where ill health is first recognized and defined and health care activities are initiated. It includes all the therapeutic options that people utilize, without any payment and without consulting either folk healers or medical practitioners. Among these options are:

- self-treatment or self-medication
- advice or treatment given by a relative, friend, neighbour or workmate
- healing and mutual care activities in a church, cult or self-help group
- consultation with another lay person who has special experience of a particular disorder, or of treatment of a physical state.

In this sector the main arena of health care is the *family*; here most ill health is recognized and then treated. It is the real site of primary health care in any society. In the family, as Chrisman[3] points out, the main providers of health care are *women*, usually mothers or grandmothers, who diagnose most common illnesses and treat them with the materials at hand. It has been estimated that about 70–90 per cent of health care takes place within this sector, in both Western and non-Western societies[4].

People who become ill typically follow a 'hierarchy of resort', ranging from self-medication to consultation with others. Self-treatment is based on lay beliefs about the structure and function of the body, and the origin and nature of ill health. It includes a variety of substances such as patent medicines, traditional folk remedies or 'old wives' tales', as well as changes in diet or behaviour. Food can be used as a form of medicine (see Chapter 3) in folk illnesses: for example, in 'high blood' in the southern USA, where certain foods are used to reduce the excess volume of blood, which is believed to cause the condition; or in parts of Latin America and Asia, where certain foods are used to counteract 'hot' or 'cold' illnesses and to restore the body to equilibrium. In both the UK and USA, self-prescribed vitamins are commonly used to restore health when one is 'feeling low'. The changes in behaviour that accompany different forms of ill health can range from special prayers, rituals, confession, fasting, or the use of talismans and charms to resting in a warm bed for a chill or cold.

The popular sector usually includes a set of beliefs about *health maintenance*. These are usually a series of guidelines, specific to each cultural group, about the 'correct' behaviour for preventing ill health in oneself and in others. They include beliefs about the healthy way to eat, drink, sleep, dress, work, pray and generally conduct one's life. In some societies health is also maintained by the use of charms, amulets and religious medallions to ward off bad luck, including unexpected illness, and to attract good luck and good health.

Most health care in this sector takes place between people already linked to one another by ties of kinship, friendship or neighbourhood, or membership of work or religious organizations. This means that both patient and healer share similar assumptions about health and illness, and misunderstandings between the two are comparatively rare[3]. The sector is made up of a series of *informal* and unpaid healing relationships of variable duration, which occur within the sufferer's own social network, particularly the family. These therapeutic encounters occur without fixed rules governing behaviour or setting; at a later date the roles may be reversed, with today's patient becoming tomorrow's healer. There are certain individuals, though, who tend to act as a source of health advice more often than others. These include:

1. Those with long experience of a particular illness or type of treatment
2. Those with extensive experience of certain life events, such as women who have raised several children
3. The paramedical professions (such as nurses, pharmacists, physiotherapists or doctor's receptionists) who are consulted informally about health problems
4. Doctors' wives or husbands, who share some of their spouses' experience, if not training
5. Individuals such as hairdressers, salespeople or even bank managers who interact frequently with the public, and sometimes act as lay confessors or psychotherapists
6. The organizers of self-help groups
7. The members or officiants of certain healing cults or churches.

All of these people may be considered as resources of advice and assistance concerning health matters by their friends or families. Their credentials are mainly their own experience rather than education, social status or special occult powers. A woman who has had several pregnancies, for example, can give informal advice to a newly pregnant younger woman, telling her what symptoms to expect and how to deal with them. Similarly, a person with long experience of a particular medication may 'lend' some to a friend with similar symptoms.

Individuals' experiences of ill health are sometimes shared within a self-help group, which may act as a repository of knowledge about a particular ailment or experience to be used both for the benefit of other members and for the rest of society. Self-help groups can bring many other benefits to members, such as sharing advice on lifestyle or coping strategies, or acting as a refuge for isolated individuals – especially those suffering from stigmatized conditions such as obesity or alcoholism.

Experiences of ill health and suffering may also be shared within a healing cult or church. For example, McGuire[5] has described some of the healing groups that are now found in middle-class suburban USA. These include movements such as Christian Science, the Unity School of Christianity, various other Christian groups (such as charismatic Catholic and Protestant Pentecostal groups), Human Potential groups (such as Scientology, EST, Progoff Process and Cornucopia), Eastern meditation and yoga groups (based on Zen or Tibetan Buddhism, Jainism or Hinduism), and the many types of spiritualist church and 'healing circles' that practise occult or psychic healing for their members. Many of these are based on the 'New Age' movement[6], which emphasizes personal development, self-care and a holistic approach to health care – encompassing mind, body, and soul. In non-Western societies too, self-help groups often have a religious basis. 'Spirit possession' cults, for example, are common in parts of Africa, especially among women. In these cults, women who have been 'possessed' and made ill by a particular spirit form what Turner[7] calls 'a community of suffering', the members of which ritually diagnose and treat those in the rest of society suffering from possession by the same malign spirit. Lewis[8] sees some of these spirit possession cults, like the Hausa

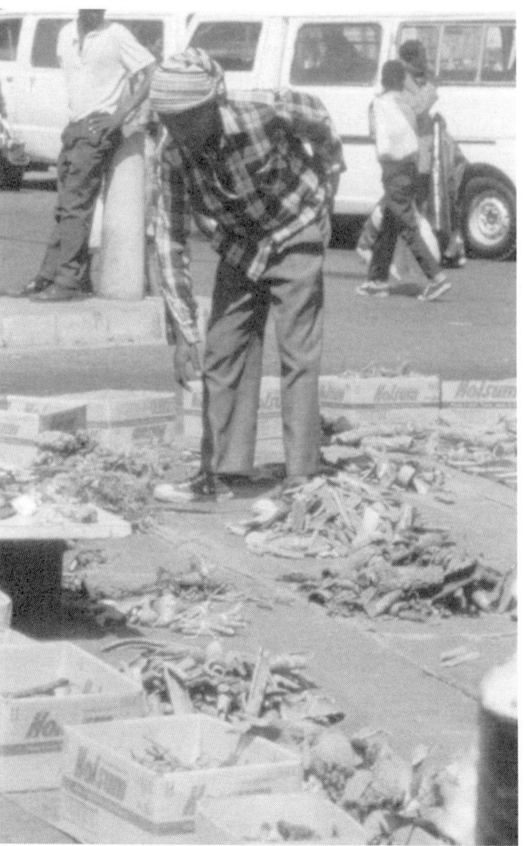

Figure 4.1 A seller of *muti*, or traditional African remedies and folk medicines, at a bus station in Langa township, Cape Town, South Africa (Source: Mthobele Guma).

bori cult in Northern Nigeria, as essentially women's protest movements against their social disadvantages. Membership of the cult brings prestige, healing power and special attention from their menfolk, who lavish gifts on them to appease the possessing spirits.

All aspects of the popular sector (and of the other two sectors as well) may sometimes have negative effects on people's mental and physical health. The family, for example, may either facilitate or impede health care. In Taiwan, according to Kleinman[9], the family's usual response to a sick member is to attempt to contain him, his sickness and the social problems that it generates within the circle of the family instead of sharing it with an outsider such as a medical practitioner.

In general, ill people move freely between the popular and the other two sectors and back again, often using all three sectors at once, especially when treatment in one sector fails to relieve physical discomfort or emotional distress.

The folk sector

In this sector, which is especially large in non-industrialized societies, certain individuals specialize in forms of healing that are either *sacred* or *secular*, or a mixture of the two. These healers are not part of the official medical system, and occupy an intermediate position between the popular and professional sectors. There is a wide variation in the types of folk healer found in any society, from purely secular and technical experts like bone-setters, midwives, tooth extractors or herbalists, to spiritual healers, clairvoyants and shamans. Folk healers form a heterogeneous group, with much individual variation in style and outlook, but sometimes they are organized into associations of healers, with rules of entry, codes of conduct and the sharing of information.

Most communities include a mixture of sacred and secular folk healers. For example, in her study of African-American folk healers in low-income urban neighbourhoods in the USA, Snow[10] has described 'herb doctors', 'root doctors', spiritualists, 'conjure' men or women, Voodoo *houngans* or *mambos*, healing ministers and faith healers, neighbourhood prophets, 'granny women' and vendors of magical herbs, roots and patent medicines. Spiritual healers, who operate out of temples, churches or 'candle shops' are particularly common, and deal with illnesses believed to be due to sorcery (hexing) or divine punishment. More secular illnesses are dealt with by self-medication, or by neighbourhood granny women or herb doctors. In practice, though, there is some overlap between their approaches and techniques. In another community, the Zulu of South Africa, there is also an overlap between sacred and secular healers. While sacred divination is carried out by female *isangomas*, treatment by African herbal medicines is by male *inyangas*; both, though, will gather information about the social background of the victim as well as details of his or her illness before making a diagnosis[11].

An example of a purely secular healer is the *sahi*, or health worker, as described by the Underwoods[12] in Raymah, Yemen Arab Republic. These healers have only appeared in Yemen in recent years, and their practice consists mainly of giving injections of various Western drugs. They have little training (usually a brief association with a health professional; in one case a month's work as a hospital cleaner), limited diagnostic skill, and they utilize few counselling or psychological skills. To the inhabitants of Raymah, however, the *sahi* practises what is considered to be the quintessence of Western medicine – 'the treatment of illness by injections'. The growing popularity of injections has been described in many Third World countries[13,14], as has the proliferation of untrained *injectionists* (also known as injection doctors, needle men or shot givers) like the *sahi*. Other examples of this trend have been described by Kimani[15] in Kenya. There, untrained bush doctors administer medicines and injections, and 'street and bus-depot doctor boys' hustle antibiotic capsules acquired through the black market.

Most folk healers share the basic cultural values and world view of the communities in which they live, including beliefs about the origin, significance and treatment of ill health. In societies where ill health and other forms of misfortune are blamed on social causes (witchcraft, sorcery or 'evil eye') or on supernatural causes (gods, spirits, ancestral ghosts or fate), sacred folk healers are particularly common. Their approach is usually a holistic one, dealing with *all* aspects of the patient's life, including relationships with other people, with the natural environment and with supernatural forces, as well as any physical or emotional symptoms. In many non-Western societies all these aspects of life are part of the definition of health, which is seen as a *balance* between people and their social, natural and supernatural environments. A disturbance of any of these (such as immoral behaviour, conflicts within the family or failure to observe religious practices) may result in physical symptoms or emotional distress, and require the services of a sacred folk healer. Healers of this type, when faced with ill health, often inquire about the patient's behaviour before the illness and about any conflicts with other people. In a small-scale society the healer may also have firsthand knowledge of a family's difficulties through local gossip, and this may be useful in reaching a diagnosis. As well as gathering information about the patient's recent history and social background, the healer may employ a ritual of *divination*. There are many forms of this world-wide[16], including the use of cards, bones, straws, shells, sticks, special stones and tea leaves, the arrangement of which is closely examined by the healer for any evidence of any underlying pattern. There is also examination of the entrails or liver of certain animals or birds, interpretation of dreams or visions, or direct consultation with spirits or supernatural beings by going into a trance. In each case, the divination aims to uncover the supernatural cause of the illness (such as witchcraft or divine retribution) by the use of supernatural techniques.

Trance divination is common in non-industrialized societies, but is becoming increasingly common in the West too, among mediums, clairvoyants, 'channellers' and the members of certain healing churches. The Zulu *isangoma,* for example, is consulted by the relatives of a sick person, who remains at home. Her diagnosis is made by going into a trance and communicating with spirits, who tell her the cause and treatment of the illness[11]. Another form of this is the *shaman,* who is found in many cultures. In Lewis's definition[17], a *shaman* is 'a person of either sex who has mastered spirits and can at will introduce them into his own body'; divination takes place at a seance, where the healer allows the spirits to enter him and through him diagnose the illness and prescribe the treatment. In some cases he may only enter his trance with the aid of powerful hallucinogenic drugs (see Chapter 8). This and other forms of divination sometimes take place in the presence of the patient's family, friends and other social contacts. In this public setting, the diviner aims to bring conflicts within a community – which may have led to witchcraft or sorcery between people – to the surface, and to resolve these conflicts in a ritual way. Sacred healers also provide explanations and treatment for subjective feelings of guilt, shame or anger by prescribing, for example, prayer, repentance or the resolution of interpersonal problems. They may also prescribe physical treatments or remedies at the same time.

Advantages and disadvantages of folk healing

For those who utilize it, folk healing offers several advantages over modern scientific medicine. One of these is the frequent involvement of the family in diagnosis and treatment. For example, as Martin[18] has pointed out, in Native American healing the patient's sickness places a responsibility on both patient and family to participate in healing rites. The focus of attention is not only the patient (as in Western medicine), but also the reaction of the family and others to the illness. The healer himself is usually surrounded by helpers, who take part in the ceremony, give explanations to the patient and his family, and answer any of their queries. From a modern perspective, this type of Native American healer with helpers, together with the patient's family, provides an effective primary health care team, especially in dealing with psychosocial problems. Fabrega and Silver[19] have examined the advantages to the patient of another type of folk healer, the *h'ilol* in Zinacantan, Mexico, over Western doctors. In particular, there is a shared world view, closeness, warmth, informality and the use of everyday language in consultations, and the family and other community members are involved in treatment. Also, the *h'ilol* is a crucial figure in the community and is believed to act for the benefit of the patient and the community as well as the gods; he can influence society at large, particularly the patient's social relationships, and he can influence the patient's future behaviour by pointing out the influence of past actions on his present illness. Finally, his healing takes place in a familiar setting, such as the home or a religious shrine. Because folk healers such as the *h'ilol* articulate and reinforce the cultural values of the communities in which they live, they have advantages over Western doctors, who are often separated from their patients by social class, economic position, gender, specialized education and, sometimes, cultural background. In particular, these healers are better able to define and treat illness – that is, the social, psychological and moral dimensions associated with ill health, as with other forms of misfortune (see Chapter 5). They also provide culturally familiar ways of explaining the causes and timing of ill health, and its relation to the social and supernatural worlds.

In many countries today such folk healers are often used in parallel with medical treatment, even though both are based on very different premises. In Mexico, for example, Finkler[20] has described the differences, as well as the similarities, between doctors and spiritual healers (who heal with the aid of spirits who possess them). She shows how people utilize *both* systems, but for different purposes. As in many other cultures, the doctors tend to tell their patients what has happened, while the healers tell them *why*. Healers explain ill health in wider, more familiar cultural terms – involving the social, psychological and spiritual aspects of their patients' lives – while doctors concentrate mainly on physical diseases and the pathogens or behaviours said to cause them. This is despite the fact that the doctors spend twice as long (about 20 minutes) with first-time patients compared to the healers. On the other hand, there are some similarities between the two approaches. Both have a dualistic view of the patient, the doctors using a mind and body approach and the healers a spirit and body approach. Both attempt to peer inside the patient's body in order to diagnose ill health, the doctors with the aid of technology and the healers by means of the spirits that possess and aid them. Their therapeutic settings, however, are very different. The healing of *Espiritualismo* takes place in a temple in the presence of family and other members of the community, while doctor–patient interactions take place in the sterile isolation of a small cubicle, occasionally in the presence of strangers such as nurses or medical students. Finkler notes also that, unlike the doctors, spiritual healers rarely give their patients a specific diagnosis but rather an assurance that the spirits know everything about their affliction. To many patients this explanation is satisfying, since on some level it matches their own expectations and subjective emotional experience of ill health. For while doctors tend to place the patient's ill health in a limited temporal frame, and to localize it in a particular part of the body, the omniscient spirits that aid the healer 'transcend time and space in the same way that the patient's sickness transcends temporal and spatial dimensions'.

Training of folk healers

In general, folk healers have little formal training equivalent to the Western medical school. Skills are usually acquired by apprenticeship to an older healer, by experience of certain techniques or conditions, or by the possession of inborn or acquired healing power. People can become folk healers in a number of ways, such as:

1. Inheritance – being born into a 'healing family', sometimes of many generations of healers.
2. Position within a family, like the 'seventh son of a seventh son' in Ireland.
3. Signs and portents at birth, like a birthmark, or 'crying in the womb', or being born with the amniotic membrane across the face (the 'caul' in Scotland).
4. Revelation – discovering one 'has the gift', which may occur as an intense emotional experience during an illness, dream or trance. In extreme cases, as Lewis[17] points out, the vocation may be announced by 'an initially uncontrolled state of possession: a traumatic experience associated with hysteroid, ecstatic behaviour'.
5. Apprenticeship to another healer – a common pattern in all parts of the world, though the apprenticeship may last for many years.
6. Acquiring a particular skill on one's own, like the Yemeni *sahi*, the Kenyan bush doctors and other forms of injectionists.

In practice, these pathways into folk healing tend to overlap; for example, someone born of a 'healing family' and with certain signs and portents at birth may still need to refine their 'gift' by a lengthy apprenticeship to an older healer. In a few cases, healers may also be qualified as nurses or other health professionals. One study[21] has estimated, for example, that in South Africa almost 1 per cent of African nurses also work part-time as traditional healers.

While most folk healers work individually, informal networks or associations of healers do exist, and these provide for the exchange of techniques and information and the monitoring of each other's behaviour. Such a network among Zulu diviners or *isangomas* is described by Ngubane[11]; meetings take place regularly between diviners to share ideas, experiences and techniques. Each diviner has the opportunity to meet the ex-students, teacher and neophyte of each of her neighbouring diviners, as well as more distant ones. It is estimated that, over a period of 3–5 years, a diviner might make contact with over 400 fellow diviners all over Southern Africa. In other settings, such as low-income black neighbourhoods in the USA, several healers might be ministers of a spiritualist church, which also acts as an association of healers. In the suburban healing circles described by McGuire[5], almost all the participants have the chance to be both healer and patient at various times; therefore these groups overlap the boundary between folk and popular healing, and also provide a venue for the exchange of information and experiences among a group of healers.

However, despite their many advantages it is important not to over-romanticize folk healers in general. Like all other health care providers, including doctors and nurses, their ranks may include those who are incompetent, ignorant, arrogant or greedy, or have a very reductionist view of ill health and how it should be treated. Furthermore, not all folk healers come from the community in which they work or are familiar with its inner social workings. Some of the techniques they use may also be very dangerous to their patients. The use of unsterilized needles by injectionists, for example, may lead to severe skin abscesses, as well as to the spread of hepatitis B or AIDS. It is important therefore to see folk healers in a balanced way, and to avoid both over-idealization and over-criticism of them. On the one hand one should avoid what Lucas and Barrett[22] term the Arcadian view – seeing them and the communities they work among as somehow natural and holistic, living in peaceful harmony with nature and with one another. On the other, the 'barbaric' view – seeing them and their communities as somehow primitive, degenerate, incompetent and underdeveloped – is also inaccurate. In most cases of folk healing, the truth lies somewhere between the two.

'Professionalization' of folk healers

The relationship between folk and professional sectors has usually been marked by mutual distrust and suspicion. Most doctors have tended to view folk healers as quacks, charlatans, witch doctors or medicine men, who pose a danger to their patients' health.

Increasingly (and often reluctantly), however, the medical authorities have recognized that, despite their shortcomings, folk healers *do* have some obvious advantages to the patient and their family, especially when dealing with psychological problems. In many developing countries, traditional folk healers are becoming incorporated into the margins of the medical system – sometimes against their will. The initiative for this has usually come from the WHO, or from national governments, or sometimes from the healers themselves. In 1978, the WHO issued its famous Alma-Ata declaration of 'Health for All by the Year 2000'. Its main proposal was for the worldwide provision of comprehensive primary health care (PHC), which would provide preventive, curative and rehabilitative services at an affordable cost[23]. However, with scarce resources, growing populations and limited medical manpower the task was almost impossible, and has recently become even more difficult due to new diseases such as AIDS. One result of this was a fresh look at traditional medicine, redefining it as a potential ally of the medical system rather than as an enemy. In 1978 the WHO recommended that traditional medicine be promoted, developed and integrated wherever possible with modern, scientific medicine[24], but stressed the necessity to ensure respect, recognition and collaboration among the practitioners of the various systems concerned. The manpower resources that WHO hoped to enlist included herbalists, Ayurvedic, Unāni or Yoga practitioners, Chinese traditional healers such as acupuncturists, and various others. Special attention has been paid to the selection and training of traditional birth attendants (TBAs)[25,26], who already deliver about two-thirds of the world's babies (see Chapter 6).

Last[27] points out that now, as a result of these two declarations, 'the potential professionalization of indigenous practitioners is firmly on the agenda'. He notes that there has been a rapid growth in the number of practitioners' organizations, especially in Africa. Some (like the Zulu *isangomas)* operate mainly as informal networks, others as pressure groups or healing churches or cults. Several – such as the Zimbabwe National Traditional Healers' Association – have become recognized by government as professional bodies in their own right, with exclusive powers to educate, evaluate, license and discipline their members.

For many folk healers, the process of forming a 'profession' (see below) has also often been a response to unequal competition from the medical system. By creating a professional association, they hope to advance their interests and those of their clients, improve standards, raise their prestige and earning power, gain official support and define an area of health care that only they can provide.

However, this is often problematic. For one thing, there is evidence that in many developing countries the actual number of traditional healers is declining, owing partially to education, urbanization and the breakdown of communities. Also, as Last[27] notes, traditional healers (especially of the sacred kind) are too diffuse a group, and their knowledge and practice too rooted in local contexts, to be effectively standardized. They also have specific notions of legitimacy, which derive mainly from the traditions of their community and their own charisma and not from some distant government bureaucracy. For many of their clients, 'the legality of a practice is less important than the practitioner's moral standing or trustworthiness'.

To some extent, this professionalization of traditional healers parallels a similar process that is happening among alternative and complementary healers in Western societies (see below). In Eastern Europe, since the eighteenth century, the Russian *feldshers* have also progressed along a lengthy road from local folk practitioners (often ex-army medics) to their more recent status as physician's assistants who often work in primary care, especially in rural areas[28]. By contrast, their equivalents in other Eastern European countries, such as the *cyruliks* of Poland, have largely disappeared[28].

Velimirovic[29] sees the WHO initiative on traditional medicine as well-intentioned but misguided. He argues that its integration into the formal (professional) sector of health care since 1978 'has contributed virtually nothing to solving the monumental health problems of the developing world', or to the attainment of 'Health for All by the Year 2000'. This is partly because, in the WHO proposal, the definition of traditional medicine was never clear or consistent. Nor was its uncritical assumption of the efficacy of traditional medicine justified, since it ignored its many failures and shortcomings – such as its inability to cure malaria, cholera, yellow fever and other diseases. In many cases, the views of traditional healers on disease, and their treatments, were so detrimental to health that they themselves were part of the problem. Furthermore, in many developing countries traditional medicine 'is often not as popular with the people themselves as health planners believe'. Given the choice, many people prefer to consult Western-style doctors rather than traditional healers or untrained community health workers – even if this involves much expense and travelling a great distance to see them.

Despite this view, it should be emphasized that there *are* examples of the successful collaboration between traditional healers and the official medical system, especially in relation to AIDS prevention[30], traditional birth attendants[26], family planning[31], the promotion of oral rehydration therapy[32], the treatment of mental illness[33] and the treatment and rehabilitation of drug addicts[34].

Traditional medicine in China and India

In countries like India and China, strong indigenous systems of healing enjoy almost the same legitimacy and popularity as Western medicine and now, with government support, offer the population parallel systems of health care. They are already to some extent 'professionalized'. In China, despite several shifts of government policy, traditional Chinese medicine – including acupuncture, moxibustion and herbal remedies – still provides a complementary system of health care for much of the population, especially in rural areas, and exists alongside biomedical clinics and other facilities. In India there are 91 recognized Ayurvedic (Hindu) and 10 Unāni (Muslim) medical schools, and Ayurvedic medicine serves a large proportion of the population. The Indian Medicine Central Council Act of 1970 set up a Central Council for Ayurveda, which established a register of qualified practitioners and oversees the training of new ones. They grant a 3-year Bachelor of Ayurvedic Medicine and Surgery degree, followed by 3 years' postgraduate study[35]. However, by the late 1980s only 12 per cent of Ayurvedic practitioners had obtained the degree of a recognized teaching institution, 54 per cent had degrees from unrecognized schools, while 33 per cent had no qualifications at all[35]. A similar process has taken place with homeopathy, which is now overseen by a Central Council for Homeopathy. This has recognized 200 000 homeopathic practitioners, and supervises 104 colleges which run undergraduate courses in the subject. Postgraduate degrees are issued by the National Institute of Homeopathy in Calcutta, and there are 130–150 homeopathic hospitals and 1500 homeopathic dispensaries in India, all supported by the government.

Srinavasan[36] noted in 1995 that Ayurveda was losing popularity to Western (allopathic) medicine in many parts of the country. One all-India survey showed that while 80 per cent of households in urban areas used allopathic medicine only 4 per cent used Ayurvedic, while in rural households 75 per cent used allopathy and 8 per cent Ayurvedic. This applied to most social classes. In Sri Lanka, by comparison, he noted that government policy has strongly encouraged traditional medicine, and that there are now 13 000 Ayurvedic physicians (1 per 1400 population) there, compared to India's 380 000 (1 per 2200 population)[36].

Alternative and complementary medicine

In most Western countries a special form of health care – alternative or complementary medicine – overlaps both folk and professional sectors. Its many types of healers usually include acupuncturists, homeopaths, chiropractors, osteopaths, herbalists, naturopaths, spiritual healers, hypnotists, massage therapists and meditation experts. This sector of health care is rapidly growing in popularity. In 1981, for example, an estimated 3.8 per cent of the population of Holland had visited an alternative practitioner, and by 1987 this had risen to 5.2 per cent[37]. In Germany, many thousands of *Heilpraktikers* (naturopaths who practise 'naturecure' and hydrotherapy) often also practise acupuncture, herbalism or chiropractic[37]. These naturopaths have been given official recognition since 1939, and according to Wirsing[38] there are about 7000 of them practising in Germany today. He also estimates that there are about 2000 physicians who practice homeopathy, and another 1000 who practice 'anthroposophic' medicine, based on the teachings of Rudolf Steiner. In the USA, Eisenberg and colleagues[39] have estimated that almost one in three people used some form of unconventional medicine in 1990, most frequently for back problems (36 per cent), headaches (27 per cent), chronic pain (26 per cent) and cancer or tumours (24 per cent). The most common treatments they used were relaxation techniques, chiropractic and massage. In most cases (89 per cent) they saw these practitioners without the recommendation of their doctors, and 72 per cent never told them. Overall, it was estimated that Americans made about 425 million visits to the unconventional practitioners in 1990, a figure exceeding the total number of visits to all US primary care physicians (388 million). Furthermore, they paid about $10.3 billion 'out-of-pocket' for these therapies, compared to the $12.8 billion they paid for all the hospital care in the USA. Most users of unconventional therapies were found to be between 25 and 49 years old, but they came from all socio-demographic groups.

The professional sector

This comprises the organized, legally sanctioned healing professions, such as modern Western scientific medicine, also known as *allopathy* or *biomedicine*. It includes not only physicians of various types and specialties, but also the recognized paramedical professions such as nurses, midwives and physiotherapists. In most countries scientific medicine is the basis of the professional sector but, as Kleinman notes, traditional medical systems may also become professionalized to some extent; examples of this are the Ayurvedic and Unāni medical colleges in India, which receive governmental support. It is important to realize that Western scientific medicine provides only a small proportion of health care in most countries of the world. Medical manpower is often a scarce resource, with most health care taking place in the popular and folk sectors. World Health Organization statistics for 1980[40] illustrated the huge variations in the availability of doctors and hospital beds throughout the world (Table 4.1).

The 1993 *World Development Report*[41], based on data from the years 1988–1992, gives a similar picture of widespread variations in the supply of medical manpower. In sub-Saharan Africa, for example, there was an average of 0.12 doctors per thousand population, compared to 0.41 in India, 1.04 in the Middle East, 1.25 in Latin America, 1.37 in China, 3.09 in the Western industrialized countries, and 4.07 in the former USSR[41].

Table 4.1 Relation of physicians and hospital beds to population in selected countries (WHO, 1980[40])

Country	*Population per physician*	*Hospital beds per 10 000 population*
Ethiopia	73 043	3.0
Malawi	47 638	174
Bangladesh	12 378	23
India	3652	7.8
Jamaica	3505	38.9
Mexico	1251	11.6
Japan	845	106.0
England and Wales	659	86.3*
France	613	63.0
United States	595	3.0
USSR	289	121.3

*Average of figures for England and Wales.

These figures, however, probably overestimate the numbers of doctors actually involved in direct patient care, as many of them work in research and administration rather than in clinical practice. In addition, the distribution of doctors is not uniform; in many non-industrialized societies they tend to cluster in cities, where facilities are better and practice is more lucrative, leaving many in the countryside to rely on the popular and folk sectors of care. In many of these countries, the proportion of doctors who work in the private sector has steadily increased, thus reducing even further the number available to provide low-cost health care by the state. In Zimbabwe, for example, 66 per cent of doctors now work in the private sector, while 59 per cent do so in South Africa and 25 per cent in Papua New Guinea[42]. Private medical practice has greatly increased in Malawi and Tanzania, following changes in government policy, while in Uganda, Bennett[42] has argued that the increase in private practitioners has 'created a culture in which good care has come to be associated with the availability of injections and other drugs, regardless of medical appropriateness'.

In most countries, especially in the Western world, the practitioners of scientific medicine form the only group of healers whose positions are upheld by law. They enjoy higher social status, greater income and more clearly defined rights and obligations than other types of healers. They have the power to question and examine their patients, prescribe powerful and sometimes dangerous treatments or medication, and deprive certain people of their freedom and confine them to hospitals if they are diagnosed as psychotic or infectious. In hospital, they can tightly control their patients' diet, behaviour, sleeping patterns and medication, and can initiate a variety of tests, such as biopsies, X-rays or venesection. They can also label their patients (sometimes permanently) as ill, incurable, malingering, hypochondriacal, or as fully recovered – a label that may conflict with the patient's perspective. These labels can have important effects, both social (confirming the patient in the sick role) and economic (influencing health insurance or pension payments).

The medical system

As stated earlier, the dominant system of health care of any society cannot be studied in isolation from other aspects of that society, for the *medical system* (or professional sector of health care) does not exist in a social or cultural vacuum. Rather, it is an expression of, and to some extent a miniature model of, the values and social structure of the society from which it arises. Different types of society therefore produce different types of medical systems and different attitudes to health and illness, depending on their dominant ideology – whether this is capitalist, welfare state, socialist or communist. One society may see free (or relatively inexpensive) health care as a basic right of citizenship, or the basic right only of the poor or the very old, while another may see medical care as a commodity to be bought only by those who can afford it. In this latter case, the pursuit of profits in health care will exclude many of those poorer members of society who do not have the resources to pay for it. Whatever the type of society, the medical system not only reflects these basic values and ideologies, but in turn helps also to shape and maintain them[43].

As an example of this, critics of the medical systems in the Western world have pointed out how the internal organization of the professional sector reflects some of the basic inequalities in those societies, especially in relation to gender, social class and ethnic background. Within the medical system most doctors are male (and usually white) and, as in the wider society, occupy many more of the prestigious, powerful and well-paid jobs than female doctors and nurses[44]. Also, the personnel within this sector are arranged in hierarchies similar to the social strata of the wider society. In its dealings with the population the medical system may reproduce many of the underlying prejudices of society, as well as cultural assumptions as to what constitutes good and bad behaviour. For example, it has been suggested that racial prejudice plays an important role in how some Afro-Caribbean patients in the UK are classified by psychiatrists as 'mad', even when there is evidence to the contrary[44] (see Chapter 10). A similar process operated in the former USSR, in state psychiatry's attitude to political dissent[45].

Other critiques of the Western medical system include that by Illich[46], who has claimed that high-tech modern medicine has become increasingly dangerous to the population's health by reducing their autonomy, making them dependent on the medical profession and damaging their health by the side effects of drugs and surgical interventions. In addition, the medical system is in a symbiotic relationship with the manufacturers of pharmaceuticals and medical equipment, and this relationship is not necessarily in the patient's interest.

Like Illich, other critics of the medical system have maintained that modern medicine, as well as controlling micro-organisms, also seeks to control the behaviour of the population, especially by 'medicalizing' deviant behaviour, as well as many of the normal stages of the human life-cycle. Stacey[47] and others have suggested that this phenomenon is particularly evident in the case of women, especially during pregnancy and childbirth (see Chapter 6). Furthermore, much of the ill health in Western society that may be caused by other factors such as poverty, unemployment, economic crises, pollution or persecution is often ignored by the medical system, because its main focus is increasingly on the *individual* patient (or even on the individual organ) and the risk factors in his or her own lifestyle[48].

Thus in understanding any medical system, one must always see it in the *context* of the basic values, ideology, political organization and economic system of the society from which it arises. In that sense, the professional sector of health care, like the other two sectors, is always to some extent 'culture-bound'.

Comparison of medical systems

One can illustrate this culture-bound aspect, in the case of Western medicine, by comparing the medical systems of different Western countries with similar levels of economic development. Obviously these countries vary in whether health care lies mainly in the private or the public sectors, in the distribution of medical resources, their arrangements for health insurance and so on, but their professional sectors are all rooted in the same tradition of Western scientific medicine, and there is considerable exchange of medical data and techniques between them.

Despite Western medicine's claim of universality, however, various studies have illustrated significant differences in the types of diagnosis given and the treatment prescribed between different Western medical systems. For example, in 1984 a comparison of the patterns of prescribing of five different European countries (the UK, Germany, Italy, France and Spain)[49] found marked variations between them – and which could *not* be explained solely by disparities in the health of their populations. The study examined the 20 leading diagnostic categories and 20 leading types of drug prescribed in each of these countries. In the UK, for example, the major group of drugs prescribed was tranquillizers, hypnotics and sedatives (8.6 per cent of the total number of prescriptions), compared to 6.8 per cent in France, 6.0 per cent in Germany, 3.1 per cent in Italy and 2.0 per cent in Spain. In the UK, neuroses were among the commonest of diagnoses (5.1 per cent of the total number of diagnoses given), compared to 4.1 per cent in France, 3.2 per cent in Italy and 1.7 per cent in

Spain. These differences may represent not only differences in morbidity between the five countries, but also major differences in nomenclature, in the criteria of diagnosis, and in *cultural* attitudes to certain types of behaviour and how they should be dealt with. Other studies, some of which are described later in this book, have shown differences between UK and US psychiatrists and between UK and French psychiatrists in the criteria they use to diagnose and treat schizophrenia (see Chapter 10); differences between UK, Canadian and US rates of various surgical operations, including Caesarean sections (see Chapter 12); and differences in the medical use of spas and hydrotherapy *(la thermalisme)* in France and in Germany (the *kur*)[50], but not in countries like the UK or the USA.

A closer look at these national differences in the perception, diagnosis, naming and treatment of disease may suggest some of the cultural values that underlie those differences. For example, Payer[51] has examined the medical systems of the USA, France, Germany and the UK. She has described some of the diagnostic categories that have no clear equivalents in other countries, such as *crise de foie* and *spasmophilia* in France, *Herzinsuffizienz* and *Kreislaufkollaps* in Germany, or chilblains or 'bowel problems' in the UK. Furthermore, in understanding these variations she has related certain medical beliefs and practices to core cultural values in each of those societies. In the USA, for example, she sees a relation between the high rate of coronary bypass operations and other types of surgery and the American view of the body as a repairable 'machine' – and one that needs to be repaired and overhauled at regular intervals. She describes the dominant attitude of US doctors to sickness as an aggressive and 'can-do' approach, part of the legacy of the frontier spirit: 'Americans not only want to *do* something, they want to do it *fast*, and if they cannot they often become frustrated.' As a result, US doctors do more diagnostic tests on their patients and perform surgery more often than do doctors from the other three countries. According to Payer, they often eschew drug treatment in favour of more aggressive surgery, and if they do use drugs, they tend to use higher doses than their European colleagues. In psychiatry, for example, the doses of some drugs used in the USA are up to 10 times higher than those used elsewhere. The reasons for these approaches to medical care are various, including the types of payment US doctors get for their services, and the threat of malpractice suits against them. However, like doctors from the three European countries, it is the underlying *cultural* values of their society that play a part in determining how ill health is diagnosed and then treated.

The medical profession

Within the medical system those who practise medicine form a group apart, with their own values, concepts, theories of disease and rules of behaviour, as well as organization into a hierarchy of healing roles; this group therefore has both cultural and social aspects. It can be regarded – like lawyers, architects and engineers – as a *profession*. Foster and Anderson[52] define a profession as being 'based on, or organized around, a body of specialized knowledge [the content] not easily acquired and that, in the hands of qualified practitioners, meets the needs of, or serves, *clients*'. It also has a *collegial organization* of conceptual equals, which exists to maintain *control* over their field of expertise, promote their common interests, maintain their monopoly of knowledge, set qualifications for admission (such as the licensing of new physicians), protect themselves from incursions or competition by outsiders, and monitor the competence and ethics of their members. Although conceptually equal, the profession is arranged in hierarchies of knowledge and power, such as professors, consultants (senior residents) and house officers (interns) in the UK. Below them are the paramedical professionals: nurses, midwives, physiotherapists, occupational therapists, medical social workers etc. Each paramedical group has its own body of knowledge, clients, collegial organization and control over an area of competence, but overall has less autonomy and power than the physicians. The doctors themselves are divided into specialized sub-professions, which duplicate on a smaller scale the structure of the medical profession as a whole. Examples of this are the surgeons, paediatricians, gynaecologists and psychiatrists. Each have their own unique perspective on ill health, their own area of knowledge and their own hierarchy, from experts down to novices.

Pfifferling[53] has examined some of the assumptions and premises underlying the medical profession in the USA. In his view, it is:

1. *Physician-centred* – the doctor, and not the patient, defines the nature and boundary of the patient's problem; diagnostic and intellectual skills are valued above communication skills; settings for health care, such as doctors' offices, are often located for the benefit of doctors, far from their patients' homes.
2. *Specialist-orientated* – specialists, rather than generalists, get the highest prestige and rewards.
3. *Credentials-orientated* – those with higher credentials can rise in the medical hierarchy, and are considered to possess greater clinical skills and knowledge.
4. *Memory-based* – feats of memory (of medical facts, cases, drugs, discoveries etc.) are rewarded by promotion and the respect of one's peers.
5. *Single-case-centred* – decisions are made on a single case of a disease, based on cumulative descriptions of previous clinical cases.
6. *Process-orientated* – evaluations of the doctor's clinical skill are made by measuring their impact on quantifiable biological processes in the patient over time (such as a fall in blood pressure).

One could add to this list the increasing emphasis on diagnostic technology rather than on clinical evaluations, and the growing influence of the corporate take-over of many hospitals throughout the country and its implications for health care. Many of these points are now beginning to apply equally to physicians in other Western countries, such as the UK.

In many industrialized countries the professional sector is also composed of local general practitioners or family physicians who, unlike many hospital doctors, are often deeply rooted within a community. There is some resemblance between these doctors (and nurses) and healers in the folk sector, particularly in their familiarity with local conditions and with the social, familial and psychological aspects of ill health, even though their healing is based on entirely different premises.

The hospital

In most countries, the main institutional structure of scientific medicine is the *hospital*. Unlike in the popular and folk sectors, the ill person is removed from family, friends and community at a time of personal crisis. In hospital they undergo a standardized ritual of depersonalization (see Chapter 9), being converted into a numbered 'case' in a ward full of strangers. The emphasis is on their physical disease, with little reference to their home environment, religion, social relationships or moral status, or the meaning they give to their ill health. Hospital specialization ensures that they are classified and allocated to different wards on the basis of *age* (adults, paediatrics, geriatrics), *gender* (male, female), *condition* (medical, surgical or other), *organ* or *system* involved (ENT, ophthalmology, dermatology) or *severity* (intensive care units, casualty departments, emergency rooms). Patients of the same sex, similar age range and similar illnesses often share a ward. All these patients have been stripped of many of the props of social identity and individuality, and clothed in a uniform of pyjamas, nightdress or bathrobe. There is a loss of control over one's body, and over personal space, privacy, behaviour, diet and use of time. Patients are removed from the continuous emotional support of family and community and cared for by staff they may never have seen before. In hospitals, the relationship of health professionals – doctors, nurses, technicians – with their patients is largely characterized by distance, formality, brief conversations and, often, use of professional jargon. Hospitals have been seen by anthropologists such as Goffman[54] as 'small societies', each with their own unique culture; their own implicit and explicit rules of behaviour, tradition, rituals, hierarchies and even language. Patients in a ward form a temporary 'community of suffering', linked together by commiseration, ward gossip and discussion of one another's conditions. However, this community does not resemble or replace the communities in which they live and, unlike the members of self-help groups, their afflictions do not entitle them to heal others, at least not within the hospital setting.

The hospital, like the rest of the medical system itself, does not exist in a vacuum. It too is heavily influenced by cultural, social, and economic factors, at both the local and the national levels. For example, hospitals in North America and northern Europe, and the care they provide, tend to be more socially separated from the communities they serve than elsewhere in the world. With the exception of some paediatric and obstetric wards, members of the patient's family or community are rarely allowed to stay over in the ward with a sick person, provide

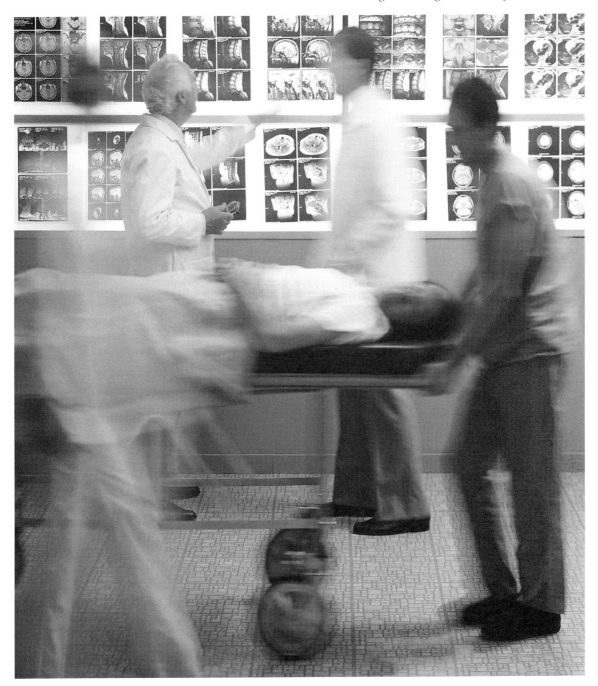

Figure 4.2 With its emphasis on diagnostic technology and the treatment of severe diseases, the hospital is the main institution of modern, scientific medicine (Source: Digital stock, MED 025).

them with food, wash and dress them, or contribute to their nursing care. In most cases they are only allowed to visit the patient at rigidly scheduled visiting hours, under the watchful eye of nurses and doctors. By contrast, in many parts of southern Europe, Asia and Africa, the boundary between hospital and community is much more porous; family members often spend many hours around the sick bed, washing, feeding and tending to the patient's intimate needs. In hospitals in the USA and northern Europe, these roles are usually carried out exclusively by nurses as part of the temporary quasi-family (nurse = mother, doctor = father, patient = child) of health professionals[55] described in Chapter 6.

There are many different ways of viewing the hospital and the many roles it plays in different countries, cultures and communities. For example, as well as a place where disease is cured and suffering alleviated, it can also be seen as:

1. A *refuge* – offering asylum (as it did in the Middle Ages) to those unable to cope in the outside world due to mental or physical ill health or old age
2. A *factory* – an industrial institution that produces 'cured' people out of the raw material of 'sick people'
3. A *business* – orientated (especially in the private, corporate sector) to making maximum profit out of the provision of health care
4. A *temple* – dedicated to a particular religious cosmology (such as Ayurveda) or healing tradition, or to the transcendent power of science over the forces of disease and death
5. A *university* – dedicated not only to the training of doctors and nurses, but also to the moral instruction of patients, teaching them *post hoc* how their ill health was the logical result of a previous lifestyle, and what they can do to prevent it happening again
6. A *prison* – protecting society by confining those regarded as mad, dissident or very unconventional, against their will
7. A *city* – a miniature metropolis with each ward a 'suburb', and with its own administration, bureaucracy, workers, security personnel, chapels and stores, together with a constantly changing and involuntary citizenry of patients.

Whatever its local variations, and however it is viewed, the hospital remains the pre-eminent institution of biomedicine. It is, as Konner[56] terms it, a 'temple of science'. However, with their large staff and bureaucracy, and advanced diagnostic and treatment technologies, most modern hospitals are extremely expensive to run and are becoming more so. In the USA, for example, hospitals are the biggest spenders of health care money, spending about $1000 per American in 1990; nearly a quarter of hospitals' money is spent on administrative costs[57]. In 1960, in the USA, there was one administrator for every 3.17 patients, but by 1990 this had risen to one patient for every 1.43 administrators[57]. In the developing world particularly, these rising costs – and the fact that most of the huge, high-tech hospitals are sited in cities, far from the rural areas where most people live[58] – have led to a re-evaluation of the hospital's role. A modern trend has been the development of smaller district hospitals, serving a local community, often in partnership with a network of local primary health care providers (see Chapter 13); while fewer, large hospitals, with specialized skills and high technology, are reserved for more serious conditions. Despite this shift, in many countries most of the medical resources are still concentrated in large metropolitan hospitals, which are also the main sites for medical technology.

The rise of medical technology

Technology can be seen as an extension of the human senses, and of their motor and sensory functions. Just as McCluhan[59] described the media (radio, television) as 'extensions' of the central nervous system and its functions (listening, looking), so does much of medical technology also provide more efficient ways of looking and listening to the human body and to its inner processes.

In every age, and in every society, healers have always made use of some form of equipment – knives, splints, scalpels, probes, spatulas or more magical items used in rituals. However, modern Western medicine is unique in the increasingly important role, both practical and symbolic, played by technology in both its diagnosis and treatment. Despite the growing cost and complexity of these machines, this 'technological imperative' is increasing every year.

Medical technologies, as complex systems of design and function, are not just physical objects used for a particular purpose. They are also cultural products, telling us something about the social, economic and historical values that produced them at a particular time and in a particular place. They have a range of meanings for those who use them professionally, and for patients who come to depend upon them. In a

Western context, this technology expresses modern medicine's desire to master and control the body, its natural processes and its various diseases. However, in other parts of the world the same technology or equipment may have very different meanings for the people who use it, depending on the social and cultural context. In many non-industrialized societies, for example, even the simple syringe is seen by the 'injectionist' and his clients (see Chapter 4) as being, in some way, the very embodiment of modern Western medical science.

Tenner[60] has described how the growth of diagnostic equipment – from Laennec's humble stethoscope in 1816, to Roentgen's discovery of X-rays in 1895 and Herrick's invention of the electrocardiogram in 1918 – led to a greater ability to *localize* disease processes within the body. Sites of pathology could now be pinpointed with greater accuracy than ever before. Although of great benefit to both patients and clinicians, this process has also contributed to a narrowing of medical vision – to the reductionism, mind–body dualism and objectification of body so characteristic today of the disease perspective.

In other ways, too, medical technology has radically altered our sense of the human body. It has had major effects on our perceptions of the body in space, as well as in time. For example, one result of both diagnostic and life support technology is to blur the boundaries of the body; to dissolve the skin as the true border of the individual self[61]. X-rays, MRI scans, ultrasound scans, CAT scans and advanced fibre-optics have all made the body more 'transparent'. Its interior has become more visible, and in some sense exterior. One can now examine its inner structure without any need to cut through the barrier of skin. Furthermore, the increasing use of life support systems, dialysis machines, monitoring equipment and incubators – as well as the new reproduction technologies (see Chapter 6) – can also contribute towards a blurring of the boundary between self and non-self. Joined to the body, these machines can help create temporary or permanent *cyborgs* – becoming, in effect, external organs (lungs, heart, kidneys) of the body, and extending it beyond the borders of skin. Commonly this process is linked to the modern metaphor of the body as a machine; one kept healthy by spare-part surgery[61]. The effects of this machine-dependency, and particularly its violation of the normal body boundaries, has been movingly described by Kirmayer[62] in the case of a haemodialysis patient. Here the patient has to witness his own blood leaving his body, then travelling through plastic tubes into the depths of the machine. Somehow in this electronic being it is mysteriously 'transformed', before once again being returned into the privacy of the body. In a sense the body is turned inside-out; that which is normally inside is now put outside it. A private, hidden physiological process – the circulation of the blood – is now on full public view. The boundaries between self and non-self are no longer as clear as they once were.

In obstetrics, Davis-Floyd[63] has also noted the negative effects of this process (see Chapter 6). She argues that obstetric hospitals in the USA have become like high-tech factories, dedicated to the mass production of perfect babies. In this environment, the overuse of technology conveys a message to the pregnant woman that her own body is merely a defective machine – one that needs to be controlled and directed by (medical) technicians, but not by herself. This in turn can have major emotional consequences for her. Despite this process, Browner[64] notes that many American women still remain ambivalent about the value of technology in their own pregnancies and childbirth.

In terms of time, some technologies can widen the gap between social and biological birth and death (see Chapter 9). For example, the development of ultrasound scans for prenatal diagnosis can help create a social identity for the foetus, in the eyes of its parents and doctors, many months before its actual delivery. Social birth can thus precede biological birth, reversing the normal order of events, and this in turn has had an effect on the abortion debate. By contrast, in the care of the dying, life support systems can extend the gap between biological death (increasingly defined as brain death) and social death (the final death of personhood). In this comatose state, and until the life support system is switched off, the body can be maintained for months or even years. Konner[65] argues that in the case of the very elderly this can create an ethical dilemma – extending the *quantity* of life, but often only at the expense of the quality.

Modern medical technology has thus had major social and economic costs for those who utilize it. Furthermore, it is increasingly expensive to buy, operate, maintain and repair. It is labour intensive, and requires specially trained technicians, maintenance workers, repairers and supervisors, as well as a constant supply of electricity and a reliable source of spare parts. As these machines become more complex and advanced, the possibility of their malfunction also increases proportionately[60]. In hospital settings, these complex technologies make health professionals increasingly dependent on outsiders – the highly paid community of experts and engineers who service, maintain and repair them. When introduced into any clinical environment, the machines often require major adjustments in people's behaviour and how they relate to one another. For example, Barley[66] has described the introduction of CT scanners into two hospitals in Massachusetts, USA, and the problems this caused for radiologists, technicians, and patients. Technical breakdowns and malfunctions required numerous social, behavioural and psychological changes, including new rituals, superstitions, and explanatory models for breakdowns, in order to integrate them into daily hospital life.

In poorer, developing countries, the purchase of these expensive technologies can have major impacts on public health policy. They may force a shift of scarce resources away from longer-term preventive medicine and health promotion towards high-tech solutions to social and health problems; from a community-based approach and district hospital system (see Chapter 13) utilizing more 'appropriate' and smaller-scale technologies, towards a focus on acute care in an expensive metropolitan hospital. In countries that cannot afford to maintain or repair them, these technologies may thus be completely inappropriate – often creating dependence on the large overseas companies who produce and maintain them and supply their spare parts.

Diagnostic technology has also led to the creation of a new tier of 'patients'. These are the products of technology – such as strips of ECG (EKG) paper, X-ray plates or printouts of blood tests. Sometimes they are the focus of more medical attention than the patients themselves. For some health professionals these 'paper patients' are as interesting – or even *more* interesting – than the patients themselves. They are easier to interpret, control, quantify and monitor over time, and there is no danger of their being uncooperative. They are also free of such ambiguous, unpredictable aspects of illness as cultural or religious health beliefs. In many cases, though, the increasing overuse of medical technology has been forced on doctors, especially by the fear of being accused of medical malpractice.

A final and paradoxical effect of diagnostic technology is that, in some cases, it may make diagnosis, treatment and communication with patients, more difficult to achieve[67]. This has resulted from the shift, noted by Feinstein[68], in how doctors make a medical diagnosis. In the past, doctors diagnosed disease based on what the patient told them about their symptoms (the history) and what they found on physical examination (the examination), as well as on the results of certain tests they performed. To make a complete diagnosis, they often also added in information they had gathered about the patient's lifestyle, family and social background. In contemporary medicine, however, the process of diagnosis has increasingly shifted from this collection of subjective or clinical information (gathered by listening, looking, touching, feeling) towards the use of notionally objective or 'paraclinical' information (gathered by the machines of diagnostic technology). Abnormalities can now be detected by these machines at the cellular, biochemical or even molecular level, even when patients have no abnormal symptoms at all and no subjective sense of anything being wrong with them. This has led to a widening gap (and increased possibilities for conflict) between medical definitions of *disease* and patients' subjective definitions of *illness* – a process described further in Chapter 5. Furthermore, doctors trained mainly to detect paraclinical disease may be less competent to interpret the complex, changing, clinical presentations found in real patients, in real life[67]. This complexity is partly due to the fact that the *same* paraclinical disease as revealed by technology (such as AIDS, cancer, or hypertension) may manifest itself in a variety of *different* clinical forms (such as weakness, pain, swelling, headaches, loss of appetite). Also, different paraclinical diseases (such as hiatus hernia and coronary artery disease) may present with almost identical clinical pictures (such as retrosternal chest pain). For all these reasons, therefore, knowledge of how to interpret both clinical *and* paraclinical data is essential for successful diagnosis, though the over-emphasis on the latter may mitigate against this.

Thus medicine's many new technologies have had major impacts, both positive and negative, on how it is practised. They have influenced how doctors diagnose and treat ill health, and how they relate to their patients. They may also have contributed, in some ways, towards alienation between patients and health professionals. In 1983, an Editorial[69] in the *Journal of the American Medical Association* posed the question: 'Has the machine become the physician?' It was suggested – as many others have since agreed – that this was, in fact, slowly happening (especially in the USA), and that it was having a major emotional effect on patients. The message the patient was now receiving was that of an 'impersonal, technology-dominated (medical) system'. Furthermore:

> The fact that the health care provided in the system may be improved as a result of the technology does not have as much impact as the subtle and hidden message that the machine has become the physician: the definitive adviser. The specialist-physician is metamorphosing into a technocrat and a businessman. The physician retreats behind the machine and becomes an extension of the machine.[69]

Despite any such disadvantages, however, what Koenig[70] terms the 'technological imperative' of modern medicine still remains, especially in Western societies. In some ways it may also have contributed to the crisis of contemporary medicine.

The 'crisis' in Western medicine

Although it is the dominant ideology of healing world-wide, many believe that biomedicine is in crisis – at least in the Western world[56,60,71]. This is despite its many successes in preventing and treating disease, alleviating suffering, and increasing life expectancy. In recent years a growing public dissatisfaction has been reflected in increasing complaints against doctors, and litigation, media campaigns against the medical profession, and the increased popularity of non-medical and alternative healers.

There are several reasons for this. Paradoxically, some are due to the very success of medicine itself. Over the last century, medicine has largely eradicated the major killer infectious diseases in most Western countries, such as smallpox, diphtheria, polio, tetanus, measles and many bacterial infections. Infant and maternal mortality has dropped, and life expectancy increased. As a result, more people are now living long enough to suffer from the *chronic* diseases – a situation that Tenner[60] terms 'revenge of the chronic'. These diseases include diabetes, hypertension, arthritis and Parkinson's disease, as well as other conditions that, like cancer, are diseases of later life. In most cases, a 'quick-fix' cure for these conditions is simply not possible. Instead, one needs a longer-term *care* model. This in turn requires a more cooperative approach to health care; one very different from the current rather authoritarian 'disease' perspective. In chronic diseases such as diabetes, patients have to become *co-healers*, monitoring their own condition and treating themselves on a daily basis, in collaboration with health professionals.[72] This increases the need for increased patient education,[73] and for a deeper understanding of the patient's needs, health beliefs and the realities of their daily lives.

At the same time, the costs of medical care are growing due to the escalating costs of hospitals, technology, drugs, medical bureaucracies, staff salaries, training, litigation and malpractice insurance. In most societies these rising costs exaggerate the effect of the already unequal distribution of health resources in the population, dividing them even further into those who can afford full medical care and those who cannot[71]. Also, the emphasis on more expensive, high-profile curative procedures – such as heart transplants – rather than on cheaper, more long-term health promotion campaigns to prevent heart disease in the first place, adds to the overall cost of the medical system.

Biomedicine's *iatrogenic* effects are now widely known to the public via the media. In addition to the thalidomide tragedy, many other drug side effects have recently been reported, as well as a growing dependence on prescribed psychotropic and other medications. In hospital settings, more complex operations and diagnostic procedures all now increase the risk of complications and unwanted side effects[60]. These include infections from antibiotic-resistant bacteria (which infect about 6 per cent of all hospitalized patients in the USA[60]), and many other adverse events. One detailed study[74,75] of over 30 000 hospital records in New York in the 1980s showed that adverse events occurred in 3.7 per cent of them. They were mainly due to drug complications (19 per cent), wound infections (14 per cent) and technical complications (13 per cent). Of these adverse events, 70.5 per cent gave rise to disability lasting less than 6 months, 2.6 per cent to permanent disability and 13.6 per cent to death. The study estimated that, among the 2 671 863 patients discharged from New York hospitals in 1984 during the study period, there were 98 609 adverse effects, 27 179 of them involving negligence.

In terms of treatment, a growing range of infectious diseases cannot be cured by medicine and its 'magic bullets'. These include *viral* diseases, such as HIV/AIDS, hepatitis B and C, Creutzfeld-Jacob disease (CJD) and some forms of influenza; *parasitic* diseases such as new strains of drug-resistant malaria; and *bacterial* diseases such as multidrug-resistant tuberculosis, resulting from the overuse of antibiotics in the past[60], and other drug-resistant bacteria. The rapid diffusion of infective agents or their vectors through jet travel and mass tourism has also made this situation much worst.

At the present time, control of diseases such as HIV/AIDS and malaria can only be successfully achieved by altering patterns of human behaviour (see Chapter 13), rather than by vaccines or antimicrobial drugs. This is especially relevant, since in most industrialized societies there is now an increasingly diverse patient population, especially in urban areas. This includes tourists, immigrants, foreign students, expatriate workers, immigrants and refugees, as well as the followers of different cults, religions and lifestyles. Each of these groups often has its own specific view of health and illness, and of how it should be treated. In socially and culturally mixed societies, therefore, a single inflexible model of health education and biomedicine may no longer be acceptable. For these reasons, medicine has to become more of an applied social science as well as an applied medical science.

Doctors in Western medical systems are undergoing major changes in their traditional roles and in what is expected of them. Like other health professionals, they are now expected to be competent in a wide variety of roles. These include those of manager, educator, computer specialist, bureaucrat, government (or medical insurance company) employee, technologist, writer, financial expert, businessman, judge, ethical expert, advocate for patients, family friend and confidant, as well as that of healer. Many feel that their clinical autonomy has been reduced by the growing pressures of government bureaucracies, insurance companies, hospitals, medical schools and health maintenance organizations[76]. The historical successes of medical science, together with the decline in organized religion, has also led to exaggerated expectations of doctors. Often they are expected to behave as secular 'priests', in their own 'temples of science'[56], even when they have no pastoral training to do so. A further issue for the medical profession is that of *information overload*. According to Haines[77], there are currently over 20 000 medical journals world-wide, and they publish a total of two million articles each year. (If stacked on top of another, the pile would be 500 m high.) He estimates that a general physician would have to digest 19 original articles *every day* in order to keep up to date in his subject.

All these factors add up to major changes in the contemporary medical system, how it is perceived, and the role it plays in any situation of health care pluralism. If the critics of biomedicine are correct, and the system *is* in crisis, then a very different paradigm for the practice of medicine will be required in the future.

Therapeutic networks

In any society, people who become ill and who are not helped by self-treatment make choices about who to consult in the popular, folk or professional sectors for further help. These choices are influenced by the context in which they are made, including the types of helper actually available, whether payment for their services has to be made, whether the patient can afford to pay for these services, and the Explanatory Model that the sick person uses to explain the origin of the ill health. This Model, which is described fully in Chapter 5, provides explanations for the aetiology, symptoms, physiological changes, natural history and treatment of the illness. On this basis, patients choose what seems to be the appropriate source of advice and treatment for the condition. Illnesses such as colds are treated by relatives, supernatural illnesses (such as 'spirit possession') by sacred folk healers, and natural illnesses by physicians – especially if they are very severe. If, for example, the ill health is ascribed to divine punishment for a moral transgression, then, as Snow[10] points out, 'Prayer and repentance, not penicillin, cure sin' – though both may be used simultaneously: a doctor is used for physical symptoms, a priest or faith healer for the cause.

In this way, ill people frequently utilize several *different* types of healer and healing at the same time, or in sequence. This may be done on the pragmatic basis that 'two (or more) heads are better than one'. For example, Scott[78] describes the case of an African-American woman from South Carolina, living in Miami, Florida. Believing that she had been 'fixed' (bewitched), she treated herself with olive oil and drops of turpentine on sugar cubes. When this failed to relieve her symptoms (abdominal pain), she consulted: two 'root doctors', who gave her magical powders, and candles to burn, and prayed over her; a 'sanctified woman', who massaged her and prayed for her; and two local hospitals, for X-rays and gastrointestinal tests to 'find out what is down there'. At one stage she was following the advice of all three folk healers simultaneously. As Scott points out, her contacts with doctors were not for curative purposes, but rather 'to check the effectiveness of the folk therapy' at each stage. Each of these healers may redefine the patient's problem in their own idiom, such as 'peptic ulcer' or 'witchcraft'. This simultaneous use of multiple forms of therapy is very common in most complex societies, especially in the presence of serious illness. Many people diagnosed as having cancer, for example, tend to change their behaviour and their diets, increase their intake of vitamins, pray more, join a self-help group, and consult with alternative or traditional healers[79] *in addition* to their biomedical treatment.

Ill people are at the centres of therapeutic *networks,* which are connected to all three sectors of the health care system. Advice and treatment pass along the links in this network – beginning with advice from family, friends, neighbours and friends of friends, and then moving on to sacred or secular folk healers, or physicians. Even after advice is given it may be discussed and evaluated by other parts of the patient's network, in the light of their own knowledge or experience. As Stimson[80] has noted, a doctor's treatment is often evaluated 'in the light of his past performance, with what other people have experienced, and compared with what the person expected the doctor to do'. In this way ill people make choices, not only between different types of healer (popular, professional or folk), but also between diagnoses and advice that *make sense* to them and those that do not. In the latter case the result may be non-compliance, or a shift to another part of the therapeutic network.

Health care pluralism in the UK

In the UK, as in other complex industrial societies, there is a wide range of therapeutic options available for the alleviation and prevention of physical discomfort or emotional distress, and popular, folk and professional sectors of health care can be identified. This section will concentrate mainly on the popular and folk sectors. The professional sector has already been examined in detail by medical sociologists such as Stacey[81] and Levitt[82]. An overview of the three sectors of health care in the UK illustrates the full range of options available for the management of misfortune, including ill health.

The popular sector

The two studies by Elliott-Binns[83,84] that are quoted below are among the few dealing with lay therapeutic networks in the UK. Other studies have concentrated on the phenomenon of self-medication. For example, in Dunnell and Cartwright's[85] large study in 1972, the use of self-prescribed medication was twice as common as the use of prescribed medicines. Self-medication was most commonly taken for temperature, headache, indigestion and sore throats. These and other symptoms were common in the sample, but while 91 per cent of adults reported one or more abnormal symptoms during the previous 2 weeks, only 16 per cent of them had consulted a doctor for this. Self-medication was often used as an alternative to consulting the doctor, who was expected to deal with more serious conditions. The idea of using a particular self-prescribed patent medicine came from a number of sources, including: spouses (7 per cent), parents and grandparents (18 per cent), other relatives (5 per cent), friends (13 per cent) and the doctor (10 per cent). Fifty-seven per cent of the sample thought the local pharmacist a good source of health advice for many conditions. This is confirmed in Sharpe's[86] study of a London pharmacy where, in a 10-day period, 72 requests for advice were received, especially for skin complaints, respiratory tract infections, dental problems, vomiting and diarrhoea. In another study by Jefferys and colleagues[87] in a working-class housing estate, two-thirds of people interviewed were taking some self-prescribed medication, often in addition to a prescribed drug. Laxatives and aspirins were most commonly prescribed. The aspirins, and other analgesics, were used for many symptoms, including 'arthritis and anaemia, bronchitis and backache, menstrual disorders and menopausal symptoms, nerves and neuritis, influenza and insomnia, colds and catarrh, and of course for headaches and rheumatism'.

The hoarding and exchanging of medication, both patent and prescribed, is common in the UK. People who have been ill sometimes act as what Hindmarch[88] terms 'over-the-fence physicians', sharing their prescribed drugs with a friend, relative or neighbour with similar symptoms. Warburton[89] found that 68 per cent of young adults in his study in Reading admitted having received psychotropic drugs from friends or relatives. In his study in Leeds, Hindmarch also found that an average of 25.9 prescribed tablets or capsules *per person* were hoarded by people living in a selected street. Decisions whether to take prescribed drugs are also part of popular health culture, and lay evaluation of the drug as 'making sense' or not may, as Stimson[80] suggests, influence non-compliance. The rate of this phenomenon has been estimated by him at 30 per cent or more.

Few studies have been done on the efficacy of popular health care in the UK. Blaxter and Paterson[90], in their study of working-class mothers in Aberdeen, found that common children's illnesses (such as a discharging ear) were often ignored if they did not interfere with everyday functioning. However, in another study by Pattison and colleagues[91] the findings were very different, and it was found that mothers were able to recognize their babies' illnesses and seek medical help, even with their first children.

An important component of the popular sector is the wide range of *self-help groups* that have blossomed in the UK since the Second World War. Like other parts of the popular sector, members' *experience*, not education, is important, especially experience of a specific misfortune. The total number of members of these groups is not known, though they number many thousands. The medical magazine *Pulse*[92] has listed 335 groups loosely labelled 'self-help' in the UK or Eire, and there are several other directories of groups available. These groups can be classified on the basis of why people join them, that is:

1. *Physical problems* (British Migraine Association, Laryngectomy Clubs, Back Pain Association, Body Positive)
2. *Emotional problems* (Depressives Associated, Phobics Society, National Schizophrenia Fellowship)
3. *Relatives* of those with physical, emotional or addiction problems (Association of Parents of Vaccine Damaged Children, Al-Anon, Adult Children of Alcoholics)
4. *Family problems* (Family Welfare Association, Parents Anonymous, Organization for Parents under Stress)
5. *Addiction problems* (Alcoholics Anonymous, Accept, Gamblers Anonymous)
6. *Social problems*, including:
   a. *Sexual non-conformity* (Lesbian Line, Gay Switchboards)
   b. *One-parent families* (Gingerbread, Families Need Fathers, National Council for the Single Woman and her Dependants)
   c. *Life changes* (Pre-retirement Association, National Association of Widows)
   d. *Social isolation* (Friends by Post, Solo Clubs, Meet-a-Mum Association)
7. *Women's groups* (Women's Health Concern, Rape Crisis Centres, Mothers' Union)
8. *Ethnic minority groups* (Caribbean House Group, Cypriot Advisory Service, Asian Women Community Workers' Group).

Most self-help groups have, as Levy[93] notes, one or more of the following aims or activities:

- information and referral
- counselling and advice
- public and professional education
- political and social activity
- fund-raising for research or services
- provision of therapeutic services, under professional guidance.
- mutual supportive activities in small groups.

Many groups are 'communities of suffering', where experience of a type of misfortune is the credential for membership. For example, the Depressives Associated describe themselves as 'a self-help organization run for the depressed by those who have been depressed and know better than most what it's like to have one's mind temporarily out of order'[64]. In Levy's[93] study of 71 groups, 41 had membership reserved for people suffering a particular affliction, while in eight membership was mainly composed of relatives of those afflicted. Some groups overlap with the professional sector, like the Psoriasis Society; its 4000 members include sufferers and their relatives, doctors, nurses, and cosmetic and pharmaceutical companies[94]. Others are hostile to orthodox medicine, and have an anti-bureaucratic and anti-professional stance.

Robinson and Henry[95] give a number of reasons for the growth of these groups in the popular sector, including the perceived failure of the existing medical and social services to meet people's needs, the recognition by members of the value of mutual help, and the role of the media in publicizing the extent of shared problems in the community. Other reasons might be the nostalgia for community (especially the caring community of the extended family) in an impersonal, industrialized world, as a coping mechanism for those with stigmatized conditions or marginal social status, and as a way of explaining and dealing with misfortune in a more personalized way.

The folk sector

In the UK, as in other Western societies, this sector is relatively small and ill defined. While local faith healers, gypsy fortune tellers, clairvoyants, psychic consultants, herbalists and 'wise women' still exist in many rural areas, the forms of diagnosis and healing characteristic of the folk sector are more likely to be found in urban areas, especially in alternative or complementary medicine. All estimates of the total number of consultations per year with alternative practitioners agree that the number is steadily rising[96]. One study, in 1985, estimated these consultations at 11.7–15.4 million consultations per year, and that about 1.5 million people (2.5 per cent of the total UK population) received some form of unconventional therapy during the course of a year, compared with the 72 per cent of the population that consult their GP during a year[97]. Of the people consulting with alternative practitioners, 33 per cent were at the same time receiving treatment from their medical practitioners[97]. As in non-Western societies, many alternative/complementary practitioners aim at a holistic view of the patient, which includes psychological, social, moral and physical dimensions, as well as an emphasis on health as balance. For example, a pamphlet from the National Institute of Medical Herbalists[98] states: 'The herbal practitioner regards disease as being a disturbance of the physiological and mental/emotional equilibrium which is the state of good health and, being aware of the forces of healing within the body, directs the treatment towards restoring that balance'. And similarly, from the Community Health Foundation[99]: 'Health is more than just the absence of pain or discomfort. Good health is a dynamic relationship between the individual, friends, family and the environment within which we live and work'.

Herbalism, faith healing and midwifery probably have the deepest roots in Britain. The first description of herbal remedies dates from 1260 AD, and numerous other 'herbals' have been published in the past 400 years. In 1636, for example, a herbal compiled by John Parkinson contained details of the medicinal use of 3800 plants[100]. Midwifery, another traditional form of health care, has been absorbed into the professional sector, especially since their compulsory registration under the 1902 Midwives' Act. Other forms of healing have been imported from abroad, such as acupuncture, homeopathy and osteopathy.

The folk sector includes both sacred and secular healers. An example of the former is the National Federation of Spiritual Healers (NFSH), who define spiritual healing as 'all forms of healing the sick in body, mind and spirit by means of the laying-on of hands or by either prayer or meditation whether or not in the actual presence of the patient'[101]. Since 1965, under an agreement with more than 1500 National Health Service hospitals, NFSH healer members may attend those patients in hospital who request their services. In addition, there are a number of Spiritualist Churches and healing circles in Britain that practise spiritual healing through prayer or the laying-on of hands; these include Christian Science Churches and some Caribbean Pentecostalist Churches. Christian healing is encouraged by the Christian Fellowship of Healing, the Churches' Council of Health and Healing, and the Guild of St Raphael[102]. An unknown number of *Wicca* or white magic groups or covens practise magical healing; writing in *Doctor* magazine, de Jonge[103] has claimed that there are 7000 'covens' in Britain, with a total membership of 91 000.

As a form of alternative healing, *homeopathy* has a special position in the UK. The principles of homeopathy were first enunciated in Germany by Samuel Hahnemann in 1796, and the first homeopathic hospital in Britain was founded in London in 1849. There has been a long association between the British Royal Family and homeopathy; in 1937 Sir John Weir was appointed homeopathic physician to King George VI, and this link with Royalty remains. In 1948 the homeopathic hospitals were incorporated into the National Health Service. There are now NHS homeopathic hospitals in London, Liverpool, Bristol and Tunbridge Wells, and there are two in Glasgow. It was estimated that in 1971 there were about 383 available beds in homeopathic hospitals, and 51 037 attendances at homeopathic medical outpatients clinics[104]. These hospitals are staffed by doctors qualified in orthodox medicine, who undertake postgraduate training in homeopathy. In addition, in 1996 there were two professional associations for non-medically qualified homeopaths and 21 training schools[105]. Although it is based on different premises from orthodox medicine, homeopathy in the UK enjoys greater legitimacy than other forms of alternative healing. Like other forms of alternative/complementary medicine, it spans both folk and professional sectors of health care.

There is a two-way influence between these two sectors. Many orthodox doctors, for example, practise one or more forms of alternative healing. They are organized into collegial organizations such as the British Homeopathic Association, The British Society of Medical and Dental Hypnosis, the Chiropractic Medical Association, the Osteopathic Medical Association, the Psionic Medical Society, and the British Association for the Medical Application of Transcendental Meditation. Similarly, alternative healers have been influenced, to a variable degree, by the training, organization, techniques, credentials and self-presentation of orthodox doctors, and are increasingly becoming 'professionalized' – forming professional organizations with an educational structure, and registers of accredited members. Some are organized on a collegial basis, like other British professions – for example, the British Acupuncture Association, the National Institute of Medical Herbalists, the Society of Homeopaths, and the General Council and Register of Osteopaths. In 1979, the British Acupuncture Association offered a 2-year training for a Licentiate, and a further year's study for a Bachelor's degree in acupuncture. It had 100 students in the UK, with 33 medically qualified and 420 non-medically qualified members on its register[106]. Over the last decade, pressure for professionalization has come not only from the healers themselves but also from the British Government, the European Union, the medical profession and the consumers themselves[105,107].

At the other end of the spectrum are the more individual forms of folk healing, including clairvoyants, astrologers, psychic healers, clairaudientes, palmists, Celtic mediums, Tarot readers, Gypsy fortune tellers and Irish seers, whose advertisements appear in the popular press, magazines, handouts and such publications as *Prediction*, *Horoscope* and *Old Moore's Almanack*. Many of these act as lay counsellors or psychotherapists: 'Do you have a health worry that you cannot get help on? Have you a personal or family worry you need advice on? Then maybe I can help you with both. I was born the 7th Son of a 7th Son'[108]. The majority of this group utilize some form of *divination*, using coins, dice, tea leaves, crystal balls or Tarot cards to decipher supernatural and cosmic influences on the individual and reveal the causes of unhappiness, ill health or other misfortune. From the patient's perspective, this approach may have the advantage of placing responsibility for misfortune beyond the individual's control; fate, bad luck or birth sign, not the patient's behaviour, are the causes of misfortune. Some of these healers are also undergoing professionalization. For example, since it was founded in 1976, the British Astrological and Psychic Society has promoted a variety of esoteric, spiritual and New Age teachings, and its members offer a wide range of 'interpretive and divinatory arts'[109]. The forms of divination they offer include astrology, palmistry, numerology, aura readings, graphology, trance mediumship, I Ching, Tarot cards, clairvoyance, clairaudience, clairsentience and psychic art. It publishes a National Register of Consultants, has defined criteria for entry, has a Code of Ethics and Conduct, and offers courses and certificates in different forms of divination. Its booklet states that its 'consultants are competent in several disciplines and can move between them in order to fulfil a client's given needs'[109].

Many ethnic minorities and immigrants in Britain continue to consult their own traditional healers, at least under certain circumstances. These include Muslim *hakims* and Hindu *vaids* from the Indian subcontinent (one estimate is that there are about 300 of them in the UK[110]), practitioners of traditional Chinese medicine (including herbalism and acupuncture), African *marabouts* and *obeah men*, and West Indian spiritual healers.

One fairly new group of healers – in the broadest sense of the word – are those involved primarily in improving their client's physical appearance, and thereby their psychological state. Throughout the UK there has been a proliferation of 'beauty clinics', staffed by 'beauty therapists'. Both the setting and atmosphere of these clinics is quasi-medical, with consultations, white coats, rows of bottles, complex machines and impressive diplomas on the wall. They are all part of a much wider phenomenon; the gradual 'medicalization' of all aspects of the human body, including its appearance.

In recent years, as there has been growing criticism of conventional medicine in some quarters, so has there been a parallel increase in all forms of complementary and alternative medicine – and a burgeoning of organizations connected with it. For example, the Council for Complementary Medicine was founded 'to promote and maintain the highest standards of training, qualification and treatment in complementary and alternative medicine to facilitate the dissemination of information relating to it'[111]. The Research Council for Complementary Medicine, as well as fostering research in this area, aims to raise standards of training and to develop 'a policy for eventual integration of such methods with existing medical services'[112]. The Institute for Complementary Medicine now has 80 professional organizations affiliated to it, and is developing a register of trained practitioners[113]. The British Holistic Medical Association, one of the oldest of these organizations, has 1159 members, both medical and lay, about two-thirds of whom are practising health professionals (such as doctors, nurses, social workers and complementary practitioners). The BHMA sees the emergence of holistic medicine as representing 'an attempt to heal medical science itself by re-integrating psychological and spiritual dimensions into healthcare'[114].

No precise statistics exist about the total numbers of non-orthodox healers in the UK and the total number of consultations with them. One major study, privately commissioned by the Threshold Foundation[115], was done in the early 1980s. They estimated that in 1980–1981 there were 7800 full- and part-time professional alternative practitioners in Britain, and about 20 000 men and women who practised spiritual and religious healing. There were also 2075 doctors who practised one or more alternative therapies although, with the exception of homeopathy, their training was 'minimal'. The alternative healers (both medical and lay) included 758 acupuncturists, 540 chiropractors, 303 herbalists, 360 homeopaths, 630 hypnotherapists and 800 osteopaths. They also estimated that alternative practitioners spend, on average, eight times longer with their patients than do orthodox doctors. Many of these practitioners practise more than one form of therapy. In a study in 1984 of 411 practitioners, 51 per cent practised a second therapy and 25 per cent a third.

In 1989, The Institute for Complementary Medicine[116] estimated that there were about 15 000 alternative practitioners in the UK in professional practice. They defined a 'practitioner' as an individual who is 'in full time practice, who is a member of a professional organization with a code of ethics and practice and a disciplinary committee to enforce them, and who is covered by personal indemnity and a third party liability'. On this basis, their figures included 7000 spiritual healers, 1500 osteopaths, 1500 acupuncturists, 1000 massage practitioners, 500 hypnotherapists, 350 nutritionists, 350 chiropractors, 300 reflexologists and 250 aromatherapists.

Training schools and professional associations for non-medically qualified healers continue to proliferate. For example, by 1996 the (non-medically qualified) homeopaths had two professional associations and 21 training schools, while the reflexologists had 13 professional organizations and over 100 schools[105].

In 1993 The British Medical Association published a detailed report into alternative medicine in the UK[117], and their conclusions were cautiously positive: 'It is clear that there are many encouraging initiatives currently taking place in the field of non-conventional therapy, and it is to be hoped that good practice can be extrapolated for general use'. However, they recommended that, before making use of it, potential clients should inquire:

1. Whether the therapist is registered with a professional organization
2. Whether that body has a public register of members, a code of practice, effective disciplinary procedures and sanctions and a complaints mechanism
3. The type of qualifications the therapist has, and where they were obtained
4. How long he or she has been practising
5. Whether the therapist is covered by any form of malpractice insurance.

Also in 1993, by virtue of the Osteopaths Act, osteopathy joined the ranks of the recognized health care and paramedical professions for the first time – just as the pharmacists had done in 1852 and 1868, the dentists in 1878, and the midwives in 1902.

However, not all alternative healers want to become 'professions', under the direct or indirect control of the government or the medical system. Many are ideologically opposed to all aspects of the medical model and what they see as its limitations and dangers; thus they see themselves as truly *alternative*, rather than complementary, to it. Nevertheless, many forms of alternative medicine in the UK besides osteopathy – especially chiropractic, homeopathy, herbalism and acupuncture – are gradually undergoing the same process of professionalization as is happening to traditional folk healers in parts of the developing world[105,107].

The professional sector

This includes the wide range of medical and paramedical professionals, each with their own perceptions of ill health, forms of treatment, defined areas of competence, internal hierarchy, technical jargon and professional organizations. The Office of Health Economics[118] estimated the numbers of all health professionals within the NHS in 1980 as 23 674 general practitioners, 31 421 hospital medical staff, 301 081 hospital nursing staff, 17 375 hospital midwives, 32 990 community health nurses and 2949 community health midwives. In 1981 the community nurses included 9244 health visitors[119]. By 1990 the total number of nurses and midwives had risen to 505 250, over 50 per cent of the total staff employed by the NHS[120]. In addition there are a large number of chiropodists, physiotherapists, occupational therapists, pharmacists and hospital technicians. Each of these categories offers some form of defined professional care, but they may also be called upon for informal advice about illness as part of the popular sector.

Despite its large size, it has been estimated[121] that about 75 per cent of abnormal symptoms are treated *outside* the professional sector – which sees only the tip of the 'iceberg of illness' – and the rest are dealt with in the popular and folk sectors of health care.

In the UK, there are two complementary forms of professional medical care, the National Health Service and private medical care, though there is an overlap of personnel between the two.

The National Health Service

Since 1948 the National Health Service (NHS) has offered free and unrestricted access to health care in the UK, at both the general practitioner and hospital levels. These two forms of medical care have different genealogies and different perspectives on ill health. The precursors of the general practitioners were specialized tradesmen called apothecaries. From 1617 they were licensed only to sell drugs prescribed by physicians. By 1703 they were entitled to see patients and prescribe for them. They became the GPs of the poor and middle classes. Physicians had a higher status initially than surgeons or apothecaries, and for centuries were the only 'real' doctors. Both physicians and surgeons enhanced their position during the growth of the hospital sector, which began in about 1700. To some extent the split and difference in status between GP and hospital medicine still persists, and is reflected in the allocation of resources. In England and Wales in 1972, for example, more than half the NHS budget was spent on the hospital sector, even though only 2.3 per cent of patients were actually cared for as hospital inpatients[122]. The NHS remains one of the largest employers in the country, with about 1 million employees; of these, in 1990, 57 900 were medical or dental staff and 505 250 were nurses or midwives[120].

The hospital sector

Many of the organizational and cultural aspects of hospitals have already been described, especially that of specialization. In 1974, according to Levitt[123] there were 42 recognized clinical specialties within the NHS hospital service. There are also numerous specialty hospitals, such as eye, ENT, heart or maternity hospitals. The hospital is the place where 99 per cent of people in the UK are born[124] and most will die. Between those two points, many people associate it with the more severe forms of ill health that cannot be dealt with by GPs or by the popular or folk sectors. As in other Western societies, the emphasis is on the individual patient as a case or problem to be solved in as short a time as possible and with maximum efficiency. To a large extent, the social, familial, religious and economic aspects of the patient's life are invisible to the hospital staff, though attempts are made to gather this information via social workers. The emphasis is mainly on the identification and treatment of physical disease, though this is less true of psychiatric hospitals. Looked at in perspective, the hospital service deals mostly with acute, severe or sometimes life-threatening episodes of ill health, as well as birth or death. It is less orientated towards dealing with the subjective meanings associated with illness, which are usually dealt with in the popular or folk sectors, or by ministers of religion.

The general practitioner service

Unlike the USA, this area of health care is largely separated from hospital medicine. For example, of the 482 782 hospital beds allocated in England, Scotland and Wales in 1976, only 13 665 (2.8 per cent) were 'general practitioner beds', and 5406 of these were obstetric beds[125]. In 1978, in England and Wales, there were only 350 GP-run cottage hospitals, with an average of 20–40 beds each[126]. While GPs can visit the wards and discuss management of their patients with the hospital medical staff, most of the responsibility for medical care rests with the hospital.

In 1976 each GP had, according to Levitt[127], an average of 2347 patients on his or her list, although this number has now dropped to about 1700. In 1997 there were 38 886 GPs in the UK, a 12.5 per cent increase since 1984[128]. The proportion of female GPs has also increased from 17.4 per cent to 31.5 per cent, in England and Wales, in the period 1983–1997. In the whole UK, 32 per cent of all GPs are now women[128].

General practice medicine is home- and community-based, and social, psychological, and familial factors are considered relevant in making a diagnosis. As Harris[129] puts it, 'all diagnoses have a social component, whether or not there are social problems', and 'in general practice it is easy to appreciate how a patient's illness and social circumstances are related, because the social circumstances are visible'. Similarly, Hunt[130] believes that GPs should 'put care of the patient's mind before that of his body', and 'the family doctor's awareness of what patients think and feel is vitally important for the whole of his or her work'. Unlike most hospital doctors, the British GP is often a familiar figure in the community. Most live locally, take part in local community activities, dress in civilian clothes and use everyday language in their consultations. As well as caring for ill people, they are associated with many of the natural milestones of life; they do antenatal and postnatal examinations, perform check-ups on infants, give immunizations and contraceptive advice, carry out cervical smears, deal with marital and school problems, and counsel bereaved families. Unlike hospital doctors (and most folk healers) they do home visits, and also deal with more than one generation of a family. And, in distinction from the hospital sector, the illnesses they do deal with tend to be relatively minor; in one study of the morbidity of 2500 patients in an NHS family practice in one year,

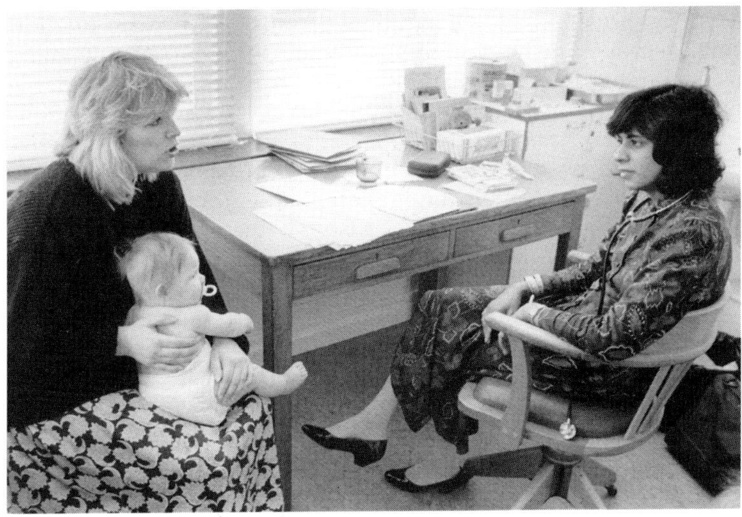

Figure 4.3 Consultation between a general practitioner and her patients in Greenwich, south London, England (Source: Philip Wolmuth/Panos Pictures).

1365 had minor illnesses, 588 chronic illness, and only 288 major illness[131].

According to Levitt, the GP is the first point of contact for about 90 per cent[131] of those who do seek professional medical help under the NHS, though consultations only last about 5–6 minutes on average[132].

Increasingly, NHS GPs now work as part of 'primary health care teams'[133]; these usually include receptionists, practice nurses and counsellors employed directly by the GP, as well as health visitors, district nurses, community psychiatric nurses, community midwives and social workers employed by the NHS. GPs, in association with their primary health care team, share some of the attributes of the folk sector, particularly the emphasis on 'illness' (see Chapter 5) – that is, the social, psychological and moral dimensions of ill health – and on the normal milestones of human life.

The nursing service

Nurses and midwives form the largest professional group within the NHS. As noted above, in 1990 they comprised over 50 per cent of its total personnel[120]. The majority of the nursing service is female, while the majority of doctors are male. However, about 10 per cent of the nursing staff in NHS hospitals are now male (the percentage is even higher in psychiatric hospitals), but very few male nurses work in the community[134]. Most of the nurses work in the hospital sector, the remainder in the community. Within the hospitals, nurses spend many more hours in direct patient care than any of the medical hierarchy, and yet have a lower income and prestige than doctors. Like the medical staff, the nurses are organized into their own professional hierarchies. In many British hospitals, this hierarchy ranges from Director of Nursing down through the various grades of Senior Nurse Manager, Clinical Nurse Specialist, Ward Sister/Ward Manager, Staff Nurse, Enrolled Nurse and Nursing Auxiliary/Health Care Assistant. Many hospital nurses specialize in different areas of care, such as ophthalmics, orthopaedics, accident and emergency, coronary or intensive care, and have extra qualifications in addition to their basic training. Various specialist nurses – Clinical Nurse Specialists – have a liaison role between the hospital and the community; for example, those working in palliative care, or with diabetic or stoma patients, or as incontinence advisers. Within the community some nurses, also with extra qualifications, work as District Nurses, others as Community Midwives, Health Visitors, School Nurses, Practice Nurses (working within a GP practice), or as hospital-based Community Psychiatric Nurses. Unlike in the USA, the emerging and important role of Nurse Practitioners is not yet formally recognized in terms of a specific qualification. Despite this they now work in a variety of contexts, in some cases carrying out tasks previously dealt with by doctors.

Some of the features of the nursing profession are described further in Chapter 6.

Private medical care

This form of health care preceded the NHS, and now co-exists with it. Encouraged by the government, it is rapidly growing, due partly to cutbacks in the NHS that have reduced the number of hospital beds and increased waiting lists for operations and outpatient appointments (by 1990 there were 710 300 people, or 1 per cent of the UK population, on waiting lists for inpatient admissions to NHS hospitals[135]). However, private medical care still provides the minority of health care. In 1983 it was estimated that only 7 per cent of the population were insured for private medical care, only 6 per cent of all hospital beds were in private hospitals, and only 2 per cent of hospital beds for acute cases were in private hospitals[8]. By 1991, though, the total number of people covered by private medical insurance had risen to 6 524 000, almost 12 per cent of the total UK population. In England in 1987, 27 per cent of those in professional occupational groups had private medical insurance, but only 1 per cent of unskilled manual labourers[136]. There is a considerable overlap in personnel between private and public medical care, though some doctors practise private medicine only. There are several private hospitals and clinics, and a number of large health funds. Also, with the exception of homeopathy and, occasionally, acupuncture, all forms of alternative or folk healing are in the private sector. From some patients' perspective, private medicine offers more control over time and choice of treatment when they are ill. Consultation times are longer in the private sector, and this provides more time for explanations of the diagnosis, aetiology, prognosis and treatment of their condition. There are also

Table 4.2 Professional, folk and popular healers in the UK

Hospital doctors (NHS)
General practitioners (NHS)
Private doctors (hospital or GP)
Nurses (hospital, school and community)
Midwives
Health visitors
Social workers
Physiotherapists
Occupational therapists
Pharmacists
Dieticians
Opticians
Dentists
Hospital technicians
Nursing auxiliaries
Medical receptionists
Local authority health clinics
Clinical psychologists and psychoanalysts
Counsellors (marriage, child guidance, pregnancy, contraception)
Alternative psychotherapists (Gestalt, bioenergetics, primal therapy etc.)
Group therapists
Samaritans and other 'phone-in' counsellors
Self-help groups
Yoga and meditation groups
Health food shops salespeople
Media healers (advice columnists in newspapers and magazines, TV and radio doctors)
Ethnic minority healers
- Muslim *hakims*
- Hindu *vaids*
- Chinese acupuncturists and herbalists
- West Indian healing churches
- African *marabouts*

Healing churches and cults
Christian healing guilds
Church counselling services
Hospital and other chaplains
Probation officers
Citizens' Advice Bureaux
Alternative healers (lay and medical)
- Acupuncture
- Homeopathy
- Osteopathy
- Chiropractic
- Radionics
- Herbalism
- Spiritual healing
- Hypnotherapy
- Naturopathy
- Massage etc. Diviners
- Astrologers
- Tarot readers
- Clairvoyants
- Clairaudientes
- Mediums
- Psychic consultants
- Palmists
- Fortune tellers etc.
- Lay health advisers (family, friends, neighbours, acquaintances, voluntary or charitable workers, salespeople, hairdressers, etc.)

shorter waiting lists for consultations with specialists or for surgical operations, and the patient has a choice of specialist and of hospital. Control over time and choice when ill is largely confined to those with a sufficient income to afford private health insurance, or those who work for large organizations that provide their employees with such insurance.

The NHS and private sectors are not watertight; as with other areas of the health care system there is a considerable flow of ill people between them, and many doctors work within both systems.

The health care system in the UK

To view the UK health care system in perspective, most of the available sources of health care or advice are listed in Table 4.2.

'Healer' here refers to all those who, either formally or informally, offer advice and care for those suffering from physical discomfort and/or psychological distress, or who advise on how to maintain health and a feeling of wellbeing. This list therefore spans all three sectors of health care in Britain – popular, folk and professional.

Case study: Sources of lay health advice in Northampton, UK

Elliott-Binns[83] studied 1000 patients attending a general practice in Northampton, UK. The patients were asked whether they had previously received any advice or treatment for their symptoms. The source, type and soundness of the advice were noted, as well as whether the patient had accepted it. It was found that 96 per cent of the patients had received some advice or treatment before consulting their GP. Each patient had had an average of 2.3 sources of advice, or 1.8 excluding self-treatment; that is, 2285 sources of which 1764 were outside sources and 521 self-advice. Thirty-five patients received advice from five or more sources; one boy with acne received it from 11 sources. The outside sources of advice for the sample were: friend, 499; spouse, 466; relative, 387; magazines or books, 162; pharmacists, 108; nurses giving informal advice, 102; nurses giving professional advice, 52. Among relatives and friends, wives' advice was evaluated as being among the best and that from mothers and mothers-in-law the worst. Male relatives

continued

usually said 'go to the doctor', without offering practical advice, and rarely gave advice to other men. Advice from impersonal sources, such as women's magazines, home doctor books, newspapers and television was evaluated as the least sound. Pharmacists, consulted by 11 per cent of the sample, gave the soundest advice. Home remedies accounted for 15 per cent of all advice, especially from friends, relatives and parents.

Overall, the best advice given was for respiratory complaints, the worst for psychiatric illness. One example of the patient sample was a village shopkeeper with a persistent cough. She received advice from her husband, an ex-hospital matron, a doctor's receptionist and five customers, three of whom recommended a patent remedy 'Golden Syrup', one a boiled onion gruel, and one the application of a hot brick to the chest. One middle-aged widower had come to see the doctor complaining of backache. He had consulted no one because he 'had no friends and anyway if I got some ointment there's no one to rub it in'.

Elliott-Binns[84] repeated this study 15 years later, on 500 patients in the same practice in Northampton. Surprisingly, the pattern of self-care and lay health advice had remained largely unchanged; 55.4 per cent of patients treated themselves before going to the doctor, compared to 52.0 per cent in 1970. The only significant changes were an increase in impersonal sources of advice on health, such as home doctor books and television, and a decline in the use of traditional home remedies (although they still accounted for 11.2 per cent of health advice). In addition, the use of advice from pharmacists increased from 10.8 per cent in 1970 to 16.4 per cent in 1985. Overall the study suggests that, in Britain, self-care still remains the chief source of health care for the average patient.

Recommended reading

Sectors of health care

Kleinman, A. (1980). *Patients and Healers in the Context of Culture*, Chapters 2 and 3. University of California Press.

Folk and popular sectors

Eisenberg, D. *et al.* (1993). Unconventional medicine in the United States. *N. Engl. J. Med.*, **328**, 246–52.

Finkler, K. (1994). Sacred healing and biomedicine compared. *Med. Anthrop. Q.* (new series), **8**, 178–97.

Fulder, S. (1988). *Handbook of Complementary Medicine.* Oxford University Press

Janzen, J. M. (1978). *The Quest for Therapy: Medical Pluralism in Lower Zaire.* University of California Press.

McGuire, M. B. (1988). *Ritual Healing in Suburban America.* Rutgers University Press.

O'Connor, B. B. (1995). *Healing Traditions.* University of Pennsylvania Press.

5 Doctor–patient interactions

Doctors and their patients, even if they come from the same social and cultural background, view ill health in very different ways. Their perspectives are based on very different premises, employ a different system of proof, and assess the efficacy of treatment in a different way. Each has its strengths, as well as its weaknesses. The problem is how to ensure some *communication* between them in the clinical encounter between doctor and patient. In order to illustrate this problem, the differences between medical and lay views of ill health – between, that is, 'disease' and 'illness' – will be described in some detail.

'Disease' – the doctor's perspective

As described in the previous chapter, those who practise modern scientific medicine form a group apart, with their own values, theories of disease, rules of behaviour and organization into a hierarchy of specialized roles. The medical profession can be seen as a healing 'sub-culture', with its own particular world view. In the process of medical education, students undergo a form of *enculturation* whereby they gradually acquire a perspective on ill health that will last throughout their professional life. They also acquire a high social status, high earning power and the socially legitimated role of healer, which carries with it certain rights and obligations. Some of the basic premises of this medical perspective are:

1. Scientific rationality
2. The emphasis on objective, numerical measurement
3. The emphasis on physicochemical data
4. Mind–body dualism
5. The view of diseases as entities
6. Reductionism
7. The emphasis on the individual patient, rather than on the family or community.

Medicine, like Western science generally, is based on scientific rationality; that is, all assumptions and hypotheses must be capable of being tested and verified under objective, empirical and controlled conditions. Phenomena relating to health and sickness only become 'real' when they can be *objectively* observed and measured under these conditions. Once they have been observed, and often quantified, they become clinical 'facts', the cause and effect of which must then be discovered. All 'facts' have a cause, and the task of a clinician is to discover the logical chain of causal influences that led up to this particular fact. For example, iron-deficiency anaemia may result from loss of blood, which may be the result of a bleeding stomach tumour, which may have been caused by certain carcinogens in the diet. Where a specific causal influence cannot be isolated, the clinical fact is labelled 'idiopathic' – that is, it *has* got a cause, but that cause has yet to be discovered. Where a phenomenon cannot be objectively observed or measured, for example a person's beliefs about what caused an illness, it is somehow less 'real' than, say, the level of the patient's blood pressure or white cell count. Because blood pressure and white cell count can be measured and agreed upon by several observers, they form the sorts of clinical 'facts' upon which diagnosis and treatment will be based.

These 'facts', therefore, arise from a *consensus* among the observers, whose measurements are carried out in accordance with certain agreed guidelines. The assumptions underlying these guidelines – that determine which phenomena are to be looked for, and how they are to be verified and measured – is termed a conceptual *model*. As Eisenberg[1] points out, models 'are ways of constructing reality, of imposing meaning on the chaos of the phenomenal world' and 'once in place, models act to generate their own verification by excluding phenomena outside the frame of reference the user employs'. The model of modern medicine is mainly directed towards discovering and quantifying physicochemical information about the patient, rather than less measurable social and emotional factors. As Kleinman and colleagues[2] put it, the modern Western doctor's view of clinical reality 'assumes that biologic concerns are more basic, "real", clinically significant, and interesting than psychological and sociocultural issues'.

This emphasis on physiological facts means that a doctor confronted with a patient's symptoms tries first of all to relate these to some underlying physical process. For example, if a patient complains of a certain type of chest pain, the doctor's approach is likely to involve a number of examinations or tests to try to identify the physical cause of the pain – perhaps coronary heart disease. If no physical cause can be found after exhaustive investigation the symptom might be labelled 'psychogenic' or 'psychosomatic', but this diagnosis is usually only made by excluding a physical cause. Subjective symptoms, therefore, become more 'real' when they can be explained by objective, physical changes. As the Goods[3] describe it:

> Symptoms achieve their *meaning* in relation to physiological states, which are interpreted as the referents of the symptoms. Somatic lesions or dysfunctions produce discomfort and behavioural changes, communicated in a patient's complaints. The critical task of the physician is to 'decode' a patient's discourse by relating symptoms to their biological referents in order to diagnose a disease entity.

These somatic or biological referents are discovered by the doctor's examination and sometimes by the use of specialized tests, often using diagnostic technology.

As described in the previous chapter, Feinstein[4] has pointed out the shift in recent years in how doctors collect information about underlying disease processes. The traditional method was by listening to the patient's symptoms and how they developed (the history), and then searching for objective physical signs (the examination). Increasingly, though, modern medicine has come to rely on diagnostic technology to collect and measure clinical facts. This implies a shift from the subjective (the patient's subjective symptoms, the physician's subjective interpretation of the physical signs) towards the notionally objective forms of diagnosis. The underlying pathological processes are now firmly identified by blood tests, X-rays, scans and other investigations, usually carried out in specialized laboratories or clinics (see Chapter 4). One result of this is the increasing use of *numerical* definitions of health and disease. Health or normality are defined by reference to certain physical and biochemical parameters, such as weight, height, circumference, blood count, haemoglobin level, levels of electrolytes or hormones, blood pressure, heart rate, respiratory rate, heart size or visual acuity. For each measurement there is a numerical range – the 'normal value' – within which the individual is considered normal and 'healthy'. Above or below this range is 'abnormal', and indicates the presence of 'disease'. Disease, then, is seen as a deviation from these normal values, accompanied by abnormalities in the structure or function of body organs or systems. For example, lower than the normal value of thyroid hormone in the blood is *hypo*thyroidism, above it is *hyper*thyroidism; between the two the thyroid is functioning normally.

The medical definition of ill health, therefore, is largely based on objectively demonstrable physical changes in the body's structure or function, which can be quantified by reference to 'normal' physiological measurements. These abnormal changes, or *diseases*, are seen as 'entities', each with their own unique 'personality' of symptoms and signs. Each disease's personality is made up of a characteristic cause, clinical picture (symptoms and signs), results of hospital investigations, natural history, prognosis and appropriate treatment. For example, tuberculosis is known to be caused by a particular bacillus, to reveal itself by certain characteristic symptoms, to display certain physical signs on examination, to show up in a particular way on chest

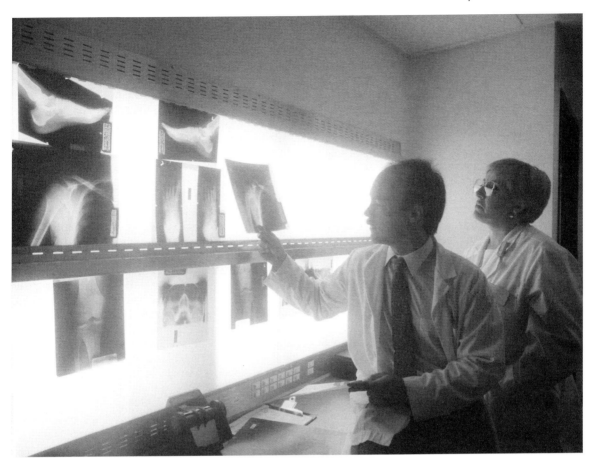

Figure 5.1 Advances in diagnostic technology have helped shift medicine towards an increased focus on *physical* abnormalities – rather than on the patient's symptoms, their psychological state, or their social and cultural background (Source: © Digital Stock MED 028).

radiographs and sputum tests, and to have a likely natural history, depending on whether it is treated or not. As Fabrega and Silver[5] point out, the medical perspective assumes that diseases are 'universal in form, progress, and content', and that they have a recurring identity; that is, it is assumed that tuberculosis will be the same disease in whatever culture or society it appears. It will always have the same cause, clinical picture, treatment and so on. However, this perspective does not include the social, cultural and psychological dimensions of ill health, and the context in which it appears, which determine the *meaning* of the disease for the individual patients and those around them. Because medicine focuses more on the physical dimensions of illness, factors such as the personality, religious belief, culture and socio-economic status of the patient are often considered largely irrelevant in making the diagnosis or prescribing treatment. Engel[6] sees this approach as further evidence of 'mind–body dualism', a medical way of thinking that focuses on identifying physical abnormalities while often ignoring 'the patient and his attributes as a person, a human being'. Reducing him, that is, to a set of abnormal physiological parameters. This conceptual dualism can be traced back at least to Descartes in the seventeenth century, who divided man into 'body' (to be studied only by science), and 'mind' or 'soul' (to be studied by philosophy and religion). In more recent times, 'mind' has been handed over to psychiatrists and behavioural scientists to study (rather than priests), while 'body' – seen increasingly as an animated machine – has been handed over to medical science and its diagnostic technology. Thus, in modern medicine the basic dualism still remains.

A further point is that modern medicine is often very *reductionist*. Increasingly its focus is less on the actual patient than on a particular diseased organ, system, group of cells or bodily part. This is partly due to advances in equipment and diagnostic technology, which can now reveal changes at the cellular, biochemical or even molecular levels and can exactly localize the site of pathology. As mentioned in the previous chapter, this has led to the development of a new group of 'patients': the products of diagnostic technology, such as X-ray plates, scans, print-outs of blood test results or the strips of paper from an electrocardiogram. The development of these 'paper patients' as a growing feature of clinical consultations, case conferences and hospital grand rounds is a further step towards medical reductionism. Furthermore, many doctors now diagnose and treat abnormalities of only a small part of the human body. Their professional aim is, in a sense, to know more and more about less and less (and often this results in knowing less and less about more and more). In modern medicine these hyper-specialists tend to have a higher status and a higher income than many generalists, such as general practitioners. In addition, those specialists who are publicly seen to 'cure' have a higher status than those who merely 'care'. Treating a small area of the body in a relatively short period of time and with a clearly defined outcome has a much higher status than dealing with those conditions where no short-term cure is evident or even possible. Thus surgeons generally have a higher status than doctors working in geriatrics, psychiatry, physical disability, terminal illness, chronic disease or preventive medicine.

The range of medical models

The medical model should not, therefore, be seen as homogeneous and consistent. In understanding doctor–patient interactions, one should always ask: '*which* doctor?', or perhaps 'which *type* of doctor?' There is really no such thing as a uniform 'Western' or 'scientific' medicine; as illustrated in Chapter 4. Although it is now international, there are enormous variations in how Western medicine is practised in different parts of the world. This applies in different Western countries, and even within those countries themselves. Furthermore, the medical model is always to a large extent culture-bound, and varies greatly, depending on the context in which it appears. Even within the same society, huge differences in perspective exist between different branches of medicine – between, say, the perspectives of surgeons[7], psychiatrists, epidemiologists, general practitioners and public health specialists. Furthermore, when a particular doctor trained in modern scientific medicine makes a diagnosis, he or she usually employs a number of *different* models or perspectives, each of which looks at the problem in a particular way. As the Goods[3] note, 'any physician or medical discipline has a repertoire of interpretative models – biochemical, immunological, viral, genetic, environmental, psychodynamic, family interactionist and so on', each with its own unique perspective on the disease. In some cases these perspectives, or models, might be very different from one another. In psychiatry, for example, Eisenberg[1] points out that 'multiple and manifestly contradictory models' are used by different psychiatrists in explaining the psychoses. These include:

1. The *organic* model, which emphasizes physical and biochemical changes in the brain
2. The *psychodynamic* model, which concentrates on developmental and experiential factors
3. The *behavioural* model, where psychosis is maintained by environmental contingencies
4. The *social* model, with its emphasis on disorders in role performance.

Whatever specialty they choose to work in, it should be noted that physicians themselves are also part of the 'folk' world for most of their lives – both before and after graduating from medical school. Both as individuals and as members of a particular family, community, religion, or social class, they bring with them a specific set of ideas, assumptions, experiences, prejudices and inherited folklore, and this can greatly influence their medical practice. When they impose (often unconsciously) their own cultural values, assumptions and expectations on their patients, that phenomenon – using psychoanalytic imagery – could be termed an example of *cultural counter-transference*.

All medical and psychiatric models tend to change over time as new concepts are developed and new discoveries are made. Disease entities such as hypertension, cancer or coronary heart disease are continuously being re-examined or re-worked as new theories of aetiology are advanced and new techniques of diagnosis and treatment are invented. The different models used by clinicians in different specialties also means that they might perceive and diagnose the *same* episode of ill health in very different ways, if an ill person consults with each of them over a period of time.

Medicine as a system of morality

A final issue is that, with the decline in organized religion in many Western societies, the moral concerns of the contemporary age are increasingly being expressed in medical rather than religious terms. Medicine has always been more than a system of scientific ideas and practices; it has also been a *symbolic* system, expressing some of the basic underlying values, beliefs and moral concerns of the wider society. In a more secularized age, religious ideas of sin or immorality often seem to be replaced by ideas of health and disease. Today, medical metaphors have become part of the daily discourse, for example a 'sick society', an 'epidemic of crime', an 'ailing economy'. Whereas a few generations ago religion spoke out against a 'sinful life', medicine now condemns the 'unhealthy lifestyle' – but the punishments occur in this world, rather than in the world to come. The ancient Deadly Sins of 'gluttony' and 'sloth' have been reconceptualized as 'over-eating' and 'lack of exercise'. Because so much moral discourse is now couched in medical terms, the definitions of certain behaviours – alcoholism, illegitimacy, truancy, drug abuse and criminality – have shifted from being bad or sinful to being in some way in the domain of medicine or psychiatry.

A related phenomenon in most industrialized societies is the growth of the *insurance* industry. While it penalizes those of its clients who have an unhealthy lifestyle (who smoke or drink, for example), it does compensate individuals for unexpected illness, accident or other misfortune – events that, in previous generations (and elsewhere in the world), were dealt with by the religious system. Arguably, in those societies where organized religion is weak, the insurance industry (like the medical system itself) provides some people with a rational, secularized way of responding to misfortune and of diminishing its effects. However, both approaches focus much less on moral responsibility than does religion; despite medicine's enhanced social role, its main focus is still on the *consequences* of illness, accident or misfortune, rather than on their cause.

Despite these changes in the social and symbolic role of medicine in modern society, and variations within the medical model itself, its predominant approach in clinical practice still remains the search for *physical* evidence of disease or dysfunction – as is the use of physical treatments (such as drugs, surgery, or radiation) in correcting these underlying abnormalities.

'Illness' – the patient's perspective

Cassell[8] uses the word 'illness' to represent 'what the patient feels when he goes to the doctor', and 'disease' for 'what he has on the way home from the doctor's office'. He concludes: 'Disease, then, is something an organ has; illness is something a man has'. *Illness* is the subjective response of an individual and of those around him to his being unwell; particularly how he and they interpret the origin and significance of this event; how it affects his behaviour and his relationship with other people; and the various steps he takes to remedy the situation. It not only includes his experience of ill health, but also the *meaning* he gives to that experience. For example, people who suddenly fall ill might ask themselves 'why has it happened to *me*?' or 'have I done anything wrong to deserve this?' or even, in some societies, 'has anyone *caused* me to be ill?'. Both the meaning given to the symptoms and their emotional response to them are influenced by their own background and personality, as well as the cultural, social and economic context in which the symptoms appear. In other words, the same 'disease' (such as tuberculosis) or symptom (such as pain) may be interpreted completely differently by two individuals from different cultures or social backgrounds and in different contexts. This will also affect their subsequent behaviour, and the sorts of treatment they will seek out.

The patient's perspective on ill health is usually part of a much wider conceptual model used to explain misfortune in general; within this model, illness is only a specialized form of adversity. For example, in many societies *all* forms of misfortune are ascribed to the same range of causes – a high fever, a crop failure, the theft of one's property or a roof collapsing might all be blamed on witchcraft or on divine punishment for some moral transgression. In the latter case, they may cause similar emotions of shame or guilt, and call for similar types of treatment, such as prayer or penitence. 'Illness' therefore often shares the psychological, moral and social dimensions associated with other forms of adversity, within a particular culture. It is a wider though more diffuse concept than 'disease', and should be taken into account in understanding how people interpret their ill health and how they respond to it.

Becoming ill

Definitions of what constitutes both 'health' and 'illness' vary between individuals, families, cultural groups and social classes. In most cases, *health* is seen as more than just an absence of unpleasant symptoms. The World Health Organization[9], for example, defined it in 1946 as 'a state of complete physical, mental and social well-being and not merely the absence of disease or infirmity'. In many non-industrialized societies health is conceived of as a balanced *relationship* between people, between people and nature, and between people and the supernatural world. A disturbance of any of these may manifest itself by physical or emotional symptoms. Among Western communities, definitions of health tend to be less all-embracing, but they also include physical, psychological and behavioural aspects. Moreover, they vary between social classes. For example, Fox[10] quotes a study of 'Regionville', a town in upper New York State where members of the highest socioeconomic class usually reported a persistent backache to their physician as an abnormal symptom, while members of the poorer socioeconomic class regarded it as 'an inevitable and innocuous part of life and thus as inappropriate for referral to a doctor'. Similarly, in Blaxter and Paterson's study[11] in Aberdeen, Scotland, working-class mothers did not define their children as ill, even if they had abnormal physical symptoms, provided they continued to walk around and play normally. This functional definition of health, common among poorer people, is probably based on the (economic) need to keep working, however they feel, as well as on low expectations of medical care. These lay definitions of health can obviously differ from those of the medical profession, as will be described.

On an individual level, the process of defining oneself as being 'ill' can be based on one's own perceptions, on the perceptions of others, or on both. Defining oneself as being ill usually follows a number of subjective experiences including:

- perceived changes in bodily appearance, such as loss of weight, changes in skin colour, or hair falling out
- changes in regular bodily functions, such as urinary frequency, heavy menstrual periods, irregular heart beats
- unusual bodily emissions, such as blood in the urine, sputum or stools
- changes in the functions of limbs, such as paralysis, clumsiness or tremor
- changes in the five major senses, such as deafness, blindness, lack of smell, numbness or loss of taste sensation
- unpleasant physical symptoms, such as pain, headache, abdominal discomfort, fever or shivering
- excessive or unusual emotional states, such as anxiety, depression, nightmares or exaggerated fears
- behavioural changes in relation to others, such as marital or work disharmony.

Most people experience some of these abnormal changes in their daily lives, though usually in a mild form, and this has been demonstrated in several studies. In Dunnell and Cartwright's study,[12] 91 per cent of a sample of adults had experienced one or more abnormal symptoms in the 2 weeks preceding the study (while only 16 per cent had consulted a doctor during this time). Having one or more abnormal changes of symptoms may therefore not be enough to label oneself as being 'ill'. For example, in Apple's study[13] of middle-class Americans, abnormal symptoms were only considered an illness if they interfered with the usual daily activities, were recent in onset and were ambiguous – that is, difficult for a layman to diagnose.

Other people can also define one as being ill, even in the absence of abnormal subjective experience, by statements such as 'You look pale today, you must be ill' or 'You've been acting very strangely recently'. In the absence of behavioural changes, cultures vary as to whether a particular form of behaviour is defined as illness or not. In Guttmacher and Elinson's[14] study, different social and ethnic groups in New York City were asked whether certain types of socially deviant behaviour (such as transvestism, homosexuality or getting into fights) were evidence of illness. The Puerto Rican group was found to be less likely to describe these as illness than other groups such as the Irish, Italians, Jews or Blacks. In most cases, though, a person is defined as being 'ill' when there is agreement between his perceptions of impaired wellbeing and the perceptions of those around him. In that sense, becoming ill is always a *social* process which involves other people besides the patient. Their cooperation is needed in order for him to adopt the rights and benefits of the 'sick role'; that is, of the socially acceptable role of an 'ill person'. People who are so defined are temporarily able to avoid their obligations towards the social groups to which they belong, such as family, friends, workmates or religious groups. At the same time, these groups often feel obligated to care for their sick members while they are ill. The sick role therefore provides, as Fox[10] pointed out, 'a semi-legitimate channel of withdrawal from adult responsibilities and a basis of eligibility for care by others'. In most cases this role is most potent when validated by a doctor or some other health professional. This care usually takes place within the popular sector of health care, and especially within the family, where the patient's symptoms are discussed and evaluated and decisions made about whether they are ill or not and, if so, how they should be treated.

The process of 'becoming ill' involves, therefore, both subjective experiences of physical or emotional changes and, except in the very isolated, the confirmation of these changes by other people. In order for this confirmation to take place there must be a *consensus* among all concerned about what constitutes health and abnormal symptoms and signs. There must also be a standardized way in which an ill person can draw attention to these abnormal changes so as to mobilize care and support. As Lewis[15] puts it:

> in every society there are some conventions about how people should behave when they are ill ... in most illness there is some interplay of voluntary and involuntary responses in the expression of illness. The patient has some control of the way in which he shows his illness and what he does about it.

Both the presentation of illness and others' response to it are largely determined by sociocultural factors. Each culture (and to some extent each gender, social class, region and even family) has its own *language of distress*, which bridges the gap between subjective experiences of impaired wellbeing and social acknowledgement of them. Cultural factors determine *which* symptoms or signs are perceived of as abnormal; they also help *shape* these diffuse emotional and physical changes into a pattern that is recognizable to both the sufferer and those around him. The resultant pattern of symptoms and signs may be termed an 'illness entity', and represents the first stage of becoming ill.

The Explanatory Model

Kleinman[16] has suggested a useful way of looking at the process by which illness is patterned, interpreted and treated, which he terms the *Explanatory Model* (EM). This is defined as 'the notions about an episode of sickness and its treatment that are employed by all those engaged in the clinical process'. EMs are held by both patients and practitioners, and they 'offer explanations of sickness and treatment to guide choices among available therapies and therapists and to cast personal and social meaning on the experience of sickness'. In particular, they provide explanations for five aspects of illness:

1. The aetiology or cause of the condition
2. The timing and mode of onset of symptoms
3. The pathophysiological processes involved
4. The natural history and severity of the illness
5. The appropriate treatments for the condition.

These models are marshalled in response to a particular episode of illness, and are not identical to the general beliefs about illness that are held by that society. According to Kleinman, lay EMs tend to be 'idiosyncratic and changeable, and to be heavily influenced by both personality and cultural factors. They are partly conscious and partly outside of awareness, and are characterized by vagueness, multiplicity of meanings, frequent changes, and lack of sharp boundaries between ideas and experience'. He contrasts this with physicians' EMs, which are also marshalled to deal with a particular illness episode but are mostly based on 'single causal trains of scientific logic'. Explanatory Models, therefore, are used by individuals to explain, organize and manage particular episodes of impaired wellbeing. Consultations with a doctor are actually transactions between lay and medical EMs of a particular illness. However, Explanatory Models do not exist in isolation. They can only be fully understood by examining the specific *context* in which they are employed, since this usually has a major influence upon them. The context of an EM may include the social and economic organization and dominant ideology (or religion) of the society in which a particular individual got ill, and in which they consulted a doctor. For example, ill people's assessment of how serious an illness is (and how it will affect their life) may depend not only on their explanation of the origin of their condition, but also on whether they are able to afford to miss work, whether they can afford private health insurance, and whether the state will provide them with free health care and disability payments while they remain unfit to work. The social and economic context will also influence the types of treatment that patients can afford for their illness, and whether these take place mainly in the popular, folk or professional sectors. Finally, the gender, age group and stage of the life cycle of different individuals will greatly influence the EMs that they employ; those of children, the elderly, new mothers and family bread-winners are all likely to be very different from one another.

The ways that lay and medical EMs interact in the clinical consultation are influenced not only by the physical context in which they occur (such as a hospital ward, or doctor's office)[17], but also by the social class, gender and age of the two parties involved. The *power* invested in clinicians by virtue of their background and training may allow them to mould the patient's EM to make it fit into the medical model of disease, rather than allowing the patient's own perspective on illness to emerge.

Another way of looking at lay explanations of ill health is to examine the sorts of questions that people may ask themselves when they perceive themselves as being ill[18] (or when they suffer from any other misfortune), and how they weave the answers to these questions into the story or *narrative* of their ill health. These questions include:

1. *What has happened?* This includes organizing the symptoms and signs into a recognizable pattern, and giving it a name or identity.
2. *Why has it happened?* This explains the aetiology or cause of the condition.
3. *Why has it happened to me?* This tries to relate the illness to aspects of the patient, such as behaviour, diet, body build, personality or heredity.
4. *Why now?* This concerns the timing of the illness and its mode of onset, sudden or slow.
5. *What would happen to me if nothing were done about it?* This considers its likely course, outcome, prognosis and dangers.
6. *What are its likely effects on other people (family, friends, employers, workmates) if nothing is done about it?* This includes loss of income or of employment, or a strain on family relationships.
7. *What should I do about it – or to whom should I turn for further help?* This includes strategies for treating the condition, including self-medication, consultation with friends or family, or going to see a doctor.

For example, someone suffering from a 'head cold' might answer these questions as: 'I've picked up a cold. It's because I went out into the rain on a cold day, directly after a hot bath, when I was feeling low. If I leave it, it may go down to my chest and make me more ill. Then I might have to stay at home for a long time, and lose a lot of money. I'd better go see the doctor, and get some medicine for it'. Before these questions can be asked or answered, the patients must see their symptoms or signs – such as muscular aches, shivering or a runny nose – as 'abnormal', before grouping them into the recognizable pattern of 'a cold'. This implies a fairly widespread belief in the patient's community about what 'a cold' is and how it can be recognized, though the EM of a particular cold is likely to have personal, idiosyncratic elements. Where many people in a culture or community agree about a pattern of symptoms and signs, and its origin, significance and treatment, it becomes an 'illness entity' or *folk illness*, with a recurring identity. This identity is more loosely defined than medical 'diseases', and is greatly influenced by the socio-cultural context in which it appears.

Folk illnesses

Rubel[19] has defined folk illnesses as 'syndromes from which members of a particular group claim to suffer and for which their culture provides an aetiology, a diagnosis, preventive measures and regimens of healing'. Anthropologists have described dozens of these folk illnesses from around the world, each with its own unique configuration of symptoms, signs and behavioural changes (see Chapter 10). Some examples are: *susto*, throughout Latin America; *amok* in Malaysia; *windigo* in north-eastern America; *narahatiye qalb* ('heart distress') in Iran; *dil ghirda hai* ('sinking heart') in the Punjab, India; *koro* in China; *brain fag* in parts of Africa; *tabanka* in Trinidad; *nervios* in much of Latin America; *vapid unmada* in Sri Lanka; *crise de foie* in France; *high blood* in the USA; *colds* and *chills* in much of the English-speaking world; and many others. Each of these is a 'culture-bound syndrome' in the sense that it is a unique disorder, recognized mainly by members of a particular culture, and treated by them in a culturally specific way. One is dealing with a culture-bound folk illness when as Rubel puts it, 'symptoms regularly cohere in any specified population, and members of that population respond to such manifestations in similarly patterned ways'.

Folk illnesses are more than specific clusterings of symptoms and physical signs. They also have a range of *symbolic* meanings – moral, social or psychological – for those who suffer from them. In some cases they link the suffering of the individual to changes in the natural environment, or to the workings of supernatural forces. In other cases, the clinical picture of the illness is a way of expressing, in a culturally standardized way, that the sufferer is involved in social conflicts, such as disharmony with family, friends or neighbours.

Case study: 'Heart distress' in Maragheh, Iran

Good[20] has described an example of this type of folk illness, *narahatiye qalb* or 'heart distress', in Maragheh, Iran. This is a complex folk illness that usually manifests itself by physical symptoms, such as trembling, fluttering or pounding of the heart, and feelings of anxiety or unhappiness, also associated with the heart ('my heart is uneasy'). This illness is 'a complex which includes and links together both physical sensations of abnormality in the heartbeat and feelings of anxiety, sadness, or anger'. The abnormal heartbeat is linked both to unpleasant affective states and to experiences of social stress. It is more frequent among Iranian women, and expresses some of the strains and conflicts of their lives. 'Heart distress' often follows quarrels or conflict within the family, the deaths of close relatives, pregnancy, childbirth, infertility and the use of the contraceptive pill (which is seen as a threat to fertility and lactation). It is primarily a self-labelled folk illness that expresses a wide range of physical, psychological and social problems at the same time. The label 'heart distress' is an image that draws together a network of symbols, situations, motives, feelings and stresses that are rooted in the structural setting in which the people of Maragheh live. The basic presentation of this illness, however, is in the form of common physical symptoms associated with the heart.

Case study: 'Sinking heart' among Punjabis in Bedford, UK

Krause[21] described a similar syndrome among both Hindu and Sikh Punjabis living in Bedford, England. The image of *dil ghirda hai* ('sinking heart') links together physical sensation, emotions and certain social experiences into one illness complex, which has specific meanings for the community. 'Sinking heart' – certain physical sensations in the chest – can happen repeatedly to the same individual, and may eventually result in heart 'weakness', heart attacks or even death. Among its many causes are: excessive heat from food or climate or from excessive emotions (such as anger) that make the body 'hot'; other emotional states such as shame, pride, arrogance or worry about one's fate, which are all seen as evidence of self-centredness; and hunger, exhaustion, old age and poverty, which all make people 'weak' and therefore unable to fulfil their moral obligations – which may in turn result in worry and sadness. 'Sinking heart' is thus especially linked to 'a profound fear of social failure', and to cultural values that stress the importance of carrying out social obligations, being able to control one's personal emotions, being altruistic and not too worried and self-absorbed and, for men, being able to control the sexuality of their female relatives. Failure in any of these – for example, being unable to prevent the disrespectful and promiscuous behaviour of one's daughters – may result in a loss of *izzat* (honour or respect) in the community, and in *dil ghirda hai*. Like many folk illnesses, therefore, the syndrome blends together physical, emotional and social experiences into a single image.

A feature of many folk illnesses is that of *somatization* (see Chapter 10), which Kleinman[22] defines as 'the substitution of somatic preoccupation for dysphoric affect in the form of complaints of physical symptoms and even illness'. That is, unpleasant emotional states (such as depression) or the experience of various social stresses is mainly expressed in the form of physical symptoms. In Taiwan, for example, Kleinman[22] describes how depression is commonly presented in the form of physical symptoms and signs. In Taiwanese culture mental illness is heavily stigmatized, as is the use of psychotherapy, and therefore stress from family problems or financial difficulties is often expressed by physical symptoms. Although these symptoms do not necessarily appear in a standardized form, they are more easily recognized by Chinese folk healers (who are more familiar with this mode of presenting personal problems and conflicts) than by Western-trained physicians.

Folk illnesses can be 'learnt', in the sense that a child growing up in a particular culture learns how to respond to, and express, a range of physical or emotional symptoms or social stresses in a culturally patterned way. Children see relatives or friends suffering from a condition and gradually learn to identify its characteristic features, both in themselves and in others. Frankenberg[23] notes how people's experience of a particular form of ill health is also shaped by much wider cultural and social forces, such as television, advertisements, newspapers and novels, as well as by the dominant ideology and social structure of the society in which they live.

A health professional working in any culture or society should therefore be aware how folk illnesses are generated, how they are acquired and displayed, and how this may affect patients' behaviour and the diagnosis of ill health.

Metaphors of illness

In most of the industrialized world a large number of folk illnesses still persist, many of them largely untouched by the medical model and still rooted in traditional folklore. In addition, certain serious and life-threatening diseases (such as cancer, heart disease or AIDS) have also become folk illnesses, though of a particular and powerful type. Often these conditions are linked in the public imagination with traditional beliefs about the moral nature of health, illness and human suffering. These diseases (especially those that are difficult to treat, explain, predict or control) come to symbolize many of the more general anxieties that some people have – such as a fear of the breakdown of ordered society, of invasion or of divine punishment. In the minds of many of the population these diseases become more than just a clinical condition; they become *metaphors* for many of the terrors of daily life.

Susan Sontag[24] has described how historically certain serious diseases – especially those whose origin was not understood and whose treatment was not very successful – became metaphors for all that was 'unnatural' and socially or morally wrong with society. In the Middle Ages, epidemic diseases such as plague were metaphors for social disorder and the breakdown of the religious and moral order. In the past two centuries, syphilis, tuberculosis and cancer have all been used as contemporary metaphors for evil. In the twentieth century particularly, cancer has been described (in the media, literature and popular discourse) as if it were a type of unrestrained and chaotic evil force, unique to the modern world, which is composed of 'primitive', 'atavistic', 'chaotic' and 'energetic' cells that behave completely without inhibitions and always destroy the natural order of the body (and of society). According to Sontag, a result of this moral model of cancer is that, for many sufferers, the disease is 'often experienced as a form of demonic possession – tumours are "malignant" or "benign", like forces – and many terrified cancer patients are disposed to seek out faith healers, to be exorcised'. In the media too, crime, terrorism, drug abuse, strikes, immigration and even political dissent have all been described as 'a cancer', a demonic force gradually destroying the very fabric of society.

Metaphors, as Kirmayer[25] notes, are creative of meaning. Their use 'involves a process of discovery or invention'. They are, in a sense, *new* ways of viewing and experiencing the world we live in. In the case of ill health, however, these metaphors – particularly when they attach to serious conditions as cancer – carry with them a range of symbolic associations that can have serious effects both on how sufferers perceive their own condition and how other people behave towards them. For example, Peters-Golden[26] has described how the stigma associated with breast cancer can cause other people to avoid the sick person and withdraw their social support from her. In her study of 100 women with breast cancer, 72 per cent of the sample said that other people treated them differently after they knew the diagnosis; 52 per cent found they were avoided or feared, 14 per cent felt they were pitied, and only 3 per cent thought people were nicer to them than they had previously been. One reason for this may be the fear that cancer is, in some way, 'contagious'. Herzlich and Pierret[27], in their study of French illness beliefs, found further evidence for this: for example, one woman with breast cancer asked her doctor whether it was contagious, and whether she could cause any harm to her daughter by sharing her plate.

Similarly, Gordon's study[28] in Italy found that many women described breast cancer as an epidemic, a 'plague', a malevolent force that somehow invaded them from outside. To one woman 'it is a thing in the air ... It plants itself in a part of the body, then begins to eat the whole person', to another 'I see it as something that comes from outside that disturbs something perfect that is inside of me ...'. Others saw it as 'an animal', 'a beast' or 'a monster' that invades and then devours the woman's body. Seeing cancer as something originating outside the body – an idea that draws on more ancient imagery of the plague, or of possession by malevolent spirits – inevitably reinforces the sense of it being dangerous, or contagious, to those in contact with one of its victims.

Hunt's study[29] in southern Mexico showed further how women with cancer struggled to deny this sense that the disease was arbitrary. To try to restore the 'sense of a general orderliness to life', they blamed it on previous events in their personal lives. These included emotional upsets, worrying too much, improper sexual behaviour, infidelity by a spouse, failure to reproduce, or a physical blow (*golpe*) to the body, as well as environmental pollution. Thus 'the illness did not just happen, it happened for a reason'. These explanations imply, therefore, that cancer has a moral element, and that responsible behaviour can often avert the disease.

Weiss[30], in a study in Israel, has compared the metaphors used for cancer, AIDS and heart disease. Cancer metaphors were those of flux and transformation, of the destruction of boundaries both within the body and beyond it. The disease was described as an alien 'thing' – an 'amoeba', 'octopus', 'spider', 'worm' or 'parasite' – that 'eats up' the victim's body from within ('Cancer eats up your body...It eats whatever it comes across. It has an open mouth with teeth and it bites off everything'). Yet although it was alien, it somehow originated within the person. By contrast, AIDS (see below) was not as an isolated 'thing', but an all-embracing part of the self ('it's his whole body that's infected, not a single discernible organ of it'). Unlike cancer, it was seen as originating completely outside the individual ('AIDS attacks you from without ... Cancer, from within'), and was linked to notions of outside pollution. Metaphors of both cancer and AIDS suggested 'an entity beyond culture'; a sense of something that belongs 'outside' yet somehow has become incorporated 'inside' both body and self (and society) and is now destroying it. By contrast, the metaphors for heart disease were much less dramatic. They described it in less symbolic but more familiar and mechanical terms. It was seen as essentially 'a problem in plumbing', and heart attacks as simply a 'pump' that suddenly fails.

All these illness metaphors are not just phenomena of language. They are also, in a sense, *embodied* or internalized by those that use them. They become part of the way that individuals experience events – both within their own bodies and beyond it – and the meanings that they give to those experiences. Metaphors often come into play at times of vulnerability due to illness, pain, anxiety or other forms of suffering. Such metaphors are often a feature, as Becker[31] has noted, of 'disrupted lives' – of sudden, traumatic interruptions in the normal flow of human events. Under these circumstances, therefore, some of the metaphors of severe illness may well contribute towards the *nocebo* effect (see Chapter 8), with damaging consequences for the physical or mental health of the person concerned as well as those around them[32].

Metaphors of AIDS

One of the most serious diseases of our age is the Acquired Immunodeficiency Syndrome (AIDS; see Chapter 13). According to Mann and colleagues[33], 484 163 cases of AIDS had been reported from 164 countries to the World Health Organization by 1992. Overall, an estimated 12 875 450 people had been infected with the HIV virus (over two-thirds of them in sub-Saharan Africa), and Mann *et al.* predicted that, by 1995, 17 454 000 would be infected. Like the plague, cancer and tuberculosis before it, AIDS in the popular perception has become a metaphor – or rather a cluster of metaphors – and a vehicle for expressing many of the fears and anxieties of modern life.

In the past few years, particularly in the lurid headlines of the popular press, a number of recurrent images or metaphors of AIDS can be identified, including the following:

1. AIDS: as a *plague* (sometimes even called 'the gay plague'[34]). This image echoes those of medieval pestilence or plague mentioned above; that is, of an invisible, spreading destructive force that brings with it chaos, disorder and the breakdown of ordered society, family life and interpersonal relationships.
2. AIDS as an invisible *contagion*. In this image, apparently based on older folk models of infectious diseases, AIDS is viewed as an unseen influence transmitted by virtually any contact with an infected person – whether this contact is with the body surface, body wastes or even with the air that they breathe. This invisible influence can occur at work, school, home, or even at church. Like medieval theories of disease, it is as if the sufferer were surrounded by an infected miasma, or cloud of poisonous 'bad air', which causes disease in others nearby. Implicit in this image is the idea that the sexual lifestyles of sufferers from the disease might also be contagious to those around them.
3. AIDS as *moral punishment*. In this image, victims of the disease are usually divided into two groups: those who are 'innocent' (the accidental recipients of blood transfusions, such as haemophiliacs and children, and the spouses of those who are bisexual or who engage in extramarital sex); and those who are 'guilty' (such as homosexual men, bisexuals, promiscuous people, prostitutes and intravenous drug users)[35].This image of AIDS is still prominent in popular press coverage of the disease.
4. AIDS as *invader*. This is an image that usually includes themes of xenophobia and foreign invasion, since it often involves prejudices against foreigners, immigrants and tourists, especially Africans, Haitians and others.
5. AIDS as *war*. This image may be linked with the previous one, where AIDS is seen as a war waged on conventional society by immoral lifestyles, promiscuity, foreign influences and stigmatized minorities (such as gays, prostitutes, immigrants or drug abusers); here, heterosexual victims of the disease have sometimes been depicted as if they were innocent civilian casualties caught up in the crossfire of a war[36].
6. AIDS as a *primitive* or pre-social force or entity. This is a similar image to that of cancer described above, but characterized more by images of childlike hedonism and unrestrained and unconventional sexuality.

These metaphors, attached in the media and in popular discourse to the very word 'AIDS', mean that it is no longer only a serious physical disease but has also become one of the major folk illnesses of our time.

Furthermore, these metaphors have often been used for political purposes, especially to stigmatize even further certain groups in society, such as homosexuals, immigrants and drug abusers. However, from a medical anthropology perspective, these metaphors are dangerous for many reasons – and especially because they may impede any *rational* assessment of the risks of the disease and how it is to be recognized, controlled, prevented and treated. Watney[37] has noted how the 'moral panic' and prejudice in most media commentary on AIDS makes any rational evaluation of the disease very difficult, since these prejudices 'heavily overdetermine all discussion of the virus'. Cominos and colleagues[38] also pointed out that the only way to prevent person-to-person transmission is by education, 'which is only effective if predicated upon in-depth understanding of prevailing knowledge, attitudes and practices related to HIV infection in diverse societies and subgroups'. However, such research on the transmission of AIDS will not be possible if the stigmas and metaphors attached to it make many people unwilling to come forward for diagnosis and treatment.

Another danger of AIDS metaphors is that the media imagery of moral punishment and the over-emphasis on stigmatized subcultures such as gay men or intravenous drug users may prevent AIDS patients from getting the compassionate care and medical treatment that they deserve. For example, Cassens[34] has described the serious social and psychological consequences that gay men diagnosed as having AIDS often have to suffer, including rejection by family or others. At a time of major psychological stress they may also have to undergo what may be termed a 'social death' of isolation, and the withdrawal of social support (see Chapters 9 and 11).

Therefore, as the examples of AIDS and cancer illustrate, under some circumstances certain serious medical *diseases* can also become forms of *folk illness*, and this can seriously impair the recognition, diagnosis, management and control of these conditions.

Lay theories of illness causation

As noted above, lay theories about illness are part of wider concepts about the origin of misfortune in general. They are also based on beliefs about the structure and function of the body and the ways in which it can malfunction. Even if based on scientifically incorrect premises, these lay models frequently have an internal logic and consistency, which often helps the victim of illness 'make sense' of what has happened and why. In most cultures they are part of a complex body of inherited folklore, which is increasingly influenced – especially in industrialized countries – by concepts borrowed from the media, the Internet and the medical model.

In general, lay theories of illness place the aetiology or causation of ill health in one of the following sites:

1. Within the individual
2. In the natural world
3. In the social world
4. In the supernatural world.

This is illustrated in Figure 5.2. In many cases, illness is ascribed to combinations of two or more causes, or to interactions between these various worlds.

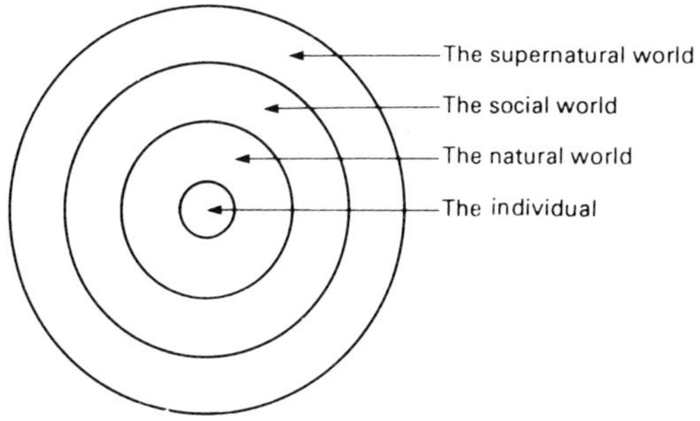

Figure 5.2 Sites of illness aetiology

As a very broad generalization, social and supernatural aetiologies tend to be a feature of some communities in the non-industrialized world (especially in rural areas), while natural or patient-centred explanations of illness are more common in the Western industrialized world, though the division is by no means absolute. For example, Chrisman[39] has described eight groups of lay aetiologies that are commonly reported among patients in the USA. They are:

1. Debilitation
2. Degeneration
3. Invasion
4. Imbalance
5. Stress
6. Mechanical causes
7. Environmental irritants
8. Hereditary proneness.

As in other Western countries, most of these aetiologies are patient-centred and do not invoke either supernatural or social explanations of why people get ill[40]. These and other lay aetiologies will be discussed in more detail below.

The individual

Lay theories that locate the origin of ill health within the individual deal mainly with malfunctions within the body, sometimes related to changes in diet or behaviour. Here the *responsibility* for illness falls mainly (though not completely) on the patients themselves[35]. This belief is especially common in the Western world (where it is often encouraged by government health education campaigns), and where ill health is increasingly blamed on not taking care of one's diet, dress, hygiene, lifestyle, relationships, sexual behaviour, smoking and drinking habits, and physical exercise. Ill health is therefore evidence of such carelessness, and the sufferer should feel guilty for causing it. This applies especially to stigmatized conditions such as obesity, alcoholism, sexually transmitted diseases and, as mentioned earlier, to some extent to AIDS. Other more common conditions are also ascribed to incorrect behaviour; in the UK, colds and chills can be caused by 'doing something abnormal' such as 'going outdoors when you have a fever', 'sitting in a draught after a hot bath', or 'walking barefoot on a cold floor'. Wrong diet can also cause ill health; for example, as described in Chapter 2, 'low blood' and low blood pressure in the southern USA are thought to result from eating too many acid or astringent foods, such as lemons, vinegar, pickles, olives and sauerkraut, while 'high blood' results from eating too much rich food, especially red meat[41]. In another study[42], a quarter of the women interviewed believed one should eat differently during menstruation so as to avoid causing ill health. For example, sweets were said to keep the menstrual flow 'going longer', while other foods caused it to stop – resulting in menstrual cramps, sterility, strokes or 'quick TB'. Similar dietary prohibitions applied to pregnant women. Other examples of personal responsibility for ill health are some traumatic injuries (also ascribed to carelessness), or injuries which are clearly self-inflicted, such as unsuccessful attempts at suicide. Finally, one's moods, feelings and emotional state can be blamed for ill health, and the responsibility of the individual is to avoid worry, sadness and despair[27] and cultivate feelings of happiness and contentment. As one French woman put it, 'I have the impression it is because I am happy that I am no longer ill'[27].

Whether people perceive ill health as resulting from their own behaviour, diet or emotions depends on a number of factors. Pill and Stott[43], in their study of 41 working-class mothers in Cardiff, Wales, found that the extent to which people believed their health was determined by their own actions (as opposed to luck, chance or powerful external forces) correlated with socio-economic variables such as education and home ownership. Those people who had most economic *control* over their own lives accepted more responsibility for ill health causation than those who perceived themselves as socially and economically powerless. In this latter group, illness was believed to result from external forces over which the victim had no control, and for which he or she felt no responsibility.

Other aetiological factors are believed to lie within the body but to be outside the victim's conscious control. This includes notions of personal *vulnerability* – psychological, physical or hereditary. Personality factors include the 'type of person one is', especially if over-anxious or easily worried. In Pill and Stott's study[43], this is illustrated in quotes like: 'Well, I think something you bring on yourself, like nerves or anything like that, it's partly down to you, I would think – to what sort of person you are. Like I'm a little bit highly strung, you know'. Physical vulnerability is based on lay notions of *resistance* and *weakness*. Some people in the sample were believed to be more resistant to illness than others ('I think some people have a better body resistance than somebody else. I don't really know why – whether it's to do with the blood grouping')[43] . This resistance could be strengthened by proper diet, clothing, tonics and so on, but was often seen as being inherited and constitutional ('Some people are born resistant to colds and things'). Similarly 'weakness' can be inherited or acquired; in the UK, some 'weaknesses' are thought to 'run in families' ('all our family have weak chests'), but people who have been severely penetrated by environmental cold may also retain a permanent weakness or gap in their defences in that part of their body ('a weakness of the chest'). Similarly, in Chrisman's[39] classification, *debilitation* – a weakness of the body which results from overworking, being 'run down', a chronic disease or a 'weak spot' in the body – was a common lay aetiology. There was also *hereditary proneness,* which is the genetic transmission of a particular illness, quality or trait, which includes 'weakness'. In addition he describes *degeneration* in the structure or function of body tissues or organs, such as occurs in the process of aging, and *invasion,* which in the USA spans the 'individual' and 'natural' zones of aetiology. Here, illness is due either to external invasion by a 'germ' or other object, or internal spread from an existing problem such as cancer. The other common 'individual' aetiologies are: *imbalance,* perceived as a state of disequilibrium (excess or depletion) within the body, such as 'vitamin deficiency' or 'a lack in the blood'; and *mechanical causes,* such as abnormal functioning of organs or systems ('bad circulation'), damage to parts of the body, 'blockage' of organs or blood vessels, and 'pressure' inside organs or parts of the body.

Explanations for ill health that are individual-centred are thus important in determining whether people take responsibility for their health, or whether they see the origin and curing of ill health as lying largely outside their own control.

The natural world

This includes aspects of the natural environment, both living and inanimate, which are thought to cause ill health. Common in this group are climatic conditions such as excess cold, heat, wind, rain, snow or dampness. In the UK, for example, areas of environmental cold are believed to cause colds or chills if allowed to penetrate the boundary of skin; cold draughts on the back cause a 'chill on the kidneys', cold rain on the head causes 'a head cold'. In Morocco, excess environmental heat (as in sun stroke) can enter the body and expand the blood vessels to cause a fullness and throbbing in the head – 'the blood has risen to my head', and, as in the UK, cold air, cold draught and getting wet are the cause of 'colds' *(berd)* or 'chills' *(bruda)*[44]. Other climatic conditions include natural disasters such as cyclones, tornadoes or severe storms.

The supposed influences on health of the moon, sun and planetary bodies, which is a common feature of societies where astrology is practised, could be included here – and astrological birth signs can also be seen as a form of hereditary proneness to health or illness. Other 'natural' aetiologies include injuries caused by animals or birds and, at least in the Western world, infections caused by micro-organisms. In the UK, infectious 'fevers' are ascribed to penetration of the body by living entities called, interchangeably, 'germs', 'bugs' or 'viruses', which are commonly thought of as being 'insect-like' ('a tummy bug'). In some cases, as noted above, cancer is conceived of as invasion of the body by an external living entity, which then grows and 'eats up' the body from within. Parasitic infestations, such as round- or threadworms, also form part of this group, as do accidental injuries. In Chrisman's classification, *environmental irritants* such as allergens, pollens, poisons, food additives, smoke, fumes and other forms of pollution were commonly ascribed causes of illness in the USA. In France, Herzlich and Pierret[27] found that the 'air, climate and seasons' were all blamed for causing ill health, and that modern notions of environmental pollution were, in many cases, a return to more traditional theories of *miasmas*, or 'dirty air', as a cause of disease.

The social world

Blaming other people for one's ill health is a common feature of smaller-scale societies, where interpersonal conflicts are frequent. In some non-industrialized societies, the commonest forms of these are witchcraft, sorcery and the 'evil eye'. In all three, illness (and other forms of misfortune) is ascribed to interpersonal malevolence, whether conscious or unconscious. In *witchcraft* beliefs, which are particularly common in Africa and the Caribbean, certain people (usually women) are believed to possess a mystical power to harm others. As Landy[45] points out, this power is usually an intrinsic one, and is inherited either genetically or by membership of a particular kinship group. Witches are usually 'different' from other people, either in appearance or behaviour; often they are ugly, disabled or socially isolated. They are usually the deviants or outcasts of a society, on whom all the negative, frightening aspects of the culture are projected. Their malevolent power, however, is often unconsciously practised, and not all 'witches' are observably deviant.

Anthropologists have pointed out that witchcraft accusations are more common at times of social change, uncertainty and social conflict. Competing factions within a society, for example, may accuse each other of causing their misfortunes by practising witchcraft. Under these circumstances, the identity of the witch may need to be exposed in divinatory ritual and its negative effect exorcised. Witchcraft beliefs were common in Europe in the Middle Ages; in England, illness was often ascribed to a witch's *maleficium*, and thousands of women were condemned as witches in the sixteenth and seventeenth centuries. This belief system has largely disappeared, but traces of interpersonal conflicts causing ill health still persist in the language – 'He broke her heart' or 'She caused him much pain' – or in modern psychiatric concepts such as the 'schizophrenogenic mother'.

Sorcery, defined by Landy[45] as 'the power to manipulate and alter natural and supernatural events with the proper magical knowledge and performance of ritual', is different from witchcraft. It is also extremely common in some non-Western societies. The sorcerer exerts his or her power consciously, usually for reasons of envy or malice. He causes illness by certain spells, potions or rituals. For example, in a study[46] of health beliefs among low-income African-Americans, ill health was often ascribed to sorcery – known variously as 'voodoo', 'hoodoo', 'crossing up', 'fixing', 'hexing' or 'witchcraft'. Sorcery is often practised among the social world of friends, family or neighbours, and is often based on envy; as one informant put it, 'Put on a few little clothes and some people get begrudged-hearted'. The daughter of another informant had been 'killed by sorcery' practised by her in-laws, who were jealous of her pretty face, attentive husband and nice home'. In other cases sorcery was used to control the behaviour of others, such as a wife using spells to prevent her husband leaving her. Illnesses that were ascribed to sorcery included a range of gastrointestinal conditions, as well as general changes such as anorexia or weight loss.

Sorcery beliefs of this type usually occur in groups whose lives are characterized by poverty, insecurity, danger, apprehension and a feeling of inadequacy and powerlessness.

The *evil eye* as a cause of illness has been reported throughout Europe, the Middle East and North Africa. In Italy it is the *mal occhia*, in Hispanic cultures it is *mal de ojo*, in Arabic cultures the *ayn*, in Hebrew the *ayin ha-ra* and in Iran the *cašm-e šur*. It is also known as 'the narrow eye', 'the bad eye', 'the wounding eye' or simply as 'the look'. Spooner[47] describes how it is found in the Middle East among all the communities there, whether Islamic, Jewish, Christian or Zoroastrian. He defines the main features of the evil eye as 'it relates to the fear of envy in the eye of the beholder, and [that] its influence is avoided or counteracted by means of devices calculated to distract its attention, and by practices of sympathetic magic. Jealousy can kill via a look'. It can also cause several types of ill health. The possessor of the evil eye usually harms unintentionally, and is often unaware of his or her powers and unable to control them. In their study of Yemen, the Underwoods[48] point out that such a person 'is usually either a stranger or a local person whose social activity, appearance, attitudes or behaviour is to some degree unorthodox or different', especially a person who 'stares' rather than speaks. In this type of society, therefore, a tourist or health worker from overseas might be thought of as a source of illness, whatever their good intentions – especially if they were seen staring at a child and complimenting its appearance just before it got ill.

The social aetiology of illness also includes physical injuries, such as poisoning or battle wounds, inflicted by other people. In many non-industrialized societies, though, other people usually cause illness by magical means, such as witchcraft, sorcery or the evil eye. In Western society, lay notions of *stress* (see Chapter 11) often play the same role, placing the origin of ill health within other people – for example, blaming illness on spouses, children, family, friends, employers or workmates; 'I usually get a migraine if I have a row with the family' or 'I get ill whenever my boss gives me stress'. Infections can also be blamed on other people, as in 'He gave me his cold' or 'I caught his germ', or in the case of sexually transmitted diseases. It could also be argued that overuse of *litigation*, especially in the USA, is analogous to witchcraft accusations, for it displaces the blame for suffering or misfortune away from oneself and on to the malevolence or carelessness of other people. In general, though, the widespread blaming of other individuals for one's own ill health is more commonly a feature of smaller and pre-industrialized societies, mainly in rural areas rather than in more urban, Western societies.

The supernatural world

Here illness is ascribed to the direct actions of supernatural entities, such as *gods, spirits* or *ancestral shades*. In the study of low-income African-Americans[46] quoted above, illness was often described as a 'reminder' from God for some behavioural lapse, such as neglecting to go to Church regularly, not saying one's prayers or not thanking God for daily blessings. Illness was a *whuppin*, a divine punishment for sinful behaviour. On this basis, neither home remedies nor a physician were considered useful in treating the condition. A cure involves acknowledgment of sin, sorrow for having committed it, and a vow to improve one's behaviour. Here, as Snow[46] puts it, 'Prayer and repentance, not penicillin, cure sin'. Similar approaches that link ill health to divine disapproval of one's behaviour have also been described among middle-class suburban Americans.

In other societies, illness is ascribed to capricious, malevolent spirits. These have been described by Lewis[49] in some African communities, where 'disease-bearing spirits' strike unexpectedly, causing a variety of symptoms in their victims. Their invasion is unrelated to the individual's behaviour, and he or she is therefore considered blameless and worthy of sympathetic help from others. Like germs or viruses in the Western world, these pathogenic spirits reveal their identity by the particular symptoms they cause, and can only be treated by driving them out of the body. A similar form of spirit possession – the *jinn* or *ginn* – is common in the Islamic world. In the Underwoods' description[48], they are ubiquitous and capricious spirits that are 'semihuman rather than supernatural', and can also cause ill health. Another form of 'spirit possession', described by Lewis[49], occurs when individuals are invaded and made ill by the spirits of their ancestors whom they have offended. This happens when the victim is guilty of immoral, blasphemous or antisocial behaviour. Diagnosis takes place in a divinatory seance, where illness is seen as punishment for these transgressions, and the moral values of the group are reaffirmed. While such supernatural explanations for illness as divine punishment or spirit possession are less common in the industrialized world, the main equivalent is blaming ill health on bad luck, fate, the stars or 'an act of God'. However, among many Western religious communities illness is blamed on moral error, on not thinking or acting in a spiritual enough way. As one American Christian Scientist explained to McGuire[50]: 'The medical way they don't heal anyone. They just don't heal, because our sense of it is if someone is ill, it's a product of his thinking. And [doctors] don't correct thinking'.

In most cases, these lay theories of illness aetiology (like medical explanations) are *multicausal*; that is, they postulate several causes acting together. This means that individual, natural, social and supernatural causes are not mutually exclusive but are usually linked together in a particular case. For example, careless or immoral behaviour may predispose to natural illnesses, divine anger or spirit possession, or an ostentatious lifestyle may attract sorcery or the evil eye. In any specific case of illness, moreover, lay Explanatory Models vary in how they explain its aetiology; Blaxter's[51] study of working-class women in Aberdeen, UK, for example, found variation in how some common conditions were explained. Of the 30 working-class women interviewed, eight attributed bronchitis to environmental factors, two attributed it to behaviour, four to heredity, three to 'susceptibility', ten to being secondary to other conditions and three as the consequence of pregnancy or childbirth. While these were seen as discrete categories in this study, most EMs see illness as multicausal, with elements of several types of aetiology involved in a particular episode of ill health.

Classification of illness aetiologies

Foster and Anderson[52] have proposed an alternative way of classifying lay illness aetiologies, especially in non-Western societies. They differentiate between *personalistic* and *naturalistic* systems. In the former, illness is due to the purposeful active intervention of an agent, such as a supernatural being (a god), a non-human being (ghost, ancestral spirit, capricious spirits) or human being (witch or sorcerer). One could also include modern notions of 'germs' in this category, especially those causing 'fevers'. In naturalistic systems, illness is explained in impersonal, systemic terms; it can be due to natural forces or to conditions such as cold, wind or damp, or to disequilibrium within the individual or the social environment. Included in this 'disequilibrium' group are systems of illness explanation such as humoral or 'hot–cold' systems in Latin America, Ayurvedic medicine in India, and the Yin–Yang system of traditional Chinese medicine. The 'colds' and 'chills' caused by environmental cold could also be included here.

Young[53] has classified belief systems about ill health as either *externalizing* or *internalizing*. Externalizing belief systems concentrate mainly on the aetiology of the illness, which is believed to arise *outside* the sick person's body, especially in their social world. Thus, in trying to identify a cause for the individual's illness, people closely examine the circumstances and social events of his life before he fell ill – such as tracing the cause of an illness from a grudge between two people, which led to feelings of resentment, then to some pathogenic act (such as witchcraft or sorcery), which then led on to the illness itself. Many of the lay models of illness aetiology from different parts of the world and described in this chapter can therefore be described as externalizing types of explanations.

By contrast, internalizing belief systems concentrate less on aetiological explanations and more on events that occur (and arise) *inside* the individual's body – and they always emphasize physiological and pathological processes as explanations for how and why some people get ill. This is the perspective of the modern scientific medical model. Its strength lies in its detailed perception of physiological events within the individual body, but its weakness lies in ignoring the social and psychological events that preceded the onset of symptoms – while the reverse is true of the externalizing systems.

Narratives of illness and misfortune

A feature of externalizing explanations for ill health is that they often take the form of a *narrative* or story about how and why that person got ill[54]. This story may include events from the sufferer's life and even events that preceded their birth, such as 'I inherited my weak chest from my father's family'. As Brody[55] pointed out, telling such 'stories of sickness' is a way of giving *meaning* to the experience of ill health, of placing it in the context of the individual's life history. It also relates it to the wider themes of the culture and society in which they live. A narrative is thus a basic way of organizing an experience, especially a traumatic one; of 'making sense of it', and giving it meaning.

Narratives of personal suffering are not only personal. They also draw on the repertoire of language, idiom, metaphors, imagery, myths and legends provided by the culture in which that suffering took place[54]. In that sense they are usually *culture-bound* to some extent – that is, the way people tell the story of their suffering in one culture may be very different from how they tell it in another. Narratives are thus, as Becker[56] puts it, 'cultural documents'. She points out that they come into being at times of unexpected disruption in the flow of everyday life. This implies a concept of an earlier state of 'normality', which may in turn be defined largely in cultural terms. At times of illness or misfortune, therefore, narratives are usually highly personal stories, but expressed in a culturally specific way.

Many narratives are created with the help of other people – with the members of a family, for example, or of a healing cult or a self-help group. In particular, healers of every sort take a major role in helping to construct their clients' narratives. Helping to reveal and then to shape these narratives of misfortune is characteristic not only of medical care but also of most forms of symbolic healing, from shamanism to psychoanalysis (see Chapter 10), and of most religious traditions. In each case, the healer aims to impose a sense of coherent order on the chaos of the patient's symptoms and feelings. Usually this places individual suffering in a much wider context of time and place, and employs cultural, religious or scientific concepts of cause and effect. In many cases, the new form of the narrative is negotiated between healer and client during the consultation. This shared, syncretic creation is then carried back home, as a sort of 'gift' from the healer to the client. In terms of symbolic healing, the healer's explanation of what has happened and why is often more important to clients than the herbs, prescriptions or other forms of physical treatment that they have been given.

Western medicine is unique in the type of narrative structure that it seeks to impose on its patients. Usually this takes a *linear* form, in keeping with pervasive Western notions of monochronic time (see Chapter 2). This seeks to organize a patient's story – their history – into a linear form, with a clear beginning for events, a sense of duration and an ending at the present time. Questions such as 'When did the pain begin?', 'What happened next?', 'Where did it move to then?', 'What did you do then?', 'What has happened since I gave you the medicine?' all impose such a linear narrative form, sometimes inappropriately, on patients' experience. Patients who fail to produce a clear oral history are often branded a 'poor historian'. In Western medicine, the doctor's narrative of the patient's experience now takes a standardized form, found in every medical journal, where it is known as the 'case history'.

Unlike in many traditional societies, the patient in Western medicine, as in psychoanalysis, does most of the talking, with the healer asking only the occasional question for clarification. In traditional healing systems, however, the situation is often reversed. The patient offers the healer only a small amount of information – their date and time of birth, for example, or the content of a particular dream – and the healer does most of the talking. In these systems, therefore, the sign of a good healer is one who quickly 'knows' the diagnosis, sometimes with the aid of divination. Their diagnosis is made without having to ask numerous questions, or eliciting a lengthy narrative from the client. To people from these communities, therefore, the sign of a good doctor may be someone who asks very *few* questions – since they should already 'know' the diagnosis by other means.

Many narratives of suffering are *non-verbal*. Personal suffering may be acted out in terms of a specific pattern of behaviour – for example, withdrawal, silence, substance abuse or even violence – over a period of time. Often this performance aspect of narrative is played out more as a mime than as a spoken play. It may take the form of behaviour changes, such as constantly missing medical appointments, losing prescriptions or always taking the wrong dose of medication, which can only be 'decoded' over time. In some societies narratives are commonly acted out in the form of a standardized culture-bound syndrome (see Chapter 10), its meaning clearly understood by other members of the group, but often not by outsiders. In clinical and psychotherapeutic practice, narratives often take the form of particular patterns of physical symptoms revealed over time – especially in the case of *somatization*, or psychosomatic disorders. Part of the task of the clinician then is to understand both the personal and the cultural meanings hidden within these patterns of symptoms. That is, to decode the somatic language in which the narrative of illness may be couched.

Thus, whatever the form they appear in, whether verbal or non-verbal, understanding narratives is an intrinsic part of understanding the nature of human suffering and the many dimensions of illness.

In the following case studies, two folk illnesses, one from the USA and one from the UK, are briefly described. In both cases the folk illness is a cluster of symptoms and signs which are subject to individual and contextual variations.

Case study: 'Hyper-tension' in Seattle, USA

Blumhagen's study[57], carried out in Seattle at the Veterans' Administration Medical Center, was on patients suffering from hypertension. He discovered a lay EM, held by many of the patients about their condition, termed 'hyper-tension'. The majority saw their condition as arising from stress or tension in their daily lives – hence hyper-*tension*. In 49 per cent of the sample, chronic external stresses such as overwork, unemployment, 'life's stresses and strains' and certain occupations were blamed for the condition; 14 per cent blamed chronic internal stress, such as psychological, interpersonal or family problems. Fifty-six per cent of the total sample thought the condition could be precipitated by acute stress, such as anxiety, excitement or anger. In this model, 'hyper-tension' is characterized by subjective symptoms such as nervousness, fear, anxiety, worry, anger, upset, tenseness, overactivity, exhaustion and excitement. It is brought on by stress, which makes the individual susceptible to becoming 'hyper-tense'. In many cases, patients did not perceive that 'hyper-tension' was the same as high blood pressure, since their model emphasized the psychosocial origin and manifestations of the condition. A smaller number saw 'hyper-tension' as resulting from hereditary or physical factors, such as excess salt, water or fatty foods. Overall, though, 72 per cent believed that 'hyper-tension' is 'a physical reflection of past social and environmental stressors, which are exacerbated by current stressful situations', and this allowed them to withdraw from familial, social or work obligations – which they saw as sources of tension. They also labelled themselves as 'hyper-tense', even in the absence of medical evidence for hypertension.

Case study: 'Colds', 'chills' and 'fevers' in London, UK

The author's own research[58] dealt with a set of commonly held beliefs about 'colds', 'chills' and 'fevers' in a London suburb. 'Colds' and 'chills' are caused by the penetration of the natural environment (particularly areas of cold or damp) across the boundary of skin and into the human body. In general, damp or rain (cold/wet environments) cause cold/wet conditions in the body, such as a 'runny nose' or a 'cold in the head', while cold winds or draughts (cold/dry environments) cause cold/dry conditions, such as a feeling of cold, shivering and muscular aches. Once they enter the body, these cold forces can move from place to place – from a 'head cold', for example, down to a 'chest cold'. 'Chills' occur mainly below the belt ('a bladder chill', 'a chill on the kidneys', 'a stomach chill'), and colds above it ('a head cold', 'a cold in the sinuses', 'a cold in the chest'). These conditions are caused by careless behaviour, by putting oneself in a position of risk *vis-à-vis* the natural environment – for example, by 'walking barefoot on a cold floor', 'washing your hair when you don't feel well' or 'sitting in a draught after a hot bath'. Temperatures intermediate between hot and cold; where the former gives way to the latter, such as going outdoors after a hot bath, or autumn, where hot summer is giving way to cold winter, are specially conducive to 'catching cold'. Because colds and chills are brought about primarily by one's own behaviour, they provoke little sympathy among other people; individuals are often expected to treat themselves by rest in a warm bed, eating warm food ('feed a cold, starve a fever') and drinking hot drinks.

By contrast, 'fevers' are caused by invisible beings called 'germs', 'bugs' or 'viruses', which penetrate the body by its orifices (mouth, nose, ears, anus, urethra, nostrils) and then cause a raised temperature and other symptoms. The causative agents are conceived of as unseen, amoral, malign entities, which exist in and among people, and which travel between people through the air. Some, like 'tummy bugs', are thought of as almost insect-like,

continued

though of a very small size. Germs have 'personalities' of symptoms and signs, which reveal themselves over time ('I've got that germ, doctor, you know – the one that gives you the dry cough and the watery eyes'). Unlike with colds, the victims of a fever are blameless, and can mobilize a caring community around themselves. The germs responsible for these conditions can be flushed out by fluids (such as cough medicines), starved out by avoiding food or killed in the body by antibiotics, though in the latter case no differentiation is made between 'viruses' and 'germs'. These lay beliefs about the colds/chills/fevers range of illnesses can affect behaviour, self-medication and attitudes towards medical treatment in both adults and children.

Children's perception of illness

Within any community, different groups – depending on age, gender, education, ethnicity, religion and social position – often have very different perceptions of illness. Recent research has focused on *children* and on how they perceive and experience illness and medical care.

The research suggests that, despite their age, children *do* have their own unique understandings of illness, what causes it and how it should be treated. Like adults, they speculate about why and how it has happened to them, and why at that particular time. Their Explanatory Models are usually a blend of ideas derived from personal experience and family influences, from school and the media. In most cases these perceptions of illness duplicate those of adults, but sometimes they are very different.

In Europe, a considerable amount of data on the subject has come from a large multinational study carried out between 1990 and 1993 on children aged 7–12 years, and funded by the European Union. Known as the COMAC Childhood and Medicines Project[59,60], it examined children's experience of illness and medicines in nine European countries. The research methods included a drawing-interview, where the children were each asked to make a drawing of the last time that they were ill and then interviewed about the content and meaning of the drawing. The results showed interesting differences, but many similarities, between the different countries.

The most common symptoms described by the children were those associated with fever, headache, dizziness or rash. Their drawings portrayed themselves as the central figure in the drama of illness, often surrounded by familiar persons or objects. Trakas[61] pointed out that their drawings often give a sense of isolation or loneliness, or of boredom, anxiety or sadness. They show a solitary figure lying in bed, 'entirely alone, seemingly passively waiting for "something" to change their state'[61]. Unlike adults, however, the children's experience of illness was not all bad. Although they described a series of negative sensations (such as pain, or fever) associated with the illness, they also described many positive experiences (such as watching television or videos, getting sweets and toys, having visitors and getting a lot of attention). While visitors were generally welcome, too many caused anxiety, as they were seen as a sign that the illness was serious. In almost all cases, the children emphasized the key role of their mother as the main care-giver. In Botsis and Trakas's study[62] in Athens, Greece, for example, their mothers were drawn 'serving hot tea, asking if juice was wanted, holding thermometers in their hand, and bringing flowers'. By contrast, fathers were hardly ever portrayed (a similar finding to the Spanish study). However, the doctor – whether male or female – was a prominent figure in many of the drawings.

Like adults, the children theorized about why they got ill. Illness was seen as something sudden and unexpected, that 'just happens', often without any reason. Their explanations for its origin – often complex and multicausal – showed how many cultural models (such as the germ theory) they had already absorbed from the adult world around them. These included concepts of the role of 'germs', contagion, cold weather, diet, and their own lifestyle or behaviour. Social causes were only occasionally mentioned, although one girl in Athens speculated that she had got stomach ache because of a spoiled cheese pie given to her by an aunt who disliked her mother. Unlike adults, though, the children usually did not ascribe their illness to supernatural, religious or similar causes[63].

Climate and the weather were often blamed for causing illness. In their study of 100 children in Spain (Madrid and Tenerife), Aramburuzabala and colleagues[64] found that cold weather was frequently seen as a cause of illness – especially after doing 'something wrong', such as 'walking without my shoes'. Ideas of contagion were also common, and terms like 'germs' and 'viruses', and 'picking up a germ' were freely used: 'Someone coughs and he gives me his germs; when you breathe, germs get into your body through your nose and mouth; germs are little animals that get inside and make you sick... colds and things like that'.

In Finland[63], the 7–10-year-olds interviewed in Jyväskylä also revealed how far they had adopted the adult microbiological model, often blaming their illness on contagion by invisible entities called 'bacteria', 'viruses' or 'bugs' – terms which they used interchangeably. One child described bacteria as 'such little things that we people do not see as they are too small'. Like other European children, they also related illness to their own behaviour ('staying too long out in the cold') as well as climatic conditions (cold, damp, rain, snow). Although illness was seen as an interruption in their normal social relationships, it also brought them closer to their parents and got them more attention.

In Holland (Amsterdam and Groningen), Gerrits and colleagues[65] also found close agreement between the views of schoolchildren and those of their parents. Both shared an emphasis on body temperature and the central role of fever in defining whether a child was ill or not and whether to call the doctor. However, the parents differed among themselves in what level was dangerous, the range varying between 38.5°C and 41°C (101.3–105.8°F).

Overall, Vaskilampi and colleagues[63] pointed out that the children's view of health is a holistic, multidimensional one, incorporating physical, psychological and social elements in it. For this reason they tended to see illness in functional terms: as not being able to *do* things.

The COMAC study revealed that children's attitudes to *medication* – both prescribed and over-the-counter – varies quite widely, although usually it is quite positive. As one Spanish child put it, 'Medicine advances and kills the microbes, which are bacteria. You get the bacteria and it harms your body; the medicine kills them'. The researchers believed that this attitude matches what, in their view, is the overuse of medication in many Spanish households[64]. Elsewhere in Europe, and especially in Holland[65], some children were more sceptical about medication than their parents. Some thought taking medicines was less important for their recovery than resting, while others were afraid of their side effects ('A lot of medicines are not right. Something gets better, but at the same moment something else gets worse').

Reviewing the COMAC study, Van der Geest[66] noted four themes common to most of the European studies:

1. Children's experiences of illness are expressed by how they describe the medicines they were prescribed. For example, they remember a sweet taste if their experience of illness was positive (such as being pampered and spoilt), but a bitter taste if they were bored and lonely.
2. In many of their accounts of their illness, children never mentioned that they were given medicines. Other aspects of treatment, such as rest and attention, are more important to them. Usually they see illness in *social* terms; as a time when they enjoy special care and attention from other people. Thus, unlike adults, they often welcome the increased dependency of ill health, which gets them more care then they are usually entitled to.
3. In illness, medicines communicate to children the powers that adults hold over them. As substances forbidden to children, except with adult supervision, they are ways of representing the boundary between child and grown-up – symbols of power and adulthood.
4. The thermometer, as a ritual symbolic object, plays an important part in marking the boundary between health and illness.

Other recent studies have indicated that a major difference between adults and children lies in the perception of *time*, since both experience life within very different timeframes. James and colleagues[67], and others, have pointed out the many ways that adults impose their own timeframes on children and how, in the home, the temporal rhythms of the child are dictated by family routines, which impose mealtimes and bedtimes on them. Beyond that, there is also the annual cycle of birthdays, major family events, vacations, and national and religious festivals. Later on, numerous other rhythms will impose themselves on the child, often against his or her will. These include the cycle of childhood vaccinations, and then of school timetables, with their rigid control by linear (or monochronic[68]) clock time (see Chapter 2). Also, children's notions of the future and the past are very different from those of adults. One reason why health promotion campaigns about not smoking, drinking or practising safe sex often have very little impact is because children's ideas of 'distant time' (when these 'bad behaviours' will begin to affect then) are so blurred that they have such little reality for them.

Illness therefore highlights these differences in the perception of time. Parents (and doctors) see illness in discrete timeframes, which they use as a way of measuring its danger and severity. These notions determine when to call the doctor if there is no improvement: 'take this aspirin, and let's see if you feel better in half an hour'. By contrast, 'young children's conception of sickness is ... primarily an experience without time limits; whether it is of short or long duration, it is the event of sickness itself, with its associated dramas, which is important'[67]. Because illness has an immediate effect, the child wants immediate relief. In some ways, this experience of illness time is similar to Hall's model[68] of 'polychronic' time (see Chapter 2), where time is experienced not in a linear monochronic way, but as a special point at which events and relationships converge.

Finally, other research indicates that children's perceptions of their doctors can be based on very idiosyncratic criteria. For example, one British study[69] found that children saw formally-dressed paediatricians as competent but not friendly, but casually-dressed paediatricians as friendly but not competent.

These and other studies therefore indicate that doctors and parents should acknowledge and respect children's views of their illness, even if these views are sometimes 'unexpected and amazing'[61]. Like adults, their ideas often have a very clear internal logic, even if they are not scientific. The studies indicate that, in general, children *are* able to recognize abnormal symptoms and understand much of what their doctors say to them. Children – even younger children – are not merely passive spectators of their own ill health. Where appropriate, it is important to give them explanations that make sense to them, in terms of their own unique frame of reference. As Trakas[61] concludes, 'Children who are able to communicate with their health care providers will grow into adults who can do the same'.

The doctor–patient consultation

Against this background of medical beliefs about disease, and lay beliefs about illness, three aspects of the doctor–patient interaction can be viewed:

1. Why do people decide (or not decide) to consult a doctor when ill?
2. What happens during the consultation?
3. What happens after the consultation?

Reasons for consulting, or not consulting, a doctor

Several studies have examined the reasons why some ill people consult a doctor while others with the same complaint do not. Often this is because people simply cannot afford to pay for medical care, or because medical care is not available to them; however, even when they *can* afford it there is often little correlation between the severity of a physical illness and the decision to seek medical help. In some cases this delay can have serious consequences for the person's health. Other studies have shown that abnormal symptoms are common in the population, but that only a small percentage of them are brought to the attention of doctors. There are therefore a number of *non*-physiological factors that influence what Zola[70] terms the 'pathways to the doctor'. These include:

1. The availability of medical care
2. Whether the patient can afford it
3. The failure or success of treatments within the popular or folk sectors
4. How the patient perceives the problem
5. How others around him or her perceive the problem.

Obviously the sparse availability of medical care in many parts of the world and the inability to pay for what care there is (or for medications, special diets, or transport to a clinic) are crucial in determining whether people consult a doctor or not. So is the failure of non-medical care to cure or reassure the individual patient. In this section, however, only the last two points, and the relationship between them, will be discussed.

The process of becoming 'ill' has already been described, particularly the definition of some symptoms as abnormal by patients and their families. Zola[70] has pointed out that this definition depends on how common the symptom is in their society, and whether it fits with the major values of that society or group. A symptom that is very common may be considered normal (though not necessarily good or desirable), and therefore be accepted fatalistically; for example, he found that tiredness is often considered to be normal, even though it is sometimes a feature of severe illness. In the study of 'Regionville' mentioned previously, backache was considered to be a normal part of life, at least by the lower socio-economic groups. The second point is that symptoms and signs must *fit* with society's view of what constitutes illness in order to gain sympathetic attention, and for treatment to be arranged. The same symptom or sign might be interpreted differently, therefore, by different groups of individuals – as illness in one, as normal in another. In both cases, the definition of ill health depends on the underlying concept of health, which, as noted earlier, often includes social, behavioural or emotional elements.

Zola[71] has also examined how this wider definition of health affects patients' decisions to consult a doctor. He interviewed more than 200 patients from three ethnic groups – Irish-Americans, Italian-Americans and Anglo-Saxon Protestant Americans – attending outpatient clinics in two Boston hospitals. The study aimed to find out why they had decided to consult a doctor, and how they communicated their distress to him. It was found that there were two ways of perceiving and communicating one's bodily complaints; either 'restricting' or 'generalizing' them. The first was typical of the Irish, the second of the Italians. The Irish focused on a specific physical dysfunction (such as poor eyesight or ptosis), and restricted its effect to their physical functioning. The Italians displayed many more symptoms, and a more 'global malfunctioning' of many aspects of their body, appearance, energy level, emotions and so on. In their perception, the physical symptoms (such as poor eyesight) interfered with their general mode of living, their social relationships and their occupations.

On this basis, Zola was able to identify five non-physiological 'triggers' to the decision to seek medical aid:

1. An interpersonal crisis
2. Perceived interference with personal relationships
3. 'Sanctioning'; that is, one individual taking primary responsibility for the decision to seek medical aid for someone else (the patient)
4. Perceived interference with work or physical functioning
5. The setting of external time criteria ('If it isn't better in three days ... then I'll take care of it').

The first two patterns draw attention to the symptom, by signifying that there is 'something wrong' in the patients' daily lives; this pattern was common among the Italians. The third pattern was common among the Irish, and also illustrates the social dimensions of illness ('Well I tend to let things go but not my wife, so on the first day of my vacation my wife said, "Why don't you come, why don't you take care of it now?" So I did'). The functional definition (the fourth pattern) of health was common among both Irish and Anglo-Saxon groups (cf. Blaxter and Paterson[11]). The fifth pattern was common among all the groups, and echoes the adult perception of time described above.

This study illustrates that decisions to consult a doctor may be related to socio-cultural factors, such as wider definitions of health, rather than to an illness's severity. Zola noted that in any community unexplained epidemiological differences may be due to the differential occurrence of these factors, which reflect the 'selectivity and attention which get people and their episodes into medical statistics, rather than to any true difference in the prevalence and incidence of a particular problem or disorder' (see Chapter 12).

Apple[13] pointed out the dangers of defining a symptom as illness only when it interferes with usual activities and is of fairly recent onset. It means that more chronic, insidious conditions, such as heart disease, hypertension, cancer or HIV infection, may not be defined as abnormal, provided one can carry on with daily life. Other reasons for the delay in seeking medical advice have been studied at the Massachusetts General Hospital in Boston: Hackett and colleagues[72] examined the delay between the first sign or symptom of cancer and the search for medical help in 563 patients. Only 33.7 per cent were 'early responders' and consulted within the first 4 weeks, while two-thirds waited over a month; 8 per cent of the sample avoided medical help until they could no longer function independently, and only then did they 'yield to family or community pressure and receive medical help'. The role of emotional factors was important: people who worried more about cancer tended to delay seeking help more than non-worriers, and it was hypothesized that the reason for the delay might be to avoid hearing the fatal diagnosis. The label given to the illness also affected the delay; labelling it candidly as 'cancer' led to a quicker response. In general, patients from higher socio-economic levels delayed a shorter time than those from poorer classes, although 'there is little evidence that cancer education programmes *per se* can be credited for this difference'. In a similar study, Olin and Hackett[73] studied 32 patients with acute myocardial infarction; most had explained away their chest pain as resulting from less serious conditions, such as indigestion, lung trouble, pneumonia or ulcer, despite the fact that they were familiar with the symptoms of coronary heart disease. The immediate response was denial, which was 'the consequence of an emotional crisis induced by chest pain and the menacing associations it evokes'. In the majority of cases, only increasing incapacity or the persuasion of family or friends led them to seek medical help.

Whether medical care is utilized – provided, of course, that it is available and affordable – depends also on the perceived *cause* of the condition; whether it is believed to originate in the individual, or in the natural, social or supernatural worlds. Some groups consider medicine is better at treating symptoms than eliminating the cause, especially if it is supernatural. In a study[74] of five ethnic groups in Miami, for example, patients sought symptomatic relief from a medical doctor but expected a folk healer to explain the cause in culturally familiar terms (such as witchcraft), and then to treat it by mystical means.

In all the above cases, a number of non-physiological factors (social, cultural and emotional) influence whether ill people or their families seek medical help or not. These factors also influence how this illness is presented in the doctor–patient consultation.

The presentation of illness

The way in which different social and cultural groups utilize different *languages of distress* in communicating their suffering to others, including to doctors, has been described elsewhere. A clinician who is unable to decode this language – which may be verbal or non-verbal, somatic or psychological – is in danger of making the wrong diagnosis and providing the wrong sort of treatment. For example, in Zola's[71] study, the Italian-Americans presented their illness in a more voluble, emotional and dramatic way, complaining of many more symptoms, and stressing its effect on their social circumstances. By contrast, the Irish tended to underplay their symptoms. Where no organic disease was found, the physicians tended to diagnose the Italians as having neurotic or psychological conditions, such as tension headaches, functional problems or personality disorders, while the Irish were given a neutral diagnosis such as 'nothing found on tests', without being labelled neurotic. At the same time, the Irish stoicism in the presentation of illness could lead to more serious conditions being missed. Zborowski's[75] findings were similar, in his study of responses to pain by Irish-American, Italian-American and Jewish-American patients in New York; the more emotional the language of distress, the more likely the patient was to be wrongly labelled as neurotic or overemotional.

The presentation of illness may also be learnt from doctors, as well as from the media, especially by patients with chronic diseases. They learn to display the typical clinical picture that the doctors are looking for. In the author's study[76], a man who was mistakenly diagnosed as having angina from 'heart trouble' developed psychosomatic chest pain, and this gradually came to resemble 'real' angina the more contact he had with clinicians, especially cardiologists. This 'symptom choice', in the absence of physical disease, has been described by Mechanic[77] in the case of 'medical students' disease', a form of hypochondria believed to afflict up to 70 per cent of medical students. As they learn about the various diseases, they frequently imagine they are suffering from them and even develop their typical symptoms and signs. This is because the stressful conditions of medical school cause many transient symptoms in the students, and those 'diffuse and ambiguous symptoms regarded as normal in the past may be reconceptualized within the context of newly acquired knowledge of disease'. This may influence the patterning and presentation of their symptomatology. This, then, is an example of the language of distress acquired from the medical profession – a situation that is becoming increasingly common as people become more knowledgeable about health issues.

Problems of the doctor–patient consultation

The clinical consultation, as Kleinman[16] has noted, is a transaction between lay and professional Explanatory Models. It is also, however, a transaction between two parties separated by differences in *power*, both social and symbolic. This power differential may be based on social class, ethnicity, age or gender, and is a crucial influence on any consultation.

Although the consultation is characterized by ritual and symbolic elements, its manifest functions are:

1. The presentation of 'illness' by the patient, both verbally and non-verbally
2. The translation of these diffuse symptoms or signs into the named pathological entities of medicine; that is, converting 'illness' into 'disease'
3. The prescription of a treatment regimen that is acceptable to both doctor and patient.

Some of its more latent functions, especially in relation to social control, have already been discussed in the previous chapter. In order for the consultation to be a success, there must be a *consensus* between the two parties about the cause, diagnostic label, physiological processes involved, prognosis and optimal treatment for the condition. The search for a consensus – an agreed interpretation of the patient's condition – has been called 'negotiation' by Stimson and Webb[78]. In this process, each tries to influence the other regarding the outcome of the consultation – the diagnosis given and the treatment prescribed. Patients may try to reduce the seriousness of a diagnosis, or the severity of a treatment regimen, for example. In particular, they may strive for diagnoses and treatments that make sense to them in terms of their lay view of ill health, such as the appeal for 'tonics' or vitamins in the UK, which have deep roots in traditional medicine. The consultation is also a social process, whereby the ill person acquires the social role of patient, with all the rights and obligations that this entails. It should always be remembered, however, that achieving a consensus between doctor and patient is no guarantee in itself that the diagnosis will be correct, nor that the treatment offered will be effective.

Within the consultation, one can isolate a number of recurring problems that interfere with the development of consensus. These problems, many of which have already been described, include the following.

Differences in the definition of 'the patient'

Western medicine focuses increasingly on the *individual* patient[40] (or even on an individual organ), but it may be the family, the community or even the wider society that are pathological, and not the individual. An inappropriate focus only on the individual and his or her symptoms, while ignoring wider familial, social and economic issues, may make both a consensus and a solution to the problem difficult to achieve.

Misinterpretation of patients' 'languages of distress'

These are clearly illustrated in the studies of Zola[71], Apple[13], Mechanic[77] and Zborowski[75]. This phenomenon is more likely if the doctor and patient come from different cultural or religious backgrounds, or socio-economic classes, though it can also arise if doctor and patient are of different age groups or gender. A common example is the misinterpretation of somatization (see Chapters 7 and 10) as evidence of physical disease, or hypochondria, or of an absence of psychological 'insight'.

Incompatibility of Explanatory Models

Medical and lay models may differ greatly in how they interpret a particular illness episode, especially its cause, diagnosis and appropriate treatment. For one thing, they are often based on different understandings of the structure and function of the body. For example, many Western-trained doctors working in a rural setting in the non-industrialized world may have difficulty in understanding supernatural and interpersonal explanations of ill health, or definitions of good health as moral or social 'balance'. The sometimes limited disease perspective of modern medicine, with its emphasis on quantifiable physical data, may ignore the many dimensions of meaning – psychological, moral or social – that characterize the illness perspective of the patient and those around him or her. Thus emotional states such as guilt, shame, remorse or fear on the patient's part may not be taken into account by the doctor, who concentrates only on diagnosing and treating physical dysfunction.

Disease without illness

This is an increasingly common phenomenon in modern medicine, with its emphasis on the use of diagnostic technology (see Chapter 4). Physical abnormalities of the body are found, often at the biochemical or cellular levels, but the patient does not feel ill. Examples of this are hypertension, raised blood cholesterol, cervical carcinoma *in situ*, or HIV infection, which are found on routine health screening programmes. People who are asymptomatic may not make use of these programmes, or may refuse treatment if an abnormality is found ('But I don't *feel* unwell'). This may also explain much of the reported non-compliance with prescribed medication; for example, a person prescribed a 1-week course of antibiotics may stop taking them after 2 or 3 days because they feel much better.

Illness without disease

Here the person feels that 'something is wrong' in their life – physically, emotionally, socially or even spiritually – but despite their subjective state they are told, after a physical examination and tests, that 'there is nothing wrong with you'. However, in many cases they still continue to feel unwell or unhappy. Included here are the many unpleasant emotions or physical sensations for which no physical cause can be found, many of them arising from the difficulties and strains of everyday life – the various 'psychosomatic' disorders (such as irritable colon, spasmodic torticollis, hyperventilation syndrome or Da Costa's syndrome); hypochondria (such as 'medical students' disease'); and the wide range of folk illnesses (such as 'spirit possession', *susto* or 'high blood'). In each of these cases the illness plays an important part in the patient's life and in the lives of their family, and reassurance that nothing is wrong physically may not be enough to treat it, as illustrated in the following case history.

Case study: Illness without disease, London, UK

Balint[79] described the case of Mr U, aged 35 years, a skilled workman who was partly disabled due to polio in childhood. Nevertheless, he had managed to work, 'overcompensating his physical shortcomings by high efficiency'. One day he received a severe electric shock at work and was knocked unconscious; no organic damage was found at the hospital, and he was discharged. He then consulted his family doctor for pains in all parts of his body, which were getting worse and worse, and he 'thought that something had happened to him through the electric shock'. Despite exhaustive tests, no physical abnormality was found, but Mr U still experienced his symptoms: 'They seem to think I am imagining things: I know what I've got'. He still definitely felt ill and wanted to know what condition he could have causing all these pains. Despite more hospital tests that were negative, he still felt himself to be ill. In Balint's view, he was 'proposing an illness' to the doctor, but this was consistently rejected; the doctor's emphasis was not on the patient's pains, anxieties, fears and hopes for sympathy and understanding, but on the exclusion of an underlying physical abnormality.

Problems of terminology

Clinical consultations are usually conducted in a mixture of everyday language and medical jargon. However, the language of medicine itself has become more and more technical and esoteric over the past century or so[80], and increasingly incomprehensible to the lay public. Where medical terms *are* used by either party, there is often a danger of mutual misunderstanding; the same term, for example, may have entirely different meanings for doctor and patient. Boyle[81] found that doctors and patients interpreted common medical terms such as stomach, heartburn, palpitations, flatulence or lungs in very different ways. The marked variations between the two groups could have important clinical implications, especially since many consultations include questions such as, 'Do you have pain in your stomach?' (which 58.8 per cent of the patients thought occupied their entire abdominal cavity). Similarly, a study by Pearson and Dudley[82] also showed major misunderstandings of terms such as gallbladder, stomach or liver. They pointed out that patients awaiting cholecystectomy could become extremely anxious if (like some of the sample) they believed that the gall*bladder* was concerned with the storage of urine. Blumhagen's study[57] on lay beliefs about the meaning of 'hyper-tension' also found them to be different from medical definitions of hypertension. In the study of lay beliefs about 'germs' and 'viruses' quoted above, these bore little relation to their description in microbiology; both were considered vulnerable to antibiotics, and these drugs were demanded even if the diagnosis was of a 'viral infection'. The use of the same terminology by doctor and patient is *not*, therefore, a guarantee of mutual understanding. The terms, and their significance, may be conceptualized by both parties in entirely different ways.

Patients' use of specialized folk terminology may also confuse the clinician: statements such as 'I have been hexed' or 'a spirit has made me ill' may be incomprehensible to doctors unless they are aware of lay theories of illness causation. The same applies to self-labelled folk illnesses such as *susto*, 'heart distress' or 'brain fag', especially where the clinician comes from a different social or cultural background.

Questions in the consultation that are designed to uncover emotional distress may also involve problems of terminology. For example, Leff[83], in a study in London, compared psychiatrists' and patients' concepts of unpleasant emotions. It was found that the psychiatrists clearly differentiated between anxiety, depression and irritability as discrete types of emotional distress, while the patients saw them as closely overlapping. To the patients, somatic symptoms such as palpitations, excessive perspiration or shakiness were considered to be as characteristic of 'depression' as of 'anxiety'. This would clearly influence how patients responded to specific questions such as, 'Do you feel depressed?' or 'Do you feel anxious?' Again, ignorance of how patients conceptualize and label ill health can lead to misinterpretation of symptoms during the consultation.

Problems of treatment

In order for medical treatment to be acceptable to patients, it must make sense in terms of their Explanatory Models. Consensus here about the form and purpose of treatment is as important as consensus about the diagnosis. This is particularly important if the treatment involves unpleasant physical sensations or side effects – where it induces, in effect, a form of temporary 'illness'. This is the case in surgery, injections, radiotherapy, chemotherapy and certain diagnostic tests such as biopsies and sigmoidoscopy. Prescribed medication may not be taken if it is perceived to cause illness or, as in the case of asymptomatic hypertension, if the patient does not feel at all ill. A medication may also not be taken if relatives or friends have previously had side effects from it. Another problem, mentioned elsewhere, is that the use of self-prescribed medicines is common in combination with the use of prescribed drugs; people may use both in ways that make sense to them in terms of their own view of ill health. The phenomenon of *non-compliance* has been estimated, in the UK, as 30 per cent or more[84]. In one British study by Waters and colleagues[85], out of 1611 prescriptions issued by general practitioners, 7 per cent were not even presented to pharmacists. The misuse of prescribed medication, based on specific lay beliefs, has been described by Harwood[86] among a group of Puerto Ricans in New York City (see Chapter 3); they divided all illnesses, foods and medicines into three groups: hot, cold and (sometimes) cool. Penicillin was regarded as a 'hot' drug, and was appropriate for prophylactic treatment in rheumatic heart disease (a 'cold' illness). If, however, an individual had diarrhoea or constipation ('hot' conditions), they would immediately break off penicillin treatment. In pregnancy, 'hot' foods or medications were also avoided lest they caused 'hot' illnesses, such as rashes or red skin, in the baby; because iron supplements or vitamins were 'hot', they might also be refused. Similar avoidance of certain foods or medicines classified as 'hot' have been found in many other communities elsewhere in the world.

The success of a treatment or medication is often evaluated differently by doctor and patient. The disappearance of an identifiable physical disease may not be accompanied by the disappearance of illness, though this situation can be reversed. For example, Cay and colleagues[87] examined patients' assessment of the results of surgery for peptic ulcers and compared these with the assessments of their surgeons, and found marked discrepancies between the two. Doctor-determined criteria of success, such as acid reduction, absence of diarrhoea, freedom from recurrence or completeness of antrectomy or vagotomy, differed from those of patients, who used quality of life criteria such as the effect on family life, social life, work, sex and sleeping habits. A successful operation in the eyes of the surgeon was sometimes seen as a failure by the patient, especially if it had interfered with any of these aspects of quality of life. That is, 'a bad result ... is determined more by psychosocial than physical evidence of failure'. Conversely, operations that the surgeons regarded as failures – due to residual symptoms of diarrhoea, for example – were regarded as a success by patients, and the residual symptoms 'a price worth paying' for the absence of severe and unpredictable ulcer symptoms. In both cases an underlying functional definition of health can be hypothesized, against which the success of the operation was judged.

The role of context

A final but very important source of problems in the doctor–patient consultation is the role played by the *context* of the consultation itself. There are two aspects to this context, both of which play a crucial role in the doctor–patient relationship:

1. An *internal context* of the prior experience, expectations, cultural assumptions, explanatory models and prejudices (based on social, gender, religious or racial criteria) that each party brings to the clinical encounter[88].
2. An *external context*, which includes the actual setting in which the encounter takes place (such as a hospital, clinic or doctor's office) and the wider social influences acting upon the two parties. These include the dominant ideology, religion and economic system of the society, as well as its class, gender or ethnic divisions – and all of these factors help to define who has power in the consultation and who does not. Of key importance here is the role of economic and social inequalities – the differences in power, particularly between doctor and patient.

The sum of these two types of contexts can greatly influence the types of communication possible between doctor and patient, for they help to determine what is said in the consultation, how it is said, and how it is heard and interpreted.

The doctor–patient relationship: strategies for improvement

This chapter has outlined some of the potential differences in medical and lay perspectives on ill health – between models of disease and those of illness – and some of the problems that this raises in the consultation. Six main strategies can be suggested to deal with these problems:

1. Understanding illness
2. Improving communication
3. Increasing reflexivity
4. Treating illness *and* disease
5. Respecting diversity
6. Assessing the role of context.

Understanding 'illness'

As well as searching for disease, the clinician should try to discover how patients and those around them view the origin, significance and prognosis of the condition, and also how it affects other aspects of their lives – such as their income or social relationships. The patient's emotional reactions to ill health (such as guilt, fear, shame, anger or uncertainty) are all as relevant to the clinical encounter as physiological data, and sometimes more so. The patient's Explanatory Model of their ill health, and those of their family, should be elicited by obtaining answers to the seven questions listed in the Explanatory Model section above. Information should also be gathered about the patients' cultural, religious and social background, their economic status, previous experience of ill health and hopes and fears, and, if possible, their view of misfortune in general, in order to put their explanations for ill health in a wider context.

Improving communication

The clinician should acquire knowledge of the specific language of distress utilized by the patient, especially the presentation of culturally specific folk illnesses. There should also be an awareness of the problems of terminology mentioned above, especially the misinterpretation of medical terms. The clinician's diagnosis and treatment must *make sense* to the patients, in terms of their lay view of ill health, and should acknowledge and respect the patients' experience and interpretation of their own condition. As Mechanic[77] puts it, 'The efficacy of the doctor's interpretations of his patient's problems will depend on the extent to which they are credible in terms of the patient's experience and the extent to which he anticipates the patient's experiences and ... the patient's reactions to symptoms and treatment'. However, as noted earlier, while good communication is essential, it does not in itself guarantee good medical care.

Increasing reflexivity

Successful doctor–patient communication is not really possible without a heightened sense of self-awareness (or 'reflexivity'[89]), on the doctor's part, in all clinical encounters. Whether in making a diagnosis or prescribing treatment, the clinician should always reflect on the role of his or her *own* social and personal background – especially culture, economic status, gender, religion, education, experiences, prejudices and professional power – in either improving or diminishing both communication with patients and effective health care. That is, they should be aware of, and where possible diminish, the possibility of *cultural counter-transference.* Doctors are not only the standardized products of medical schools and their disease perspective; their perceptions are personal, idiosyncratic and cultural as well as professional. For this reason it is important to emphasize that one cannot really understand other people's inner motivations and beliefs without, to some extent, understanding one's own.

Treating illness *and* disease

Medical treatment should never deal solely with physical abnormalities or malfunctions. The many dimensions of illness – emotional, social, behavioural, religious – should also be treated by adequate explanation and reassurance in terms that make sense to the patients and those around them. Where necessary, treatment may have to be shared with a psychotherapist, counsellor, priest, alternative practitioner, social worker, self-help group, community organization, housing or employment agency – even, in some settings, with a culturally sanctioned folk healer. In this way *all* dimensions of the patient's illness can be treated, as well as any physical disease.

Respecting diversity

Clinicians need to acknowledge that the Western medical model of ill health is not the only valid one available. They have to recognize that there are many other ways, world-wide, of interpreting human suffering, and many different ways of relieving it. Furthermore, some of these have distinct advantages over the biomedical model, although others do not. This should imply a respect for the diversity of health beliefs and practices found in different countries, communities and individuals. It also involves seeing biomedicine in proportion – as just one part (albeit a very successful and important part) of a world-wide system of pluralistic health care.

Assessing the role of context

In order to understand any doctor–patient interaction, the role of both the internal and external *contexts* described above should always be assessed. It is particularly important to understand those external contexts – such as social and economic factors (including poverty, discrimination, racism, unemployment, crowding and gender roles) and environmental factors (such as pollution, overcrowding, shortage of health care facilities and contaminated water supplies) – that may contribute to the origin, presentation and prognosis of ill health. A consideration of context also helps the clinician to decide who is the real patient, and whether the focus of diagnosis and treatment should be on sick individuals, their family, their community, or the wider society in which they live.

Recommended reading

Disease *versus* illness

Kleinman, A. (1980). *Patients and Healers in the Context of Culture.* University of California Press.

Lock, M. and Gordon, D. (eds) (1988). *Biomedicine Examined.* Kluwer.

Lay health beliefs

Currer, C. and Stacey, M. (eds) (1986). *Concepts of Health, Illness and Disease.* Berg Publishers.

Helman, C. G. (1978). 'Feed a cold, starve a fever': folk models of infection in an English suburban community, and their relation to medical treatment. *Cult. Med. Psychiatry,* **2**, 107–37.

Snow, L. F. (1993). *Walkin over Medicine.* Westview Press.

Narratives of illness

Becker, G. (1997). *Disrupted Lives.* University of California Press.

Kleinman, A. (1988). *The Illness Narratives.* Basic Books.

6 Gender and reproduction

All human societies divide their populations into two social categories, which they call 'male' and 'female'. Each of these categories is based on a series of assumptions – drawn from the culture in which they occur – about the different attributes, beliefs and behaviours characteristic of the individuals included within that category.

Although this binary division of humanity into two genders is universal, on closer examination it is clearly a rather more complex phenomenon, with many variations reported in how male and female behaviour is defined in different cultural groups. To illustrate this point, the following chapter will examine two separate, though inter-related, subjects: anthropological research into gender, and its relationship to health and health care; and pregnancy and childbirth in a cross-cultural perspective.

Gender

The nature versus nurture controversy

One of the basic debates of social thought, especially for the past century or so, has been the nature *versus* nurture controversy – which in anthropology has been the debate between the ideas of 'nature' and those of 'culture'. In summary, this nature/nurture debate centred on whether human behaviour and the human mind (including its intelligence and personality), as well as perceived differences between human groups (such as ethnic or religious groups, social classes or genders), were all due to *nature* or to *nurture*. 'Nature' was conceptualized as rooted in biology, and as something fixed, universal and immutable, while 'nurture' was seen as the influence of the environment (both social and cultural), and was therefore more changeable and more dependent on local contexts. This conceptual division had all sorts of political and social implications; taking the strict nature line, for example, could mean that one group of people (or another gender) was regarded as biologically inferior to another, and that this could never be altered, no matter what environmental influences were brought to bear upon them. Within the last century this approach has often been used as a justification for the persecution, colonization or exploitation of various groups of people in different parts of the world.

Today this type of debate has largely receded, at least in academic circles, and most anthropologists would reject both extreme biological determinism *and* extreme environmental determinism. In explaining human behaviour they would look instead at the complex *interaction* (within a specific environment) between culture, ecology and social structure, and the psychobiological nature of human beings[1].

The echoes of the nature/nurture debate still remain in contemporary discussions of gender. Here gender is often described as if it were the result of either nature *or* of culture (that is, of nurture). Feminist anthropologists[2] have pointed out that, in Western thought particularly, women and their sexuality have often been seen as less 'cultural' than men, and equated with 'nature' (uncontrolled, dangerous, polluting) rather than with the 'culture' (controlled, creative, ordered) of the male world. They have argued that this conceptual division of nature from culture (and the implied opposition between the two) is in itself artificial, a false dichotomy that represents a specifically Western and culture-bound way of looking at human behaviour. Furthermore, this way of thinking, and the conceptual division of the world into these two value-laden categories, is not found to the same extent elsewhere in the world.

They have also pointed out the social implications of this division, for in Western thought culture is usually seen as being superior to, and more human than, nature. At its most extreme – especially in the nineteenth century – this model provided a justification for the superiority of men, for it saw female nature as something to be conquered, transformed and then made productive by the forces of male culture.

In looking at sexual identity, though, it is reasonable to say that both biological *and* environmental influences play some part in the definition of any individual's gender. In all societies, men and women have different body shapes and different physiological cycles; women menstruate, become pregnant, give birth and lactate, while men do not. There are also emotional and behavioural differences between the two. However, it is the *cultural meanings* that are given to those physiological, psychological and social phenomena, and how these in turn influence people's behaviour and even the social, political and economic system of the society, that is of chief interest to the modern anthropologist.

Components of gender

The 'gender' of a particular individual can best be understood as the result of a complex combination of a number of elements. These include:

1. *Genetic gender*, based on genotype and the combinations of the two sex chromosomes, X and Y (XX = female and XY =male)
2. *Somatic gender*, based on phenotype (especially physical appearance) and the development of secondary sex characteristics (external genitalia, breasts, voice and distribution of body fat and hair)
3. *Psychological gender*, based on the person's own self-perception and behaviour
4. *Social gender*, based on the wider cultural categories of male and female, which define how individuals are perceived by society, how they must look, think, feel, dress, act and perceive the world that they live in.

However, at each of these levels there are areas of anomaly and ambiguity in this neat binary division of humankind. At the genetic level, for example, the division of the population into either XX or XY can be altered where certain abnormalities of the sex chromosomes occur, such as in Turner's syndrome (XO), Klinefelter's syndrome (XXY), Y polysomy (XYY) or even true hermaphroditism (XX/XY)[3]. At the somatic level, abnormalities of hormonal development can lead to secondary sex characteristics that are at variance with genetic gender. Examples include both male and female *pseudohermaphroditism*, where an individual has the genetic constitution and gonads of one sex but the external genitalia of the other[3]. People may also have both genotype and phenotype of a biological male, be defined as male by the wider society, and yet behave, dress and perceive themselves as essentially *female* – as in the case of some transsexuals.

Of all aspects of gender identity, 'social gender' is the most flexible one and that most influenced by social and cultural environment. Anthropologists who have studied the two categories of male and female in many societies throughout the world have found a great many variations in the scope and content of each of these categories. That is, they have found that behaviour considered appropriately 'male' (or 'female') in one group may often be considered more 'female' (or 'male') in another.

Gender cultures

Until comparatively recently, most of the fieldwork carried out by male anthropologists paid little attention to the 'women's worlds' of the societies that they studied[4]. Where the male and female worlds were very separate, they had virtually no access to the inner secrets of the women's worlds, especially to their beliefs and practices relating to sexuality, pregnancy, childbirth and menstruation. In recent years, however, a large number of ethnographies have been done, especially by female anthropologists, which have corrected this earlier imbalance. One of the features of this new wave of research is to highlight the role of 'nurture', or social and cultural influences, on the definitions of gender in human societies.

In all societies, the division of the social world into 'male' and 'female' categories means that boys and girls are socialized in very different ways. They are educated to have different expectations of life and to develop emotionally and intellectually in particular ways, and are subject in their daily lives to different norms of dress and behaviour. Whatever the contribution of biology to human behaviour, it is clear that *culture* also contributes a set of guidelines, both explicit and implicit, that are acquired from infancy onwards, and tell the individual how to perceive, think, feel and act as either a male or a female member of that society.

These two sets of guidelines within a particular society can be described as the *gender cultures* of that society. In some parts of the world, especially in less industrialized countries, these gender cultures may be so different from one another that men and women in that society could be described as living like 'two nations under one flag'.

As an example of this, in many societies in New Guinea, men's and women's worlds are so polarized that they actually live in separate houses in different parts of the village and, in Keesing's[5] words, 'have sexual relations infrequently in an atmosphere of tension and danger'. In some of these societies, where homosexuality is institutionalized, this adds further to the polarization of the two sexes.

In another example, Goddard[6] has described the different male and female worlds in the city of Naples, Italy, especially in relation to sexual behaviour and to the cultural values of honour and shame. As in other Mediterranean societies, very different norms (and a moral double standard) operate for each of the sexes. For example, healthy, 'normal' men are expected to have many premarital and extramarital affairs as proof of their masculinity, while women are barred from either. Men are expected actively to defend their own and their family's honour, while women's honour lies in preserving their purity and chastity. Men's honour can be damaged (and be replaced by shame) if the honour of their womenfolk is compromised in any way. However, as in other cultures, there is an ambivalence in the men's attitudes towards women – in this Mediterranean community they are seen as 'either dangerously vulnerable or eminently available and seducible'. Dunk[7] has described a similar picture among Greek villagers living in Montreal. Despite local variations, there is a general assumption in rural Greece that men's role is to protect the family honour through their self-respect or sense of honour *(philotimo)*, while women's sexual modesty or shame *(dropi)* must be protected through their carefully controlled behaviour. In order to protect their *dropi*, women must exert considerable self-control both in private and in public. Family honour and social worth are particularly important and are constantly being scrutinized by other families. Shepherd[8] describes a similar division of norms among Muslim Swahilis in Mombasa, Kenya. Women are thought (by men) to be 'sexually enthusiastic and sexually irresponsible, given the opportunity'. They are expected to be dependent on men, but at the same time the men also fear the polluting power of their menstrual blood. By contrast, men are expected to support – and therefore control – both women and children. This control is considered most effective when exerted over the virginity of their unmarried daughters, but less effective when dealing with the faithfulness of their wives. For a young girl in that community, marriage and its consummation is 'the only pathway to female adulthood'.

In each of these cases quoted above, as elsewhere in the world, the division of human society into two gender cultures is one of the basic elements of social structure, and an important part of the symbolic system of any particular society. However, part of this binary structure expresses the ambivalence with which some men regard the women of their community; at times as nurturant mothers or healers (see Chapter 4), and at other times as malevolent 'witches' (see Chapter 5) or as dangerous sources of menstrual pollution (see Chapter 2).

Variations in gender cultures

Gender roles, however, are by no means completely rigid, and they can often change and develop, especially under the influence of urbanization and industrialization. In industrial societies, as the Embers[9] have noted, 'when machines replace human strength and when women can assign child care to others, strict division of labour by sex begins to disappear'.

Although there are always certain constancies cross-culturally in the gender divisions of labour[4,9], there is also considerable evidence from anthropological research of the wide variation in gender cultures in different parts of the world. That is, what may be seen as typical of the behaviour of one gender in a particular society may not be regarded as such in the next. For example, in some societies women have only a domestic role and are restricted to the home and never allowed to work outside it (such as the *purdah* system in many Islamic societies[9]), while in other societies women play a major role in the wider economic system. In some industrial societies they are major wage earners – in the USA, for example, more than 50 per cent of married women now work outside the home[9] – while in many peasant societies, as well as their domestic role, women are also involved in the raising of livestock, the planting, cultivation, harvesting and marketing of crops and the production of clothes, pottery and various handicrafts for market.

Some anthropologists have suggested that the subordination of women (especially their relegation to the domestic rather than the public sphere of life) is a universal phenomenon, and common to all human societies[10]. However, other anthropologists have argued against this concept, and have pointed out that the situation is much more complex and that each case must be evaluated differently. For one thing, in all societies men envy the biological powers of women to create life, bring it to birth and sustain it with breast milk[4], especially as this power is reinforced by the rites and religions of almost all societies. Furthermore, in many traditional societies, women – especially older married women with children – wield great personal, symbolic and economic power, have considerable autonomy and are sometimes key power brokers within that society. As Keesing[4] points out, 'women's power exercised behind the scenes may in some sense be more genuine than men's power enacted on centre stage', which in turn may merely be 'empty posturing and pageantry'.

Later in this chapter some of the relationships between the various gender cultures and health will be described, for, if the role of physiological differences between the sexes is excluded, it is possible to see how each of the two gender cultures may (depending on the context) be either *protective* of health or *pathogenic*. That is, the beliefs and behaviours characteristic of a particular gender culture may contribute to the cause, presentation and recognition of various forms of ill health.

Gender cultures and sexual behaviour

Although gender cultures lay down norms of sexual behaviour for each of the sexes, there are many variations cross-culturally in what those norms are. For example, ethnographic studies indicate that there is much variation between societies in the degree of heterosexual activity permitted before marriage, outside of marriage and even within marriage itself.

As an example of this, studies quoted by the Embers[9] indicate that extramarital sex occurs in many societies – in an estimated 69 per cent of the world's societies the men commonly have extramarital sex, and in about 57 per cent the women commonly do so. Significantly, while 54 per cent of societies say they allow extramarital sex for men, only 11 per cent say they allow it for women.

Patterns of sexual behaviour are important in the transmission of several diseases. Where promiscuity and extramarital sex is common within a society, there is a greater likelihood of the spread of sexually transmitted diseases (such as gonorrhoea, syphilis, herpes genitalis and AIDS), as well as of hepatitis B and possibly cervical cancer (see Chapter 12). A strict 'double standard' of extramarital sexual behaviour, especially with frequent recourse to prostitutes, may also contribute to the persistence and spread of these diseases. In this case, the prostitutes may act as the 'reservoirs' of the infection within the community. The recent AIDS epidemic has led to an increased emphasis by health education authorities on the importance of limiting promiscuous sexual behaviour among both heterosexuals and homosexuals. The practice of anal intercourse among adolescent heterosexuals in some societies[11], as a way of preserving female virginity, is also relevant to the spread of this disease.

Membership of a particular gender culture does not always coincide with sexual behaviour. For example, there are vast variations worldwide in whether societies are tolerant of some forms of sexual behaviour, such as homosexuality (both male and female), that transgress the usual norms of a gender culture. In some societies homosexuality is completely forbidden, but in others it is accepted or limited to certain times and to certain individuals. Among the Etoro people of New Guinea, for example, heterosexuality was prohibited for as many as 260 days a year, while homosexuality 'is not prohibited at any time and is believed to make crops flourish and boys become strong'[9].

Shepherd[8] has described male and female homosexuality among the Swahili in Mombasa, Kenya, where the rigid gender boundaries were often transgressed by the institution of homosexuality and transvestism. Both male and female homosexuality were common and were tacitly tolerated. Homosexuality among teenage boys was particularly common, though most of them would later have heterosexual relations and eventually get married. She points out that this homosexual behaviour does not weaken the rigid conceptual divisions between men and women since, whatever their sexual practices, 'their biological *sex* is much more important than their *behaviour* as a determinant of gender' (italics in original). She contrasts this with the modern UK and USA, where behaviour is more important in defining one's gender, and male behaviour that transgresses gender rules is often described as 'womanish' or effeminate.

Caplan[12] has argued that where desire for fertility and childbearing is high, sexuality and fertility are hardly separated from each other conceptually and – as described above – it is the *biological* sex of individuals that is most important in defining their gender, whatever their sexual behaviour. Where the desire for many children is less (as in the modern, urban Western world) and where contraception is more easily available, sex becomes gradually divorced from fertility, and sexual practices that do not lead to pregnancy (such as homosexuality) are more tolerated; gender in these modern societies is therefore defined less by biological criteria and more by social and sexual behaviour. It has also been suggested[9] that societies more tolerant of homosexuality are those with population pressure – that is, too many people for their resources – and where an increase in population from heterosexual sex is therefore less desirable.

Gender cultures and health care

As described earlier in this book, in almost every culture most primary health care takes place within the family, and in the *popular* sector the main providers of health care are usually women – often mothers and grandmothers. Also within the popular sector, women have often organized themselves into *healing* cults, circles or churches, which act as either self-help groups for their members (such as the *Dertlesmek* or 'sharing of sorrow' groups described by Devisch and Gailly[13] among Turkish immigrants to Belgium) or as groups which combine self-help with the healing of outsiders (such as the *zar* possession cults in Africa, described by Lewis[14], or the churches and cults practising ritual healing in the middle-class suburbs of the USA[15]). Within the *folk* sector, women have always played a central role, from the village 'wise woman' and the several types of female medium or spiritual healer in Britain to the many female folk healers in the non-industrialized world and the traditional birth attendants (TBAs) that still provide the majority of the obstetric care in those countries.

Within the *professional* sector of modern medicine, however, while the majority of health care professionals (nurses and midwives) are still female, the higher paid and higher prestige jobs are usually held by male physicians. As described in Chapter 4, the medical profession is always, to some extent, an expression of the dominant social ideology and economic system of that society, including its division into social strata and its sexual division of labour. Thus medicine, until quite recently, was a predominantly male profession in most Western countries. For example, in the UK in 1901 there were only 212 female doctors out of a total of 36 000 registered medical practitioners[16]. Medicine remained a predominantly male profession until the 1970s, since when more women have been admitted into medical schools, and by 1985 about 23 per cent of all British registered medical practitioners were women[17]. Within the National Health Service (NHS) in the UK about 75 per cent of personnel are women, but these are mostly found in its lower echelons, as nurses, ancillary workers, caterers and cleaners[17]. Most of the administrators and most of the doctors are male. For example, in 1981, 89 per cent of hospital consultants (specialists) and 75 per cent of junior hospital doctors were male[18]. In general practice the picture was different; figures from England and Wales in 1983 showed that 82.6 per cent of general practitioners were male and only 17.4 per cent female (many of whom worked part-time). By 1999, however, the proportion of female GPs in England and Wales had almost doubled to 31.5 per cent of the total[19].

The nursing profession

From an international perspective, there is a wide variation in the numbers of nurses available to the population in different parts of the world. In 1990, the population per nurse ranged from 5470 in Tanzania and 5040 in Pakistan to 380 in Malaysia and 70 in Austria. There was also variation in the ratio of nurses to doctors. In the years 1988–1992 this varied from, for example, 13.1 in Mozambique and 11.3 in Niger, down to 5.1 in Sri Lanka, 3.9 in Malaysia, 2.8 in the USA, 2.0 in the UK, 0.5 in Venezuela and 0.1 in Brazil[20].

In the UK, the nursing profession (including midwives) is the single largest group of health professionals within the NHS, and in 1990 made up over 50 per cent of its total personnel[21]. Despite the fact that over 90 per cent of nursing staff in the UK are female, there is a disproportionately high number of men (30–40 per cent) in senior nursing management positions[22].

Most nurses work within the hospital sector where, like most other institutions in Western society, many of the basic gender divisions of the wider culture are recreated. Gamarnikow[23] has argued that the relation of doctors to nurses still mirrors the gender divisions of the Victorian family, in the days when Florence Nightingale developed her model of nursing. This means that, within the hospital structure, the equation is still doctor = father, nurse = mother and patient = child. In terms of power relationships in the provision of health care, the nurse's sphere is separate but still subordinate to that of the male doctor. This view is supported by some of the family-imagery still used in the UK hospital structure, where the various ranks of the nursing profession were, until very recently, designated as either 'nurses', 'sisters' or 'matrons'.

Also, a nurse's job, like that of the mother of a young infant, still involves intimate contact with the patient's body (particularly with its surface) and with its various waste products. By contrast, doctors, who spend relatively little time in the company of patients and have virtually no contact with their bodily wastes, have a specialized knowledge mainly of the inner biological secrets and workings of their patients' bodies. Because gender divisions of labour within the medical profession continue to persist, despite major social changes this century, two anomalous types of health professionals are gradually becoming more common: the ambiguous roles of the 'male nurse' and the 'lady doctor'.

Stacey[16] has described how the nursing profession in the UK grew out of religious orders and how, when hospitals were established in the eighteenth and nineteenth centuries, nurses were incorporated largely to do the domestic work and watch over the sick. From the nineteenth century onwards nursing gradually emerged as a profession in its own right, but still remained subordinate to the medical profession. The College of Nursing was founded in 1916, a Register of nurses was established in 1918, and the 1943 Nurses' Act established a Roll of nurses in addition to the Register. Since then, training within the nursing profession has become increasingly specialized, and in both Europe and the USA many nurses now have postgraduate training within a range of specialties and subspecialties. Nursing is now well established as an independent health profession in its own right.

Case study: Advertisements in medical and nursing journals in the USA

Krantzler[24] has analysed advertisements in medical and nursing journals in the USA. She points out how in recent years the adverts have shown a gradual reduction of the traditional medical symbols used by doctors (such as the white coat and stethoscope). Instead, this symbolic display of science-in-action is now more frequently seen in nursing journals, and it is nurses who now are more frequently shown using the healing symbols previously associated only with physicians. In many of the adverts they are still associated with the older key symbols of nursing – the white uniform and cap – but increasingly these adverts suggest that nursing symbols and behaviour have come to mimic those of physicians. She speculates that this 'reflects the desire not merely for respectability but for professional status'. In these nursing adverts, male physicians now tend to be peripheral and 'nurses are shown alone, with other nurses or with patients'. She notes that in the USA, this 'direct relationship with a client, unmitigated by a third party, is an important symbol of professionalization'.

Littlewood[25] has suggested that, although nursing education still takes place within a biomedical framework, nurses are much better placed than physicians to understand and to deal with the problems of 'illness' as well as 'disease' (see Chapter 5). She notes the crucial role of nursing in assessing and managing chronic illnesses, disability, pregnancy and the health problems of the elderly. In each of these cases, the 'quick fix' of the medical model is either inappropriate or of little benefit. In the case of the chronically sick and disabled, who in this society are marginal people 'with discredited social identities', nursing can have a major impact on the quality of life and in understanding the meanings patients give to their life and suffering. She therefore sees the nurse as the health professional best placed to 'negotiate between the goals of the doctor ... and the goals of the patient'.

Medicalization

In recent years the concept of *medicalization* has been put forward by critics of modern medicine, such as Illich[26], as well as by many medical sociologists. Gabe and Calnan[27] define medicalization as 'the way in which the jurisdiction of modern medicine has expanded in recent years and now encompasses many problems that formerly were not defined as medical entities'. These include a wide variety of phenomena, such as many of the normal phases of the female life cycle (menstruation, pregnancy, childbirth and menopause) as well as old age, unhappiness, loneliness and social isolation, and the results of wider social problems such as poverty or unemployment.

There are many explanations for medicalization. Many medical sociologists have argued that modern medicine is increasingly used as an agent of social control (especially over the lives of women)[28], making them dependent on the medical profession and on its links with the pharmaceutical and other industries[29]. It has also been seen as a way of controlling socially deviant behaviour, by defining those who do not conform to social norms as 'ill' or 'mad', rather than as 'evil' and 'bad'. Perhaps most importantly, the decline of a religious world-view and the gradual replacement with health as a moral model of the universe have meant the spread of medical explanations into areas of life and its misfortunes which it was never designed to deal with. Nowadays, as described in Chapter 5, the notion of the unhealthy lifestyle resulting in ill health has replaced the earlier religious concepts of sinful behaviour leading to divine retribution. This process has probably been aided by the undoubted successes of technology and science (including medical science) in improving the expectation and quality of life in many ways. Medicalization is probably also more likely if the body is conceptualized as a 'machine', and one that is only viewed stripped of its social and cultural context (see Chapter 2). A final possible reason for the growth of medicalization was suggested earlier, in the discussion of the nature/nurture controversy. If some men still see women and their physiology as representative of nature – that which is uncontrolled, unpredictable and dangerously polluting – then medical rituals and medical technology become a way of taming the uncontrolled (especially in the age of feminism) and making it more 'cultural' in the process.

In describing cases which some sociologists and anthropologists have cited as examples of medicalization, this section will focus on:

1. Aspects of the life stresses of women, and their relation to psychotropic drug prescribing
2. Aspects of the female physiology and life cycle, such as menstruation, menopause and, later in this chapter, childbirth.

Women and psychotropic drug prescribing

The widespread use of psychotropic drugs in the industrialized world as a solution to personal and social problems will be discussed in Chapter 9. However, studies in several Western countries have all indicated that *women* are prescribed psychotropics roughly twice as often as men[28]. The reasons why doctors prescribe more of these drugs for women than for men are complex, but they include the influence of the advertisements from the pharmaceutical industry, promoting these drugs as solutions for women s life stresses and role conflicts. In contrast, alcohol and tobacco rather than psychotropic drugs seem to be the main chemical comforters used by men in many societies.

Case study: Psychotropic drug advertisements in the UK

Stimson[30] studied advertisements for psychotropic drugs in British medical journals, and found that images of women in the adverts outnumbered men by 15 to 1. In the adverts, the women's place in society was predominantly shown 'as one which generated stress, anxiety, and emotional problems'. Images of the tired and tearful 'harassed housewife' in a cluttered kitchen, surrounded by crying children, were common. According to Stimson, these adverts reveal that women's role problems and conflicts are increasingly defined only in medical terms, and the message of the adverts is that 'certain life events put people in a position where the prescription of a drug might be appropriate'. Furthermore, the descriptions of the drug always showed the individual adapting to the situation with the aid of medical help rather than by changing the social situation itself.

This medicalization of the stress and anxieties of some women's lives is part of a wider medicalization of social and personal problems such as bereavement, loneliness, divorce, political upheaval, poverty and unemployment. It is also part of the growing trend towards 'chemical coping', and the search for a stressless and painless utopia, as a modern way of life (see Chapter 8).

The female physiology and life cycle

In looking at the concept of 'medicalization' put forward by many critics of modern medicine, it should always be remembered that many women have not seen this process as necessarily a bad thing[27]. Instead they have welcomed the development of medical treatments for the premenstrual syndrome, dysmenorrhoea, menopausal symptoms and some of the pain and difficulties of childbirth.

Menstruation

Menstruation is a normal part of female physiology from the menarche until the menopause. Nevertheless, it is often a process surrounded by a variety of taboos and special behaviours designed to protect symbolically the menstruating woman from harm during this vulnerable period, and also to protect men from the dangerous polluting power of her menstrual blood.

Women in Western industrial countries, especially in urban areas, have very different experiences of menstruation to women in many developing countries. In developing countries, especially in rural areas, menstrual periods are relatively uncommon for a number of reasons – just as they were a century ago in the Western world. This is because of a number of major changes in women's lives that have occurred in the industrialized countries over the past hundred years. These include a fall in the birth rate, a reduction in the average number of pregnancies per woman, a lowering of the age of menarche, a decline in infant and maternal mortality, and increased life expectancy and therefore a greater proportion of women who live to the menopausal age[31]. In the 1890s the average British working-class woman spent 15 years in a state of pregnancy and in nursing a child for its first year of life, while the time so spent today would only be 4 years[31], so many more years of menstruation are likely. In the developing world, two other factors may also contribute to amenorrhoea or to infrequent periods; first, prolonged breast-feeding after birth, which is common in many of those countries, and secondly inadequate nutrition, which may have the same effect. Nutrition is particularly important, since women require at least 17 per cent of their body weight as fat in order to have menarche, and 22 per cent in order to have regular cycles[32].

In recent years one aspect of menstruation, the *premenstrual syndrome* (PMS), has increasingly been seen not as a physiological phenomenon but as a problem of pathology and hormonal deficiency. Dalton[33], for example, has described PMS as 'the commonest endocrine disorder', and one that is due to a deficiency of progesterone. This is in contrast with menopause, which has also been defined by some clinicians as a deficiency disease, though this time of oestrogen (see below).

Gottlieb[34] has described the symbolic nature of the premenstrual syndrome in contemporary US culture. She sees the negative moods (such as irritability and hostility) that define the PMS as the opposite of what is normally expected of women in the USA, a form of symbolic invasion of the idealized behaviour expected of them the rest of the month (to be always nice, quiet, kind, selfless and compassionate to others). Women are permitted, and even encouraged, to oscillate between these two extremes of personality within certain times of the month. According to Gottlieb, many American women have internalized this split model of feminine behaviour. However, their monthly 'ritual of reversal' of these values has a largely conservative effect, since it turns women's experience against themselves because they 'in effect choose, however unconsciously, to voice their complaints at a time when they know their complaints will be rejected as illegitimate'.

Johnson[35], too, sees the PMS (and the ways that it is described in American women's magazines) as a 'culture-bound syndrome' (see Chapter 10). He argues that in modern industrial society women's roles are changing, and they are increasingly placed in situations of role conflict – expected to be 'both productive and reproductive; to have both careers and families'. However, at the same time society criticizes them if they exclusively choose either of these options, or if they try to do both at the same time. PMS thus symbolizes and encapsulates this role conflict between productivity and generativity by simultaneously denying the possibility of each: 'in menstruating, one is potentially fertile but obviously nonpregnant; in having incapacitating symptomatology one is exempted from normal work role expectations'. In this way, the cultural idiom of PMS is a symbolic cultural safety valve which recognizes the need for women to turn away simultaneously – at least temporarily – from both of these conflict-laden alternative role demands. In the process, however, it also solidifies stereotypes of women being delicate and fragile, and thus incapable of assuming male roles in the public domain.

As well as the PMS, menstruation itself may be medicalized; in some cases this may act to disguise more traditional beliefs about the vulnerability of the menstruating woman to outside forces, and the polluting or poisonous properties of menstrual blood (see Chapter 3). For example, in their study of menstrual beliefs in Taiwan, Furth and Shu-Yueh[36] found that traditional images of the vulnerable menstruating woman's unclean or shameful menstrual blood were couched – especially among younger women – in the language of health or cleanliness. Most of them took 'health precautions' during their periods, to avoid invasion by infection and 'germs'. These precautions included herbal medicines, keeping warm, not washing one's hair, and avoiding baths, heavy exercise, iced or raw foods. Sexual intercourse during menstruation was thought to be dangerous to women ('It can cause a fever in the womb') and also to men.

Menopause

Like regular and frequent menstrual periods, the menopause is more a feature of modern, industrialized societies, where women have a longer life expectancy and most now live to the menopausal age and beyond.

Lock[37] has pointed out significant changes in the way menopause has been defined over the past century or so by Western medicine. In the nineteenth century, for example, menopause was thought to *cause* disease, but since the mid-twentieth century it has itself been redefined *as* a disease. Thus a normal feature of the female life cycle has increasingly become medicalized, though there are often important differences between lay and medical models of menopause.

Kaufert and Gilbert[38] noted that the biomedical definition of menopause as primarily an *endocrine* disorder (oestrogen deficiency) often leads to the defining as 'menopausal' of only those symptoms that can be attributed to an oestrogen deficiency (such as hot flushes, night sweats, osteoporosis and atrophic vaginitis), while ignoring those symptoms (especially social or psychological ones) that are not easily corrected by hormone replacement therapy (HRT). A further problem of seeing menopause as primarily a medical condition is that once it is defined as a hormonal deficiency disease, it can only be diagnosed by a physician and by laboratory tests, treatment can only be prescribed by a physician, and thus it often becomes 'a permanent condition to be permanently managed' by the medical system.

However, as Lock[37] points out, the medical model itself is not uniform, and there is much dispute within the medical literature on the defining symptoms and appropriate treatment of the menopause, as well as on the relation of oestrogen deficiency to both symptoms and other pathological changes (such as osteoporosis). There is also disagreement about other, more vague, menopausal symptoms, such as irritability, depression, tiredness, headaches, dizziness and loss of libido, and whether these are due to a hormonal deficiency or not. There is of course a physiological change – the end of the menses and of fertility – that occurs at this time. However, this also coincides with a series of socio-cultural events in the woman's life (hence it is often called a 'change of life'); these are often associated with other social transitions, such as retirement, children leaving home (the 'empty nest syndrome') or ill health, and may also be responsible for some of the symptoms associated with menopause.

In her own study, carried out in Montreal, Canada, Lock[37] found that the medical management of menopausal symptoms was often very variable, and while some doctors always prescribed HRT, others hardly ever did. In some cases the decision to prescribe HRT seemed to be determined by the context in which consultation took place, as well as by the personality, training, age, sex and experience of the clinician and the social and cultural attributes of the patient herself. Similar findings, also from Canada, are illustrated in the following case history.

Case study: Medicalization of the menopause in Manitoba, Canada

Kaufert and Gilbert[38] studied 2500 women in Manitoba, Canada, aged between 40 and 59 years. Thirty-seven per cent were premenopausal, 14 per cent perimenopausal and 30 per cent postmenopausal; 19 per cent had previously had a hysterectomy. They found that in this sample of women, menopause was much less medicalized than anticipated. Overall, just under half the women said they had never discussed their menopausal status with a physician. Kaufert and Gilbert concluded that, within the sample, the experience of menopause was not a highly medicalized process, and was one in which some women involved their physicians not at all. This was unlike childbirth, which is highly medicalized in Canada; childbirth is a publicly visible process with little choice over whether to disclose it, unlike menopause. In Canada, the culture of pregnancy usually includes seeing a physician and, like the USA, nearly all births involve some form of medical intervention. However, North American society attaches a relatively light weight to menopause, as compared to childbirth, and this may explain why it has only been partially medicalized.

In the case of both the premenstrual syndrome and menopause, it can be argued that two of the natural physiological events of women's lives have been redefined by some clinicians as 'endocrine deficiencies', or 'diseases'. This medicalization means that some women have become more dependent on the medical profession and its treatments than their mothers ever were. However, as mentioned earlier, many women have also welcomed the development of those medical treatments that have relieved the unpleasant symptoms of both menstruation and menopause.

Gender cultures and health

The gender roles prescribed by a particular gender culture may, like other cultural beliefs and behaviours, be either protective of health or pathogenic, depending on the context. This section will briefly describe how being allocated at birth to the social category of either 'male' or 'female' may, under some circumstances, have a negative effect on an individual's health. Those conditions where the beliefs, expectations and behaviours inherent in a particular gender culture can be said to contribute towards ill health may be termed *diseases of social gender.*

Diseases of male social gender

Several aspects of male gender culture can be said to contribute to men's ill health, or to the risk of such ill health developing. For example, in comparison with women, men are encouraged to drink more alcohol, smoke more cigarettes, to be more competitive and take more risks in their daily lives. In almost all cultures, both warfare and hunting are exclusive male pursuits, and men's health – particularly that of younger men – is often put at risk by the dangerous and competitive sports, bodily mutilations, rituals of initiation and public trials of manhood and 'machismo' characteristic of so many cultures.

In the face of suffering and pain men are usually expected to have an unemotional language of distress; to be stoical and uncomplaining, and thus to have a high threshold for consultation with a doctor or other health professional (especially if they are also male). In many cases this stoicism may be counterproductive to health, for it may lead some men to ignore early symptoms of serious disease, or to the doctor underestimating the seriousness of that disease.

Another example of the relation of male gender cultures to ill health is the Type A behaviour pattern (TABP), which is described in more detail in Chapter 11. This is a type of competitive, ambitious and time-obsessed behaviour, which has been found to increase the risk of coronary heart disease (CHD) in some individuals. Waldron[39] has explained the fact that death rates in the USA from CHD are twice as high for men as for women as due partly to cultural factors, especially to different American child rearing practices. Competitiveness, ambition and other features of the TABP are more likely to be encouraged and rewarded in men than in women. Men are expected to succeed in the occupational sphere while women are expected to succeed in the domestic sphere, and each sphere requires different behavioural adaptations if success is to be achieved. Later in life this type of socialization may be protective of women, but not of men, in contributing to the development of CHD.

Diseases of female social gender

Some of these have already been discussed in Chapter 2 in the context of the many alterations of body image that occur world-wide, especially among women. In the Western world these include mammoplasty, rhinoplasty and other forms of plastic surgery – all of which carry with them the risks inherent in surgery and anaesthesia, as well as of post-operative infection. Other more exotic changes in the body surface and appearance, such as foot-binding, scarification, tattooing and lip-piercing, all carry with them clear risks to health. More recent fashions of clothing and body adornment can also be damaging to health; for example, orthopaedic problems may result from wearing platform heels and high-heeled shoes, and contact dermatitis or urticaria can follow the use of cosmetics, bath salts, deodorants and hair dyes. Furthermore, major changes in body shape to conform to current cultural images of female beauty may lead to 'food fads' and 'diet fads', which can be dangerous for nutrition and health. In some individuals, the cultural emphasis on female slimness may even contribute to the development of anorexia nervosa[40]. It may also lead to depression and a poor self-image among those women with obesity or those whose bodies do not conform to the current cultural images of female beauty.

By contrast with males, women are socialized to have a low threshold for consultation with a doctor, and to display a more emotional language of distress, such as the various forms of 'nerves' described by anthropologists in different parts of the world[41] (see Chapter 11). This in turn may lead to a misdiagnosis of hysteria or hypochondria by male clinicians[42], to the medicalization of their life events and physiological changes, and to the unnecessary use of drug therapy (especially psychotropic drugs). On the other hand, frequent consultations with a doctor may sometimes aid in the early recognition of certain diseases.

Finally, in modern industrial societies many women are increasingly the focus of contradictory influences from their gender culture. On the one hand their domestic role is emphasized and they are expected to remain at home with their families, but on the other hand they are expected at the same time to follow careers and to contribute towards the wider economy. These role conflicts have greatly increased the stresses in the lives of many modern women.

Reproduction and childbirth

Anthropologists have reported widespread differences in the perceptions of conception, pregnancy and birth among different cultural groups. This inherited belief system, which Hahn and Muecke[43] call the *birth culture* of a particular society, 'informs members of a society about the nature of conception, the proper conditions of procreation and childbearing, the workings of pregnancy and labour, and the rules and rationales of pre- and postnatal behaviour'.

Many of these 'birth cultures', from both the industrial and non-industrialized worlds, have been described by anthropologists. In modern middle-class Europe and the USA, for example, pregnancy and birth – like menopause and menstruation – have increasingly been seen as medical conditions, and thus the proper subjects for medical diagnosis and treatment.

Western birth culture

In all cultures, women giving birth are assisted during the labour by one or more helpers. These people may be female relatives or friends, a traditional midwife or birth attendant or, in a hospital setting, a medically qualified obstetrician.

Stacey[44] has described how in the UK midwifery was an exclusive female profession until the seventeenth century, when a few men-midwives (or *accoucheurs*) began to appear. Much of the knowledge of the traditional midwives came from their own experience of pregnancy and childbirth. Although many physicians were opposed to the idea, during the latter half of the nineteenth century midwives were gradually incorporated into the medical system, though they were only allowed to attend 'normal' births. Their position as practitioners in their own right was eventually formalized in the Midwives Act of 1902, though they still remained subordinate to the medically qualified obstetricians. According to Leavitt[45], a similar process has taken place in the USA. Before 1880, women giving birth were aided mainly by female relatives and birth attendants. Only occasionally were doctors called in to help with difficult labours, but even then the power to make decisions about the birth remained with the woman, her family and friends. From 1880 to 1920, however, although most births still took place at home, the medical profession gradually increased its authority over the birth process and how it was to be managed. By the 1930s, for the first time, childbirth took place more often in hospital than at home. In this new hospital setting, control over the management of the birth process became almost exclusively a medical matter.

The growth of hospital obstetrics

In 1959 one in three of all births in the UK took place at home or in a nursing home, while today 99 per cent of births take place in a National Health Service hospital[18]. In the USA, too, approximately 98 per cent of births take place in a hospital setting[45]. The decline of home deliveries in the UK, and the gradual shifting of childbirth into a hospital environment, is shown by the changes in the numbers of hospital midwives and those still working in the community; between 1974 and 1980, hospital midwives increased from 15 002 to 17 163, while the number of community midwives declined from 4237 to 2773[18].

In the past half-century or so, modern obstetrics has achieved notable successes in reducing both maternal and neonatal mortality and morbidity, preserving the lives of premature infants, diagnosing congenital abnormalities *in utero*, and successfully treating infertility with *in vitro* fertilization (IVF) and other techniques. However, for all its technical success, the birth culture of Western society – like other aspects of modern medicine – has been criticized by many women on a number of counts. These include:

- its overemphasis on the physiological, rather than the psychosocial, aspects of pregnancy and birth
- its tendency to medicalize a normal biological event, turning it into a medical problem, and thus converting the pregnant woman into a passive and dependent patient.

In particular, as in the distinction between disease and illness described in the previous chapter, medicine has been criticized for ignoring the meanings that women give to both their pregnancy and their childbirth experiences.

This overemphasis on birth as a technical problem often seems to imply a 'plumbing' model of the woman's body, as described in Chapter 2. In the minds of some obstetricians, birth seems to be seen as merely the technical problem of getting a living object (the baby) from one tube (the uterus) down another (the birth canal) and then out into the hands of the physician.

The origins of Western 'birth culture'

What are the origins of the birth culture of modern Western obstetrics? Davis-Floyd[46] traces it to the seventeenth century image, developed by Descartes, Bacon and Hobbes, of a mechanistic universe, following predictable laws, which could be discovered by science and controlled by technology. The Cartesian model of mind–body dualism led to the metaphor of the body as a machine, and the conceptual divorce of body from soul removed the body from the purview of religion and placed it firmly in the hands of science. Davis-Floyd argues further that Christian theology held that women were inferior to men and closer to nature. Consequently, the men who established the idea of body-as-a-machine also firmly established the male body as the prototype of this machine; in so far as the female body deviated from the male standard, so it was regarded as inherently abnormal, defective, dangerously unpredictable and under the influence of nature, and in need of constant manipulation by men. The demise of midwifery and the growth of the metaphor of the female body as a defective machine formed the philosophical basis for modern obstetrics. A further feature, especially in American obstetrics, is the hospital as a high-tech factory, dedicated to the production of perfect babies; 'the most desirable end product of the birth process is the new social member, the baby; the new mother is a secondary by-product'.

Furthermore, the conceptual separation of mother and infant is basic to this technological model of birth. The baby is removed from the mother and handed to a nurse, who inspects, tests,

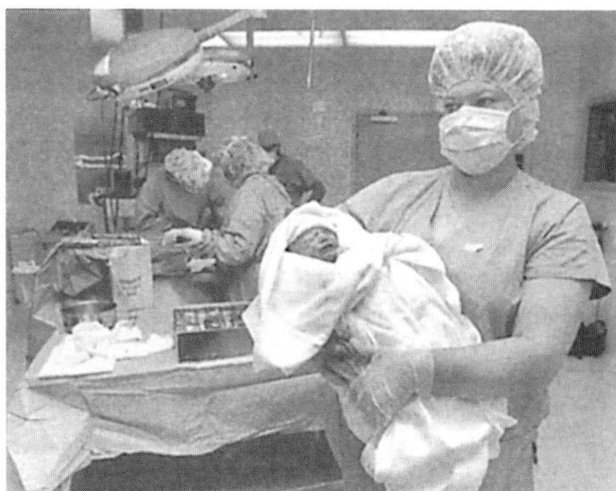

Figure 6.1 Despite its success in reducing maternal and infant mortality, modern obstetrics has been criticized for 'medicalizing' birth, and transforming 'even the most natural of childbirths into a surgical procedure' (Source: © Digital Stock 129056).

bathes, diapers and wraps the newborn, administers a vitamin K injection and antibiotic eye drops, then – having been 'properly encultured' or 'baptized' into the world of technology – the baby is handed back to its mother for a short time before being placed in a plastic bassinet for 4 hours of observation and then returned to its mother. To Davis-Floyd, therefore, 'the mother's womb is replaced, not by her arms but by the plastic womb of culture'. This separation is further intensified by assigning a separate doctor – the paediatrician or neonatologist – to the newborn infant.

She describes how during the birth itself, the mother lies surrounded by medical technology: by external and internal foetal monitors, intravenous drips, charts and instruments. To the woman, 'her entire visual field is conveying one overwhelming perceptual message about our culture's deepest values and beliefs: technology is supreme, and you are utterly dependent on it and on the institutions and individuals who control and dispense it'. This impression is strengthened by the frequent use of an episiotomy, which 'transforms even the most natural of childbirths into a surgical procedure'.

The medicalization of birth

As Davis-Floyd[46] describes, medicine (including obstetrics) has increasingly defined health and ill health mainly in terms of physiological dysfunction (see Chapter 5). As it has done so, the gap between lay and obstetrical birth cultures seems to have widened considerably and the possibility of a 'culture clash' between them seems more likely than before. This is especially true in many parts of the industrialized world, where some women have expressed considerable dissatisfaction with certain aspects of the medical management of birth.

For example, Graham and Oakley[47] have described some of the fundamental differences between doctors' and mothers' perspectives on childbearing, particularly whether it is a natural or a medical process. This conflict is part of the wider differences in perspective inherent in all doctor–patient interactions. The medical view of pregnancy abstracts it from the rest of the woman's life experience, and treats it as an isolated medical event. The patient enters medical care at the onset of pregnancy, and leaves medical care after giving birth. For the mother, on the other hand, it is integrated with *other* aspects of her life, for she acquires (with a first birth) a new social role, as well as profound changes in her financial situation, marital status, housing situation and personal relationships. There are also differences in how she and the obstetrician assess the quality of the childbearing experience, how they measure a successful outcome, and how they decide who should control the method and pace of the birth itself. Thus there is an inherent clash between the obstetricians – clinicians (usually male) who have a specialized knowledge of childbirth – and the mothers, whose expertise 'stems not primarily from medical science but rather from a woman's capacity to sense and respond to the sensations of her body'.

As well as having a technical purpose, many of the procedures of modern obstetrics can also be described as rituals of social transition or *rites de passage*, which will be described later in Chapter 9. For the purposes of this section, however, it is important to note that in all human societies pregnancy and childbirth are more than just biological events. They are also part of an important transition of the woman from the social status of 'woman' to that of 'mother'. As with all social transitions, during the dangerous journey from one status to another the individual must be *protected* from harm by the observance of certain ritual beliefs and behaviour. In many of these transitions the person concerned goes through a temporary period of withdrawal from ordinary life, before being 're-born' into their new social status; as Kitzinger[48] observes, the initiate often 'goes through an act of infantilization, in which he or she is reduced to the state of a small, dependent, submissive child', and 'it is as if only by going back to the beginning can re-birth take place'. The practice in some hospitals of shaving women's pubic hair and giving them an enema before they give birth can also be seen as part of this infantilization, or at least of returning the woman to a pre-pubertal state. However, as Davis-Floyd[46] has argued above, many of the rituals of obstetrics are also ways of transmitting some of society's most basic values to the woman undergoing childbirth. According to her, these values include her powerlessness in the face of patriarchy, the 'defectiveness' of her female body, the need of medicine to control her natural processes, her dependence on science and technology, and the enduring importance of institutions and machines over individual beliefs and meanings. This type of cultural message is more likely to be transmitted to the new mother in the impersonal atmosphere of a hospital obstetric unit than when the birth takes place in the familiar atmosphere of the home. As Kitzinger[48] has put it, 'in large centralized, hierarchical institutions existing outside and apart from the family there is a special likelihood of these rituals being used to reinforce the existing system and maintain the power structure'.

Despite this, Browner[49] notes that many pregnant women in the USA are deeply ambivalent about the value of medical technology, especially in prenatal care and diagnosis. Although they trust their own experience and 'embodied knowledge', few reject the findings of medical science. She predicts that as the role of clinical technology in childbirth grows, so will the consensus that biomedicine alone holds 'authoritative knowledge', especially in the domain of prenatal care.

Non-Western birth cultures

Hahn and Muecke[43] described the discrepancies between the birth culture of middle-class USA and those of some of the social and ethnic groups in that country, such as working-class blacks, Mexican-Americans, Chinese and the Hmong (from Laos). In each case, some of the basic assumptions of white middle-class obstetricians – for example, that the husband should be present at the birth – may *not* be shared by the members of those groups (or by men from other groups in society, as well). Among some traditional Chinese groups, for example, women and their bodily products are regarded as dangerous and polluting for men, who therefore avoid the scene of birth and any contact with the woman in the month following the birth. As with other traditional groups, female obstetricians and birth attendants may be preferred to males.

In many cultures in the non-industrialized world, giving birth in the lithotomy or supine position favoured by Western obstetrics is not at all common. In her review of the literature on the subject, MacCormack[50] states that 'throughout the world, in Latin America, northern Thailand, India, Sri Lanka and West Africa, women either stand, squat or sit reclining against something or someone in the latter stages of labour'. In the second stage of labour, the midwife is often seated on the floor in front of the labouring woman. With breach or transverse presentations, traditional birth attendants are often skilled at manipulating the baby into the cephalic position by external massage.

Reviewing the literature covering Vietnam, Thailand, Burma, India, East and West Africa, Jamaica, Guatemala and Brazil, MacCormack[50] points out that, unlike in Western obstetrical practice, the umbilical cord is usually cut *after* the placenta is expelled, and not before. In some areas, dung is rubbed into the infant's umbilicus to stop bleeding, and this can increase the risk of neonatal tetanus[50].

After the birth, women in most cultures observe a special postpartum rest period, during which they have to follow certain dietary and other taboos and are cared for mainly by other women. This period of rest and seclusion usually lasts between 20 and 40 days. Among Tamils in Sri Lanka, for example, the period of 'childbirth pollution' is 31 days, followed by special rituals which purify the house, as well as a ritual bath for the mother and the shaving of the child's head[51]. Pillsbury[52] describes how in rural Chinese communities, in both the People's Republic of China and Taiwan (where it is called the *tso yueh*), 'doing the month' involves 1 full month of postpartum convalescence, during which time the woman is confined to her home, looked after by relatives, and has to eat a special diet and observe special taboos. She points out how, by contrast, the 'lying in' period of Western birth culture has given way to the puerperium, which does not have the same symbolic importance and 'no longer connotes the specificity of behaviour that continues to characterize "doing the month"'. A further important aspect of the postpartum period is that many cultures prohibit sexual relations between husband and wife for a period of time after the birth. In some cases this may last for several months; among many traditional Chinese in the USA, for example, sexual contact is sometimes proscribed for anything up to 100 days postpartum[43].

Traditional birth attendants (TBAs)

By contrast with the modern, technological model of birth, most babies world-wide – especially in rural areas of the developing world – are delivered in a very different way, usually by female birth attendants such as the *parteras* of Mexico, the *comadronas* of Puerto Rico, the *nanas* of Jamaica, the *dais* of India and the *dayas* of Egypt.

In Africa and in rural India, an estimated 80 per cent of women are assisted during birth by traditional birth attendants (TBAs). World-wide, it has been estimated by the World Health Organization that about 60–80 per cent of babies are delivered by TBAs[53].

TBAs are found in almost every village and in many urban neighbourhoods throughout Africa, Asia, Latin America and the Caribbean. As well as delivering babies, they also supervise antenatal and postnatal care, perform important rituals during pregnancy and birth and, in some parts of the world, carry out female circumcisions. In 1978 and 1992, WHO reports[54,55] supported the further training of traditional birth attendants. The WHO's aim has been to increase their numbers and further training, and also consultation with them, so as eventually to integrate them into the overall health programmes in developing countries whilst ensuring at the same time the continuation of the traditional art and respect for their roots in traditional cultures. After training, it was intended that they would take on other roles in the community, such as providing first aid, giving advice on family planning, and distributing oral rehydration solution (ORS) in cases of infantile diarrhoea. As community health educators, they were to give advice on nutrition, the prevention of HIV infection, the importance of personal and environmental hygiene, and the need to bring babies and children to health clinics to monitor their development and get them vaccinated[55].

In countries where TBAs are recognized by the authorities, considerable numbers have been trained and used in basic health services during the past 30 years, including in Ghana, Indonesia, Malaysia, Pakistan, the Philippines, Sudan and Thailand. In Egypt, for example[56], where 80–90 per cent of babies are still delivered by *dayas*, the training programme has had four main objectives:

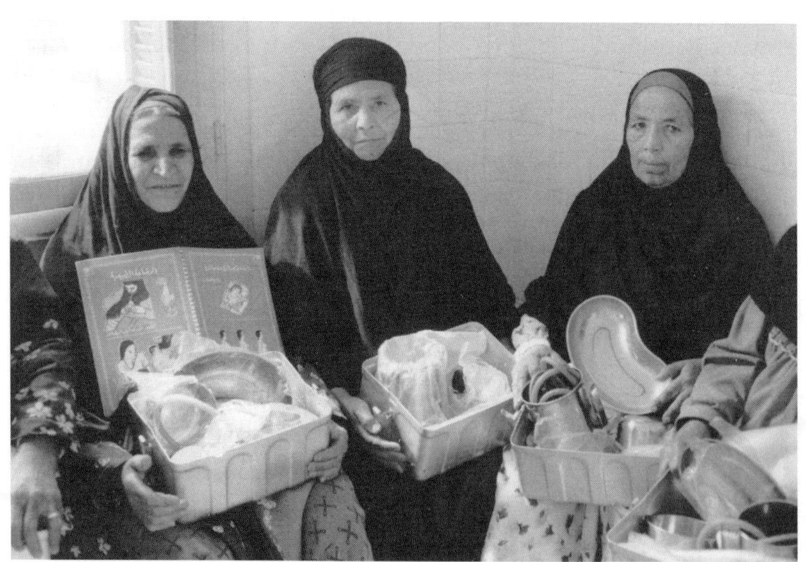

Figure 6.2 Traditional birth attendants or *dayas* in the Nile Delta, Egypt, holding equipment kits and pamphlets given to them by UNICEF (Source: Sean Sprague/Panos Pictures, no. Egy 220).

1. To expand the scope of their practice
2. To increase the safety of their techniques
3. To increase their referral to hospitals of babies and mothers who are at risk
4. To increase cooperation between them and local health staff.

Despite their lack of formal training, and the shortcomings of some of their techniques, TBAs therefore offer the possibility of non-technological birth care, at little or no cost, in many parts of the non-industrialized world.

Case study: The *nana* in Jamaica

Kitzinger[48] described an example of a traditional birth attendant, the *nana* or folk midwife of Jamaica. She estimated that about 25 per cent of Jamaican babies, especially in rural areas, are delivered by a *nana*. Because these women are not legally recognized by the state, most of these births are registered as 'born unattended' or 'delivered by mother' (or by a friend or relative). In the villages, the *nana* is a person of high standing and great authority, 'a key figure in the cohesion of women in Jamaican rural communities'. Together with the village schoolteacher and the postmistress, she forms 'the political centre' or core of the social networks that tie the community together. *Nanas* are familiar figures, deeply rooted in their communities, and are often called upon for help in a variety of family crises. The midwifery skills of the *nana* are handed down within families, from mother to daughter. *Nanas* are always mothers themselves, for 'to be a *nana* is really an extension of the mothering role, so all *nanas* are mothers who are seen to be successful in their role'. They see their role as shepherding the women safely from conception to birth by facilitating their natural processes, and in doing so assisting in the drama of 'the re-birth of a woman as a mother'. Their care usually continues from pregnancy until the ninth day postpartum. The *nanas* supervise all the many rituals and taboos of pregnancy and birth (see Chapter 9) that mark the woman's transition from pregnancy to motherhood, and which help give meaning to her experience, by placing it in the context of the wider cultural values of her religion and community. Kitzinger contrasts this intimate, culturally familiar approach with the Western-style, technological birth procedures used in many Jamaican hospitals, where nurses and midwives value 'efficiency, speed of delivery of the patient, hospital routines concerning hygiene and order, and the suppression of emotional factors in childbirth so that they can get on with the work in an organized way, and treat the greatest number of patients in the shortest possible time'.

According to Kitzinger, the Jamaican *nanas*, who do things in 'the old time way', tend to be derided both by the medical profession and the educated middle-class as inefficient and harmful to health, and as echoes of a past of slavery and subjugation. However, she points out that the *nanas* are very experienced in the techniques of midwifery, are keen to learn more from modern obstetrics and are quick to call in a trained midwife or send the woman straight to hospital if anything goes wrong with the birth. Many rural women now use *nanas* during pregnancy and the first stage of labour, and then transfer to a qualified midwife for the birth itself.

Although they are still active in the countryside, a more recent study by Sargent and Bascope[57] suggests that the use of *nanas* is in overall decline in Jamaica, especially in urban areas. This is partly due to government policy and health education campaigns. Increasingly, pregnant women are placing their trust in hospital obstetrics, especially in the government nurse-midwives based in those hospitals.

Fertility and infertility

Fertility is a universal human concern, as is anguish over infertility, whatever its cause. Most cultures include a series of rituals or prayers or special precautions to help a woman successfully conceive, and to carry her through to a safe delivery. Where a woman fails to conceive, a wide variety of cultural explanations usually come into play to explain her infertility and how to deal with it. As described in the previous chapter, such lay explanations for misfortune usually lay the blame on the individual's behaviour, on the natural world, on the malevolence of other people, or on supernatural forces or gods. In addition, they often draw on deep cultural images of what constitutes 'a woman' and what 'a man'. Becker[58] has described the poignant narratives of American women who have found that they are infertile. She shows how this knowledge strikes at the very sense of their own identity, unravelling their basic understanding of who they are. In the USA, as elsewhere, the ability to nurture others, and thus to be fertile, is the very basis of womanhood. The women compared themselves repeatedly to this cultural ideal of the 'natural mother': 'one who nourishes her child with the riches of her body'. While the pregnant body – 'a body that is nurturant, natural, and healthy' – stands as the very embodiment of the cultural values of womanhood, their own infertile bodies seemed somehow 'abnormal' by comparison.

Concepts of fertility and infertility are also partly dependent on how people conceptualize the inner workings of their bodies and the processes of conception and birth. For example, Cosminsky[59] has described how in a Guatemalan village some of the traditional midwives believed that infertility was caused by a 'cold womb', which was not 'hot' enough to receive the semen. One form of treatment was to administer 'hot' herbal teas, and to 'warm the womb' in a special sweatbath. If, however, the villagers believed that the sterility was caused by divine intervention, then the midwife was not expected to cure it.

In small-scale societies particularly, a 'barren woman' is often a marginalized figure, and seen as someone both personally unfulfilled and socially incomplete. In most traditional societies, blame for the infertility is usually placed on the *woman*. In many communities world-wide, producing a child – especially a son – is considered to be public proof of a man's virility, as well as of his adulthood. As a result, men are often reluctant to admit to any responsibility for infertility. According to McGilvray[51], among Tamils in Sri Lanka and throughout most of South Asia, infertility is seen as primarily a problem with the woman and not the man. Sometimes a supernatural cause for the infertility is suggested, but rarely is the potency of the husband questioned, and most men would never acknowledge the possibility of their own sterility. In this type of setting, the very suggestion that they and not their wives, are sterile may be very threatening to many men. For example, Palgi[60] describes the case of a Yemenite man from a traditional background who had emigrated to Israel. When his first wife failed to produce a child, he divorced her. When the second marriage was also childless, and doctors told him that *he* was the sterile one, he suffered a severe emotional collapse, with fearfulness, insomnia and a feeling of being tormented by evil spirits. Palgi links this reaction to cultural beliefs in his community that a man's dignity and respect are linked to the number of his progeny, especially sons. Furthermore, a common belief was that if there were no heirs to pray for a father's soul after death, then 'his peaceful life after death is endangered'.

It should be noted, however, that such definitions of who is responsible for the infertility are not static. They often undergo significant changes during westernization, migration, urbanization and other major social changes.

Assisted reproduction: the new reproductive technologies

In recent decades, in most industrialized countries, there have been major advances in the medical treatment of infertility, both male and female. Although they have helped many infertile couples to conceive, the new reproductive technologies (NRTs) remain controversial. This is largely because they have challenged the very notions of family, kinship and parenthood, especially the relationship between social and biological parenthood. They have also altered perceptions of the physical functions and boundaries of the individual body, particularly the female body.

Despite this, their popularity continues to grow. By 1994 it was estimated that about 40 000 children had been born from *in vitro* fertilization world-wide[61]. In some countries such as Japan, however, there has been both public and official opposition to the use of these procedures[61].

Although a whole range of NRTs is now available, and in different combinations[62], the best known of them are:

1. *In vitro fertilization* (IVF), involving ovum or sperm donation, either by the spouse of the infertile person or by an anonymous donor
2. *Surrogate motherhood*, whereby one woman carries a baby on behalf of another, and then gives it to her once it is born. Here the foetus may be either the surrogate mother's own child by the husband of the infertile woman, or the implanted, fertilized egg of another couple.

Before the development of the NRTs, ovulation, fertilization and pregnancy were events that all took place within the same woman's body. Now one or more may take place outside her body, or even in the bodies of three different women. In 1983, Snowden and colleagues[63] divided the maternal role into three parts: 'the genetic mother, the carrying mother, and the nurturing mother'. A woman who performs all three roles they described as a 'complete mother'. As a result of the development of IVF and surrogate motherhood, however, it is now possible for each of these roles to be carried out by a different woman – one providing the egg (also known as the 'commissioning mother'), another bearing the child (the 'carrying mother') and a third caring for the baby once it is born. Does the child therefore have one mother, or two, or even three? And which one, from its point of view, is the 'real' one?

A potential effect of the NRTs is thus to widen the split between biological and social parenthood. This does not apply only to motherhood; already it has been estimated that about 20 per cent of children born in the UK are not biologically related to their 'fathers'[62], and the use of IVF with sperm donation is likely to increase this percentage. Another result has been the creation of new and complex webs of kinship between, for example, 'carrying mothers' and 'commissioning mothers', children and their unknown genetic 'mothers' or 'fathers', couples and the anonymous donor of their child's ovum or sperm, and grandparents and grandchildren who are not genetically related to one another. Konrad[64], for example, has described the sense of 'relatedness' felt by both ova donors and recipients, even if they never meet one another in person.

In Western societies, where nuclear families are often the rule, social and biological parenthood usually coincide – except in the case of adoption, or where remarriage takes place following divorce or death of a spouse. Although the new forms of kinship created by the NRTs, appear novel and unusual to Western culture, anthropologists have described many examples of what amounts to 'surrogate parenthood' – of social and biological parenting being provided by different people. This is particularly common in traditional societies where large extended families are the rule and children may be cared for by a variety of adults – aunts, uncles, grandparents, older siblings and neighbours – as well as by their own biological parents. For example, Evans-Pritchard[65], in the early 1950s, described unusual patterns of kinship and marriage among the Nuer people of the Sudan. Here, the failure to have any children, especially males to carry on the name, was regarded as a great tragedy by every Nuer family, and they adopted various strategies to overcome this problem. For example, in 'ghost marriage' – which occurs when a man dies without legal male heirs – a kinsman of his (such as brother or nephew) marries the widow 'in the name of his dead kinsman'; as a result, the children of that union are regarded as belonging to the dead man, and the sons will carry his name. The woman is known as *ciekjooka*, the wife of a ghost, and her children are *gaatjooka*, children of a ghost. In another pattern, 'woman marriage', a barren woman 'marries' another woman and then arranges for a male kinsman or friend to make her pregnant. The children of this union become part of the 'husband's' family (who would not otherwise have any descendants); she is regarded as their legal father, they will carry her name, and sometimes they even refer to her as 'father'.

Both 'ghost marriage' and 'woman marriage' among the Nuer can be regarded as analogous to the sperm donation of IVF, though the donor, of course, is not anonymous. Ovum donation, however, was technically impossible until recent developments in reproductive technology. Overall, though, the growth of the NRTs in most Western countries is likely to result in a gradual weakening of the neat equation between biological and social parenthood, and in new definitions of family and kinship.

Contraception, abortion and infanticide

Different attitudes to contraception, abortion and infanticide, all of which can be seen as forms of population control, seem to vary widely between cultures. Part of the reason for a society practising infanticide, for example, may be the size of the population, its food supply and the particular ecological niche that it occupies. In some cases the infants of one gender may be killed, but not the other – as in the case of the Tenetehara, a Brazilian Indian tribe, who believed that a woman should have three children, but not all of the same sex; if she had two daughters (or two sons) and gave birth to a third, then the baby would be killed (see Chapter 12). Overall, as Keesing[66] notes, in the past 'there is little doubt that peoples with finite space and resources in many parts of the world practised infanticide, of both sexes or of females, so as to restrict population numbers'. Infanticide of female babies still persists in different parts of the world, especially in rural areas. The reasons for this are a complex mixture of cultural values, economic imperatives, government policy and sexist ideology. For example, Miller[67] has described female infanticide, as well as the fatal neglect of some female children, in a society with a strongly patriarchal culture in the Punjab, northern India. A similar situation has been reported for many years from parts of rural China, even before the government's current 'one-child' policy[68].

The particular 'population policy' of a culture may include a widespread tolerance of abortion, acceptance of abortion under certain limited circumstances, or strict taboos against it at any stage of pregnancy or for any reason. In the Western world, the debate on abortion centres both on whether the woman is entitled to control over her own body and fertility, and on whether the foetus is regarded as a 'person', with the same rights as other members of the society, or merely as an organ or collection of cells.

Males and pregnancy

Although pregnancy and childbirth are female events, both physically and socially, most men are deeply involved in the birth of their children. In many cultures this emotional involvement is recognized by a series of rituals that the men must carry out during their wives' pregnancy, birth and postpartum period.

Heggenhougen[69] has reviewed much of the literature on the role of fathers in the birth of their children. He points out that in most modem middle-class Western industrial cultures, the husband has only a minimal role to play – usually that of anxious spectator – in the birth of his child. Overall, the majority of human cultures exclude men from the scene of birth. However, this is not true of certain Native American, Eskimo, African and Maori groups.

Where the father is present at the birth, his presence is almost always functional, and the role and rituals that are prescribed for him are believed to be integral to the actual birth process. He has certain tasks to perform which are designed to protect mother and child and make the delivery easier, and which may be termed the *ritual couvade.* In many non-industrialized cultures he is expected to follow certain strict taboos; in Java the husband follows many of the same taboos as his wife, and supports her during labour, and this is also found in some Guatemalan communities, among the Catiguan villagers of the Philippines and in parts of northern Europe. In the Lan tsu Miao tribe of Kweichew, South China, the husband not only takes to his bed during his wife's labour, but also takes care of and 'mothers' the baby. In the Buka, Ashanti and Chickchee tribes, men perform rituals to fool evil spirits and attract their attention until the child is safely born. Among the Arapesh people of New Guinea, the verb 'to bear a child' is used indiscriminately for either man or woman, and childbearing is believed to be as heavy a drain on the man as on the woman. Among the Hopi Indians of the USA and the Chiriguano Indians of Paraguay, both husband and the last-born child go into couvade during the wife's pregnancy. In the modern Western world, largely under the influence of the women's movement and the trend towards 'natural childbirth', men tend to be more involved in their partner's pregnancy and are often present at the actual birth, but they lack the protection of a ritually prescribed role (see Chapter 9) characteristic of more traditional societies.

In many cultures, especially those where the ritual couvade is not practised, men have often been reported as suffering from physical and/or psychological symptoms during their wife's pregnancy, birth and postpartum period. This is known as the *couvade syndrome* (from the Basque word *couver,* to brood or hatch), and has been reported from many parts of the world. According to Heggenhougen[69], one can view this couvade syndrome as 'a subconscious form of participation or perhaps even competition, with the wife', while ritual couvade is 'a conscious participation, though it may have a subconscious base'.

A contemporary illustration of this syndrome, from the USA, is described in the following case history.

Case study: Couvade syndrome in Rochester, New York, USA

Lipkin and Lamb[70]carried out a study on the couvade syndrome, in Rochester, New York. They defined this syndrome as the occurrence of new physical or psychological symptoms in the mates of pregnant women, for which they sought medical care, and which were not otherwise objectively explained. In their study of 267 mates of postpartum women, 60 (22.5 per cent) of the men were found to have suffered from this syndrome. This translates to a prevalence rate of 225 of 1000 husbands at risk due to their wife's pregnancy. Many of their symptoms were vague and non-specific, such as 'feeling rundown', 'feeling lowdown' and 'weakness', as well as more 'pregnant' symptoms such as backache, genital burning, water retention (not confirmed on physical examinations), retrosternal burning, groin pain, dizziness and abdominal cramps. One patient complained of a chest pain that felt like 'something was pushing out'.

Whatever the cause, the evidence is that men are physically, as well as emotionally, deeply involved in the birth of their children. Clinicians should therefore be aware of the possibility of unexplained symptoms – both physical and psychological – in many expectant fathers.

Recommended reading

Davis-Floyd, R. E. (1992). *Birth as an American Rite of Passage*. University of California Press.

Hahn, R. A. and Muecke, M. A. (1987). The anthropology of birth in five US ethnic populations: implications for obstetrical practice. *Curr. Probl. Obstet. Gynecol. Fertil.*, **10**, 133–71.

Heggenhougen, H. K. (1980). Fathers and childbirth: an anthropological perspective. *J. Nurse-Midwifery*, **25(6)**, 21–6.

Lock, M. (1998). Menopause: lessons from anthropology. *Psychosom. Med.*, **60**, 410–19.

MacCormack, C. P. (ed.) (1982). *Ethnography of Fertility and Birth*. Tavistock.

7 Pain and culture

Pain, in one form or another, is an inseparable part of everyday life. It is probably also the commonest symptom encountered in clinical practice[1], and is a feature of many normal physiological changes such as pregnancy, childbirth, or menstruation as well as of injury and disease. Many forms of healing or diagnosis also involve some form of pain; for example, surgical operations, injections, biopsies or venesection. In all of these situations there is more to pain than merely a neurophysiological event; there are social, psychological and cultural factors associated with it that also need to be considered. In this chapter some of these factors will be examined in order to illustrate the following propositions:

1. Not all social or cultural groups may respond to pain in exactly the same way
2. How people perceive and respond to pain, both in themselves and in others, can be influenced by their cultural and social background
3. How, and whether, people communicate their pain to health professionals and to others can also be influenced by social and cultural factors.

Pain behaviour

From a physiological perspective, pain can be thought of as 'a type of signalling device for drawing attention to tissue damage or to physiological malfunction'[2]. Pain arises when a nerve or nerve ending is affected by a noxious stimulus, either from within the body or from outside it. It is therefore of crucial importance for the protection and survival of the body in an environment full of potential dangers. Because of this biological role it is sometimes assumed that pain is culture-free, in the sense of there being a universal biological reaction to a specific type of stimulus such as a sharp object or extremes of hot or cold. However, the two forms of reaction can be differentiated into:

1. An *involuntary*, instinctual reaction, such as pulling away from the sharp object
2. A *voluntary* reaction, such as
   a. removing the source of pain, and taking action to treat the symptom (by taking an aspirin, for example)
   b. asking another person for help in relieving the symptom.

Voluntary reactions to pain that involve other people are particularly influenced by social and cultural factors, and will be described below in more detail, with examples.

As Engel[3] puts it, pain thus has two components: 'the original sensation, and the reaction to the sensation'. This reaction, whether voluntary or not, has been called *pain behaviour* by Fabrega and Tyma[4], and includes certain changes in facial expression, grimaces, changes in demeanour or activity, as well as certain sounds made by the victim, or words used to describe his condition or appeal for help. It is possible, though, to exhibit pain behaviour in the absence of a painful stimulus or, conversely, not to exhibit such behaviour despite the presence of the painful stimulus. To clarify this point, it is useful to identify two types of pain behaviour or reactions to pain: *private* pain and *public* pain.

Private pain

Pain, as Engel[3] points out, is 'private data'; that is, in order for us to know whether a person is in pain we are dependent on that person signalling that fact to us, either verbally or non-verbally. When that happens, the private experience and perception of pain become a social, public event; private pain becomes public pain. Under some circumstances, however, the pain may remain private; there may be no outward clue or sign that the person is experiencing pain, even when it is very severe. This type of behaviour is common among societies that value stoicism and fortitude, such as the Anglo-Saxon 'stiff upper lip' in the presence of hardship. It is more likely to be expected of men, particularly younger men or warriors. In some cultures the ability to bear pain without flinching – that is, without displaying pain behaviour – may be one of the signs of manhood, and part of initiation rituals marking the transition from boyhood to manhood. For instance, among the Cheyenne Indians of the Great Plains, young men who wanted to display their manhood and gain social prestige would undergo ritual self-torture in the Sun Dance ceremony – for example, suspending themselves from a pole by hooks passed through the skin of their chests, and accepting the pain without complaint[5]. Other less dramatic forms of a lack of pain behaviour occur in those who are semiconscious, paralysed, or too young to articulate their distress, or in situations where such behaviour is unlikely to bring a sympathetic response from other people. Therefore, an absence of pain behaviour does not necessarily mean the absence of private pain.

Public pain

Pain behaviour, especially its voluntary aspects, is influenced by social, cultural and psychological factors. These determine *whether* private pain will be translated into pain behaviour, and the *form* that this behaviour takes, and the social settings in which it occurs.

Part of the decision about whether to translate private into public pain depends on the person's interpretation of the *significance* of the pain; whether, for example, it is seen as 'normal' or 'abnormal' pain – the latter being more likely to be brought to the attention of others. An example of normal pain is dysmenorrhoea. In two American studies quoted by Zola[6], women from both lower and upper socio-economic groups were asked to keep a calendar in which they recorded all bodily states and dysfunctions. Only a small percentage even reported the dysmenorrhoea as a 'dysfunction', and among the lower income group only 18 per cent even mentioned the menses or its accompaniments. Definitions of what constitutes an 'abnormal' pain, and which therefore requires medical attention and treatment, tend to be culturally defined, and to vary over time. As Zola notes, 'the degree of recognition and treatment of certain gynaecological problems may be traced to the prevailing definition of what constitutes the necessary part of the business of being a woman'. This in turn may be influenced by the social and economic context in which the women's lives are embedded, such as the need to care for children or carry on working despite being in pain. Other definitions of abnormal pain depend on cultural definitions of body image, and the structure and function of the body[7]. Commonly held beliefs that 'the heart' occupies the entire chest or example, may lead to an interpretation of all pains in this area as 'heart trouble' or a 'heart attack'. Elsewhere the case was described of a man with psychosomatic chest pains who clung to the idea that he had 'trouble with the heart', despite numerous diagnostic tests that excluded cardiac disease, because he still had 'pain over my heart'[8].

Zborowski[9] has pointed out that a cultural group's *expectations* and acceptance of pain as a normal part of life will determine whether it is seen as a clinical problem that requires a clinical solution. Cultures that emphasize military achievements, for example, both expect and accept battle wounds, while more peaceful cultures may expect them, but not accept them without complaint. Similarly, he notes how in Poland and in some other countries labour pains are both expected and accepted by women giving birth, while in the USA they are not accepted and analgesia is frequently demanded. These attitudes towards pain are acquired early in life, as part of growing up in a particular family and community, and are an essential part of any culture's child-rearing practices.

Although physical pain is a particularly vivid and emotionally laden symptom, it can only be understood in a cultural context by seeing it as part of the wider spectrum of *misfortune*. Pain, like illness generally, is only a special type of human suffering. As such, it can provoke the same types of questions in the victim as do other forms of misfortune: 'Why has it happened to me?', 'Why now?' or 'What have I done to deserve this?'. Where pain is seen as divine punishment for a behavioural lapse, the victims may be unwilling to seek relief for it. Experiencing the pain without complaint becomes, in itself, a form of expiation. Alternatively, they may demand more painful treatments from a physician, such as a surgical operation or an injection. If pain is seen as the result of moral transgressions, the response might also be self-imposed penitence, fasting or prayer, rather than consultation with a health professional. If interpersonal malevolence, such as sorcery, witchcraft or 'hexing' are thought to have caused a pain, the strategy for pain relief may be an indirect one – by a ritual of exorcism, for example.

In many cultures, because pain is seen as only one type of suffering within the wider spectrum of misfortune, it is *linked* with other forms of suffering in a number of ways. These include having a common cause (such as divine punishment or witchcraft), and therefore requiring a similar form of treatment (prayer, penitence or exorcism). This wider view of pain is common in non-Western societies, and members of these societies may find the secular Western treatment of pain – the prescribing of a pain-relieving drug – both incomplete and unsatisfying. Although Western medicine does acknowledge the existence of 'psychosomatic' or 'psychogenic pain', its attitude to organic pain does not take into account the social, moral and psychological elements that many people associate with pain. Nevertheless, the idiom of pain in modern English does still show linkages to other forms of suffering, including emotional distress, interpersonal conflicts and unexpected misfortune. These are often described using the metaphor of physical pain, for example 'I was sore at him', 'she hurt him deeply', 'a biting comment', 'a painful experience', 'a mere pinprick', 'it was a blow to me', 'tortured soul' and 'heartsore'. In more traditional societies, the link between physical pain and the social, moral and religious aspects of everyday life is likely to be much more direct, and to influence closely how people perceive their own ill health.

Case study: The language of pain in North Indian culture

Pugh[10] described the many meanings of pain in North Indian culture, and the metaphors used to express it. In the absence of Western mind–body dualism, neither traditional practitioners (*hakims*) nor their patients see pain (*dard*) solely in physical terms. When talking about pain, they draw on a shared reservoir of words, images and metaphors derived from local culture and everyday life. The metaphors they use (such as a 'burning', 'gripping', or 'stabbing' pain) blend together physical and emotional experiences into a single image. Thus the same word, phrase or metaphor often conveys the meaning of physical *and* psychological suffering at the same time. For example, the metaphors used for physical pain can also be used to describe certain emotional states; sadness and grief, like 'hot' foods, can make the heart 'burn', and Urdu poets describe 'the burning ache of the heart', and the 'wonderful feelings of love-pain'. Such metaphors for pain as 'hot' or 'burning' reflect, as Pugh puts it, 'the integrated mind–body system of Indian culture'. Thus 'physical pain in Indian culture incorporates psychological malaise, while emotional distress manifests itself simultaneously in both mind and body'.

Furthermore, many of the words used to describe different types of pain suggest both its cause and its probable cure. On the basis of 'like causes like', the description of 'hot' or 'burning' pains implies their causation by 'hot' or 'burning' foods, or by hot weather, or by certain 'hot' emotional states (such as anxiety or anger). Their treatment is by remedies that cause 'cooling', such as cool packs, or cold musk medicine that 'provides psychophysical relief for pain, palpitations, and anxiety by "cooling" the body's heat and "calming" the heart'.

Finally, the metaphors 'which imbue pain with its sensory qualities draw on the familiar surroundings of house, field, and workshop', and the experiences of daily life. A 'burning pain' of the stomach, chest or throat is often said to be accompanied by a 'sour' (*khatta*) or 'bitter' (*katu*) taste. Both these tastes are also found in most people's diet: sourness in limes, pomegranates and tamarind; bitterness in mustard-seed oil, certain lemons and turmeric. Thus the experience of pain, and the meanings given to that experience, are linked to many other aspects of local culture, cuisine, language and tradition. Because different types of pain, at different times, in different places, and in different parts of the body, all carry with them so many associations – physical, emotional, social, spiritual, dietary and climatic – the Western model of pain as mainly a physical event may be inappropriate. Pugh concluded that this is because North Indian cultural patterning depicts pain 'not as a single, fixed entity but rather as a fluid, context-sensitive constellation of meanings'.

The types and availability of potential healers or helpers also determine whether a person will display pain behaviour, and in what settings. For example, such behaviour is more likely to bring sympathetic help from a hospital doctor or nurse than from a punitive army sergeant. The personality and idiosyncrasies of the clinician, as well as whether they come from a similar culture and social class to the sufferer, may influence the decision to display it or not. Such behaviour may be displayed to one clinician but not to an unsympathetic colleague, leading to different evaluations of the patient's condition by the two clinicians.

A further factor determining whether private pain is made public is the perceived *intensity* of the pain sensation itself. There is some evidence that this perception (and pain tolerance) can be influenced by culture. In a review of the literature on culture and pain, Wolff and Langley[11] point out the paucity of adequately controlled experimental studies in this area. However, those studies that have been done confirm that 'cultural factors in terms of attitudinal variables, whether explicit or implicit, do indeed exert significant influences on pain perception'. Also, as Lewis[12] has noted, the intensity of a pain sensation does not follow automatically from the extent and nature of an injury. Beliefs about the meaning and significance of a pain, the context in which it occurs and the emotions associated with that context can all affect pain sensation: 'Fear of implications for the future may intensify awareness of pain in the surgical patient, or, by contrast, the hope and likely chance of escape from deadly risks of battle may diminish the injured soldier's sense of pain and his complaints, though the injury be similar in both cases'. A common example of this is soldiers who only notice that they have been wounded once the battle is over; the intensity of emotional involvement in the battle may divert attention, at least temporarily, from a painful wound. In certain states of religious trance, meditation or ecstasy, the intensity of pain perception can also be reduced, although the physiological reasons for this are not well understood. Examples of this phenomenon are the *yogis* and *fakirs* of India, or the fire-walkers of Sri Lanka, who all undergo self-inflicted pain or discomfort, apparently without experiencing the full intensity of the pain.

Attitudes and expectations of a particular healer or treatment can also influence the intensity of pain, as in placebo analgesia; here, a pharmacologically inactive drug in which the patient 'believes' causes subjective pain relief in the sufferer. Levine and colleagues[13] have suggested that the release of endorphins or endogenous opiates within the brain is the physiological mechanism underlying placebo analgesia, since it can be counteracted by the use of nalorphine. Whatever the underlying mechanism, the perception of the intensity of a pain, as well as the meanings associated with it, may influence whether a privately experienced pain is shared with other people.

The presentation of public pain

Each culture and social group, even sometimes each family, has its own unique 'language of distress'; its own complex idiom by which ill or unhappy individuals make other people aware of their suffering. There is a specific, often standardized way of signalling, both verbally and nonverbally, that they are in pain or discomfort. The *form* that this pain behaviour will take is largely culturally determined, as is the *response* to this behaviour. As Landy[14] puts it, this depends, among other factors on 'whether their culture values or disvalues the display of emotional expression and response to injury'. Some cultural groups expect an extravagant display of emotionality in the presence of pain; others value stoicism, restraint and the playing down of their symptoms. Zola[6], in his study of reactions to pain by a group of Italian-Americans and Irish-Americans, pointed out that the Italian response was marked by 'expressiveness and expansiveness', which he saw as a defence mechanism (dramatization) – a way of coping with anxiety 'by repeatedly over-expressing it and thereby dissipating it'. By contrast, the Irish tended to ignore and underplay their bodily complaints; for example, 'I ignore it like I do most things'. They tended to deny or play down the presence of pain – 'It was more a throbbing than a pain ... not really pain, it feels more like sand in my eye'. Zola sees this denial as a defence mechanism against the 'oppressive sense of guilt' that he, and other researchers, see as a feature of rural Irish culture. These two different languages of distress may have negative effects on the types of medical treatment that these patients are given, especially by clinicians from different cultural backgrounds. The Italian-Americans, for example, might be dismissed as over-emotional or hypochondriacal by a clinician who values stoicism and restraint, and the Irish-Americans might have their suffering ('private pain') ignored as they continually underplay it. Zola warns that this might perpetuate their suffering by creating a 'self-fulfilling prophecy'.

Pain behaviour may be *non-verbal*, and this too can be patterned by culture. In his study of bodily gestures, Le Barre[15] has pointed out that while gestures differ cross-culturally they can only be interpreted by taking into account the context in which they appear. For example, in the Argentine, shaking one of the hands smartly so that the fingers make an audible clacking sound, can mean 'wonderful', but also signify pain when one says '*Ai yai*' following an injury. Therefore, non-verbal languages of distress include not only gestures but also facial expressions, bodily posture and exclamations, all of which take their meaning from the context in which they appear. They may also include other changes in behaviour, such as withdrawal, fasting, prayer or recourse to self-medication. Thus, as noted in Chapter 4, different types of pain behaviour can be an intrinsic part of a non-verbal narrative of suffering – one displayed over time to family, friends or health professionals.

Because pain behaviour, whether verbal or not, is often standardized within a culture, it is open to imitation by those who wish to get sympathy or attract attention, by displaying public pain without any underlying private pain. Examples of this are the hypochondriac, the malingerer and the actor. People with Munchausen's syndrome, for example, may exactly mimic real pain behaviour and therefore undergo repeated surgical operations or investigations before being discovered[16]. Pain behaviour may also mask an underlying psychological state, such as an extreme anxiety state or depression, as in somatization (see Chapter 10). In this case, the primary symptom complained of will not be anxiety or depression, but rather physical symptoms such as weakness, breathlessness, sweating or vague aches and pains. This type of somatization is said to be more common among low-income groups in the Western world; however, it is also a feature of many other higher socio-economic groups, as well as of other cultures world-wide. For example, in Taiwan the open display of emotional distress is not encouraged; instead this state is usually expressed in a mainly somatic or physical language of distress. Kleinman[17] notes that in Taiwan, Chinese culture 'defines the somatic complaint as *the* primary illness problem', even if psychological symptoms are also present. In one period, 70 per cent of the patients who visited the Psychiatry Clinic at the National Taiwan University Hospital initially complained of physical symptoms[17]. In this and other cultures, a depressed person may complain of vague fleeting pains, or 'pains everywhere', for which no physical cause can be found. Just as culture can influence somatization, so can the personality and background of the clinician. A doctor orientated towards purely physical explanations of ill health, for example, may only acknowledge somatic symptoms, in contrast to a colleague more interested in psychodynamic or social processes.

How pain is described is influenced by a number of factors, including language facility, familiarity with medical terms, individual experiences of pain, and lay beliefs about the structure and function of the body (seen in the 'glove-and-stocking' distribution of hysterical pain or anaesthesia). The use of technical terms borrowed from medicine to describe a pain may also confuse the clinician; the person who says, 'I've had another migraine, doctor', may be using the term to describe a wide variety of head pains, not only migraine. The cues from clinicians that help shape a diffuse, especially psychosomatic, pain into a recognizable medical form, are questions like: 'Does it travel down your left arm?', 'Does it come on when you climb stairs?' or 'Does it feel like a tight band across your chest?'. Medical history-taking, examinations, diagnostic tests and health education campaigns may all unwittingly train patients to identify and describe the characteristic form of a particular type of pain, such as angina, colic or migraine[8]. Clinicians should therefore be aware of this process and the difficulties it poses for reliable diagnosis.

Social aspects of pain

Public pain implies a *social* relationship, of whatever duration, between the sufferer and another person or persons. The nature of this relationship will determine whether the pain is revealed in the first place, how it is revealed, and the nature of the response to it. Lewis[12] notes how the *expectations* of sufferers are important here, particularly the likely response to their pain and the social costs and benefits of revealing it: 'Possibilities of care, of sympathy, the allocation of responsibility for sickness in others, affect how people show their illness'. People will receive maximum attention and sympathy if their pain behaviour matches the society's view of how people in pain should draw attention to their suffering, whether by an extravagant display of emotions or by a quiet change in behaviour. As Zola[6] puts it, 'It is the "fit" of certain signs with a society's major values which accounts for the degree of attention they receive'. There is thus a dynamic between the individual and society (illustrated in Figure 7.1) whereby pain behaviour, and the reactions to it, influence each other over time.

The types of permissible pain behaviour within a society are learned in childhood and infancy. Engel[3] points out that pain plays an important role in the total psychological development of the individual: 'It is ... intimately concerned with learning about the environment and its dangers .... and about the body and its limitations'. It is integral to all early relationships: in infancy, pain leads to crying, which leads to a response from the mother or another person. In early childhood, pain and punishment become linked; the adult world inflicts pain for 'bad' behaviour. Pain may therefore signal to the individual that he or she is 'bad', and therefore should feel guilty; it may too become an important medium for the expiation of guilt. Pain is also part of relationships of aggression and power, and of sexual relationships. Engel has described the 'pain-prone patient' who is particularly liable to 'psychogenic pain', and whose personality is characterized by strong feelings of guilt. In his view, this patient is more likely to complain of pains of one sort or another as a means of self-punishment and atonement; penitence, self-denial and self-deprecation may all be used as forms of self-inflicted punishments to ease the feelings of guilt. One could hypothesize that cultures characterized by a pervasive sense of guilt are also those that value 'painful' rituals of atonement and prayer, including fasting, abstinence, isolation, poverty and even self-flagellation.

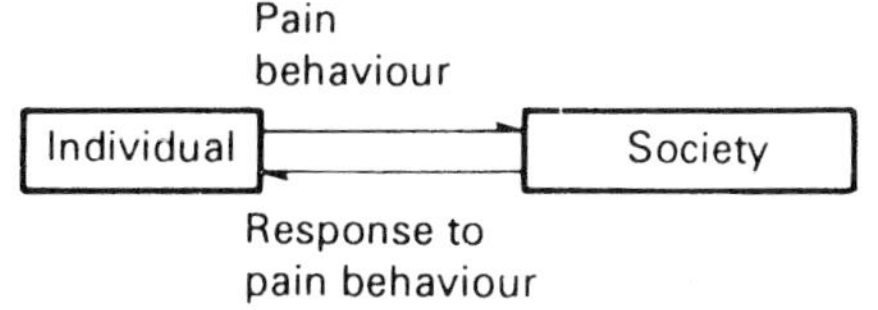

Figure 7.1 Pain behaviour relationship between the individual and society

Child-rearing practices help shape attitudes towards and expectations of pain later in life – particularly, as Zborowski[9] notes, the cultural values and attitudes of parents, parent-substitutes, siblings and peer groups. In his 1952 study described below, a group of Jewish-American and Italian-American parents manifested 'over-protective and over-concerned attitudes towards the child's health, participation in sports, games, fights, etc.'. The child was often reminded to avoid colds, injuries, fights and other threatening situations. Crying in complaint was quickly responded to with sympathy and concern. In Zborowski's view, the parents thereby fostered an over-awareness of pain and other deviations from normal, as well as anxiety about their possible significance. By contrast, 'Old American' Protestant families were less overprotective; the child was told 'not to run to mother with every little thing', to expect pain in sports and games, and not to react in too emotional a way to them. All these culturally defined languages of distress will influence how private pain is signalled to others, and the types of reaction expected from them. Problems might arise, however, if the sufferer and those around them have different cultural origins, or come from different social classes, with different expectations of how a person in pain should behave and how they should be treated.

In some cultural groups, individual sufferers are encouraged to turn their private pain into public pain within a ritual context of healing. This is seen in some of the public rites of healing in Africa and Latin America, described in Chapter 4, but is also true of some religious groups in the West where, in a ritual setting, pain becomes a means of personal and spiritual transformation. Skultans[18], for example, describes how women in a Welsh Spiritualist church are encouraged to share their painful symptoms with one another, and to each become 'possessed' by the pain of an ill member, thus helping to lessen her private pain by sharing it amongst themselves. Similarly, Csordas[19] describes how a healer in the Catholic Charismatic Renewal movement in the USA often 'embodies' the pain of a sufferer, as part of the ritual of diagnosis and healing. For example, an intense pain in the healer's heart means a 'heart healing' is taking place in the patient, while the healer may detect headache or backache in a supplicant 'through the experience of a similar pain during the healing process'. McGuire[20], in her study of ritual healing in suburban USA, describes how some Episcopalian communities see pain as a *positive* phenomenon, a type of lesson by which they can learn more about life and come closer to God. 'You ask the Lord what you're supposed to learn from this', one woman said, while another commented: 'Pain and illness aren't the end. You wouldn't know goodness and joy, if you hadn't experienced pain'. Members of some Eastern meditation groups also see pain as a potentially useful lesson or message to the individual. As one yoga adherent explained: 'Pain is your body's way of saying, "Hey, something's wrong, do something about it, don't block it out". It can be a way of turning your life around'. On a more individual level, the psychoanalyst McDougall[21] has described several cases of severe psychosomatic disorders where the experience of pain or other discomfort can play an important psychological role in reassuring certain patients, reminding them of their personal identity, the borders of their body, or even of their own existence. As she puts it: 'A body that suffers is also a body that is alive.'

Chronic pain

One particular type of pain, chronic pain, poses unique problems for the sufferers and for those around them. As Brodwin[22] points out, chronic pain is truly a 'private disorder'. Unlike acute pain, which begins suddenly and lasts a short time only, the 'visibility' of chronic pain to other people tends to disappear over time, despite the individual's continued suffering. 'Even when it begins with a traumatic accident or major illness, it continues long after these events have faded from people's memory'. Often few visual clues, such as a bruise, bandage, scar, or plaster cast, remain to remind family or friends of the pain and how it originally began. Brodwin[22] describes how in this situation chronic pain sufferers may evolve ways of displaying their private pain in a public performance to those around them, in order to get help and attention. Within families, particularly, their recurrent 'rhetoric of pain' may become an integral part of the family dynamics. It can also apply in relations with their employers and co-workers, since 'this rhetoric helps chronic pain sufferers communicate their wants and needs in crucial social relationships, especially when the use of other languages is not sanctioned'.

Chronic pain is often intimately linked with social and psychological problems. Interpersonal tensions, for example, may cause someone to develop chronic pain, and *vice versa.* In many families and cultural groups, a 'performance' of pain may be the only way of signalling personal distress, whatever its cause. This is an example of somatization (see Chapter 10), and may take many forms, from 'pain everywhere' to recurrent pain in a particular organ or body part. As Kleinman and colleagues[23] put it, 'Depression and anxiety, serious family tensions, conflicted work relationships – all conduce to the onset of or exacerbation of chronic pain conditions and, in turn, may be worsened by chronic pain'.

Case study: Cultural components of pain in New York, USA

Zborowski[9], in 1952, examined the cultural components of the experience of pain among three groups of patients at a veterans' hospital in New York City: Italian-Americans, Jewish-Americans and mainly Protestant 'Old Americans'. Marked differences in pain behaviour and in attitudes towards pain were found between the groups. Both Italian-Americans and Jewish-Americans tended to be more emotional in response to pain and to exaggerate their pain experience, leading some of the doctors to conclude, quite wrongly, that they had a lower threshold of pain than other groups. However, this emotional display, although similar in the two groups, was based on different attitudes towards pain.

The Italians were mainly concerned with the immediacy of the pain experience, especially the pain sensation itself. They complained a great deal, drawing attention to their suffering by groaning, moaning, crying and so on, but once they were given analgesics, and the pain wore off, they quickly forgot their suffering and returned to normal behaviour. The anxieties of the Italian patients had centred on the effects of the experience upon their immediate situation, such as occupation and economic situation. By contrast, Jewish patients were mainly concerned with the meaning and significance of the pain 'in relation to their health, welfare and, eventually, for the welfare of the families'. Their anxieties were concentrated on the implications for the future of the pain experience. Several of the Jewish patients were reluctant to accept analgesia, as they were anxious about its side effects and concerned that the drug only treated the pain and not the underlying disease. Even after the pain was relieved, many continued to display the same depressed and worried behaviour 'because they felt that though the pain was currently absent it may recur as long as the disease was not cured completely'. Some also tended to over-exaggerate their physical symptoms, not as an indication of the amount of pain experienced but as a means of ensuring that the pathological causes of the pain would be adequately taken care of. By contrast, the Italians seemed more trusting that the doctor would acknowledge their pain and take steps to relieve it; their emotional display was designed to mobilize efforts towards relieving the immediate pain sensation.

From these data, Zborowski concluded that:

1. 'Similar reactions to pain manifested by members of different ethnocultural groups do not necessarily reflect similar attitudes to pain'
2. 'Reactive patterns similar in terms of their manifestations may have different functions and serve different purposes in various cultures'.

By contrast to these two groups, the 'Old Americans' – those who had been Americanized for several generations – tended to be less emotional in reporting pain, and to adopt a detached air in describing their pain, its character, duration and location. They saw no point in over-exaggerating their pain, because 'it won't help anybody'. Withdrawal from society was a common reaction to severe pain. This group often had a more idealized picture of how a person should react to pain, and what the appropriate American response should be. As one patient put it, 'I react like a good American'. In hospital, they tended to avoid being a 'nuisance' and to cooperate closely with the ward staff (who also often had 'Old American' attitudes). Like the Jewish-Americans, their anxiety was future-orientated, though they tended to be more optimistic. They were more positive towards hospitalization – unlike the other two groups, who were 'disturbed by the impersonal character of the hospital and by the necessity of being treated there instead of at home'.

Although this study was one of the first to indicate how pain behaviour and cultural background may be related, many of its findings are no longer relevant to patient populations in the USA from any of these cultural or religious backgrounds. Furthermore, Zborowski[9] himself emphasized that these variations in pain behaviour between different groups of Americans have tended to disappear over time: 'the further is the individual from the immigrant generation the more American is his behaviour'. Kleinman and colleagues[23] have therefore warned of the dangers of using ethnic stereotypes in understanding how and why different individuals respond to pain. They emphasize the need to understand and to empathize with 'the peculiar qualities of the sting and throb of pain affecting a particular person – with a unique story, living in a certain community and historical period, and above all with fears, longings, aspirations'.

Thus, although health professionals should be aware of cultural influences when evaluating people in pain, each case should always be assessed individually and generalizations or the use of stereotypes avoided in predicting how a person from a particular social, cultural or religious background will respond to being in pain.

Recommended reading

Engel, G. L. (1950). 'Psychogenic' pain and the pain-prone patient. *Am. J. Med.*, **26**, 899–909.

Good, M. D., Brodwin, P. E., Good, B. J. and Kleinman, A. (eds) (1992). *Pain and Human Experience: An Anthropological Perspective.* University of California Press.

Pugh, J. F. (1991). The semantics of pain in Indian culture and medicine. *Cult. Med. Psychiatry*, **15**, 19–43.

Wolff, B. B. and Langley, S. (1977). Cultural factors and the responses to pain. In: *Culture, Disease, and Healing: Studies in Medical Anthropology* (D. Landy, ed.), pp. 313–19. Macmillan.

8 Culture and pharmacology

In many cases, the effect of a medication on human physiology and emotional state does not depend solely on its pharmacological properties. A number of other factors, such as personality, social or cultural backgrounds, can either enhance or reduce this effect, and are responsible for the wide variability in people's response to medication. This chapter examines some of these *non*-pharmacological influences, in relation to placebos, psychotropic and narcotic drugs, alcohol and tobacco.

The 'total drug effect'

Claridge[1] has pointed out that the effect of any medication on an individual (its 'total drug effect') depends on a number of elements *in addition* to its pharmacological properties. These are:

1. The attributes of the *drug* itself (such as taste, shape, colour, name)
2. The attributes of the *recipient* of the drug (such as their age, experience, education, personality, socio-cultural background)
3. The attributes of the *prescriber* or supplier of the drug (such as their personality, age, attitude, professional status, or sense of authority)
4. The physical *setting* in which the drug is prescribed or administered – the 'drug situation' (such as doctor's office, a hospital ward, a laboratory, or a social occasion).

To extend this model a step further, the physical setting of drug can be termed the *micro-context*, which can be differentiated from what can be called the *macro-context*. This is the whole social, cultural, political and economic milieu in which use of the drug takes place, and includes:

- the moral and cultural values attached to it, which either encourage or forbid its use
- the prevailing socio-economic climate, such as levels of poverty or unemployment
- the role of economic forces in producing, advertising and selling the drug
- the social grouping in which drug use actually takes place – such as a family, group of friends, members of a healing cult, or even a sub-culture of heroin addicts.

In each case of drug use (and irrespective of what the drug is), the cultural values and economic realities of the macro-context will always, to some extent, impinge on the micro-context. For example, they may help validate a particular type or appearance of drug, a particular way of using it, or the attributes of the individual who actually supplies it (such as a doctor or nurse).

Thus Claridge's model, which originally dealt mainly with medically prescribed drugs or placebos, can be extended to include all forms of drug use. It can be applied equally to the analysis of the placebo and nocebo effects, and to the use of psychotropic drugs or hard drugs, recreational drugs such as alcohol and tobacco, and the hallucinogenic drugs used by certain religious and cultural groups. Based partly on Claridge's model, Figure 8.1 summarizes all the *non*-pharmacological influences on the use of any particular drug, whether medically prescribed or not.

Because the 'total drug effect' is thus dependent on the mix of these many influences in any particular case, there can be wide variation in how different people respond to the same drug or medication. In the case of very powerful

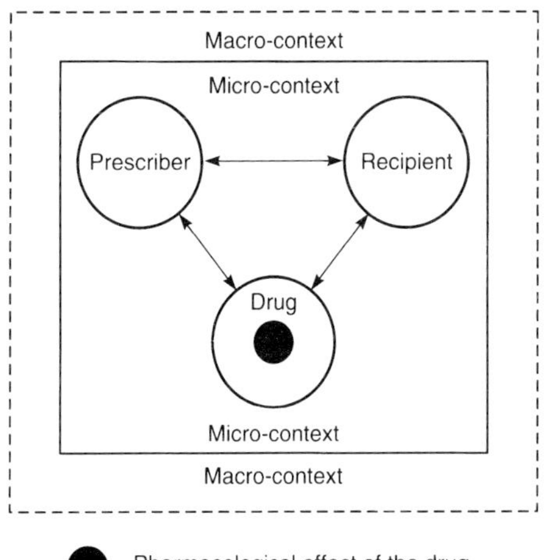

Figure 8.1 The 'total drug effect'

drugs, though, such as certain poisons, the effect is entirely due to its pharmacological actions.

The placebo effect

The placebo effect can be understood as the 'total drug effect', but *without* the presence of a drug. Much research has been carried out in recent years into this phenomenon. This research, carried out mainly in medical settings, has also shed light on other phenomena such as drug addiction and habituation, alcoholism and the therapeutic effects of healing rituals in many cultures. In the medical literature, placebos are often viewed merely as pharmacologically inert substances administered as part of a double-blind trial of a new drug. Other writers have pointed out that the placebo effect is much wider than this. Wolf[2], for example, defines it as 'any effect attributable to a pill, potion or procedure, but not its pharmacodynamic or specific properties'. For Shapiro[3] it is 'the psychological, physiological or psychophysiological effect of any medication or procedure given with therapeutic intent, which is independent of or minimally related to the pharmacologic effects of the medication or to the specific effects of the procedure, and which operates through a psychological mechanism'. It is therefore the *belief* of those receiving (and/or administering) a placebo substance or procedure in the *efficacy* of that placebo or procedure that can have both psychological and physiological effects.

In one review of the literature, Benson and Epstein[4] point out that placebos may affect practically any organ system in the body. Placebos have been reported to provide relief in a variety of conditions, including angina pectoris, rheumatoid and degenerative arthritis, pain, hay fever, headache, cough, peptic ulcer and essential hypertension. Their psychological effects include the relief of anxiety, depression and even schizophrenia.

Other studies indicate that, depending on people's expectations, placebos can even cause side effects (such as drowsiness)[5] or psychological dependence on them[5]. Both these phenomena are examples of the *nocebo* effect; that is, the negative effects on health of belief and expectations (see Chapter 11). Hahn[6] points out that 'beliefs can make us sick as well as healthy'. In his comprehensive review of the subject, he cites numerous studies that show that a patient's negative expectations of a particular medical treatment or procedure can seriously affect many aspects of their mental and physical health.

While the power of the placebo effect has been widely reported, its exact mechanism is still not clearly understood. Some attempt, though, has been made to explain placebo analgesia from a scientific perspective. In a study by Levine and colleagues[7], for example, post-operative dental pain was relieved by placebos, but this effect disappeared when the patients were given naloxone. It was hypothesized that placebo analgesia was mediated by endogenous opiates, or endorphins, whose effect was counteracted by the naloxone. Other physiological effects of placebos are still being investigated.

For the placebo effect to occur, a certain atmosphere or setting is required. Placebos, whether medications or procedures, are generally *culture-bound*; that is, they are administered within a specific social and cultural setting that validates both the placebo and the person administering it. Placebos that work in one cultural group or context may not, therefore, have any effect in another.

According to Adler and Hammett[8], the placebo effect is an essential component in *all* forms of healing, and from a wider perspective it is an important component of everyday life. They see all forms of therapy, cross-culturally, as having two characteristics:

1. Participation by all those taking part (patient, healer, spectators) in a shared cognitive system
2. Access to a relationship with a culturally sanctioned parental figure (the healer).

The shared cognitive system refers to the cultural world-view of the group – how they perceive, interpret and understand reality, especially the occurrence of ill health and other misfortunes.

In some societies this world-view is rationalistic, in others it is more religious or mystical. In either case, the perspective on ill health is part of their wider view of how the world operates or how things 'hang together'. This world-view 'enables man to locate himself spatially and historically', and 'provides a conceptual–perceptual structure beyond the limits of which few men transgress even in imagination'. This cognitive system, shared with other members of one's culture or society, makes the chaos of life (and of ill health) understandable, and gives a sense of security and *meaning* to people's lives.

The other component of the placebo effect is the emotional dependence of members of society on prominent people, such as healers. Whatever their form, sacred or secular, the healers occupy a social niche of respect, reverence and influence comparable with the parental role. The therapeutic potency of this relationship is probably due to 'a reactivation of the feelings of basic trust adherent to the original mother–infant dyad'. In Adler and Hammett's view[8], both these aspects 'are the necessary and sufficient components of the placebo effect'; what people take from a placebo may be what they need from life – a sense of meaning and security derived from membership of a group with a shared world-view, and a relationship with a caring, parental-type authority figure. Both these aspects are also part of Western healing rituals, such as the doctor–patient consultation, and of most forms of symbolic healing (see Chapter 10).

All medications prescribed in this specialized setting are likely to have some placebo effect. In Joyce's[9] view, there is a placebo or symbolic element in *all* drugs prescribed by doctors, whether they are pharmacologically active or not. He estimates that nearly one in five of all prescriptions written by general practitioners in the UK are for their placebo or symbolic functions, and that there are at least 500 000 people in the UK who each year are 'symbol-dependent' patients. In his view, any drug given for more than 2 years has a large symbolic component for the individual taking it. Any drug prescribed by a doctor can be seen as a 'multi-vocal' symbol, having a range of meanings for the individual patient. Some of these are discussed below, in the section on drug dependence.

The placebo effect of the drug itself has been studied by several researchers. For example, Schapira and colleagues[10] studied the effect of the *colour* of drugs used for treating anxiety in 48 patients at a psychiatric outpatient department. It was found that anxiety symptoms and phobic symptoms seemed to respond best to green tablets, while depressive symptoms responded best to yellow. The yellow tablets were least preferred by patients for alleviating their anxiety. The authors conclude that one 'cannot ignore any ancillary factor which might enhance the response of patients to drug treatment'. In another study, by Branthwaite and Cooper[11], self-prescribed analgesic tablets used for headaches were found to vary in their effectiveness, depending on whether the analgesic was labelled as a well-known, widely marketed proprietary analgesic. Patients found these branded or labelled analgesics much more effective in relieving headaches than unbranded forms of the same drug. The *brand name* can be seen as having a symbolic aspect for those that take it, and to stand for a drug with a general reputation for efficiency over many years. Another example of the potency of branded drugs in the eyes of their users was shown by Jefferys and colleagues[12] in their study of self-medication on an English working-class housing estate. Aspirins were found to be widely used for a range of complaints, including insomnia, anxiety and 'nerves'. In the author's study[13] of a group of long-term users of psychotropic drugs, 36 per cent said they would take a proprietary analgesic (such as Aspro, Panadol or Veganin) for the relief of insomnia or anxiety if their psychotropic was withdrawn or unobtainable. Colour and name are not the only attributes of a drug that may influence its effect: size, taste, texture and overall appearance should also be considered. This applies as much to coffee, tea, alcohol, cigarettes and 'hard drugs' as to conventional medications.

The attributes of the *patient* receiving the drug can also influence the placebo response. Among these are, as Claridge[14] puts it, the patient's 'attitude towards and knowledge of drugs, [and] what he has been told about the particular drug he is taking'. Also relevant is whether he is part of the same shared cognitive system as the prescriber, and certain traits of his personality. Various attempts have been made to define a 'placebo type' of personality, who is more likely to show this response. Among the attributes mentioned are over-anxiety, emotional dependency, immaturity, poor personal relationships and low self-esteem. As Adler and Hammett have noted above, the placebo may supply some of what is lacking in their lives; a sense of meaning, security, belonging and a caring relationship with a 'parental' prescriber. One should note, however, that *all* ill people display some of these characteristics to a lesser or greater extent, especially in the presence of severe illness. This sense of anxiety, vulnerability and dependence may enhance the placebo effect in a ritual of healing.

The characteristics of the *prescriber* or healer are crucial to the placebo effect, especially if their healing role is validated by their society. This validation is likely to be displayed by the use of certain ritual symbols, such as a white coat, stethoscope or prescription pad. By manipulating these potent symbols in a healing context, the prescriber is both expressing and reaffirming certain basic values of the society, and enhancing a feeling of security and continuity on which the placebo effect depends (see Chapter 9). Their age, appearance, clothing, manner and air of authority are also relevant here, as are their own beliefs and expectations of the drug or procedure. As Claridge points out, the authority of the prescriber can also be used to manipulate *how* people respond to a particular drug: 'Deliberately manipulating the individual subject's motives or expectations is one way ... in which drug effects can be enhanced, diminished or reversed'[15].

Rapport, mutual confidence and understanding between prescriber and patient also contribute to the placebo effect. For this effect to be maximized there must be a congruence between the doctor's approach to therapy and the patient's attitudes towards illness and expectations from treatment. This atmosphere of prescribing is complemented by the social environment (the 'micro-context') in which *ingestion* of the medication actually takes place. The patient's perception of other people's behaviour with whom they are interacting may affect their response to the drug. This type of response is more clearly seen in the public healing rituals of some small-scale non-Western societies, where the patient is surrounded by a crowd of friends and relatives who share expectations of the treatment's efficacy. However, even in a Western setting the experience and expectation of a patient's family and friends of a particular drug (or doctor) may influence the degree of the placebo response.

The placebo effect is also intrinsic to the effect of recreational drugs, such as tobacco, alcohol or hard drugs. In these settings, the attributes of the 'prescriber' – whether waiter, barmaid or drug dealer – are likely also to contribute some influence to the total drug effect, as is the atmosphere in which ingestion takes place, whether it is a restaurant, café, bar, pub or addicts' 'shooting gallery'.

In summary, the placebo effect may be seen with either pharmacologically inactive *or* active preparations, though its effects have been more vividly described with the former. It is also a feature of double-blind trials of new drugs, where about one-third of the sample usually respond to a placebo. It is fashionable for some doctors, trained to look only for physiological data and to explain the reasons for every physical change, to dismiss this phenomenon as only 'the placebo effect' (and therefore not *real* medicine). This is in marked contrast to most folk healers in non-industrialized countries (and to many alternative healers in the West), who see the placebo effect as an ally, not an enemy, in any successful treatment.

It should therefore be noted that the therapeutic effects of belief, expectations and a good healer–patient relationship have been utilized by healers in every human culture, in all parts of the world, and throughout human history.

Case study: Placebo effect in angina pectoris

The placebo effect depends on the beliefs and expectations of physicians, as well as those of patients. This was illustrated in a study by Benson and McCallie[16] of the effectiveness of various types of therapy for angina pectoris. Many of these have been tried, only to be abandoned later on. They include heart muscle extract, various hormones, X-irradiation, anticoagulants, monoamine oxidase inhibitors, thyroidectomies, radioactive iodine, sympathectomies and many other treatments. When each of these has been introduced, their proponents (or 'enthusiasts') have reported remarkable successes in their initial trials of treatment. Most of these non-blind or single-blind trials fail to control the strong placebo effect evoked by the investigators' expectations of success. Later, when more controlled trials are done by 'sceptics' (more sceptical investigators who operate under circumstances that minimize the placebo effect), the therapy is found to be no better than inert, control placebos. Quantitatively, there is a consistent pattern of a 70–90 per cent success reported initially by the enthusiasts, which is reduced in the sceptics trial to 30–40 per cent baseline placebo effectiveness. This 30 per cent, as already mentioned, is the usual proportion of placebo types in a group, or the degree of placebo effect from any drug or procedure.

continued

Benson and McCallie analysed the results of five erstwhile treatments for angina pectoris, all of which 'are now believed to have no specific physiologic efficacy, yet at one time all were found to be effective and were used extensively'. These were the xanthines, khellin, vitamin E, ligation of the internal mammary artery, and implantation of this artery. Vitamin E, for example, was introduced as a therapy for angina in 1946. Initial enthusiastic reports noted that 90 per cent of 84 patients benefited from several months' treatment with it. Over the years, several more trials were carried out which found a gradually reduced level of effectiveness. By the 1970s, controlled trials were showing it to be no better than placebo pills. That is, 'the discrepancy between the results of advocates and sceptics may be attributed, in part, to the greater degree of placebo effect evoked by the enthusiasts'. More than 80 per cent of patients initially reported subjective improvement in symptoms, from any of these five treatments. There were also objective improvements, such as increased exercise tolerance, reduced nitroglycerin usage and improved electrocardiograph results. In some cases these lasted up to 1 year.

The authors pointed out that 'the placebo effect will most likely persist as long as the psychologic context in which it was evoked remains unchanged. Patient and physician belief in the efficacy of the therapy and a continuously strong physician–patient relation should maintain the effects for long periods'. This can even occur in the presence of angiographically verified coronary-artery disease. They also point out that the history of angina treatments demonstrates that the advent of a 'new' procedure may impair the effectiveness of an old one, and that the expectation of better results transfers the placebo effect to the new procedure. In conclusion, they quote Trousseau's remark that: 'You should treat as many patients as possible with the new drugs while they still have the power to heal'.

Drug dependence and addiction

Drug dependence

Psychological dependence on drugs has been defined by Lader[17] as:

> The need the patient experiences for the psychological effects of a drug. This need can be of two types. The patient may crave the drug-induced symptoms or changes in mood – a feeling of euphoria or a lessening of tension, for example. Or the patient may take the drug to stave off the symptoms of withdrawal.

Both personality and socio-cultural factors are as important as the pharmacology of the drug used, in both psychological dependence and physical addiction. In some cases the pharmacology can be irrelevant, as in psychological dependence on a placebo, or on a drug taken for years that no longer has a significant physical effect. In understanding these phenomena, the social and cultural contexts in which drugs are prescribed, administered or taken – all of which contribute to the total drug effect – need to be taken into account.

Some of these factors have been examined in the case of psychotropic drugs, such as tranquillizers and sleeping tablets. From the early 1960s onwards, these drugs formed the single largest group of drugs prescribed each year in the Western world. Recently their numbers have begun to decrease, while prescriptions for antidepressants, such as Prozac (fluoxetine), have greatly increased. In the UK from 1965 to 1970, prescriptions for tranquillizers increased by 59 per cent and for non-barbiturate hypnotics by 145 per cent[18]. In 1972, 45.3 million prescriptions for psychotropics were issued by NHS general practitioners in England alone (17.7 per cent of the total number of prescriptions)[19]. In the USA in the 1970s, benzodiazepine psychotropics were the most commonly prescribed drugs[20], and in 1973 it was estimated that prescriptions for one of these, diazepam (Valium), was increasing at a rate of 7 million annually[21]. Ever since 1987, when Prozac was first launched, its popularity has risen throughout the industrialized world. By 1990 it was the drug most commonly prescribed by psychiatrists in the USA, and by 1994 it was the second most commonly prescribed drug in the world (after Zantac)[22].

Many psychotropic drugs are given by regular repeat prescriptions or 'refills', and are taken for many years. In Parish's[23] study in Birmingham, 14.9 per cent of the patient sample had taken psychotropics regularly for 1 year or more, and 4.9 per cent for 5 years or more. Yet Williams[24], of the Institute of Psychiatry in London, quotes studies showing that most hypnotics lose their 'sleep-promoting properties' within 3–14 days of continuous use by the patient, and that there was little convincing evidence that benzodiazepines were effective in the treatment of anxiety after 4 months' continuous treatment. It would therefore seem that many people are taking psychotropics for reasons other than their pharmacological effect. The symbolic *meaning* of the drug for the individual taking it is an important component of the phenomenon of psychological dependence.

Both the psychotropic drug and the prescription for it can be viewed as 'multi-vocal' ritual symbols (see Chapter 9), the power of which is conferred in the ritual of prescribing, and which signify many different things for the patient and for those around them. Ostensibly the drug is meant to have a particular physical effect (its 'manifest function'), but it may have other dimensions of meaning ('latent functions') for those ingesting it. It may symbolize, for example, that the person is ill; that all personal failures are due to this illness (or to the drug's side-effects); that they deserve sympathy and attention from family and friends; that the doctor – a powerful, respected, healing figure – is still interested in them; and that modern science (which produced the drug) is powerful, reliable and efficient. Smith[25], in reviewing the literature on this subject, lists 27 of these latent functions, as well as seven more manifest ones. Perhaps most importantly, the drug carries with it some of the healing attributes of the doctor who prescribed it.

Psychotropic drug use is embedded in a matrix of *social* values and expectations – a crucial part of the 'macro-context'. In this setting, the drug can be used to improve social relationships by bringing one's behaviour (and emotions) into conformity with an idealized model of 'normal' behaviour. In the author's study[13] of 50 long-term users of psychotropics, for example, the drugs were often taken for their believed effect on relationships with others. With the drug, the patient was 'normal', self-controlled, good to live with, nurturing, non-complaining, sociable and assertive. Without it the opposite would occur, with damaging effects on their relationships. Without the drug, 'I'd be nervy, impatient with other people', 'I'd be nasty, jumpy, not nice to live with', 'I wouldn't want to see people', 'I couldn't help those I love'.

At a study at the Addiction Research Foundation in Toronto carried out by Cooperstock and Lennard[26], the findings were similar. Tranquillizers were taken as an 'aid in the maintenance of a nurturing, caring role', especially by women in role conflicts between work and home. Men saw tranquillizers particularly 'as a means of controlling somatic symptoms in order to perform their occupational role'. In both these studies, psychotropic drugs were seen as a means (both pharmacological and symbolic) of meeting social expectations, whether at work or within the family. These expectations include the culture's view of what constitutes 'normal', acceptable behaviour, and how this is to be attained. Several authors have pointed out that in Western industrialized society there is widespread social support for what Pellegrino[27] terms 'chemical coping' – that is, the regular use of medications (including alcohol, tobacco and psychotropics) to improve one's emotional state and social relationships and help one to conform to societal norms. Warburton[28] has called this phenomenon 'the chemical road to success'.

Social acceptance of psychotropic drug-taking as a normal part of life can lessen the stigma of psychological dependence on them. In the author's study[13], for example, 72 per cent of the sample knew of another person taking the same drug, and 88 per cent were known by others to be taking a psychotropic. Only 18 per cent reported disapproval by others, 10 per cent reported approval and 29 per cent said that those who knew they took the drug did not care either way. In this sample, at least, psychotropic drug ingestion took place openly, and in the absence of any major moral disapproval. This climate of acceptance makes possible 'fashions' in drug taking, and facilitates the exchange of drugs between people. In Warburton's[28] study in Reading, England, 68 per cent of young adults interviewed admitted receiving psychotropics from friends or relatives.

This 'normalization' of drugs, as part of the macro-context of Western culture, is illustrated by lay beliefs about what is, and what is not, 'a drug'. In Jones's [29] study, for example, while 80 per cent of patients interviewed agreed that heroin was 'a drug', only 50 per cent classified morphine, sleeping tablets and tranquillizers as such, while only one-third saw aspirin as a drug. While 84 per cent of patients in the author's study[13] saw psychotropics as 'drugs', they were at pains to point out that they were *not* powerful or 'hard' drugs – that is, something they had little control over, and which interfered with consciousness: 'It's just a calmer, a help. I can cut it off when I want to', and 'It's soft, sweet. It's different. It's softer' (than other drugs).

The social values that support this normalization may partly be *learned* from doctors, who in turn may be influenced by colleagues, and by the advertising of the pharmaceutical industry.

Parish[23] has suggested that in prescribing these drugs for personal problems, doctors are communicating a model on how to deal with these problems, not by confronting them but by taking a drug. The issuing of repeat prescriptions or 'refills' can also be interpreted by patients as tacit approval of psychological dependence. People's experiences of taking psychotropics with medical sanction can have cumulative effects. As Joyce pointed out, 'People who have had one favourable outcome from drug treatment will more probably experience such an outcome on subsequent occasions as well', and this can lay the foundations for future dependence. In Tyrer's[30] view, this dependence on psychotropics is more likely if the drug is prescribed in a fixed dosage regimen (where it becomes a fixed point around which the day is organized), and for a long period of time.

The 'chemical road to success'

Overall, the widespread acceptance in Western, industrialized society of the 'chemical road to success', and the growing use of 'chemical comforters' (whether legal or illegal), means that in Western society the cultural formula for 'success' has become:

Individual + Chemical = Success

where 'success' can be defined in mental, physical, social, sexual or economic terms. The 'chemical comforters' used range from vitamins, nutriceuticals, tea, coffee, tobacco and tranquillizers through to alcohol, marijuana, cocaine, heroin, and the newer 'designer drugs' such as Ecstasy. This formula, and the pursuit of the 'success', can increasingly be applied to many different aspects of modern life. These include personal life, relationships, marriage, work activities, leisure pursuits and even sport – where the use of anabolic steroids as 'performance-enhancing drugs', is increasingly common in international competitions[31]. Increasingly, the definition of 'success' now also seems to include the absence of any anxiety, worry, guilt, anger and grief – emotions that were considered to be a normal part of human life in all previous generations.

Drug addiction

In *physical dependence*, or *addiction*, social and cultural factors also play an important role. Claridge[32] pointed out that the distinction between psychological and physical dependence may be more theoretical than real: 'Medically recognized addiction is only the pathological end-part of a continuum of drug-taking that involves us all. Even the most upright of citizens have their chemical comforters, most of which are psychologically harmless when taken in small quantities'. These 'chemical comforters' include tea, coffee, tobacco, psychotropic drugs and, of course, alcohol. Cultures differ on what particular comforter is most commonly used, and under what circumstances, and there are usually tacit rules controlling their use. Historically, too, there have been many shifts in the ways that different chemical comforters have been regarded; several of them regarded as dangerous, addictive or immoral in one century have been considered harmless in another. In Europe, for example, chocolate, tea, coffee and snuff have all been regarded with moral horror at one time or another[33]. 'Among the many disorders which the intemperance of mankind has introduced that shorten life, one of the greatest, I believe, is the use of chocolate', wrote G. B. Felici of Florence in 1728[34]. The Spanish, and every other nation which goes to the Indies, once they become accustomed to chocolate, its consumption becomes such a vice that they can only with difficulty leave off from drinking it every morning', wrote the explorer Franceso Carletti in 1701[34]. It has been argued that what has freed chocolate, coffee and tea from being defined as addictive substances in modern industrial societies is not that they are completely harmless, but that – unlike 'hard' drugs – they do not stop their users from working[34].

In the case of the 'hard' drugs, such as heroin or morphine, the socio-cultural matrix in which drug taking occurs also has its tacit rules and sanctions. Addicts often form an *outcast subculture*, with their own particular view of the world[35]. These sub-cultures may play an important part in the spread of certain disease, such as infectious hepatitis. Recently there has been increased research on the role of needle sharing among intravenous drug users in the spread of AIDS. In Edinburgh, Scotland, for example, it has been estimated that about 60 per cent of injecting drug users in the city are now HIV-positive[36], while a study in Spain[37] has also related the spread of AIDS to the growing numbers of intravenous drug users in the country.

The extent to which individual addicts are integrated into this sub-culture may determine whether they are able to give up hard drugs or not. If for any reason the sub-culture is dismantled, then addicts may overcome their physical addiction with unexpected ease. For example, Robins and colleagues[38] conducted a follow-up study of drug use by US servicemen returned from Vietnam. They studied 943 men who had returned to the United States from Vietnam in 1971, 8–12 months after their return. Four hundred and ninety-five of these had tested positive in urine tests for opiates at the time of departure from Vietnam, and three-quarters of these felt that they had been addicted to narcotics whilst there. In the 8–12 months after their return, one-third had had more experience with opiates, but only 7 per cent of the group showed signs of physical dependence. Almost none of the urine-positive group expressed a desire for treatment or addiction rehabilitation programmes. As Robins and his colleagues pointed out, this result is surprising 'in the light of common belief that dependence on narcotics is easily acquired and virtually impossible to rid oneself of, [yet] most of the men who used narcotics heavily in Vietnam stopped when they left Vietnam and had not begun again 8–12 months later'. Part of the explanation for this is probably that the *milieu* or macro-context in Vietnam – psychologically, socially and economically – was favourable towards the persistence of an addict sub-culture without, as the authors put it, 'the deterrents of high prices, impure drugs, or the presence of disapproving family'.

Physical addiction, therefore, is *not* just a physical phenomenon; it also requires certain social or cultural factors for its persistence. A further example of this is a case quoted by Jackson[39], from St Louis, Missouri, in the mid-1960s. Here the lifestyle and activities of heroin addicts remained, unexpectedly, unchanged when the supply of heroin in the city dried up. It was temporarily replaced by metamphetamine – the pharmacological effect of which is the polar opposite of heroin – but the addicts carried on behaving exactly as before: 'They went to the same shooting galleries to shoot up, scored from the same connections, and bought the magic white powder (metamphetamine instead of heroin) in the same little glassine envelopes they knew so well'. As Jackson concludes, 'The addicts maintained the heroin sub-culture on a metamphetamine metabolism; obviously the sub-culture had had powerful and spectacular magic working for it'.

Case study: Addict sub-culture in Lexington, Kentucky, USA

The power and nature of an addict sub-culture was studied by Freeland and Rosensteil[40] at the Clinical Research Center in Lexington, Kentucky. They found that self-defined groups, such as narcotic addicts, 'tend to justify their own way of life by stereotyping the behaviour of others in a negative fashion'. The power of culturally based stereotypes to influence a person's life and perceptions depends on how committed the person is to that way of life. In the case of the narcotic addicts, this commitment was intense and all-embracing. Their cultural (or rather sub-cultural) belief system embodied a strong we–they dichotomy. 'They' were the 'squares', whose lives were seen as being boring, passive, hypocritical, fear-ridden and subordinate. This negative picture was contrasted with their own idealized self-image as 'hustlers', a hustler being 'an active, dominant, capable, self-motivated person who is highly aware of his surroundings and in control of them'. They saw themselves as living 'the fast life'; a hustler first and an addict second. Hustlers were seen as having a specialized type of knowledge about the world which 'maximizes one's abilities as a predator'. In the researchers' view, the maintenance of this we–they dichotomy, and the stereotypes of 'square' and 'hustler', tend to minimize the impact of any therapeutic or rehabilitative programmes directed towards the addicts.

As a strategy to overcome this situation, they organized lengthy discussions on these stereotypes between the addict group and a group of 'squares'. The aim was to reduce the addicts' tendency to stereotype by reducing their ethnocentrism – that is, by providing them with alternative ways of seeing the world, derived from other groups. The 'squares' included medical staff and students, as well as others from churches and schools. Both groups were encouraged to discuss the stereotypes of the others, and to examine how these stereotypes affected their interactions. The addicts were also shown films of other societies, and it was pointed out that stereotyping was a universal human feature, although it could be dangerous and inhibit communication. The outcome of this process was to convince the addict group that they could modify their lifestyle 'without being doomed to a life of subservience, boredom, inactivity, and passivity', and this was a major step in their rehabilitation into everyday life. It was also helpful in enhancing rapport between addict patients and medical staff.

Case study: 'Crack' cocaine sub-culture in Spanish Harlem, New York City, USA

Bourgois[41] studied the violent street culture of 'crack' cocaine dealers and their clients in Spanish Harlem, New York City. He described the bleak lives of the residents of this poor, inner-city area, many of them Puerto Ricans, and the role played by the underground economy of drug dealing, distribution and consumption within the community. He pointed out that in order to understand the origins of this violent and crime-ridden drug sub-culture, larger social issues, such as the 'objective, structural desperation of a population without a viable economy, and facing systematic barriers of ethnic discrimination and ideological marginalization', cannot be ignored.

However self-destructive their lives, Bourgois did not see the drug dealers as propelled by an 'irrational cultural logic distinct from that of mainstream USA'. On the contrary, although completely excluded from the mainstream economy and society, many of their values are ultimately derived from it. The participants in the underground crack economy are frantically pursuing their own, distorted version of the American dream. As in conventional society, their ambitions include rapid upward economic mobility, the respect of their peers and the accumulation of flashy consumer objects.

Faced with the prospects of unemployment, low wages and discrimination in the outside world, some of the residents of Spanish Harlem have chosen to become aggressive, self-employed private entrepreneurs – like Papito, who owns a 'string of crack franchises' run by street sellers. People like him are, wrote Bourgois, 'the ultimate rugged individualists braving an unpredictable frontier where fortune, fame and destruction are all just around the corner'. Much of the crack economy is run on conventional business lines, with a recognizable hierarchy of bosses, wholesalers, messengers and street salesmen (who have to meet sales quotas set by their bosses). However, the entire crack economy is based on violence and a culture of terror and, ultimately, on self-destructiveness. Dealers have to be tough and violent enough to intimidate competitors, impress their clients and cement partnerships with other dealers. As a result, homicides, woundings, robberies and high rates of crack addiction are common in the community.

Despite their violent, and ultimately doomed lifestyle, Bourgois emphasized that for these marginalized inner-city young men, employment (or even better, self-employment) in the underground crack economy 'accords a sense of autonomy, self-dignity and an opportunity for extraordinary rapid short-term upward mobility'.

These studies, like the others mentioned above, stress the importance of the *non*-pharmacological variables in producing and maintaining drug addiction, and the complexity of trying to deal with it. In any individual addict, these variables will always include a mix of socio-cultural, economic, geographical and personality factors. For this reason, drug addiction – and the culture of drug production and drug-dealing that feeds upon it – is very difficult to change. This is especially so because the 'chemical road to success' has become so imbedded in modern daily life. Solutions to drug addiction cannot, therefore, be based solely on the treatment of individuals. In the long term, wider economic, social and cultural issues must also be addressed in order to reduce demand for these drugs, as well as their supply[42].

In the short term, however, a variety of approaches to reducing drug addiction have been tried, some of them making positive use of the cultural milieu in which the addict lives. In several cases, traditional healers or religious figures have been used to help people come off hard drugs and change their lifestyles. These include *curanderos* in Latin America, Buddhist monks in Thailand, acupuncturists in the Far East, and many religious and missionary groups in the Western world. In Malaysia, for example, the traditional Malay folk healer or *bomoh* has been found to be effective in treating some forms of mental illness[43]. However, since the 1970s, many of the 200 000 *bomohs* in the country have also been used to help prevent addiction and to treat and rehabilitate heroin addicts[44]. During their treatment, the addicts live in a controlled environment within the *bomoh's* compound. There they are treated with a mixture of herbal remedies, purificatory baths and religious rituals. *Bomohs* are said to have their own familiar 'spirits' (*hantu raya* or *pelisit*) to help them in their treatments, and some former patients have stated that the reasons for their continued abstinence after treatment was fear of this 'spirit', and the punishment it might bring if they were to relapse. In many cases, *bomoh* therapy has proved to be as effective, or even more effective, than orthodox medical treatments of addiction[44].

Alcohol use and abuse

Excessive alcohol usage is a feature of many groups and individuals world-wide, especially those of lower social status and income. Alcohol abuse – and its many social, economic, and psychological effects – is now one of the major public health problems world-wide[45].

Various studies of the problem have indicated that the incidence of alcoholism, and the regular consumption of alcohol on ritual and other occasions, differs markedly between cultural groups and social groups, even within the same society. In the USA, for example, Italian-Americans and Jewish-Americans have low rates of alcoholism, while Irish-Americans[46] and some Native Americans[47] have very high rates. In the UK, alcohol consumption is relatively low among some immigrant and ethnic minority groups – Afro-Caribbeans, Indians, Pakistanis and Bangladeshis – but is rising in some sections of the Sikh community[48]. Among the many reasons for these differences must be the ways that alcohol intake is embedded in the matrix of *cultural* values and expectations of different groups.

A number of anthropological and other social science theories, some of which are outlined below, have been advanced in order to explain how and why some cultural and social groups drink more than others. Although they are useful, their predictive value at the individual level is limited. They can never fully explain why one particular person from a particular group has an alcohol problem, while another from the same group does not. In each case, the reasons for alcohol use and abuse are always a complex mix of influences, not all of which can be explained by the social sciences.

At the level of the individual drinker, the effect of alcohol depends, as with all 'total drug effects', on a number of factors; physical, psychological and socio-economic. The physical factors include the body build of the drinker, the presence or absence of liver damage, whether drinking took place on an empty stomach or not and, possibly, an inherited intolerance of alcohol. They also include the pharmacological properties of the drink itself, especially its volume, type and concentration. These physical and pharmacological factors are not enough, however, to explain how and why people drink, and how it affects their behaviour. One should also consider the *socio-cultural* characteristics of drinkers, their family and friends, and the setting in which drinking takes place. In particular, the attitudes of their cultural group towards two different types of drinking –'normal' and 'abnormal' – should be examined. Furthermore, the *economic* status of the drinker is an important factor, since the stress of poverty is often associated with alcohol abuse. Finally, the *psychological* influences on an individual drinker need always to be considered, including the drinker's personality, early experiences and current emotional state (especially depression).

'Normal' and 'abnormal' drinking

'Normal' drinking refers to the everyday use of alcohol at mealtimes, or on social and ritual occasions. In these cases, the moderate use of alcohol is an accepted part of daily life. However, the type and amount of alcohol, and when and by whom it is consumed, are strongly *controlled* by cultural rules and sanctions. In 'abnormal' drinking, these mores are transgressed and there is frequent and excessive intake of alcohol, with resultant uncontrolled, drunken behaviour. Cultural groups vary in how and under what circumstances abnormal drinking takes place, and in how they define the behavioural characteristics of drunkenness. The boundary between normal and abnormal drinking is not clear-cut, however. In an Irish wake, for example, drunkenness is sometimes acceptable, but it is considered abnormal in other contexts. O'Connor[49] has pointed out that, 'If one looks at the patterns and attitudes of drinking in a society, one may come to some understanding of drinking pathologies or alcoholism'. That is, one should look at the culturally defined 'normal' drinking behaviour of a group in order to understand the 'abnormal' forms of drinking that may be found within it.

On this basis, O'Connor has classified cultures, in relation to drinking, into four main groups:

1. Abstinent cultures
2. Ambivalent cultures
3. Permissive cultures
4. Over-permissive cultures.

This classification refers to attitudes towards drinking as a normal part of everyday life, and towards drunkenness. In *abstinent* cultures the use of alcohol is strictly prohibited under any circumstances, and there are strong negative feelings towards alcohol use. Examples of this are the Muslim cultures of North Africa and the Middle East, and certain Protestant ascetic churches in the Western world (such as Baptists, Methodists, Mormons and Seventh Day Adventists). While normal drinking is rare in these cultures, problem (abnormal) drinking is slightly higher here than in more permissive cultures, especially as a result of personal problems. O'Connor quotes studies that show that, in the American South, which has a strong abstinence tradition, 'a relationship was found between parental disapproval of drinking and an increase in the percentage of problem drinkers'. Similarly, another study showed a high incidence of heavy drinking and intoxication among a group of Mormon students; because drinking by members of abstinent groups is not controlled by any drinking norms, therefore alcoholism is more likely among such groups.

'Drinking norms' are tacit rules about who can drink, in whose company, in which settings, and how much can be consumed. 'Alcoholism', therefore, is the overuse of alcohol, and behaviour *uncontrolled* by social norms. The implication here is that in some cultures people are more familiar with how to drink as an ordinary part of everyday life. They know when to drink, the amounts to drink safely, and when to stop. In other groups, though, unfamiliarity with alcohol means that if they start drinking, they do so in a chaotic, uncontrolled and potentially dangerous way.

Ambivalent cultures have two, mutually contradictory attitudes towards alcohol. O'Connor applies this label to the Irish. On the one hand, drinking is a normal part of Irish life: 'From the womb to the tomb the Irish were seen to use drink at christenings, weddings and funerals. All social and economic life was centred around the use of alcohol'. On the other hand, there has been strong disapproval of all drinking by various abstinent temperance movements in the past 150 years. This has led to the absence of a consistent, generalized and coherent attitude in Ireland towards alcohol intake. In this situation, 'the culture does not have a well integrated system of controls, the individual is left in a situation of ambivalence which may be conducive to alcoholism'.

In a *permissive* culture, by contrast, there are norms, customs, values and sanctions relating to drinking which are widely shared by the group. Everyone is allowed to drink, but only in a controlled way and on certain occasions. In this type of culture, the moderate intake of alcohol at mealtimes, and on certain social or festive occasions, is encouraged as being normal, though there are strong sanctions against drunkenness or other forms of uncontrolled drinking behaviour. In these groups, such as Italians, Spaniards, Portuguese and orthodox Jews, the rate of alcoholism is low. For example, as Knupfer and Room[46] pointed out, Italian-Americans see wine as a type of food, to be consumed only as part of a meal, while among orthodox Jews wine is an integral part of many religious rituals. Both groups tend to despise drunken behaviour. Among both, intoxication is regarded as a personal and family disgrace, and the use of wine between meals is frowned upon. France, too, is a permissive culture towards drink, though in O'Connor's view it is *over-permissive*. While less wine is taken in France than in Italy, alcoholism is much higher in France, and the pattern of drinking in the two countries is very different. Not only are French attitudes towards normal drinking favourable, but cultural attitudes 'are also favourable to other forms of deviant behaviour while drinking'. Drinking is also associated with virility, and 'there is widespread social acceptance of intoxication as fashionable, humorous or at least tolerable'.

In general, therefore, both 'permissive' and 'over-permissive' cultures, where drinking is allowed (but only in a controlled form), have lower rates of alcoholism – that is, abnormal, uncontrolled drinking behaviour – than either 'abstinent' or 'ambivalent' cultures. These sociocultural patterns are passed on from generation to generation, and partly determine whether a particular member of the society is likely to seek solace in drink at times of crisis or unhappiness.

However, while O'Connor's model of different cultural macro-contexts is useful, it is limited in its applicability. As noted at the beginning of this book, cultures are never homogeneous: particularly in complex modern industrial societies. Within the same society, for example, there may be very different attitudes, among different groups of people, towards what constitutes normal or abnormal forms of drinking. These attitudes towards drink may be influenced by a variety of factors, including education, gender, age group, religious faith, social class, or even region. Nevertheless, the model does highlight the value of looking at 'normal' drinking patterns before trying to understand the origins of alcohol problems within a community.

Ethnic, religious and cultural variables

The differences in alcohol use and abuse among ethnic and cultural groups in the USA have been examined in detail by Greeley and McCready[50], using data gathered by the National Opinion Research Center. The study was based on almost 1000 families of Irish, Jewish, Italian and Swedish origin. They developed a model to examine how children learn drinking behaviour, and to explain much of the ethnic diversity in drinking patterns that has been found. In their view, five variables, from both the individual's upbringing and their present situation, can influence drinking behaviour, both 'normal' and uncontrolled:

1. *Family drinking* – that is, whether and how frequently both parents drank; a 'drinking problem' within the family; and parental approval of their children drinking.
2. *Family structure* – in particular, the decision-making style in the home, that is, whether decisions regarding the children are made by one parent or jointly by both; and also the degree of explicit affection and mutual support within the family.
3. *Personality variables* – particularly orientations towards achievement, efficacy and authority. It has been suggested that an authoritarian family structure produces men with a particular type of personality, especially a great need to be the only (and powerful) decision-maker, and that this attitude may predispose to problem drinking.
4. *Spouse's drinking behaviour* –alcoholism is more likely if a spouse drinks heavily as well.
5. *Drinking environment* in which the person lives – that is, the prevalence of drinking and the availability of drink in their socio-cultural environment, including on social, ritual or festive occasions.

These five groups of variables, taken together, account for many of the differences in drinking patterns and rates of alcoholism among ethnic and cultural groups; they may also help in understanding why an individual in a particular group is at risk of becoming a problem drinker. However, the socio-economic environment of different groups should also be included, since poverty, unemployment and a sense of helplessness may also predispose to the overuse of alcohol.

O'Connor[49] has developed a similar model to show 'that for groups that use alcohol to a significant degree, the lowest incidence of alcoholism is associated with certain habits and attitudes'. These attitudes include:

1. Exposing the children to alcohol early in life, within a strong family or religious group
2. Use of alcohol in a very diluted form (to give low blood-alcohol levels)
3. Alcohol being viewed mainly as a 'food', and usually consumed with meals
4. Parents presenting an example of moderate drinking
5. Drinking not being given any moral importance, as either a virtue or a sin
6. Drinking not being considered proof of adulthood or virility
7. Abstinence being socially acceptable
8. Drunkenness being socially unacceptable and not considered 'stylish, comical or tolerable'
9. Wide agreement among members of the group on 'the ground rules of drinking' – that is, the norms governing drinking behaviour.

The setting of alcohol use

A further factor governing drinking behaviour is the *setting* (micro-context) in which it takes place (such as a pub, club, bar, *taverna*, restaurant or home), and the social function performed by these settings. An important aspect of this is whether drinking takes place in private or public, and whether in what is culturally defined as a 'male' or 'female' space. Whichever setting it takes place in, each has its own implicit rules governing the drinking behaviour that takes place within them, including how and what to drink and who drinks with whom. Drinking patterns in public settings, such as bars or clubs, are often independent of the drinkers' socio-cultural background (though there are more ethnic settings, such as 'Irish pubs'). For example, Thomas[51] studied public drinking in bars and taverns in an urban working-class community of 50 000 people in New England, with the pseudonym 'Clyde Cove'. He found that these 'laboring-men's bars' functioned mainly as social clubs after work, where working-class men could meet together in an atmosphere of relative equality and mutual acceptance. In this setting, alcohol was merely a social lubricant and not the main reason why the men came together. As Thomas puts it: 'In the after-work hours of 4–6 pm, nothing more is derived from bar life than a light form of *communitas* and a short period of time-out from the workaday world'. There were implicit rules governing their normal drinking behaviour; drunkenness or problem drinking was very infrequent, and was considered to be deviant behaviour within the bar. The bar customers were drawn from many ethnic groups, but ethnicity did not affect the content of bar life, and in many bars blacks and whites drank freely together. In Mars's study[52] of longshoremen in Newfoundland, drinking played the role of a badge of identity; defining and strengthening the boundaries of one group of men ('regular men'), while excluding the members of another ('outside men'). 'Regular men' – those with secure jobs unloading the boats – always drank beer together in taverns near the waterfront. Groups or 'gangs' of these men who worked together provided mutual help and 'insurance facilities' for their members, collecting funds for a sick member or donating blood for an injured one. They also formed a collective unit for bargaining with employers. Although ostensibly a leisure activity, drinking only took place with other members of one's work gang. Thus drinking together, and buying each other drinks, acted to strengthen the relationships between fellow workers, while linking the world of work with that of leisure. By contrast, 'outside men' – those without regular employment, who were only hired to work erratically and on a temporary basis – never drank in the taverns. Marginal to the waterfront economy, and excluded from these mutually supportive groups of workmates, they tended to drink in the street or in parked cars, sharing the same bottle of cheap wine or rum with different men each time. Similarly, in a study of the small Irish fishing community of 'Clontarf', Peace[53] has shown how social drinking also plays a crucial role both in the creation of masculine identity and in relation to the world of work. Drinking heavily together in the village pubs every weekend gives men the opportunity to display their physical toughness to their mates, and to show that they can 'hold their beer well'. It helps to create and cement the bonds between men, many of whom will work together during the week, while at the same time clearly separating them from the world of women.

Thus, as Gefou-Madianou[54] has described in detail, alcohol often plays an important part in creating gender identity in many different cultures, both in Europe and elsewhere. Reviewing studies from Greece, Spain, France, Hungary, Sweden and Ireland, she illustrates the very different ways that men and women consume alcohol. Whatever the cultural milieu, they generally obey different drinking norms, consume different types of alcohol, in different amounts, and drink in very different settings. Although in Mediterranean societies such as Greece alcohol is often consumed together by men and women, on religious occasions or at family gatherings, their behaviour differs markedly from when they drink in single-sex settings, such as the males-only *taverna* or local café.

From an anthropological perspective, therefore, alcohol intake should always be viewed against its social, cultural and economic backgrounds. These include patterns of 'normal' and 'abnormal' drinking, the role of gender and social background, the settings in which it occurs and the values associated with these factors. Other relevant factors are the economic interests involved in alcohol production and marketing (see below), and the meaning given to drinking by individuals or groups – such as proof of virility, manhood, adulthood or rebelliousness. *All* these elements, in addition to personality traits and socio-economic status, should be taken into account in understanding why and how a particular individual abuses alcohol.

Case study: Social uses of alcohol in two pubs in Cambridgeshire, UK

Hunt and Satterlee[55] described the different social uses of alcohol in two pubs in a village in Cambridgeshire. One pub, 'The Griffin', was frequented mainly by newcomers to the village, who were predominantly upwardly mobile and middle-class, and about one-third of them were women. Here alcohol was a way of creating and sustaining new relationships, especially by the ritual of 'round buying', which involved taking turns to buy drinks for as many as 20 people in the group. Much of their bonhomie spilled over into social events in one another's homes, either before or after visiting the pub. By contrast, the clientele of 'The Three Barrels' were predominantly male, mainly working-class and middle-aged. Most of them had been born in the village, lived nearby, had known one another for many years, and were often related to one another. In this ambience, 'round buying' was rare and unnecessary, since group cohesion was already maintained by a shared history, shared kinship and shared neighbourhood. In each pub, therefore, the same form of alcohol had a different meaning, and played a different social role in maintaining the cohesion of the group of drinkers.

Smoking behaviour

Tobacco, like tea, coffee, alcohol and psychotropic drugs, is a commonly used 'chemical comforter'. It was first brought to Europe in the fifteenth century, after the discovery of the Americas. As with the other 'comforters', the widespread psychological dependence on smoking cannot be explained only by reference to the pharmacological properties of nicotine or tobacco. Socio-cultural factors also play an important role in determining who smokes, under what circumstances and for what reasons. As with alcohol use, it is important to understand the symbolic meanings of tobacco smoking – for the individual smoker and for those around him. In some cases, cultural background may *protect* against smoking and its effects. For example, studies in the UK indicate that among immigrants from the Indian subcontinent, smoking is still rare among men and almost unknown among women[56].

In the USA, cigarette smoking is believed to be the single largest cause of disease and death[57], responsible for about 400 000 deaths per year[57], and the annual cost of morbidity from smoking-related diseases has been estimated at 27 billion dollars[58].

There are several studies that examine the demographic characteristics of these smokers, especially their age, sex, education, marital state and socio-economic position, and from these data some of the influences on smoking behaviour can be inferred. Reeder[59] reviewed most of the available literature on this subject. He pointed out that, in the US and Europe, consumption of cigarettes has increased three-fold since 1930, despite anti-smoking propaganda. While the proportion of adult smokers in the USA has dropped, that of teenagers has risen. The proportion of smokers has been declining among males, but increasing among females. Men and women who were 21 years old in the late 1970s now smoke at equal rates, but many men in their fifties have given up the habit. Smoking rates are lowest among better-educated groups, but this is less true for women. In general, there is a greater prevalence of smoking among women employed outside the home as compared to housewives, and female white-collar workers are more likely to smoke than women in other occupations. Men in upper income categories are less likely to smoke, while women in the same bracket are more likely to be current smokers. Reeder related these contradictory statistics to the changing sex roles of females, a greater proportion of whom (in the US) have a college education and paid employment. There is a general trend towards equality 'in virtually all domains of social and economic life', and smoking rates reflect this equality. However: 'In the case of socio-economic status the pattern is delayed, so that the smoking behaviour may be perceived as in some way an indicator of increased social power and/or independence – even before there is equality in economic status'. Tobacco smoking is also an increasing problem among the young, and early onset of the habit can lead to longer-term problems. In a 1994 report, the US Surgeon General noted that nearly all first use of tobacco occurred before high school graduation, and that if adolescents could be kept tobacco-free until that time, most of them would never start smoking[60].

Some studies[59] relate heavy smoking to a perception of powerlessness by the smokers, and a sense of 'anomie' and futility in the daily lives. Other correlations of high adult smoking rates were a drop in socio-economic status (in men) and experience of divorce or separation. Among teenagers, those less academically successful or from one-parent families were more likely to smoke. As with alcohol, teenagers were more likely to smoke if parents, siblings and friends already did so, the likely mechanisms in this case being imitation and role-modelling behaviour.

Considerable numbers of people still continue to smoke, despite all the health warnings from government and other agencies about its dangers. Some studies indicate that many smokers still do not believe that smoking could damage their health. For example, Marsh and Matheson[61] studied beliefs about smoking among 2700 British smokers and 1200 non-smokers aged 16–66 years. Forty-five per cent of the smokers rejected outright the concept that they were more liable to heart disease due to their smoking, and 33 per cent that smoking made them more prone to lung cancer. Overall, only 14 per cent completely accepted the idea that smoking causes heart disease, and 11 per cent that it causes lung cancer.

Doherty and Whitehead[62] suggested that cigarette smoking may also persist because it can be a way of communicating a wide range of social messages, especially among family and friends. Among other messages, smoking may signal to other people 'let's talk', 'let's relax together', 'I need to be alone' or 'I'm not going to tell you how I'm feeling'. Smoking, like alcohol, may therefore play a variety of social roles, and may help define a sense of social cohesion or of social withdrawal.

Economic aspects of tobacco use

Cigarette smoking does not, however, only persist because of smokers' anomie, ignorance or use of cigarettes as a social message. An overall picture of smoking must include the *economic* interests involved in tobacco production, advertising and use. Nichter and Cartwright[63] estimated that, world-wide, the tobacco industry spends about $12.5 billion annually on advertising and promotion ($2.5 billion of it in the USA). This figure contrasts markedly with the amount spent by governments urging people to avoid smoking. In the UK, for example, the government's Health Education Authority (HEA) spends £5.5 million a year urging people not to smoke, while the tobacco industry spends about £130 million telling them that they should smoke[64]. The HEA estimated in 1991 that each year 284 159 people are admitted to National Health Service hospitals with smoking-related illnesses, that 110 703 premature deaths are caused in the UK annually by these diseases, and that the cost to the NHS in inpatient bills alone is £437 million per year[64].

In 1986, the *Bulletin of the Pan American Health Organization*[65] reviewed tobacco use world-wide, based on data from the World Health Organization. It pointed out that tobacco is

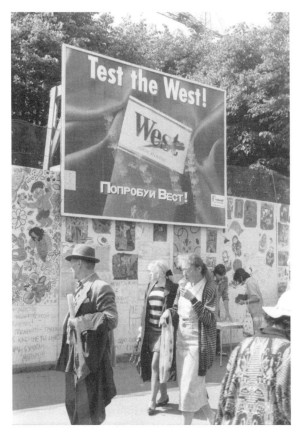

Figure 8.2 Advertisement for cigarettes in a street in St Petersburg, Russia (Source: Sean Sprague/Panos Pictures, No. Rus: 36).

produced in about 120 countries, and that the contribution of developing countries to world tobacco production increased from 50 per cent in 1963 to 63 per cent in 1983. The major tobacco producing and consuming countries are China, the USA, the CIS (formerly the USSR), India and Brazil. About 37 per cent of the world's cigarettes are produced by state-controlled industries in centrally planned countries, and a further 17 per cent are manufactured by state monopolies whose aim is to maximize government revenue. The remainder of the market is dominated by seven international conglomerates. In many countries the tobacco industry provides thousands of jobs, and it also provides income for the advertising industry, tax revenue for governments, and foreign currency for nations short on foreign exchange. Against this economic background, the *Bulletin* deplores 'the common government reluctance to act on tobacco, which is demonstrably a cause of avoidable disease and death on a scale unmatched by any other currently available product for human consumption'.

The 'legal addictions'

Both tobacco and alcohol have been termed 'legal addictions' by anthropologists Baer and colleagues[66]. They argued that, in the USA, both are sanctioned by society in ways that other 'chemical comforters' (such as heroin or marijuana) are not. The reason why they are the 'most commonly used non-medical legal drugs in US society' is partly because of pressure from the tobacco and alcohol industries. These firms, often multinational corporations, have not only tried to prevent these substances being classified as drugs, but have also often denied that they are addictive or harmful (although in the case of tobacco, recent court cases in the USA have ruled otherwise). Over the years their advertising campaigns and sponsorship activities have had a major impact on sales of their products, especially on the young. In addition, both alcohol and tobacco products are increasingly being exported from Western countries into the developing world – like the pharmaceuticals described below. For example, studies quoted in the *World Mental Health* report in 1995[45] indicate that the expansion of mainly Western alcohol conglomerates into low-income countries, and their dominance of the markets there, is advancing swiftly. The countries of Africa, Asia and Latin America are now one of the fastest-growing import regions for both hard liquor and beer, with 15 per cent and 25 per cent respectively of the global import totals. An estimated 15–20 per cent of adults in Latin America are said to be alcoholics or excessive drinkers, and there is increasing alcohol consumption in parts of China[45].

Thus on both a local and an international level, any fuller understanding of these legal chemical comforters must always take this macro-context of economic issues and profit motives into account.

Western pharmaceuticals in developing countries

In recent decades, a significant development has been the huge influx of pharmaceutical products, mainly manufactured by Western multinational firms, into the developing world. There is now a growing dependence on these imported drugs in many Third World countries, and this has important implications[67].

Ferguson[68] describes how these drugs are produced by a relatively small number of firms (50 per cent of the world's pharmaceuticals are supplied by only 25 firms), based in a small number of countries – mainly in the USA, Europe and Japan. Furthermore, these firms 'tend to manufacture medications designed to meet the health needs of populations in the developed countries', rather than those of the poorer countries. Despite this, enormous quantities of expensive pre-packaged medications are being exported to the Third World, backed by advertising campaigns that stress their advantages over both traditional remedies and locally produced pharmaceuticals. Imported drugs are now a major drain on the finances of the less developed countries, where 75 per cent of the world's population live. The Director General of the WHO points out that these poor countries account for only 20 per cent of the world consumption of pharmaceuticals, but it costs them annually about $170 000 million, and still about 'half the world's population lacks regular access to the most-needed 57 medicines'[69].

These imported drugs significantly influence how people regard and treat their own ill health. Anthropologists have shown how, in different cultures, and in different groups within those cultures, the same drugs may be conceptualized and used in very different ways[67]. Embedded in local cultural and social contexts, their use is often based more on inherited folklore and traditional beliefs than on medical criteria[70]. They have described the large 'informal sector' of pharmaceutical use in many Third World societies, parallel to their more 'formal' use by the medical profession, although there is often overlap between the two. In many developing countries, drugs that are only available on prescription in the Western world can be bought over-the-counter (often at relatively high cost) from local pharmacies, shopkeepers or street vendors, or administered by traditional practitioners or untrained folk healers (such as the 'injectionist').

Many Western pharmaceuticals *do* have a very useful role to play in developing countries, especially in the hands of health professionals or trained primary care workers. Even in the informal sector, when bought from vendors or over-the counter, they are often useful in alleviating various symptoms and treating many common disorders[59]. Also, the informal sector helps distribute the pharmaceuticals widely, even to areas where there are no available doctors or nurses or other sources of health care[71]. In some cases people with stigmatized conditions such as sexually transmitted diseases may even prefer the anonymity of treatment by some itinerant injectionist to a consultation with a local health professional; sometimes it may also be cheaper.

However, as well as their high cost, these imported drugs carry with them many dangers, especially when used as self-medication. These include: severe side effects, drug allergies, self-poisoning, accidental overdoses, inappropriate use (treating viral infections with antibiotics, for example), and the development of drug-resistant strains of microbes or parasites – like tuberculosis and malaria. Furthermore, in many parts of the world they have stimulated a growth in the number of injectionists, with all the dangers associated with this (see Chapter 4). Overall, anthropologists have argued that the massive inflow of pharmaceuticals into Third World countries contributes towards a gradual 'medicalization' of ill health and suffering[68] – moving away from more social, holistic or indigenous approaches to illness towards an emphasis on only one form of therapy, drug treatment. That is, towards the 'chemical road to success' outlined above.

In many developing countries, the main retail outlet for imported pharmaceuticals is local pharmacies. For example, in her study of the town of Asuncion, El Salvador, Ferguson[68] found that these pharmacies were also the main source of health care for poorer people, providing them with advice and information as well as over-the-counter medicines. However, most of the time the pharmacies in Asuncion were actually run by unqualified, sometimes illiterate, pharmacy clerks. Often the advice given by them was inappropriate, or a blend of folk and biomedical modes of treatment – for example, advising clients with a mild viral infection to avoid certain behaviours or 'cold' foods or drinks, but at the same time selling them tetracycline or another strong antibiotic.

The Essential Drugs programme

To deal with this chaotic situation, and to ensure a more rational and fairly distributed use of drugs world-wide, the World Health Organization has since 1977 developed a 'Model List of Essential Drugs' (now numbering about 250), which is regularly updated[72]. These are the basic drugs that should be available to any population, and the list excludes many of the more expensive or exotic patented drugs available in the West. A further step, in 1981, was the establishment of the WHO's Action Programme on Essential Drugs to help member countries develop national drugs policies for 'selecting, procuring, storing and distributing essential drugs, and through training and monitoring to see that drugs are used properly'[73]. Above all, the policy aimed to ensure 'regular supplies of affordable drugs of good quality'[61]. Many of these would be locally produced, or else bought cheaply in bulk from pharmaceutical firms in their generic forms (that is, without brand names and expensive packaging). As well as improving the quality of available drugs and reducing their price, the aim was to achieve a more rational use of drugs and greater coverage of the world's population.

Opposition to this programme has come not only from sections of the pharmaceutical industry, but also from local populations. In many Third World communities, these beautifully packaged imported drugs, adorned with internationally renowned brand names, seem to offer greater healing power to consumers than the cheaper, poorly packaged, locally produced alternatives on a government's Essential Drugs list. In El Salvador, for example, Ferguson[68] describes how, as a result of the penetration of these expensive imported drugs into local markets, there has been a marked shift towards them and away from the use of equally effective but much cheaper pharmaceuticals produced by Salvadorean firms, as well as from self-treatment with home remedies (which are sometimes also very effective).

As with the psychotropic drugs and other chemical comforters described earlier, belief in the 'quick fix' of a tablet (or of an injectionist's needle) may not provide an adequate solution to the social and psychological stresses faced by many Third World countries. Although these drugs do have a role in treating or preventing, ill health, many of the health problems of these poor communities cannot be solved solely by expensive antibiotics or other drugs. Overall, there is the danger that an overemphasis on drug treatment – especially on treating the symptoms of disease rather than their cause – 'fosters the notion that the solution to illness resides in the consumption of medicines rather than improvements in living conditions'[68]. In other words, the cultural formula of 'drugs + individual = success', mentioned above, may in its medical forms spread to include much of the non-Western world.

Case study: Distribution of Western pharmaceuticals in South Cameroon

Van der Geest[71] described the formal and informal distribution of pharmaceuticals in an area of South Cameroon. In the formal sector, medicines are provided without charge by state-run hospitals and health centres and issued by hospital pharmacies. Private non-profit institutions, usually church-run hospitals, health centres and primary care projects, also prescribe medicines, but make a charge for them. In addition, private commercial pharmacies (of which there were 76 in the whole country) sell large numbers of these medications over-the-counter and without prescriptions. In general, these pharmacies are only situated in urban areas, since the pharmacists 'are entrepreneurs who only settle in areas with a high purchasing power'. They are highly profitable, with a high turnover; in 1978, the value of medicines distributed by this commercial sector was 50 per cent greater than those distributed by the entire public sector. Parallel to these officially sanctioned outlets, there is an enormous informal sector of pharmaceutical distribution in South Cameroon. It consists of many hundreds of people who sell pre-packaged medications to the public, in towns and villages throughout the country. These include:

- shopkeepers, who sell medicines as well as general provisions (in one town there were 75 general stores that also sold at least one or two types of medicine)
- market vendors, who sell these drugs alongside their other products
- hawkers, who travel from village to village during the cocoa harvest season, selling medicines as well as other articles
- traders who specialize in selling medicines, and who carry a much larger assortment than the other groups
- the personnel of medical institutions who illegally sell medicines that should be provided to patients free of charge (he estimated that up to 30 per cent of state-supplied medicines do not reach patients, but are sold privately by the health workers themselves).

The informal retail trade therefore obtains many of its drugs from the formal sector. While some are smuggled across the border from Niger, most are bought from pharmacists or hospital personnel – indicating how closely interwoven are the formal and informal sectors. In one example of this inter-relationship he describes how, in one hospital, because patients had to wait a long time before seeing a doctor, they sometimes bought their medications (such as analgesics) while they were waiting from a medicine vendor who had set up his stand in the hospital grounds right next to the polyclinic.

In all, Van der Geest found 70 different drugs circulating in the informal sector, especially analgesics (13 types), antibiotics (12 types),

continued

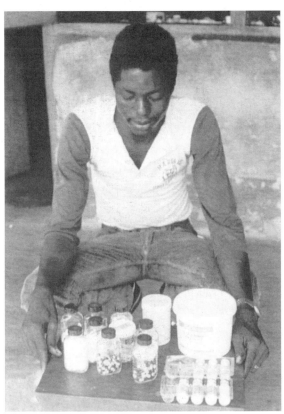

Figure 8.3 Selling Western pharmaceuticals to the public: a street vendor in Ghana (Source: WHO/Goldschmidt, *World Health*, No. 3, May–June 1998, page 26).

cough and cold remedies, laxatives, vitamins, worm remedies, remedies for anaemia and anti-malarials. He pointed out that while this sector does have advantages – for example, making drugs available locally at prices lower than at pharmacies – it can also be very detrimental to health. Despite this, it would be impractical to try to dissolve the informal sector, since this would deprive much of the population of their only source of modern medicines. Therefore, the aim should be to reduce the importation of drugs, thereby excluding dangerous or useless drugs from this sector, as well as improving the knowledge of vendors and clients as to the proper use of medicines.

Sacramental drugs

In many cultures, drugs are used as sacramental substances, intrinsic to the rituals of religion, divination and healing, and to certain social interactions. Like the 'social foods' described in Chapter 3, their ingestion may contribute to the continuity and cohesion of a particular group of people. World wide, the most common ritual drug is obviously *alcohol*, and some of its social and religious uses have been described above. Other common substances important to the rituals of social encounters are the chemical comforters of tobacco, tea and coffee.

In some cultural groups hallucinogenic drugs are used to obtain states of transcendence and fervour, and in their trance state those who take them are 'possessed' by the power inherent in the drug. Such rituals may take many hours or even days to perform. Sometimes the drug is used only by a shaman or ritual healer, whose visions will reveal the source of individual or collective misfortune. Dobkin de Rios[74], for example, described the use of the hallucinogen *ayahuasca* by folk healers (*ayahuasqueros*) in an urban slum in Iquitos, Peru. As part of the ritual of healing the healer imbibes the *ayahuasca*, and the visionary content of his drug experience helps to identify the cause of the individual's illness (such as witchcraft, evil eye, or *susto*), and how it should then be dealt with.

In Medieval Europe, certain hallucinogens were used as part of 'witches' brew' or as unguents rubbed into the skin. They included belladona (*Atropa belladona*), henbane (*Hyoscyamus niger*), mandrake (*Mandragora officinarum*) and the fly agaric mushroom (*Amanita muscaria*).

Although most hallucinogenic drugs have powerful pharmacological effects on individuals, the cultural context of their use also influences the drug experience. In a ritual of divination, for example, it will influence the structure and timing of the ritual itself and the expectations and behaviour of its participants, as well as shaping the content of the shaman's visions and how they are communicated to those around him.

Among the more well-known hallucinogenic drugs used in a ritual context today are:

- marijuana (*Cannabis sativa* and *Cannabis indica*), known as *hashish* or *kif* in the Middle East and North Africa, as *dagga* in Southern Africa and as *ganja* among Rastafarians in the Caribbean[75]
- psilocybin (*Psilocybe mexicana Heim*), used by some Mexican Indian groups
- peyote cactus (*Lophophora williamsii*), used by Native Americans in the southwestern USA and members of the Native American Church (which claims about 250 000 members)[76]
- *ayahuasca* or *yagé* vine (*Banisteriopsis caapsis* and *B. inebrians*), a hallucinatory drink used by South America Indians (especially in Brazil, Ecuador, Peru and Colombia)[77]
- morning glory seeds (*Rivea corymbosa* and *Ipomoca violacca*), used by Mexican Indians in healing and divinatory rituals
- iboga (*Tabernanthe iboga*), used as a hallucinogen in parts of Zaire and Gabon
- jimson weed (*Datura stramonium*), used among the Algonquin Indians in the northeastern USA, and other species of *datura* used in parts of South America, Africa and Asia[78].

In Yemen, leaves of *qat* (or khat) (*Catha edulis Forssk.* and *Catha spinosa Forssk.*) are chewed for their stimulant or hallucinogenic properties. *Qat* is also used in parts of Ethiopia, Somalia and Kenya (where it is known as *miraa* or *marongi*)[79]. Cola nuts (*Cola nitada* or *Cola acuminata*) are also widely chewed for their stimulant and hunger-relieving effects in parts of West Africa, especially in Senegal, Sierra Leone, Ivory Coast, Ghana and Nigeria[80]. Sometimes they are seasoned before use with pepper, salt, ginger or tobacco flowers. Coca (*Ethroxylum coca*) is grown in highland areas of Peru, Ecuador and Bolivia[80].

Mixed with lime paste, the leaves are commonly chewed to alleviate the symptoms of hunger, thirst and fatigue, as well as for their stimulant effect. Its use in rituals dates back to the time of the Incas. Among its producers, it is rarely used in either the form or dosage preferred by those addicted to its derivative, cocaine. In Melanesia, including parts of New Guinea, the Solomon Islands, Fiji and Vanuatu, kava (from the shrub *Piper methysticum*) is either chewed or drunk as an infusion. It induces feelings of tranquillity and wellbeing[80]. Pituri (from the shrub *Duboisia hopwoodii*) is chewed by Australian Aborigines as a hallucinogen, or to alleviate the symptoms of pain, fatigue and hunger, but it also played an important role in certain male initiation rituals[80,81].

In recent years, use of many of these hallucinogenic plants has spread beyond their groups of origin and their original ritual context. In the industrialized world, many have been used as recreational drugs, in either their original or synthetic forms. In some susceptible individuals they are known to have caused addiction, habituation, acute psychosis, suicidal behaviour and various other disorders. Even in those groups that have traditionally used sacramental drugs in a controlled way, their overuse and abuse is now becoming more common. This is now true of drugs such as cannabis, *qat*, coca and, of course, alcohol.

Recommended reading

Benson, H. and Epstein, M. D. (1975). The placebo effect: a neglected asset in the care of patients. *JAMA*, **232**, 1225–7.

Douglas, M. (ed.) (1987). *Constructive Drinking*. Cambridge University Press.

Gefou-Madianou, D. (ed.) (1992). *Alcohol, Gender and Culture*. Routledge.

Hahn, R. A. (1997). The nocebo phenomenon: concept, evidence, and implications for public health. *Prev. Med.*, **26**, 607–11.

Helman, C. G. (1981). 'Tonic', 'food' and 'fuel': social and symbolic aspects of the long-term use of psychotropic drugs. *Soc. Sci. Med.*, **15B**, 521–33.

Nichter, M. and Cartwright, E. (1991). Saving the children for the tobacco industry. *Med. Anthropol. Q.* (new series), **5**, 236–56.

Rudgley, R. (1993). *The Alchemy of Culture: Intoxicants in Society*. British Museum Press.

9 Ritual and the management of misfortune

Rituals are a feature of all human societies, large and small. They are an important part of the way that any social group celebrates, maintains and renews the world in which it lives, and the way it deals with the dangers and uncertainties that threaten that world. Rituals occur in many settings, take on many forms and perform many functions, both sacred and secular. This chapter will describe the type of rituals that relate to health and illness and the management of misfortune.

What is ritual?

Anthropologists have defined the various attributes of ritual in a number of ways, and they have pointed out that, for those that take part in it, ritual has important social, psychological and symbolic dimensions. A key characteristic of any ritual is that it is a form of repetitive behaviour that does not have a direct overt technical effect. For example, brushing the teeth at the same time each night is a repetitive form of behaviour, but it is not a ritual; it is designed to have a specific physical effect – the removal of food and bacteria from the teeth. If, however, this action is accompanied by others that do not directly contribute towards the effect, such as always using a toothbrush of a particular colour or saying certain words or prayers before, during or after brushing the teeth, then these extraneous actions can be thought of as having a private ritual significance for the person. In some cases, *all* actions in a repetitive pattern of behaviour have no technical effect – as in private prayers or religious observance, or in some of the actions of the obsessive compulsive neurotic. In general, though, this form of private ritual behaviour is of less interest to anthropologists than the public rituals that take place in the presence of one or more other people.

Loudon[1] has defined these public rituals as 'those aspects of prescribed and repetitive formal behaviour, that is those aspects of certain customs, which have no direct technological consequences and which are symbolic'. That is, 'the behaviour or actions say something about the state of affairs, particularly about the social conditions of those taking part in the ritual'. In a social setting, rituals both express and renew certain basic values of that society, especially regarding the relationships between people, between people and nature, and between people and the supernatural world – relationships that are integral to the functioning of any human group. As Turner[2] puts it, 'ritual is a periodic restatement of the terms in which men of a particular culture must interact if there is to be any kind of coherent social life'. He sees two functions of ritual; an expressive function and a creative function. In its *expressive* aspect, ritual 'portrays in a symbolic form certain key values and cultural orientations'. That is, it expresses these basic values in a dramatic form, and *communicates* them to both participants and spectators. Leach[3] and other anthropologists see this aspect of ritual as being the most important. For them ritual has some of the properties of a language, which can only be understood within a specific cultural context and by those who can decode its meaning. As Leach[3] puts it, 'we must know a lot about the cultural context, the setting of the stage, before we can even begin to decode the message'. In its *creative* aspect, ritual, according to Turner[4], 'actually creates, or recreates, the categories through which men perceive reality – the axioms underlying the structure of society and the laws of the natural and moral orders'. It therefore restates, on a regular basis, certain values and principles of a society and how its members should act *vis-à-vis* other men, gods and the natural world, and it helps to *re*create in the minds of the participants their collective view of the world.

The symbols of ritual

These two functions of ritual, expressive and creative, are achieved by the use of *symbols*. These include certain standardized objects, clothing, movements, gestures, words, sounds, songs, music and scents used in rituals, as well as the fixed order in which they appear. Turner[2] has examined the forms and meanings of ritual symbols, particularly those used in healing rituals. He points out that, especially in pre-literate societies, rituals have the important function of storing and transmitting information about the society; each ritual is an aggregation of symbols, and acts as a 'storehouse of traditional knowledge'. He sees each symbol as a 'storage unit' into which is packed the maximum amount of information. This is because ritual symbols are 'multivocal', that is, they represent many things at the same time. Each symbol can be regarded as a multifaceted mnemonic, with each facet 'corresponding to a specific cluster of values, norms, beliefs, sentiments, social roles and relationships within the cultural system of the community performing the ritual'. Therefore, to the outsider observing a ritual, there is always more to the symbols than meets the eye. Each symbol has a whole range of associations for those taking part in the ritual. It tells them something about the values of their society, how it is organized and how it views the natural and supernatural worlds. This restatement of basic values is particularly important at times of danger or uncertainty – when people feel that their world is threatened by misfortunes such as accident, famine, war, death, severe interpersonal conflicts or ill health.

As mentioned above, ritual symbols can be 'decoded' only by looking at the context in which they appear. For example, a white coat worn in a hospital setting has a different range of associations from one worn by a supermarket attendant. Although both may be worn as a hygienic measure, the context in which they are worn adds many other associations to them. The white coat worn by a doctor in a healing context (hospital or doctor's office) may be regarded as a ritual *symbol*. While it does have a technical aspect – maintaining hygiene and avoiding dirt and contamination – it also carries a number of associations with it. For those taking part in medical healing (doctors, nurses, patients) it symbolizes or represents a number of attributes associated with doctors in general. Some of these associations are shown in Table 9.1. The potency of this multivocal symbol is shown by its widespread use in television or newspaper advertisements for patent medicines, which feature an 'expert' whose white coat symbolizes 'science' and 'reliability'.

Similarly, these coats are often worn by medical secretaries and receptionists, though this is often not crucial for hygienic reasons. Here the coat symbolizes membership (however peripheral) of the healing profession, and carries with it some of the attributes of doctors. Because of the proliferation of white coats among hospital nurses, paramedical staff and technicians, however, other subsidiary symbols, such as a stethoscope, bleeper, or specially coloured name tag, are required to complete the message to others involved in the healing context.

The sum of these symbols communicates information about the wearer of the coat, and also reinforces ideas of how 'a doctor' should dress and behave. These symbols refer less to the individual doctors than to the attributes of their role as representatives of that special category of persons who constitute the official healing profession, a group that is empowered to use the forces of science or technology for the benefit of their patients. Thus individual doctors employ the potent symbols of medical science (such as a white coat or a stethoscope) in their rituals of healing in the same way that non-Western healers employ certain religious symbols or artifacts (such as certain plants, talismans, divination stones, holy texts or statuettes) that also symbolize powerful healing forces (such as gods, spirits or ancestors). In this way, the use of these symbols brings the wider values of the society directly into the doctor–patient interaction.

In Britain, unlike in the USA and some European countries, most general practitioners

Table 9.1 Some associations of the physician's white coat as ritual symbol

A training in medicine
A licence to practise medicine
Membership of the medical profession
Being answerable to a professional organization
A repository of specialized and inaccessible knowledge
Power to:
take a medical history
obtain intimate details of patients' lives and examine patients' bodies
order a wide range of tests
prescribe medication or other treatments and make life or death decisions
hospitalize patients, some against their will
control those lower in the professional hierarchy, e.g. junior doctors, nurses, medical students
Orientation towards caring, and the relief of suffering
A scientific orientation in concepts and techniques
Confidentiality
Reliability and efficiency
Emotional and sexual detachment
Cleanliness
Respectability and high social status
High income
Familiarity with situations of illness, suffering and death

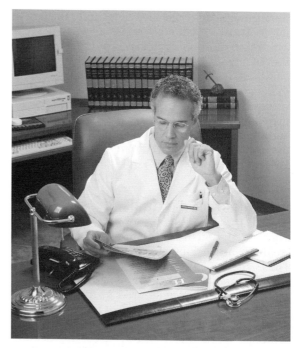

Figure 9.1 The physician's white coat: a potent ritual symbol of the healing powers of medical science (Source: © Digital Stock MED 2016).

(GPs) and many hospital doctors do not wear white coats. In these cases, *other* aspects of their dress need to play a more important ritual role. One study[5] in England found that for 64 per cent of patients, the way that their GP dressed was important in inspiring confidence in their professional skills. They preferred their family doctors not to dress too informally, but to wear more traditional, formal dress; a suit and tie in men, but a white coat in women. Another British study[6] found that while children saw formally-dressed paediatricians as competent but not friendly, they saw casually dressed paediatricians as friendly but not as competent.

Turner[4] has pointed out another attribute of ritual symbols; 'polarization of meaning'. This refers to the clustering of the associations of a particular multivocal symbol around two opposite poles. At one pole the symbol is associated with 'social and moral facts'; at the other with 'physiological facts'. This is seen in both healing rituals and rites of social transition. For example, in some societies a girl's first menstruation, the menarche, is marked by a special ritual. Some of the symbols used in this ritual are associated, in the minds of the participants, both with the *physiological* event (the menarche) and the *social* event of her new membership of the community of adult, fertile women. The ritual symbol acts as a 'bridge' linking the physiological and social stages of human life. These stages include birth, puberty, marriage and death. The symbols are a way of integrating physiological changes (especially at puberty), which might potentially be socially disruptive if left unchecked, with the laws and values that help keep society together. As Turner puts it, 'powerful drives and emotions associated with human physiology, especially with the physiology of reproduction, are divested in the ritual process of their antisocial quality and attached to components of the normative order'[4]. In the Western world, many of the rituals that used to mark life stages such as birth, puberty and death have disappeared. This means that these major life changes are not surrounded by ritual symbolism that gives meaning to the event far beyond its physiological significance. In contrast, in many non-Western societies, the symbols associated with physiological changes link these changes to wider social or cosmological events. Pregnancy, for example, is not only a physical event, but is also the social transition of 'woman' to 'mother'. Death is a physical event, but is sometimes seen as a simultaneous 'birth' into the society of ancestors. Some of these rituals will be described further in this chapter.

Case study: Colour symbolism of Zulu medicines

Ngubane's description[7] of the symbols used in healing rituals by the Zulu of South Africa illustrates the multivocal and bipolar aspects of ritual symbols. In this community, it is the *colour* of the medicines rather than their pharmacological properties that is considered the most important attribute. This colour symbolism is particularly important in medicines used for prophylactic purposes, or in dealing with illnesses thought to have a supernatural origin. The medicines are divided into three groups – black (*mnyama*), red (*bomvu*) and white (*mhlope*) – and each colour is associated with a cluster of meanings, physiological, social and cosmological. Black represents night time, darkness, dirt, pollution, faeces, death and danger. Defecation, dirt and death can be seen as antisocial elements, all of which should be absent from normal social encounters. Also, night is the time when people cannot see, when they withdraw from their usual social activities; at night, sick people become sicker and sorcerers are said to work. Ancestral spirits visit their descendants in dreams, so that sleep is a point of contact with the dead. Sleep, as Ngubane, says, 'may be regarded as a miniature death that takes a person away from the conscious life of the day'. In contrast, white symbolizes the good things of life, good health and good fortune. It represents daylight and the events that take place during it, such as eating or social interactions. During the day, people participate in social activities and live their lives. They see clearly, and there is no sense of danger. White represents the social values of life, eating and seeing. The third colour, red, symbolizes the states of transition between black and white, much as sunset and sunrise are between day and night. It represents an in-between position, slightly more dangerous than white but less so than black. It also stands for other states of transition or transformation, such as growth, regeneration or rebirth. The association of blood with states of transition (such as birth, or a fatal wound) is also relevant here. In treating an ill person the Zulu traditional healer aims to restore health, which is seen as a *balance* between the person and the environment. This is achieved by expelling from the body what is bad by the use of black and red remedies, and then strengthening the body by the use of white medicines. The medicines are always used in a fixed order – black, red, white. This is meant to achieve a transformation from illness to health, 'from the darkness of night to the goodness of daylight', from death to life, from danger to safety, from antisocial to social behaviour. As Ngubane puts it:

> the daylight represents life and good health. To be (mystically) ill is likened to moving away from the daylight into the dimness of the sunset and on into the night ... The practitioner endeavours to drive a patient out of the mystical darkness by black medicines, through the reddish twilight of the sunrise by red medicines, and back into daylight and life by white medicines.'

Types of ritual

While there are many different types of private ritual, anthropologists have described three main types of public ritual:

1. Cosmic cycle or calendrical rituals
2. Rituals of social transitions (*rites de passage*)
3. Rituals of misfortune.

Calendrical rituals

Calendrical rituals celebrate changes in the cosmic cycle, such as the changing of seasons and the division of the year into segments such as months, weeks or days, as well as certain festivals and holy days. The identity and world-view of the group is linked symbolically to events in the cosmic cycle, or to certain specified points within that cycle. Examples of this are harvest festivals, midsummer festivals, holy days such as Christmas and Easter, or commemorative days such as Thanksgiving or Remembrance Sunday. These social occasions are usually based on the cycle of the seasons, or the position of the moon, sun or planetary bodies. In many of these rituals, the symbols used link the social and cosmological dimensions and help reinforce and recreate the social organization and values of the society.

Rituals of social transition

The rituals of social transition are present in one form or another in every society. They relate changes in the human life cycle to changes in social position within the society by linking the physiological to the social aspects of an individual's life. Examples of this are rituals associated with pregnancy, childbirth, puberty, menarche, weddings, funerals and severe ill health. In each of these stages, the ritual signals the *transition* of the individual from one status to another – such as from 'wife' to 'mother' in pregnancy. As Standing[8] points out, the ritual taboos and prescriptions surrounding pregnancy in many societies help prepare the woman, in terms of her behaviour, for her future role as a mother, as well as dramatizing this change in status to the society at large. In Western society, puberty rituals (such as confirmation or *barmitzvah*) still exist, and signal the transition between child and young adult. Birth rituals such as baptism, christening or circumcision signal 'social birth' (new membership of society), shortly after biological birth.

Leach[9] sees the origin of these transition rituals in the human tendency to divide things or actions into *categories*, each with its own boundary and name (see Chapter 1). As he puts it: 'When we use symbols (either verbal or non-verbal) to distinguish one class of things or actions from another we are creating artificial boundaries in a field which is "naturally" continuous'. These 'boundaries in the continuous field of perception' are characterized by a sense of ambiguity and danger. When things lie in the no man's land between definitions or categories, when they are 'neither fish nor fowl', they provoke a sense of uneasiness, especially in those who prefer things to be more clearly defined. This process, according to Leach, applies also to the progress of the individual through various social identities during the course of their life – such as 'child', 'adult', 'mother' and 'widow'. In the period of transition between these identities, the individual is considered to be in an interval of 'social timelessness', in a vulnerable, 'abnormal' position, dangerous both to themselves and to others; for this reason, special rituals of social transition are invoked that mark the event and protect both individual and society by various ritual taboos and observances. For example, many Western wedding customs still specify that in order to avoid bad luck the bride should not be seen by her groom the night before the wedding, and she is kept protectively veiled until well into the wedding ceremony, after which she is no longer considered vulnerable. In many non-Western societies the vulnerable period of transition may last for months or even years.

In Leach's view[9], most ritual occasions in any society are concerned with this 'movement across social boundaries from one social status to another'. In these circumstances, ritual has two functions: 'proclaiming the change in status' and 'magically bringing it about', though the two are closely related. To the participants, the belief is that without the ritual the change would somehow not take place.

Stages of social transition

Van Gennep[10] has described three stages in these *rites de passage*. They are:

- separation
- transition
- incorporation.

In the first stage, the person is removed from his or her normal social life and set apart by various customs and taboos for a variable period of time. After this stage of transition, other rituals celebrate the third stage of incorporation, whereby the person is returned to normal society, and into their new social role. Often this last stage is marked by ritual bathing or other rites of symbolic purification. Based on Van Gennep's and Leach's work, the three stages of these rituals of social transition are illustrated in Figure 9.2.

Rituals of pregnancy and childbirth

In all societies, pregnancy and childbirth are more than just biological events. As described in Chapter 6, they are also social events – the transition of the woman (especially with a first birth) from the social status of 'woman' to that of 'mother'. During pregnancy, the woman is in a

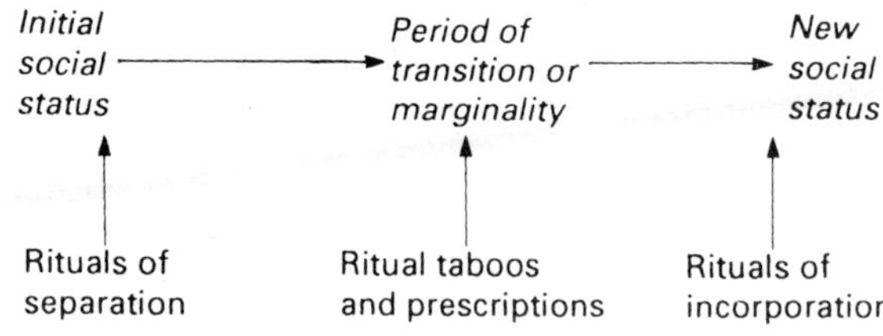

Figure 9.2 Rituals of social transition

state of transition between these two social statuses. In this state of limbo she is often considered to be in an ambiguous and socially abnormal situation, vulnerable to outside dangers and sometimes dangerous to other people. In many traditional societies pregnant women withdraw from social activities and live somewhat apart from other people, subject to certain taboos about diet, dress and behaviour. These taboos are designed to protect the pregnancy, but they are also ways of marking the transition between social statuses. In some cases these taboos may extend well into the postpartum period. Among the Zulu people of South Africa, for example, a woman is considered to still be vulnerable to outside dangers until all her postpartum bleeding ceases[11]. Furthermore, this blood is considered to be dangerous to her husband's virility, as well as to plants in the field and even to livestock.

Many of the practices and beliefs associated with modern Western obstetrics can also be seen as having an important ritual component[12], and the ritual symbols used here are those of medical science and technology. Some of the culturally specific messages transmitted to pregnant women and their families by these symbols were described in more detail in Chapter 6. Overall, pregnancy and childbirth in the Western world are as ritualized, in their own way, as they are elsewhere. As Kitzinger[13] has put it:

> Baptism, circumcision, naming ceremonies, segregation of the new mother and baby, churching of women, taboos on sexual intercourse following birth, even the postnatal checkup, are all often complicated steps in a kind of dance which continues until mother and child are safely established in their correct social places and are considered no longer at risk.

The three main stages of social transition in pregnancy and childbirth are illustrated in Figure 9.3.

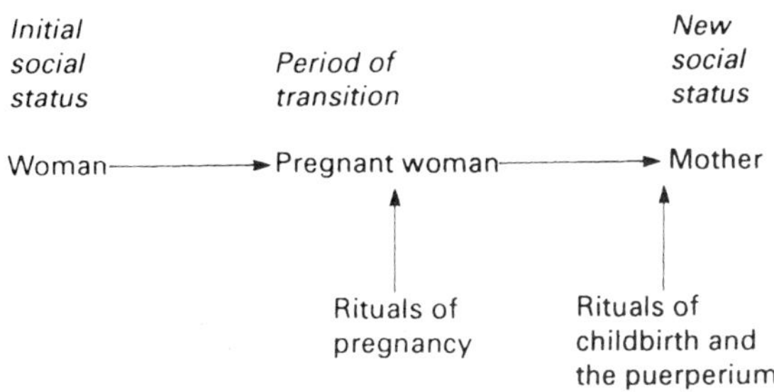

Figure 9.3 Rituals of pregnancy and childbirth

Rituals of death and mourning

Hertz[14] examined one form of rituals of social transition; those associated with death and mourning. He examined the funerary customs of many societies, and sees common themes among them. In most human societies people have, in effect, *two* types of death; one biological and the other social. Between these two there is a variable period of time, which may be days, months or even years. While biological death is the end of the human organism, social death is the end of the person's social identity. This takes place at a series of ceremonies, including the funeral, where the society bids farewell to one of its members and reasserts its continuity without him or her. Hertz points out that, in most non-Western societies, death is seen not as a single event in time but as a *process* whereby the deceased is slowly transferred from the land of the living into the land of the dead; simultaneously there is a transition between social identities from living person to dead ancestor. During the period between biological death and final social death, the deceased's soul is often considered to be in a state of limbo, still a partial member of society and potentially dangerous to other people as it roams free and unburied. In this transitional phase the soul still has some residual social rights, especially over its bereaved relatives. They have to perform certain ceremonies, act or dress in a special way, and generally withdraw from ordinary life. Like the deceased's soul, they, too, are in a socially ambiguous state between identities, dangerous both to themselves and to others. In many cultures a widowed woman is prohibited from remarrying for a specified period (sometimes forever) after her husband's death. In Hertz's model she is considered to be in a transitional state, still married to the soul of her husband, until his final moment of social death and even beyond it.

In the Malay archipelago, the corpse is given a first, temporary burial while it decomposes, before being reburied months or even years later at a final ceremony. During the period between the two funerals, 'the deceased continues to belong more or less exclusively to the world he has just left. To the living falls the duty of providing for him; twice a day till the final ceremony ... [they] bring him his usual meal'. During this period 'the deceased is looked upon as having not yet completely ended his earthly existence'. The final funeral ends this existence, and the ritual is one of incorporation, whereby the deceased is initiated or reborn into the society of dead ancestors, and the mourners reincorporated into normal society and liberated from the special taboos and restrictions of their transitional state. The final ceremony also removes the danger from the soul, which is no longer in limbo.

Eisenbruch[15] described some of the culturally patterned ways of taking leave of the deceased among different social and cultural groups in the USA, including urban African-Americans, Chinese, Italians, Greeks, Haitians, Latinos and South East Asian refugees, and showed the wide variations in their bereavement beliefs and customs. In the UK, Skultans[16] has also described some of the range of bereavement practices among different cultural and religious groups. The Irish *wake*, for example, involves watching of the corpse by relatives for several days and nights, and sometimes involves feasting and drinking. Among Greek Cypriots there is 'socially patterned weeping and wailing', followed by a defined period of mourning and wearing black. Among orthodox Jews, in Britain and elsewhere, the *shib 'ah* has a precise structure of mourning, lasting 7 days after the funeral, during which time the bereaved remain at home and are visited by consolers. Mourning dress is worn till the thirtieth day, and recreation and amusement are forbidden for 1 year. In this case the transitional period lasts from the funeral (shortly after biological death) until the tombstone is dedicated a year later and mourning officially ends. The dedication of the tombstone can be seen as the last of a series of 'funerals', during which the deceased gradually leaves the world of the living. In this group, as in many others, 'social death' takes place slowly, in a series of culturally defined stages. Also in Britain, Laungani[17] described how the bereavement practices of Hindu immigrants to Britain have changed over the years, compared to those practised back in India. This is particularly so in relation to the open display of the dead, cremation and the subsequent scattering of the ashes in a holy river (such as the Ganges). Nevertheless, compared to Christian burials in Britain, Hindu funerals are still characterized by a more communal approach and by a more public and volatile display of emotions.

In some societies, the care and preparation of the corpse is carried out only by close family members. In others, however, it is done by certain specialized individuals within the community – individuals who may be termed *traditional death attendants* (TDAs). These individuals are also familiar with all the rituals necessary for the funeral itself and subsequent mourning. Among orthodox Jews, for example, the *chevra kadisha* or Burial Society of each community, made up of volunteers, carries out this ritual role of caring for the corpse and preparing it for burial. In many cases, therefore, people who have immigrated from societies where either the family or these TDAs usually take care of the corpse may find the rather impersonal approach of professional undertakers rather difficult to accept, especially where they are unfamiliar with the cultural background of the grieving family.

To some extent, all funerary practices are influenced by a culture's view of the existence, or nature, of an after-life. In ancient Egypt, for example, prominent people were buried together with texts from the 'Book of the Dead' – a guidebook for the deceased, telling them about the world-to-come and how they should behave within it. Cultures that believe in reincarnation – who see time as circular or spiral, and expect the souls of the dead eventually to be 'recycled' back onto Earth – are likely to have very different attitudes to mourning to those without such a belief, who see death as a final, permanent event, rather than as part of a more cyclical process.

In Western society death, like birth, is increasingly 'medicalized' (see Chapter 6). The natural stages of biological dying are now often seen as being, in some way, unnatural or even pathological. In many industrialized societies, the concept of death by 'natural causes' has almost disappeared. Konner[18] has criticized this approach, which emphasizes the quantity of life expectancy rather than the quality, especially where resuscitation involves heroic, aggressive, uncomfortable and painful forms of treatment. He contrasts two poignant examples: an elderly American man, semi-comatose and subject to a variety of intense, painful treatments in Sun City, Arizona, 'his body poked full of needles and tubes surrounded by busy strangers'; and the slow, dignified, natural death of an elderly Indian woman, dying among her close family in Benares on the Ganges.

In most traditional societies the dead do not really die – at least, not in a social (or emotional) sense. In much of sub-Saharan Africa and Asia, and in parts of Latin America, they remain as an omnipresent part of the lives of their relatives and an invisible member of the family (see Chapter 10). Their death as a member of society is followed by their birth into the community of ancestors. Here they remain forever, observing, protecting and sometimes punishing those who survive them. Thus in many of these societies *ancestor worship* is common, and frequent and regular offerings are made at shrines to appease them. The ancestors may communicate with their families in dreams or visions, or as part of certain rituals, or with the aid of traditional healers. In much of sub-Saharan Africa, they remain as permanent guardians of the social order, causing ill health or misfortune to those of their descendants who break the moral code. In Mexico, their continuing membership of the family is celebrated at the beginning of each November, when a meal is 'shared' between the living and their dead relatives at the graveside as part of the annual 'Day of the Dead' (*El Día de los Muertos*)[19]. This ritual is believed by anthropologists to combine aspects of Catholicism (All Souls Day) with elements of the religion and ancestor-worship of the ancient Aztecs.

As these examples illustrate, there is a wide variation in the care of the dying, bereavement practices and beliefs about death in different social and cultural groups. Because of these differences, Eisenbruch[15] has emphasized that although there are certain constancies in how human beings grieve, it cannot be assumed that the states of grieving in different cultures all occur at the same rate, or even in exactly the same sequence.

The three main stages of social death are illustrated in Figure 9.4.

Birth and death: social and biological

The relationships described above, between biological and social birth and death, are summarized in Figure 9.5.

In most societies, *social birth* follows biological birth and can be said to extend over many years. Growing up involves a whole series of social births. At each stage individuals are 'born' into a new social identity, until finally they acquire the status of a full adult member of their community. In Western societies these stages usually begin with acquiring a name, and being christened, baptized or circumcised. Thereafter, each stage – beginning at school, going through puberty, leaving school, being allowed to drive, drink alcohol, have sexual intercourse, vote, inherit property, enter work or college, get married and have children – is a form of social birth. However, in some cases social birth can be regarded as preceding the moment of biological birth. As mentioned earlier, much of the debate around the abortion issue centres on whether the foetus is a person, with social and legal rights, or not – either from conception onwards, or from some other point during the pregnancy. For some women, viewing the ultrasound image of their growing foetus as part of an antenatal check-up may help increase the social identity of the foetus long before the actual delivery takes place.

As with social birth, *social death* usually takes place after biological death, in a series of stages – including the funeral, mourning and annual rituals of remembrance – outlined above. However, in some circumstances a form of social death can be said to *precede* biological death, often by many years. Here individuals are still alive physically, but in a subtle way less 'alive' socially, both in the eyes of the wider society and sometimes their own families. For example, those who have been confined to institutions for the rest of their lives (prisons, old age homes, geriatric wards, hospices for the terminally ill, homes for the mentally handicapped) may all be said to have undergone a form of social death long before the date of their biological death. In many societies, retirement or unemployment may also have the same effect, as may the diagnosis of a serious disease, such as AIDS or cancer. In each case, such a social death may contribute to the *nocebo* effect (see Chapter 11) and seriously affect the health of the individual. One dramatic example of social death followed shortly afterwards by biological death is 'voodoo death' or 'hex death', described in more detail in Chapter 11.

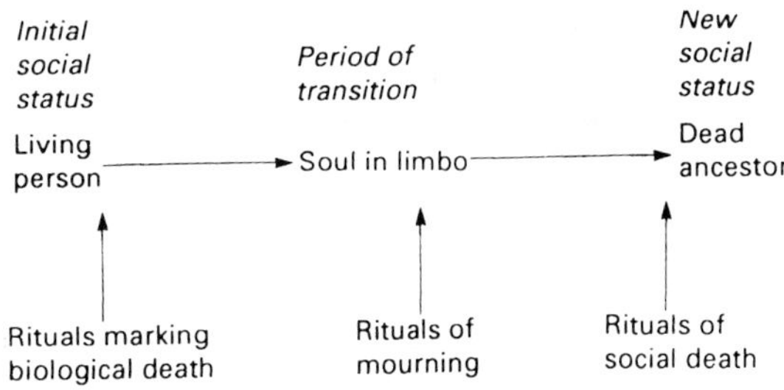

Figure 9.4 Stages of social death

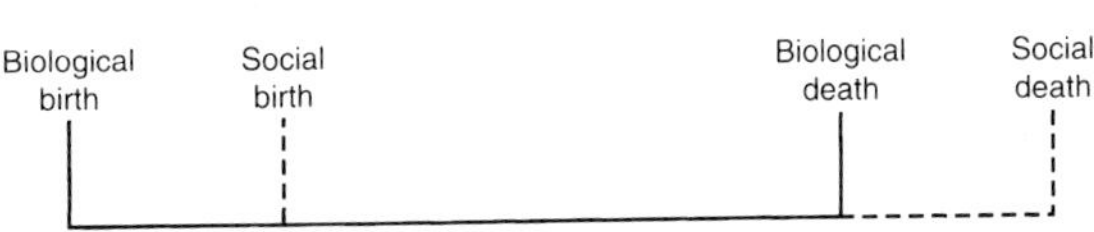

Figure 9.5 Social and biological birth and death

Modern medical technology has had an important impact on the nature of death. In some cases of severe illness or extreme old age, it now enables doctors for the first time to more-or-less control the exact timing of death. Modern life-support systems make it possible to widen the duration of biological death and postpone social death almost indefinitely. They can now convert death from a single point in time to a period of time. In the case of brain death, technology can now maintain the patient in a comatose state for months or even years – thus increasing the period of transition or liminality for them as well as for their family. This in turn may have profound emotional implications for all concerned. Technology also enables doctors to end this period, whenever they decide to do so, by switching off the machine. In coming years, the effects of these changes on our perceptions of death are likely to be profound.

Rituals of hospitalization

Many healing rituals are also rituals of social transition whereby an 'ill person' is transformed into a 'healthy person'. This often involves the patient's withdrawal from everyday life while certain treatments are followed and taboos observed. If the patient recovers he or she is ritually reincorporated into normal society, but in the phase of transition the sufferer is considered especially vulnerable, as well as dangerous to other people. To some extent, the hospital can be seen as a setting for these rites of social transition. Patients admitted to hospital leave their normal life behind and enter a state of limbo characterized by a sense of vulnerability and danger. As with other institutions, such as the army or prison, they undergo a standardized ritual of entry by which they are divested of many of the props of their social identity. Their clothing is removed and replaced by a uniform of pyjamas or nightdress. In the ward they are allocated a number, and transformed into a 'case' for diagnosis and treatment. Later, when they have recovered, they regain their own clothes and rejoin their community in the new social identity of either a 'cured' or a 'healthier' person. While hospital treatment is designed to provide intensive medical care and observation, and to remove patients with infectious disease from the community, it also follows Van Gennep's three stages of separation, transition and incorporation, as illustrated in Figure 9.6.

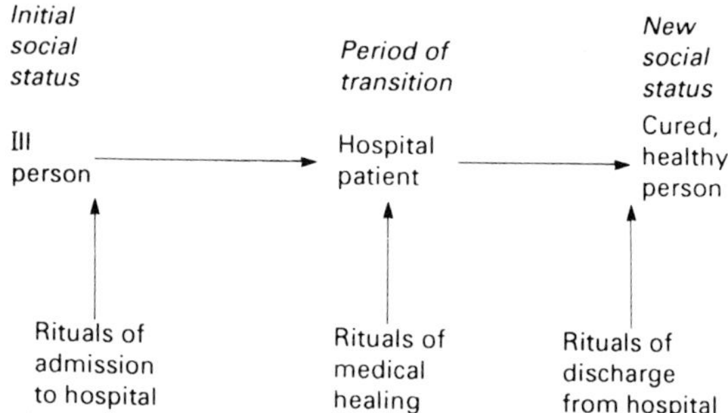

Figure 9.6 Hospitalization as a ritual of social transition

Clinicians should be aware of these social dimensions of hospitalization, especially patients' feelings of unease and anxiety about their ambiguous or abnormal social status.

Rituals of misfortune

These usually come into play at times of unexpected crisis or misfortune, such as accidents or severe ill health. Loudon[1] sees two functions of this type of ritual; a manifest function (the solution of specific problems) and a latent function ('the re-establishment of disturbed relationships between human beings'). In many small-scale non-industrialized societies they also function to repair disturbed relationships with the social and supernatural worlds. As Foster and Anderson[20] pointed out, in these societies:

> illnesses are often interpreted as reflecting stress or tears in the social fabric. The purpose of curing therefore goes well beyond the limited goal of restoring the sick person to health; it constitutes social therapy for the entire group, reassuring all onlookers that the interpersonal stresses that have led to illness are being healed.

Illness is therefore seen as a *social* event. The illness of one member, especially if blamed on witchcraft or sorcery resulting from interpersonal conflicts, threatens the cohesion and continuity of the group. The group has an interest in finding and resolving the cause of the illness, and restoring both the victim and themselves to health. As a result, such healing rituals usually take place in *public*, in marked contrast to the privacy and confidentiality that characterize doctor–patient consultations in the Western world. The aim of these public rituals is visibly to restore the harmonious relationships between man and man, man and his deities, and man and the natural world.

Rituals of misfortune usually have two consecutive phases; the phase of *diagnosis* or divination of the cause of the misfortune, and the *treatment* of the effects of the misfortune and removal of the cause. In the case of ill health, the first phase includes giving the condition a label or identity within the cultural frame of reference. This implies a concept of how misfortune is caused, its probable natural history and its prognosis, which is shared by healer, patient and spectators. There are many techniques used by different cultures to diagnose ill health, ranging from divinatory seances to the use of sophisticated diagnostic technology. Several of them have been mentioned in Chapter 4. As an example, Beattie[21] described a divinatory seance among the Nyoro people in Uganda, where the diviner goes into a trance, speaking in a small falsetto voice and using a special vocabulary 'so people knew that the spirit had come into his head, and they began to ask him questions'. These questions related to the diagnosis of a variety of misfortunes, such as marital conflicts, theft and ill health. It was the 'spirit' who diagnosed their cause and prescribed treatment, speaking publicly through the mouth of the diviner. In contrast, the private diagnosis of Western medicine refers mainly to disorders of the patient's body or emotions; in general, neither mystico-religious beliefs nor social relationships are considered major factors in diagnosis and treatment. In both cases, there is an overlap between these rituals and rites of social transition. Many involve the transition of the sufferer from the social identity of 'ill person' towards that of 'cured person', via the three stages described by Van Gennep.

Technical aspects of ritual

In looking at all forms of healing ritual, it is important to distinguish the ritual aspect from the practical or *technical* aspect that often coexists with it. In practice, the division between the two is not absolute; a purely sacred ritual can have the practical, technical effect of permanently altering people's behaviour or emotional state, for example. The technical aspect is often interwoven with the ritual, and includes such practical techniques as the use of medicines, surgical operations[22], inhalations, massages, cupping, injections and bone-setting, as well as techniques of psychotherapy and midwifery. Even in the most primitive society, where the purely ritual aspect of healing is strongest, there is likely to be a component of shrewd observations and experience on the part of the healer as to why and how people get ill, some knowledge of human nature, and a mastery of certain theatrical and practical techniques.

In Western society, medical diagnosis and treatment also take place in ritual time and ritual space – that is, at certain times and in certain settings carefully marked off from the rest of everyday life (such as a hospital clinic or a doctor's office). In this setting even the most technical treatments are influenced by the ritual atmosphere, and this is clearly illustrated in the case of the placebo effect. Also, as Balint[23] has pointed out, the most important drug that can be administered in this setting is the personality of the doctor.

Functions of ritual

Rituals fulfil many functions, both for the individual and for society. Depending on the perspective from which they are viewed, these functions can be classified into three overlapping groups; *psychological*, *social* and *protective*.

Psychological functions

In situations of unexpected misfortune or ill health, rituals provide a standardized way of explaining and controlling the unknown. The sudden onset of illness causes feelings of uncertainty and anxiety in the victims and their family. They ask: 'What has happened?', 'Why has it happened?', 'Why to me?', 'Is it dangerous?'. As Balint[24] puts it, in the consultation 'the patient is still frightened and lost, desperately in need of health. His chief problem, which he cannot solve without help, is: What is his illness, the thing that has caused his pains and frightens him?'. Part of the function of a healing ritual (as well as treating the condition) is to provide explanations for the illness in terms of the patient's cultural outlook – that is, to convert the chaos of symptoms and signs into a recognizable, culturally validated condition, whether it is pneumonia or *susto*, with a name and a known cause, treatment and prognosis. In a psychological sense, therefore, diagnosis itself *is* a form of treatment, converting the unknown into the known, and reducing the uncertainty and anxiety of patient and family. In the words of Phineas Parkhurst Quimby, a famous folk healer born in New England in 1802[25]:

> I tell the patient his troubles, and what he thinks is his disease, and my explanation is the cure. If I succeed in correcting his errors I change the fluids in the system, and establish the patient in health. The truth is the cure.[25]

Ritual also lessens anxiety at times of physiological change, such as pregnancy. These rituals, many of them public, help to control the sense of anxiety or unease associated with this vulnerable transitional state. Standing[8] has noted how it is impossible to eradicate *all* risk in pregnancy, but following prescribed rituals and taboos at least provides some kind of assurance that everything possible is being done to minimize that risk. Some diagnostic rituals can also be used to explain misfortune or failure *post hoc*, and thus lessen feelings of guilt or responsibility. For example, in some communities a woman who has given birth to a deformed child might be told that she had been bewitched by an unknown person during pregnancy, and that therefore the deformity was not her fault. However, in some cases the modern rituals of childbirth that are heavily dependent on technology may have a much more negative effect, causing the woman to feel more anxious, more helpless, and less in control of her own body at a crucial time for her[26].

At times of extreme crisis, such as bereavement, rituals usually provide a standardized mode of behaviour that helps to relieve the sense of uncertainty or loss. Everyone knows what to do and how to act under those circumstances, and this restores a sense of order and continuity to their lives. It also enables the bereaved slowly to adjust to the fact of death, and to see it not as the end of one cycle but as the beginning of another. This gradual acceptance occurs in well-defined ritual stages, which vary between cultures[15,27]. The normal phases of grieving in most Western communities (though not necessarily elsewhere), from 'numbness' to 'reorganization', described by Murray Parkes[28], can therefore be placed in a ritual context, and at each stage the mourners can be given much-needed social support and understanding. For example, in previous generations in the UK and other European countries, the status of mourner was signalled by wearing black clothes or a black armband. This marked mourners out from other people, and for a period of time ensured a special, protective attitude towards them. Skultans[16] has speculated that the increased risk of death among the recently bereaved (see Chapter 11) may be partly due to the disappearance of this type of protective ritual. She points out that in modern, middle-class Britain, while:

> some rituals are maintained at the actual time of death and funeral in that the family gathers and mourning dress is worn ... the absence of ritual is most marked during the subsequent period of mourning. Most noticeably, the bereaved are given no guidance on how to behave in their precarious position: they are not, as in non-industrialized societies, set apart from the rest of society for a prescribed period of time, nor are they given ritual protection in this severe crisis.

Today there is thus little outward change in behaviour and dress, and often grieving is seen as a 'pathological state', to be treated by antidepressants or other medication. Mourning rituals that encourage emotional displays of grief and define precisely when the mourning period ends probably limit the possibility of excessive or pathological mourning.

Rituals also provide a way of expressing and relieving unpleasant emotions; that is, they have a *cathartic* effect. This is especially true of the public rituals of small-scale, non-Western societies. As Beattie[21] puts it, 'they provide a way of expressing, and so of relieving, some of the inter-personal stresses and strains which are inseparable from life in a small-scale society'. In this setting, this 'safety valve' function benefits both the individual and society. Both diagnosis and treatment take place in the presence of all the family, friends and neighbours of the patient, and their part in the causation of the illness is openly discussed, as well as what they can do to help the patient. In Western clinical practice, as Turner[29] remarked, 'relief might be given to many sufferers from neurotic illness if all those involved in their social networks could meet together and publicly confess their ill will towards the patient and endure in turn the recital of his grudges against them'. In most cases, however, this type of emotional catharsis only takes place in private, in the presence of only one other person – whether psychotherapist, counsellor, psychiatrist or priest.

Finally, the rituals of healing can also function to reduce anxiety and uncertainty in the healers themselves. Bosk[30] has suggested that many of the occupational rituals of American physicians

– such as case conferences, grand rounds and mortality and morbidity conferences – may help the physicians to cope with their *own* sense of anxiety and uncertainty, and to make the necessary treatment decisions. Katz's detailed study[22] of surgical rituals in the USA has come to the same conclusion.

Social functions

These overlap with the psychological functions. Particularly in small-scale societies, the cohesion of the group is threatened by interpersonal conflicts. By ascribing ill health to these conflicts, the group can use this misfortune to bring conflicts into the open and publicly resolve them; this is a feature of societies where ill health and other misfortune is ascribed to interpersonal malevolence, such as witchcraft or sorcery. Illness also creates a temporary caring community around the victim, and old antagonisms are forgotten, at least for the moment. Because ill health reminds the community of its own vulnerability to death and decay, both rituals of misfortune and those of social transition (such as mourning rites) help reassert the continuity and survival of the group after the illness or death of one of its members.

Another social function of rituals is to create or recreate the basic axioms on which the society is based. By the use of multivocal symbols, the rituals dramatize these basic values and remind people of them. According to Turner[2], the way a society lives can be seen as an attempted imitation of models portrayed and animated by ritual. As such, rituals can modify behaviour towards a more sociable form, and resolve the tensions between self-interest and the interests of the group. In the colour symbolism of Zulu healing, for example, the colours are always used in the sequence black, red, white; that is, from 'anti-social' symbols, through a transitional phase towards more positive social symbols – from defecation, death and dirt towards life, eating and cleanliness. In other societies, rituals of social transition help control or tame potentially antisocial sexual impulses at puberty by restrictive taboos during the period of 'becoming an adult'.

Protective functions

Rituals dealing with ill health can protect the participants in two ways; psychologically or physically. The role of rituals in protecting against the anxiety and uncertainty associated with illness, death and other misfortune has already been described. In other ways, ritual observances can protect the ill or weak person from physical dangers such as infection. Some of the rituals surrounding pregnancy, birth or the postpartum period, for example, may protect the woman and her newborn child from sources of infection or injury, especially if they involve withdrawal from normal social life. Secluding an ill person, as part of a ritual of social transition, may also limit the spread of infectious diseases to the community, while a healing ritual held in public may have exactly the opposite effect. Other protective functions arise from cleansing and purification rites, which, although carried out for ritual purposes, may also remove dirt and bacteria and promote physical cleanliness.

This section has listed some of the main functions of ritual, psychological, social and protective, especially in rituals of illness and misfortune. If Douglas[31] is correct, and the industrialized world is moving away from ritual and 'there is a lack of commitment to common symbols', then the individual's management of misfortune, disease, death and the stages of the human life cycle might all become more difficult.

In the following case studies, three types of ritual of misfortune are contrasted: a public healing ceremony in a non-Western community; the more private diagnostic ritual in a Western society; and the ritual setting of a new type of syncretic, traditional healer – one increasingly common in many countries, whose rituals and practices utilize a mixture of Western and traditional elements.

Case study: Curative rites among the Ndembu of Zambia

Turner[29] described curative rites among the Ndembu people of Zambia in the 1960s. The Ndembu ascribe all persistent or severe ill health to social causes, such as the secret malevolence of sorcerers or witches, or punishment by the spirits of ancestors. These spirits cause sickness in an individual if his or her family and kin are 'not living well together', and are involved in grudges or quarrelling. Because death, disease and other misfortunes are usually ascribed 'to exacerbated tensions in

continued

social relations', diagnosis (divination) takes place publicly, and becomes 'a form of social analysis', while therapies are directed to 'sealing up the breaches in social relationships simultaneously with ridding the patient ... of his pathological symptoms'. The Ndembu ritual specialist or traditional healer, the *chimbuki*, conducts a divinatory seance attended by the victim, his kin and neighbours. The diviner is already familiar with the social position of the patient, who his relatives are, the conflicts that surround him, and other information gained from the gossip and opinions of the patient's neighbours and relatives. By questioning these people, and by shrewd observation, he builds up a picture of the patient's 'social field' and its various tensions. Actual divination takes place by peering into medicated water in an old meal mortar, in which he claims to see the 'shadow soul' of the afflicting ancestral spirit. He may also detect witches or sorcerers, who have caused the illness, among the spectators. The diviner calls all the relatives of the patient before a sacred shrine to the ancestors, and induces them 'to confess any grudges ... and hard feelings they may nourish against the patient'. The patient, too, must publicly acknowledge his own grudges against his fellow villagers if he is to be free of his affliction. By this process, all the hidden social tensions of the group are publicly aired and gradually resolved. Treatment involves rituals of exorcism, to withdraw evil influences from the patient's body. It also includes the use of certain herbal and other medicines, manipulation and cupping, and certain substances applied to the skin. These remedies are accompanied by dances and songs, the aim of which is the purification of both the victim and the group. Turner doubted whether the medicines he saw used in these rituals had much pharmacological effect, but he pointed out the psychotherapeutic benefits, to both the victim and the community, of the public expression and resolution of interpersonal conflicts, and the degree of attention paid to the victim during the ceremony.

Case study: Consultation with a general practitioner in the UK

The consultation between the average British general practitioner (GP) or family physician and his or her patients is markedly different from the Ndembu example, but it too is a form of healing ritual. Consultations take place at defined times and places (the office or surgery), and are governed by implicit and explicit rules of behaviour, deference, dress and subject matter to be discussed. Events take place in a fixed order: entering the surgery, giving one's name to a receptionist, sitting in a waiting room, being called in turn to see the doctor, entering the doctor's room, exchanging formal greetings, and then beginning the consultation. From this point onwards, Byrne[32] has described six stages in the procedure:

1. The establishment of rapport between GP and patient
2. The doctor discovering why the patient has come
3. The doctor's verbal and/or physical examination
4. Both parties' 'consideration of the patient's condition'
5. The doctor detailing treatment or further tests
6. The termination of the consultation, usually by the doctor.

The patient's symptoms and signs are recorded, during the consultation, on the medical card, and the present condition is seen against the background of previous illnesses recorded there. Particular attention is paid to questions like 'when did the pain begin?' and 'when did you first notice the swelling?' as part of the verbal diagnosis. As Foster and Anderson[33] point out, this historical approach is characteristic of Western diagnosis; in other cultures, the healer is expected to know all about the patient's condition without asking so many probing questions. As well as gathering clinical information by taking a history, physical examination or tests, GPs – like the Ndembu *chimbuki* – use informal knowledge gathered over the years in the community. As a result, assessment of a patient is based not only on the consultation but also on the GP's knowledge of the patient's environment, family, work, past medical history, pattern of behaviour and the culture of the neighbourhood.

The consultation is characterized by privacy and confidentiality, and usually involves only one patient and one doctor at a time. Its form is the ritual exchange of information between the two; symptoms and complaints flow in one direction, diagnoses and advice in the other. The patient receives practical advice ('Spend a day or two in bed') or a prescription for medication. The prescription form itself resembles a contract, with the name of the doctor, the name of the patient, and the prescribed medication linking the two written on it. It is assumed that the authority of the doctor extends beyond the consultation, because the drug must be taken as prescribed once the patient gets home ('Take one tablet three times a day, after meals, for seven days'). As with other healing rituals, the consultation takes place at specified times and in a setting set aside for this purpose. The GP's room, although designed for a technical purpose, includes many objects that will not be used in a particular consultation, and can therefore take on the significance of ritual symbols. These may include: a framed diploma on the wall; a stethoscope, otoscope and ophthalmoscope; a sphygmomanometer; tongue depressors; scalpels, forceps, needles and syringes; a glass cabinet full of instruments; bottles of antiseptic and other medicines; one or more telephones; a computer terminal; a bookshelf filled with impressive-looking textbooks or journals; a large desk; family photographs; sheaves of special forms or notepaper; an ink pad and rubber stamps; and a pile of previous patients' medical cards.

In this formalized setting of ritual time and place, the patient's diffuse symptoms and signs are given a diagnostic label and organized into the named diseases of the medical model. As well as prescribed medication, the most powerful drug administered in this setting is faith in the healing powers of the doctor[23].

Case study: 'Doctor John': An innovative traditional healer in Transkei, South Africa.

Simon[34] described the setting and healing rituals of 'Doctor John', a Xhosa traditional healer in rural Transkei, eastern South Africa. 'Doctor John' utilized many of the ritual symbols and practices of Western medicine, but blended them with certain aspects of traditional African healing. Situated in a village back street, his consulting room was in a small, dilapidated shack. Although without formal qualifications, a lavishly painted sign hung outside proclaiming: 'Dr John: Homeopath, Naturopath, Herbalist. Welcome'. At any one time, 20–30 people were waiting for him, some standing in the courtyard outside, others sitting in his tiny waiting room in which an assortment of herbs, bulbs, roots, dried skins, and calabashes were crammed onto makeshift shelves. Many of the bottles of herbs had labels with popular brand names, others had illegible instructions scrawled on them. Within the actual consultation room (its door labelled 'Dr John's Office'), the healer sat behind a desk, dressed in a white coat, a suit and tie, and wearing a pair of green-tinted spectacles. On the table, illuminated by two candles, lay a number of significant ritual objects: burning incense, small calabashes, beads, a stethoscope, a syringe and a stack of medical publications, ranging from scientific journals to home doctor books. His assistant was an elderly woman, who also wore a white coat. All the patients who entered the room were asked how they were feeling, and then each one was examined with the stethoscope. Then 'Dr John' announced that he would implore his *amakhosi*, or spirits, to aid in the diagnosis and discover the cause of the patient's illness. Afterwards, he told the patient that he would use a 'doctor's book' to find the most appropriate treatment for them. He then read out a passage from one of his books, translating its meaning to the patient. To strengthen the effect, he often repeated sentences aloud from it in English. He then scribbled instructions on a piece of paper (the 'prescription'), and asked the patient to hand this to his assistant, who then dispensed the appropriate herbs. Like other traditional healers in that area, he always also included one or two pharmaceutical products in the prescription – such as cough mixtures, aspirins, laxatives or milk of magnesia – which he kept in a small closet nearby. Simon noted that his syncretic mix of Western and African healing practices, his 'commitment to the parallel utilization of medical traditions, and not a singular devotion to either form of practice', had made him a popular and effective healer locally.

Whatever the success or otherwise of his treatments, the case of Dr John and his ritual setting shows that in the modern age traditional medicine is not static. 'Like any form of therapy, local (traditional) healing is a dynamic, changeable profession, with shifting ideas and practices tailored to suit the times'.

Recommended reading

Hertz, R. (1960). *Death and the Right Hand*, pp. 28–86. Cohen and West.

Katz, P. (1981). Ritual in the operating room. *Ethnology*, **20**, 335–50.

Leach, E. (1968). Ritual. In: *International Encyclopaedia of the Social Sciences* (D. L. Sills, ed.), pp. 520–26. Free Press/Macmillan.

Turner, V. W. (1974). *The Ritual Process.* Penguin.

10 Cross-cultural psychiatry

Cross-cultural psychiatry is the study and comparison of mental illness in different cultures. It is one of the major branches of medical anthropology, and has been a valuable source of insight into the nature of health and ill health in different parts of the world. Historically, research into the subject has been carried out by two different types of investigator:

1. Western-trained psychiatrists who have encountered unfamiliar, and what seemed to them bizarre, syndromes of psychological disturbance in parts of the non-Western world, and who have tried to understand these syndromes in terms of their own Western categories of mental illness, such as 'schizophrenia' or 'manic depressive psychosis'
2. Social and cultural anthropologists, whose main interests have been the definitions of normality and abnormality in different cultures, the role of culture in shaping personality structure, and cultural influences on the cause, presentation and treatment of mental illness.

Although these two approaches have led to different perspectives on the subject, they share a concern with two types of clinical problem:

1. The diagnosis and treatment of mental illness where health professional and patient come from different cultural backgrounds
2. The effect on mental health of migration, urbanization and other forms of social change.

The focus of cross-cultural psychiatry is mainly on mental illness rather than on mental disease. That is, it is concerned less with the organic aspects of psychological disorders than with the psychological, behavioural and socio-cultural dimensions associated with them. Even when the condition clearly has an organic basis, as in neurosyphilis, delirium tremens, cerebral malaria or dementia, anthropologists are more interested in how *cultural* factors affect the patient's perceptions and behaviour, the content of their hallucinations or delusions, and the attitudes of others towards them.

In general, the relationship of culture to mental illness can be summarized as:

- it defines 'normality' and 'abnormality' in a particular society
- it may be part of the aetiology or cause of certain illnesses
- it influences the clinical presentation and distribution of mental illness
- it determines the ways that mental illness is recognized, labelled, explained and treated by other members of that society.

Normality *versus* abnormality

Definitions of 'normality', like definitions of 'health', vary widely throughout the world, and in many cultures these two concepts overlap. Mention has already been made in Chapter 4 of some of the medical definitions of health that are based upon the measurement of certain physiological and other variables that lie within the normal range of the human organism. At its most reductionist, this approach concentrates mainly on the physical signs of brain dysfunction before diagnosing mental illness. In this chapter, some other ways of looking at the problem will be examined, especially the *social* definitions of normality and abnormality. These definitions are based on shared beliefs within a group of people as to what constitutes the ideal, 'proper' way for individuals to conduct their lives in relation to others. These beliefs provide a series of guidelines on how to be culturally 'normal' and – as will be described below – how also to be temporarily 'abnormal'. Normality is usually a multidimensional concept. Not only is the individuals' behaviour relevant, but also, for example, their dress, hairstyle, smell, personal hygiene, posture, gestures, emotional state, facial expression, tone of voice and use of language, all of which are taken into account – as is their *appropriateness* to certain contexts and social relationships.

Some of the many dimensions of social behaviour are illustrated in Figure 10.1. This represents the range of possible *perceptions* – by members of a particular society or culture – of a particular form of social behaviour: whether they see it as 'normal' or abnormal for their society, and whether it is controlled or not by the norms of that society. It also reflects the fact that all human groups recognize that there are certain times and places when people can be allowed to behave in an 'abnormal' way, provided that they are seen to conform to the strict guidelines (explicit or implicit) laid down by their culture for this type of situation. In this case, even if their behaviour is bizarre or unconventional, it is still to some extent controlled by social norms. By contrast, most cultures disapprove of forms of public behaviour that are obviously not being controlled by the rules of their society: and which they usually label as either 'mad' or 'bad'. Thus in Figure 10.1 there are four possible zones of social behaviour (A, B, C, D) according to the perceptions of that society, or of groups or individuals within that society.

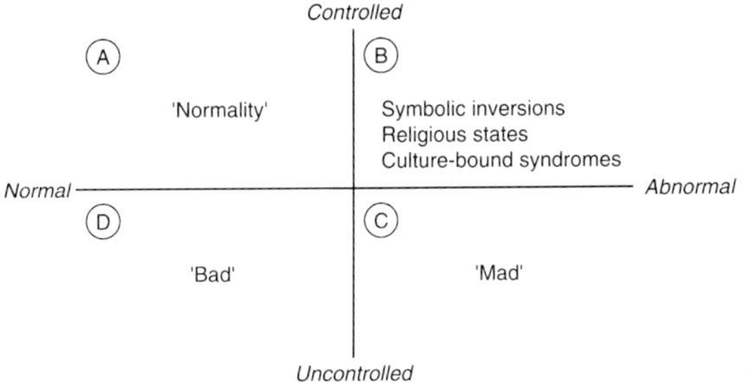

Figure 10.1 Perceptions of social behaviour

It should always be emphasized, however, that these zones, and the definitions of behaviour they encompass, are *not* static. Rather they are a series of fluid categories, a spectrum of possibilities, that are likely to change with time and circumstance and the particular perspective of the onlooker. Thus behaviour seen as 'bad' in one generation may be seen as 'mad' in the next, and 'normal' behaviour in one group of people may be regarded as 'abnormal' in another. Alcohol consumption, for example, has – at various times and places (sometimes within the same society) – been seen as normal, as morally bad, as a symptom of psychological disorder, and as an accepted part of certain ritual or religious occasions. Furthermore, these broad social categories do not necessarily take into account *individual* factors such as personality, motivation, experience, emotional state or physiology. Their focus is not primarily on an individual's perspective but rather on that of society as a whole – or, at least, of a section of that society. However, in the case of 'controlled normality' (A), 'uncontrolled normality' (D) and 'controlled abnormality' (B) it is assumed that the individual is at least *aware* (consciously or not) of what the social norms are, whether they conform to them or not. That is, that they have some degree of self-awareness, or insight, into their own behaviour.

The social definition of normality (A) is not uniform within a population. Most cultures have a wide range of social norms that are considered appropriate for different age groups, genders, occupations, social ranks and cultural minorities within the society. Attitudes towards foreigners or minorities often include stereotyped views of their normal behaviour, which may be seen as bizarre, comical or even threatening. Furthermore, most societies, especially those with rigid codes of normal behaviour, often make provision for certain specified occasions where these codes are deliberately flouted or *inverted*, and 'abnormal' behaviour becomes the temporary norm (B). Anthropologists have described many of these 'rites of reversal' or 'symbolic inversions', which Babcock[1] defines as 'any act of expressive behaviour which inverts, contradicts, abrogates, or in some fashion presents an alternative to commonly held cultural codes, values and norms be they linguistic, literary or artistic, religious, or social and political'.

These special occasions – such as certain festivals, bacchanalia, parades, *mardi gras* and carnivals (like those in Brazil, the Caribbean, southern

Europe and London's Notting Hill Gate) – sometimes involve a collective inversion of normal behaviour and roles. For example, in their study of the carnival in St Vincent, West Indies, and 'belsnickling' (a form of Christmas mumming) on La Have Islands, Nova Scotia, Abrahams and Bauman[2] described how they both involve 'a high degree of symbolic inversion, transvestism, men dressed as animals or supernatural beings, sexual licence and other behaviours that are the opposite of what is supposed to characterize everyday life'. In a Western setting, such temporarily 'abnormal' social behaviour is often found on New Year's Eve, April Fool's Day, at fancy dress balls, university 'Rags' and on Halloween, as well as on vacations far from home. Many tourists, especially those on trips to distant, poorer countries, dress and act in ways that are opposite to their normal life back home, especially in terms of sexual and drinking behaviour. Similar alterations or inversions of normal role behaviour are found in some of the spirit possession cults of African women, described by Lewis[3], where women who seek power and aspire to roles otherwise monopolized by men 'act out thrusting male parts with impunity and with the full approval of the audience'. All these forms of 'abnormal' behaviour in public by large crowds of people are, however, also strictly *controlled* by norms, since their timing and location are clearly defined and structured in advance.

On a more individual level, displays of behaviour that are 'abnormal' by the standards of everyday life must also be seen against the background of the culture in which they appear. Like the crowd behaviour at a 'rite of reversal', they are also controlled (to a variable extent) by implicit cultural norms, which determine how and when they may appear. In many cultures, especially in the non-industrialized world, individuals involved in interpersonal conflicts, or who are experiencing feelings of unhappiness, guilt, anger or helplessness, are able to express these feelings in a standardized language of distress (see Chapter 5). This may be purely verbal, coded in a language of physical symptoms, or involve extreme changes in dress, behaviour or posture. To the Western-trained observer, some of these languages of distress may closely resemble the diagnostic entities of the Western psychiatric model. For example, they may involve statements such as 'I've been bewitched', 'I've been possessed by a spirit (or by God)' or 'I can hear the voices of my ancestors speaking to me'. In a Western setting, people making this type of statement are likely to be diagnosed as psychotic, probably schizophrenic.

However, it should be remembered that in many parts of the world people freely admit to being 'possessed' by supernatural forces, to having 'spirits' speak and act through them, and to having had dreams or visions that conveyed an important message to them. In most cases this is not considered by their communities to be evidence of mental illness. One example of this is the widespread belief, especially in parts of Africa, of spirit possession as a cause of mental or physical ill health. Women especially are the victims of possession by malign, pathogenic spirits that reveal their identity by the specific symptoms or behavioural changes that they cause. In these societies, notes Lewis[3], possession is a normative experience, and whether or not people are actually in a trance, they are only possessed when they consider they are, and when other members of their society endorse this claim. That is not to say that spirit possession is 'normal', in the sense that most people expect to be possessed during their life. Rather, it is a culture-specific way of presenting and explaining a range of physical and psychological disorders in certain circumstances. In these societies:

> belief in spirits and in possession by them is normal and accepted. The reality of possession by spirits, or for that matter of witchcraft, constitutes an integral part of the total system of religious ideas and assumptions. Where people thus believe generally that the affliction can be caused through possession by a malevolent spirit (or by witchcraft), disbelief in the power of spirits (or of witches) would be a striking abnormality, a bizarre and eccentric rejection of normal values. The cultural and mental alienation of such dissenters would in fact be roughly equivalent to that of those who in our secular society today believe themselves to be possessed or bewitched[3].

Possession, then, is an 'abnormal' form of individual behaviour, but one that conforms with cultural values, and whose expression is closely controlled by cultural norms. These norms provide guidelines as to who is allowed to be possessed, in what circumstances and in what way, as well as how this possession is to be signalled to other people.

Another form of controlled abnormal behaviour is *glossolalia*, or speaking in unknown tongues. To those who believe in it, it is thought to result from a supernatural power entering into the individual, with 'control of the organs of speech by the Holy Spirit, who prays through the speaker in a heavenly language'[4]. It is a dissociative, trance-like state in which the participants 'tend to have their eyes closed, they may make twitching movements and fall; they flush, sweat and may tear at their clothes'. It is a feature of religious practices in parts of India, the Caribbean, Africa, Southern Europe, North America and among many Pentecostal churches in the UK (including those with West Indian congregations). There are believed to be about two million practitioners of glossolalia in the USA in various denominations, including some Lutheran, Episcopalian and Presbyterian churches. Glossolalia usually takes place in a specified context (the church) and at specified times during the service. It can be seen as a form of 'controlled abnormality' that, to a Western-trained psychiatrist, might seem evidence of a mental illness. However, there is no evidence that this is the case. On the contrary, there is some evidence from various cultures that 'in any particular denomination, those members of it who speak in tongues are better adjusted than those who do not'[4]. In one study, a comparison between a group of schizophrenic patients from the Caribbean and West Indian Pentecostals suggested that the Pentecostals believed that the patients 'were unable to control their dissociative behaviour sufficiently to conform with the highly stylized rituals of glossolalia in church'[4]. Although both groups might appear to practise similar glossolalia, it was the culturally *uncontrolled* form that was regarded as mental illness by members of that community.

In every society, there is a spectrum between what people regard as 'normal' and 'abnormal' social behaviour. However, as the examples of glossolalia, spirit possession and carnivals illustrate, there is also a spectrum of 'abnormal' behaviour – from *controlled* to *uncontrolled* forms of abnormality. As with the abnormal, uncontrolled drinking behaviour (drunkenness) described in Chapter 8, it is behaviour at the *uncontrolled* end of the spectrum that cultures regard as a major social problem, and that they label as either 'mad' (C) or 'bad' (D). As Foster and Anderson[5] put it, 'there is no culture in which men and women remain oblivious to erratic, disturbed, threatening or bizarre behaviour in their midst, whatever the culturally defined context of that behaviour'. According to Kiev[6], the symptoms that would suggest mental disorder include uncontrollable anxiety, depression and agitation, delirium and other gross breaks of contact with reality, and violence both to the community and to self. In one study by Edgerton[7], lay beliefs about what behaviour constitutes madness or psychosis was examined in four East African tribes; two in Kenya, one in Uganda and one in Tanzania (Tanganyika). It was found that all four societies shared a broad area of agreement as to what behaviours suggested a diagnosis of 'madness'. These included such actions as violent conduct, wandering around naked, 'talking nonsense' or 'sleeps and hides in the bush'. In each case the respondents qualified their description of psychotic behaviour by saying that it occurred 'without reason'. That is, violence, wandering around naked and so on occurred without an apparent purpose, and in the absence of any identifiable and acceptable external cause (such as witchcraft, drunkenness or simply malicious intent). Edgerton notes how this catalogue of abnormal behaviours is not markedly at variance with Western definitions of psychosis, particularly schizophrenia. In these cultures, as elsewhere in the world, behaviour is labelled as 'mad' (C) if it is abnormal, not controlled by social norms, and has no discernible cause or purpose. Rarely, the label of 'temporary madness' may be also applied – usually to cases of mass hysteria, intoxication by alcohol or drugs, or 'crimes of passion' (in some European countries).

Certain other behaviours, also uncontrolled by social norms, are still regarded by society as being 'normal', even though they are classified as socially undesirable and often illegal. These are the behaviours classified as 'bad' or 'criminal' (D); in these cases, persons convicted of a crime would be regarded as guilty but 'normal'. The issue debated in their trial by lawyers and forensic psychiatrists would be the accused's awareness (or lack of awareness) of what the social norms or laws of their society are; whether they had 'insight', were responsible for their actions and 'knew right from wrong'.

As described above, the 'abnormal' behaviours at the controlled end of the spectrum (B) frequently overlap with religious and cosmological practices, as in glossolalia, spirit possession and the use of hallucinogens in religious rituals, and also the healing rites of the *shaman* (see Chapter 8). The latter is a form of sacred folk healer who is found in many cultures. The shaman, often known as a 'master of spirits', becomes voluntarily possessed by them in controlled circumstances and, in a divinatory seance, both diagnoses and treats the misfortune (and illness) of the community. To a Western psychiatrist, the behaviour of the shaman during his trance may closely resemble that of the schizophrenic. However, as Lewis[3] points out, shamans in their ritual performances act in conformity with cultural beliefs and practices, and in the selection of shamans, frankly psychotic or schizophrenic individuals are screened out as being too idiosyncratic and unreliable for the rigours of the shamanic role.

At various points along the spectrum of 'controlled abnormal' behaviours (B), the different *culture-bound* mental illnesses can also be located. These conditions, described below, are all under the control of social norms to a variable extent. For example, their timing and setting may be unpredictable, but the clinical presentation of their symptoms and behaviour changes are not chaotic but patterned by the culture in which they appear. Also, unlike the severe uncontrolled psychosis in the East African example (C), a culturally explicable cause for them can usually be found – such as *susto* following an unexpected accident or fright, or *evil eye* resulting from, for example, an extravagant lifestyle that was bound to attract envy. These conditions do not occur in the formalized setting of temple or ritual, but cultural factors influence their presentation, recognition and treatment.

The comparison of psychological disorders

Given the marked variation in cultural definitions of 'normal' and 'abnormal' throughout the world, can meaningful comparisons be made between mental illness in different groups and societies? Landy[8] has summarized two of the questions faced by medical anthropologists and cross-cultural psychiatrists who have examined this problem:

1. Can we speak of some aspects of behaviour as normal or abnormal in a pan-human sense (that is, specific to the human species)?
2. Are the psychoses of Western psychiatric experience and nosology universal and transcultural, or are they strongly shaped by cultural pressures and conditioning?

The answers to both these questions are important, since they determine whether mental illness can be adequately diagnosed and treated cross-culturally, and whether the prevalence rates of mental illness in different cultures can be compared. They would also shed light on why some forms of mental illness seem to be more common in some parts of the world than in others.

In examining notions of 'abnormality' in the section above, most of the emphasis has been on abnormal *social behaviour* rather than on organic disorders or on emotional state. For most medical anthropologists the social and cultural dimensions of mental illness are the main areas of study. This is because cultural factors influence the clinical presentation and recognition of many of these disorders, even those with an organic basis. In addition, in many parts of the Third World (and elsewhere) mental illness is perceived as 'abnormal action' rather than 'mistaken belief'[9]. Diagnosing mental illness by psychological state, such as the presence of a delusion, may be difficult where the content of the delusion is shared by other members of the society. For example, in some cultures a person who accuses a neighbour of having bewitched him may initially be perceived as acting in an acceptable, rational way for that society. He will only be viewed as 'mad' or psychotic if his accusations are then followed by 'mal-adaptive personal violence rather than the employment of the accepted communal technique for dealing with sorcery'[9]. In this case, the diagnosis of mental illness by a Western-trained doctor would depend not only on his or her own clinical observations, based on assessment of the affected person's behaviour, biological changes (such as anorexia, insomnia and loss of libido) and response to certain psychological tests, but also on how the affected person's behaviour is perceived by his own community. The problem, therefore, in comparing mental illness in different societies, is whether to compare Western clinical evaluations of patients in different cultures, or the perceptions by various cultures of those that they regard as mentally ill.

Those who have examined this problem in more detail have tended to take one of three approaches; the *biological* approach, the *social labelling* approach, or the *combined* approach,

The biological approach

This approach sees the diagnostic categories of the Western psychiatric model as being universally applicable to mankind, despite local variations due to cultural factors, since they have a *biological* basis. In Kiev's[10] view, the forms of psychiatric disorders remain essentially constant throughout the world irrespective of the cultural context in which they appear. As he puts it, for example: 'the schizophrenic and manic-depressive psychotic disorders are fixed in form by the biological nature of man, while the secondary features of mental illness, such as the *content* of delusions and hallucinations are, by contrast, influenced by cultural factors'. On this basis, Kiev[11] proceeds to classify the various culture-bound disorders within the diagnostic categories of the Western model. For example, *koro, susto* and bewitchment are forms of anxiety; the Japanese *shinkeishitsu* is an obsessional compulsive neurosis; evil eye and voodoo death are examples of phobic states; and spirit possession, *amok* in Malaya and *Hsieh ping* in China are all examples of dissociative states. In Kiev's opinion, these conditions 'are not new diagnostic entities; they are in fact similar to those already known in the West'. This approach, which is similar to the view of diseases as universal entities (see Chapter 5), has been criticized for the primacy it gives to the Western diagnostic and labelling system[12]. In addition, Western categories of mental illness are also 'culture-bound', as well as being the product of specific social and historical circumstances, and are therefore not necessarily pan-human in their applicability. For example, Kleinman[13] has criticized the WHO International Pilot Study of Schizophrenia, which compared schizophrenia in a number of Western and non-Western societies. He points out that the study enforced a definition of schizophrenic symptomatology, and that this definition may have distorted the findings by 'patterning the behaviour observed by the investigators and systematically filtering out local cultural influences in order to preserve a homogeneous cross-cultural sample'. Applying the Western model of, say, schizophrenia to other parts of the world may therefore be an example of what Kleinman[13] terms a *category fallacy* – that is, 'the reification of a nosological category developed for a particular cultural group that is then applied to members of another culture for whom it lacks coherence and its validity has not been established'. The danger of category fallacies is therefore implicit in much of the biological approach, and in its attempt to fit exotic illnesses into a universal, diagnostic framework[14].

A further critique of the biological approach is that the *same* mental illness may play *different* social roles in different societies. For a fuller understanding of an episode of that mental illness in another culture, one must always know something of the *context* – social, cultural, political and economic – in which it has taken place. For example, in some small-scale societies a psychotic episode may be viewed as evidence of an underlying social conflict, which must be resolved by a public ritual, while the same psychosis is unlikely to play such a central role in the life of a Western, urban community.

The social labelling approach

This perspective, developed by sociologists, sees mental illness as a 'myth', essentially a *social* rather than a biological fact, and one that can appear with or without biological components. Society decides what symptoms or behaviour patterns are to be defined as deviant, or as that special type of deviance called 'mental illness'. This mental illness does not appear until it is so labelled, and had no prior existence. Once the diagnostic label is applied, it is difficult to discard. According to Waxler[15], mental illness is only defined relative to the society in which it is found and cannot be said to have a universal existence. She notes how, in Western societies, social withdrawal, lack of energy and feelings of sadness are commonly labelled 'depression', while in Sri Lanka the same phenomena receive less attention and very little treatment. The definition of mental illness is thus culture-specific. The process of labelling involves a first stage, where an individual's minor deviant behaviour is labelled as 'mental illness'. There are, however, certain culture-specific contingencies under which potential deviants are immune from this labelling, and these include the individual's power relative to the labeller (based on his or her age, sex, race, economic position etc.). Once individuals are labelled as 'mentally ill', they are subject to a number of cultural cues that tell them *how* to play their role; that is, 'the mentally ill person learns how to be sick in a way his particular society understands'. Once labelled, individuals are dependent on the society at large for 'de-labelling' them and releasing them from the sick role, and in some cases they may never be able to free themselves from this role. The value of the social labelling perspective is that it sheds light on the *social* construction and maintenance of the symptomatology of mental illness. Since this mental illness only exists by virtue of the society that defines it, 'mental illness' is a relative concept and cannot easily be compared between different societies. This perspective has been criticized for its neglect of the biological aspect of mental illness, especially in those conditions where this is a definite feature (such as brain tumours, delirium tremens, dementia or cerebral malaria). It also ignores the more extreme psychoses, which do seem to be universal in distribution.

The combined approach

This utilizes elements of both the biological *and* the social labelling perspectives, and is the one most medical anthropologists would agree with. In this view, there *are* certain universals in abnormal behaviour, particularly extreme disturbances in conduct, thought or effect. While there is wide variation in their form and distribution, the Western categories of major psychoses, such as 'schizophrenia' and 'manic depressive psychosis', *are* found throughout the world, though of course they may be given different labels in different cultures. An example of this, the similarity to Western definitions of psychosis of folk categories of 'mad' behaviour in four East African tribes, has already been described above. The major psychoses, therefore, as well as disorders arising from organic brain disease, seem to be recognized in all societies, though their clinical presentations are usually influenced by the local culture. For example, psychotics in a tribal society may say that their behaviour is being controlled by powerful witches or sorcerers, while Western psychotics may feel controlled by spacemen, Martians or flying saucers. Those who suffer these extreme psychological disorders are usually perceived by their own cultures as exhibiting 'uncontrolled abnormal' (C) forms of social behaviour. To a variable extent their clinical pictures can be compared between societies. Foster and Anderson[5] have suggested that this comparison should be between their *symptom patterns* rather than between diagnostic categories (such as schizophrenia); on this basis, the problem of trying to fit other cultures' mental illnesses into Western diagnostic categories can be overcome.

The comparison of symptom patterns can also be carried out for the culture-bound disorders described below, many of which could be classified as 'neuroses' or 'functional psychoses' in the Western psychiatric model. These conditions, especially those with a preponderance of neurotic or somatic symptoms, are probably more difficult to compare than are the major psychoses. Many of them do seem to be unique clusters of symptoms and behaviour changes, which only make sense within a particular context and within a particular culture, and have no equivalent in other societies. The specific symptom patterns of *susto*, for example, are unlikely to be found in the UK, at least not among the native-born population. Not only does culture closely pattern their clinical presentations, but the *meanings* of these conditions for the victim, their family and community are difficult for a Western observer to evaluate or quantify. Nevertheless, anthropologists like Rubel[16] believe that these folk illnesses have a fairly constant clinical presentation within a culture, and can therefore be quantified and investigated using standard epidemiological techniques (see Chapter 12).

Cultural influences on psychiatric diagnosis

Before psychological disorders can be compared, they have to be diagnosed. In recent years a number of studies have indicated some of the difficulties in standardizing psychiatric diagnoses, particularly among psychiatrists working in different countries. Variations in the clinical criteria used to diagnose schizophrenia, for example, have been found between British and American psychiatrists and British and French psychiatrists, and among psychiatrists working within these countries. Some of the diagnostic categories in French psychiatry, such as 'chronic delusional states' (*délires chroniques*) and 'transitory delusional states' (*bouffées delirantes*), are significantly different from the diagnostic categories of Anglo-American psychiatry[17]. A further example was the diagnostic category 'sluggish schizophrenia' in Soviet psychiatry, which was virtually limited to the former USSR[18]. All of these discrepancies in diagnostic behaviour among psychiatrists are important, since they affect both the treatment and prognosis of mental illness as well as the reliability of comparing morbidity statistics for these conditions between different countries.

Part of the reason for these differences lies in the nature of psychiatric diagnosis, and the categories into which it places psychological disorders. Unlike the diagnosis of medical 'diseases', there is often little evidence of typical biological malfunctioning, as revealed by diagnostic technology. Where biological evidence does exist, it is often difficult to relate this to specific clinical symptoms. Most psychiatric diagnoses are based on the doctor's subjective evaluation of the patient's appearance, speech and behaviour, as well as performance in certain standardized psychometric tests. The aim is to fit the symptoms and signs into a known category of mental illness by their similarity to the 'typical' textbook description of the condition. However, according to Kendell[19], the way that psychiatrists learn how to do this may actually make diagnostic differences among them more likely. He points out how the majority of patients encountered by trainee psychiatrists do not possess the 'typical' cluster of symptoms of a particular condition. They may have some of the symptoms but not others, or have symptoms typical of another condition. As a result, trainee psychiatrists learn how to assign diagnoses largely by the example of their clinical teachers: 'He sees what sorts of patient his teachers regard as schizophrenics, and copies them'. So while young psychiatrists see many 'typical' cases of various disorders during their studies, their diagnostic behaviour tends to be modelled on that of their teachers, rather than using the stricter criteria of their textbooks. As a result, 'diagnostic concepts are not securely anchored. They are at the mercy of the personal views and idiosyncrasies of influential teachers, of therapeutic fashions and innovations, of changing assumptions about aetiology, and many other less tangible influences to boot'[19].

Among these influences, Kendell[20] cites the personality and experience of the psychiatrist, the length of his diagnostic interview, and his styles of information-gathering and decision-making. To this list can be added the psychiatrist's social class, ethnic or cultural background (especially its definition of 'normality' and 'abnormality'), as well as prejudices, religious or political affiliations, and the context in which diagnosis takes place.

An example of how these influences work in practice was provided by Temerlin's[21] classic experiment in 1968. Three groups of psychiatrists and clinical psychologists were each shown a videotaped interview with an actor who had been trained to give a convincing account of normal behaviour. Before the viewing, one of the audiences was allowed to overhear a high-prestige figure comment that the patient was 'a very interesting man because he looked neurotic but actually was quite psychotic'. The second group were allowed to overhear the remark, 'I think this is a very rare person, a perfectly healthy man', while the third group was given no suggestions at all. All three audiences were asked to diagnose the 'patient's' condition. In the first group of 95 people, 60 diagnosed a neurosis or personality disorder, 27 diagnosed psychosis (usually schizophrenia), and only eight stated that he was mentally normal. In the second group, all 20 people diagnosed the 'patient' as normal, while only 12 of the 21 members of the third group also diagnosed normality; the other nine diagnosed neurosis or personality disorders.

Another factor enhancing the subjective element in psychiatric diagnosis is the diffuse and changeable nature of the diagnostic categories themselves. Kendell[22] points out that many of these categories tend to overlap, and ill people may fit into different categories at different times as their illnesses evolve. Each category or syndrome is made up of the 'typical' clinical features, but as he notes[22]:

> Many of these clinical features, like depression and anxiety, are graded traits present to varying extents in different people and at different times. Furthermore, few of them are pathognomonic of individual illnesses. In general, it is the overall pattern of symptomatology and its evolution over time that distinguishes one category of illness from another, rather than the presence of key individual symptoms.

However, psychiatrists differ on whether to adopt this historical approach or whether to focus mainly on the individual's current mental state – as indicated by the degree of 'insight' displayed, or behaviour at the clinical interview. There is also a difference of opinion as to what explanatory model should be used to shape this diffuse clinical picture into a recognizable diagnostic entity.

Eisenberg[23] notes that Western psychiatry is not an internally consistent body of knowledge, and that it includes within it many different ways of viewing mental illness. For example, its perspective on the psychoses includes 'multiple and manifestly contradictory models', such as the medical (biological) model, the psychodynamic model, the behavioural model and the social labelling model. Each of these approaches emphasizes a different aspect of the clinical picture, and proposes a different line of treatment. The choice of explanatory model, and of diagnostic label, may sometimes be as much a matter of temperament as of training.

Political and *moral* considerations also play a part in the choice of diagnosis. In some cases, psychiatrists may be called upon to decide whether a particular form of socially deviant behaviour is 'mad' or 'bad'. In the Western world this is common as part of the judiciary system, but has also been applied to such conditions as homosexuality, alcoholism, truancy or obesity. Szasz[24] has argued also that confining lawbreakers to psychiatric hospitals, ostensibly for treatment (that is, labelling them as 'mad' rather than 'bad'), is just another form of punishment, but without the benefits of a proper defence and trial. Psychiatrists making these decisions are likely to be under the influence of social and political forces, the opinions of their colleagues, and their own moral viewpoints and prejudices. In some societies, many forms of political dissent are labelled as mental illness. The state and its supporters are assumed to have a monopoly of truth, and disagreement with them is considered to be clear evidence of psychosis. Wing[25] has described a number of these cases in different countries where state psychiatrists have labelled dissent as 'madness', especially in the former USSR, where, according to Merskey and Shafran[18], political dissidents were often diagnosed as having 'sluggish schizophrenia'.

In their study of mental illness among immigrants to the UK, Littlewood and Lipsedge[9] also suggest that psychiatry can sometimes be used as a form of social control, misinterpreting the religious and other behaviour of some Afro-Caribbean patients (as well as their response to discrimination) as evidence of schizophrenia. By contrast with the high rate of schizophrenia among Afro-Caribbeans, depression is rarely diagnosed, and the authors suggest that 'whatever the empirical justification, the frequent diagnosis in black patients of schizophrenia (bizarre, irrational, outside) and the infrequent diagnosis of depression (acceptable, understandable, inside) validates our stereotypes'[26]. In dealing with immigrants and the poor, they warn against psychiatry's role in 'disguising disadvantage as disease'. Other researchers, however, while agreeing that ethnic and racial prejudices do exist among UK psychiatrists, dispute that this alone leads to an over-diagnosis of schizophrenia among Afro-Caribbeans. Lewis and colleagues[27], for example, in their study of 139 British psychiatrists, *did* find evidence of stereotyping and 'race-thinking' towards Afro-Caribbean patients – judging them as potentially more violent, less suitable for medication, but more suitable for criminal proceedings than white patients. Presented with identical vignettes of black and white patients, they were more likely to diagnose cannabis psychosis and acute reactive psychosis among the black patients, but *less* likely to diagnose schizophrenia. Thus, while confirming the role of prejudice in psychiatric diagnosis, they found no evidence of a 'greater readiness to detain patients compulsorily or to manage them on a locked ward merely on the grounds of "race"'. Thomas and colleagues[28], in a study of compulsory psychiatric admissions in Manchester, found that second-generation (UK-born) Afro-Caribbeans had nine times the rate of schizophrenia of whites. However, this could largely be explained by their greater socio-economic disadvantage, with poor inner-city housing and higher rates of unemployment – all of which have been correlated with high rates of schizophrenia – rather than by psychiatric misdiagnosis. They therefore suggest that 'efforts aimed at improving social disadvantage and the provision of employment for ethnic minority groups may improve the mental health of such groups'. Wesseley and colleagues[29] also found higher rates of schizophrenia among Afro-Caribbeans in south London, irrespective of their place of birth, compared to other groups, but these differences could also mostly be explained by the greater social adversity they suffered rather than by their ethnicity. However, many of these studies have not yet been replicated in ethnic minorities throughout the UK, and some aspects of their methodology can be seen as problematic. It is difficult, for example, to define the precise inter-relationships of 'race', 'culture', 'ethnicity' and 'social class' within a society. Furthermore, the classification of people by ethnic group – such as 'Afro-Caribbean', 'Asian' or 'white' – is in itself problematic, since each of these groups is not homogeneous and contains within it people from very different backgrounds. Rates of a particular psychiatric diagnosis in a particular community are also not the whole story; the political and socio-economic *context* in which this diagnosis takes place, and the *meanings* attached to it, are equally important. A final, relevant issue is the degree to which different communities have been offered equal access to treatments such as psychotherapy, and whether this psychotherapy was culturally appropriate or not.

Eisenberg[23] mentioned another example of how deviant behaviour can be given a moral (bad) or medical (mad) diagnosis. The same constellation of symptoms and signs (including weakness, sweating, palpitations and chest pain on effort) can, in the absence of physical findings, be diagnosed either as 'neurocirculatory aesthenia' or 'Da Costa's syndrome' (and thus as a medical problem), or as the symptoms of cowardice (and thus a moral problem) if they appear in a soldier during battle. This is illustrated also by the gradual shift, since the turn of the century, from moral definitions of 'cowardice' or 'weakness' among military personnel to more recent medicalized definitions such as 'shell shock', 'battle fatigue' or 'post-traumatic stress disorder' (PTSD). More recently, Blackburn[30] has also suggested that the psychiatric definition of the 'psychopathic personality' is 'little more than a moral judgement masquerading as a clinical diagnosis'.

Looked at in perspective, there are thus a number of factors that can affect the standardization of psychiatric diagnostic concepts between different societies. These include the lack of hard physiological data, the vagueness of diagnostic categories, the range of explanatory models available, the subjective aspect in diagnosis, and the influence of social, cultural and political forces on the process of diagnosis. Some of the differences in diagnosis between psychiatrists in different Western countries, and within a single country, are illustrated in the following case studies.

Case study: Differences in psychiatric diagnosis in the UK and the USA – I

Cooper and colleagues[31] examined some of the reasons for the marked variations in the frequency of various diagnoses made by British and American hospital psychiatrists. Hospitals in the two countries differ in their admission rates (as noted on the hospital records) for the condition 'manic-depressive psychosis'. In the UK, for some age groups, admission for this condition is over ten times more frequent than in US state mental hospitals. The authors posed the problem: 'Are the differences in official statistics due to differences between the doctors and the recording systems, or do both play a part?' That is, was the actual prevalence of manic-depressive psychosis different in the two cities (London and New York), or were the differences in admission rates due to the diagnostic terms and concepts used by the two groups of hospital psychiatrists? At a mental hospital in each city, 145 consecutive admissions in the age range of 35–59 years were studied. These were assessed by the project psychiatrists, and diagnosed according to objective, standardized criteria. These diagnoses were then compared with those given by the hospital psychiatrists. Hospital staff in both cities were found to diagnose 'schizophrenia' more frequently and 'affective disorders' (including manic-depressive psychosis and depressive neurosis) less frequently than did the project psychiatrists. Both these trends were more marked in the New York sample. While differences in the incidence of the various disorders *were* found by the project staff between the cities, these differences were less significant than the hospital diagnoses suggest. The hospital psychiatrists appeared to exaggerate these differences by diagnosing schizophrenia more readily in New York, and affective illness more readily in London. The study does not reveal, however, how the cultural differences between the two groups of psychiatrists affected their diagnostic behaviour.

Case study: Differences in psychiatric diagnosis in the UK and the USA – 2

Katz and colleagues[32] examined the process of psychiatric diagnosis among both British and American psychiatrists in more detail. The study aimed to discover whether disagreements among these diagnoses were 'a function of differences in their actual perception of the patient or patients on whose symptoms and behaviour they are in agreement'. Groups of British and American psychiatrists were shown films of interviews with patients, and asked to note down all pathological symptoms and make a diagnosis. Marked disagreements in diagnosis between the two groups were found, as well as different patterns of symptomatology perceived. The British saw less pathology generally; less evidence of the key diagnostic symptoms 'retardation' and 'apathy'; and little or no 'paranoid

continued

projection' or 'perceptual distortion'. On the other hand, they saw more 'anxious intropunitiveness' than did the Americans. Perceiving less of these key symptoms led the British psychiatrists to diagnose schizophrenia less frequently. For example, one patient was diagnosed as 'schizophrenic' by one-third of the Americans, but by none of the British. The authors conclude that 'ethnic background apparently influences choice of diagnosis and perception of symptomatology'.

Case study: Differences in psychiatric diagnosis in England and France

Van Os and colleagues[33] studied the concepts of schizophrenia held by a sample of 92 British and 60 French psychiatrists. They found major differences in how each group conceptualized the aetiology, diagnosis and management of the disorder. Overall, they seemed 'to have been particularly affected by the traditional divide between Anglo-Saxon empiricism and continental rationalism – between trying to reach the truth through experiment and trying to reach it through ideas'. In France, psychoanalytic theories – emphasizing the aetiological role of family dynamics and parental factors – have been more influential, while in the UK psychiatry has been more linked to physical medicine and has focused more on neurodevelopmental and genetic causes. Similarly, in treatment the British preferred more biological and behavioural approaches compared to the French. The study also found major differences in the incidence of schizophrenia in the two countries. In France, the number of first admissions to psychiatric hospitals for this condition under the age of 45 years was much higher than in England, but much lower after 45 years. Also, rates of first admission for the period 1973–1982 were rising in France but falling in England. These apparent differences in the incidence of schizophrenia could largely be explained by the cultural and conceptual differences between the two groups of psychiatrists, and differences in the diagnostic criteria used. French psychiatrists were reluctant to diagnose schizophrenia after 45 years, and before that age the French concept of schizophrenia encompassed a number of other chronic psychological states (such as *heboidophrenic* or 'pseudopsychopathic' schizophrenia), which in the UK would not be included under the diagnosis of 'schizophrenia'.

Case study: Differences in psychiatric diagnosis within the UK

Copeland and colleagues[34] studied differences in diagnostic behaviour among 200 British psychiatrists, all of whom had at least 4 years in full-time practice and possessed similar qualifications. They were shown videotapes of interviews with three patients, and asked to rate their abnormal traits on a standardized scale and to assign the patients to diagnostic categories. There was fairly good agreement on diagnoses among the sample, except that psychiatrists trained in Glasgow had a significant tendency to make a diagnosis of 'affective illness' in one of the tapes, where the choice of diagnosis was between affective illness and schizophrenia. In addition, psychiatrists trained at the Maudsley Hospital, London, gave lower ratings of abnormal behaviour on the patients than the rest, while older psychiatrists and those with psychotherapeutic training rated a higher level of abnormalities than did younger psychiatrists. The authors point out that rating behaviour as 'abnormal' is 'likely to be affected by the rater's attitude towards illness and health and what is normal and abnormal'. The survey illustrates therefore that differences in these attitudes are associated with differences in postgraduate psychiatric training, as well as with age.

Cultural patterning of psychological disorders

Each culture provides its members with ways of becoming 'ill', of shaping their suffering into a recognizable illness entity, of explaining its cause, and of getting some treatment for it. Some of the issues raised by this process, in the case of physical illness, have already been discussed in Chapter 5, and they apply equally to cases of psychological disorder. Lay explanations of these conditions fall into the same aetiological categories: personal behaviour, and influences in the natural, social and supernatural worlds. Mental illness can therefore be explained by, for example, spirit possession, witchcraft, the breaking of religious taboos, divine retribution, and the 'capture' of the soul by a malevolent spirit. Foster and Anderson[5] point out how these types of 'personalistic' explanations for mental illness are much more common in the non-Western world; by contrast, the Western perspective on mental illness emphasizes psychological factors, life experiences and the effects of stress as major aetiological factors.

As with physical illness, cultures influence the 'language of distress' in which personal distress is *communicated* to other people. This 'language' includes the many culturally-specific definitions of 'abnormality', such as major changes in behaviour, speech, dress or personal hygiene. When it includes the verbal expression of emotional distress, including the description of hallucinations and delusions, it usually draws heavily on the symbols, imagery and motifs of the patient's own cultural milieu. For example, in Littlewood and Lipsedge's[35] study, 40 per cent of their patients with severe psychoses who had been born in the Caribbean and in Africa structured their illness in terms of a religious experience, compared with only 20 per cent of the white patients born in the UK. Similarly, Scheper-Hughes[36] points out that in rural Kerry in western Ireland, psychiatric patients showed a greater tendency to delusions of a religious nature, including the motifs of the Virgin and the Saviour, than would occur among American schizophrenics, who would be more likely to have 'secular or electromagnetic persecution delusions'. While possession by a malign spirit may be reported in parts of Africa, possession by 'Martians' or 'extra-terrestrials' is more likely among Western psychotics. Each culture thus provides a repertoire of symbols and imagery in which mental illness can be articulated, even at the 'uncontrolled abnormality' end of the spectrum. As with the ritual symbols described in Chapter 9, the symbols in which mental illness is expressed show polarization of meaning. On the one hand they stand for personal psychological or emotional concerns; on the other they stand for the social and cultural values of the wider society. Where mentally ill people come from a cultural or ethnic minority, they often have to utilize the symbols of the dominant majority culture in order to articulate their psychological distress and obtain help[37]. That is, they have to internalize (or appear to internalize) the value system of the dominant culture, and to utilize the vocabulary that goes with these values. This process is illustrated in the following case study.

Case study: 'Beatrice Jackson', London, England.

Littlewood[38] described the case of 'Beatrice Jackson', a 34-year-old widow, daughter of a black Jamaican Baptist minister, who had lived in London for 15 years. She lived alone with her son, and worked at a dress factory far from home. She was often lonely and depressed, and felt guilty about her long estrangement from her father back in the Caribbean. She was very religious and frequently attended church. After her father died she became increasingly guilty, constantly ruminating over her past life. She developed pain in her womb, and persuaded a gynaecologist to do a hysterectomy, so 'clearing all that away'. The pains now shifted to her back, and she continued to ask for further operations to remove the trouble. Her psychotic breakdown was precipitated by her son's criticism of the white police during a riot, which she bitterly contested. The following day she was admitted to a mental hospital, talking incoherently and threatening to kill herself, shouting that her son was not hers because he was black, and that black people were ugly although *she* was not as she was not black. In hospital she became more attached to the white medical and nursing staff, helping them as far as she could and taking their part against the patients in any dispute. By contrast, she kept on getting into arguments with the West Indian staff, refusing to carry out requests for them which she readily agreed to if asked by a white nurse.

Closer analysis of the case revealed that she saw the world literally in black and white terms. According to Littlewood, she had internalized the dominant racialist symbolism of both colonial Jamaica and of the England she had encountered, where 'black' represented badness, 'sin, sexual indulgence and dirt'. In her religion, black also represented hatred, evil (evil people were 'blackhearted'), devils, darkness and mourning. By contrast, 'white' was associated with 'religion, purity and renunciation'; it also stood for purity and joy, and both brides and angels are dressed in white. In the Caribbean, popular magazines often advertise skin lightening creams and hair straighteners, and a lighter coloured skin is a highly valued social asset. She had internalized this dichotomy, and had hoped to become 'white inside' by strict adherence to religious values, but could not match this by social acceptance from the white world outside. She felt that part of her remained 'black' (and therefore evil, unacceptable) and located the trouble in her

continued

sexual organs, blaming these for the carnal feeling which 'is in conflict with that part of her which seems to have managed to become white'. Her son's repudiation of the police, the representatives of white society, seemed to threaten her category system of white = good, black = bad, and she could no longer reconcile her inner symbolic system, the outer social reality, and her emotional relationships. Thus 'her system collapsed'. In hospital she attempted to restate her value system, identifying once again with the white staff and blaming her psychotic episode on the machinations of the (black) devil. Littlewood suggested that, at each stage of her life problems, she attempted to adapt to and make sense of the outer reality of her life in terms of the black/white symbolic system that she had internalized. Eventually, though, it became increasingly difficult to reconcile external reality with her system of explanations, and a psychotic episode was precipitated.

Somatization

A problem frequently encountered in making psychiatric diagnoses cross-culturally is that of *somatization* (see Chapters 5 and 7) – the cultural patterning of psychological and social disorders into a language of distress of mainly physical symptoms and signs. As Swartz[39] put it, somatization is 'a way of speaking with the body'. This phenomenon has been reported from numerous cultures world-wide, and from a variety of socio-economic groups within those societies. It is particularly a feature of the clinical presentation of depression, and of personal suffering and unhappiness. In these cases, depressed people often complain of a variety of diffuse and frequently changeable physical symptoms, such as 'tired all the time', headaches, palpitations, weight loss, dizziness, 'pains everywhere' and so on. They frequently deny feeling depressed, or having any personal problems. Hussain and Gomersall[40], for example, described how depression among Asian immigrants in the UK often manifests primarily as somatic symptoms, especially generalized weakness, 'bowel consciousness', exaggerated fear of a heart attack, and concern about the health of genital organs, nocturnal emissions, and the loss of semen in urine (known as *dhat* or *jiryan*[41]) – though the presence of these specific symptoms does not, of course, always mean depression.

Kleinman[42,43] points out how different cultures and social classes sometimes pattern unpleasant effects, such as depression, in different ways. For some, somatization represents a culturally specific way of coping with these effects, and functions to 'reduce or entirely block introspection as well as direct expression'. Unpleasant effects are expressed in a non-psychological idiom: 'I've got a pain' instead of 'I feel depressed'. He points out that in the USA this tends to be more common among poorer social classes – blue-collar workers with a high school education or less, and who have more traditional life styles – while *psychologization* (seeing depression as a psychological problem) is more common among upper middle-class professionals and executives with a college or graduate school education. Overall, however, the pattern of 'speaking with the body' is probably much more common world-wide, across a wide variety of social and cultural groups, than expressing distress and anxiety in purely abstract, psychological terms[39].

In many cases, however, the distinction between somatization and psychologization is more theoretical than real. As illustrated in the case history by Ots (see below), ostensibly somatic symptoms may actually carry a powerful *emotional* message, clearly understood by both healer and patient. In a study in the UK, Krause[44] found that although Punjabi immigrants tended to somatize, they *were* able to articulate their distress in psychological terms, and even where somatic symptoms were present these were considered to express psychological as well as physical distress. Furthermore, even though psychologization – the use of abstract psychological terms or concepts to describe subjective mental states – is the notional opposite of somatization, it is also often couched in a somatic or non-psychological idiom. In everyday English, for example, emotional distress is often expressed in a somatic idiom: examples of this include 'broken hearted', 'a pain in the neck', 'full of joy', 'can't stomach something', 'a painful experience' and 'hungry for attention'. In the author's study[45] in Massachusetts, USA, patients with psychosomatic disorders often described their emotions and feelings as if they were tangible 'things' that somehow entered them and caused damage to their bodies: 'I tend to hold lots of things inside ... Anger, tension, hostility, any kind of fear – I think of them as being crammed into my colon', 'I put negative feelings inside myself ... Doctors often say anger gets stored in the colon'. This Western view of certain emotions (especially antisocial ones such as anger, fear or envy) as 'pathogens' or 'forces' that cause ill health or unhappiness, and which originate either within the self or in the outside world, has become increasingly common. In many cases they are believed to somehow accumulate within the individual, causing distress or illness in a particular part of the body, unless they 'can get it all out'. In its modern form this echoes the remark by Henry Maudsley, the famous nineteenth century anatomist, that 'The sorrow that has no vent in tears makes other organs weep'[46].

In Taiwan, Kleinman[42] describes how somatization is extremely common. In both Hokkien and Chinese, the two languages spoken on the island, there is an impoverishment of words referring to psychological states, and often words meaning 'troubled' or 'anxious' express these emotions in terms of bodily organs. Self-scrutiny is not encouraged, and as an American psychiatrist working there he found it 'extremely difficult to elicit personal ideas and feelings' from his Taiwanese patients.

Kirmayer and Young[47] have summarized the different ways that clinicians, psychiatrists and anthropologists have interpreted the phenomenon of somatization. Depending on their interpretive stance, they have seen such somatic symptoms as indicating one or more of the following:

- an index of disease or disorder
- a symbolic expression of intrapsychic conflict
- an indication of a specific psychopathology
- an idiomatic expression of distress
- a metaphor for experience
- an 'act of positioning' within a local world
- a form of social commentary or protest.

They point out both the complexity and widespread occurrence of somatization, and how our understanding of it may be a reflection of Western cultural ways of thinking – especially of our mind–body dualism.

Overall, the use of somatization as a language of distress (expressing psychological or social disorders) across so many cultures illustrates how important it is to understand it from a holistic point of view. In any interpretation of somatization the complex interweaving of psychological, physical and social states, in different contexts, must be taken into account in order to understand why some people somatize while others do not.

Two examples of somatization from China – one from Hong Kong, the other from Nanjing – are illustrated below.

Case study: Depression in Hong Kong

Lau and colleagues[48] studied 213 cases of depression (142 females, 71 males) presenting to a private general practice in Hong Kong over a period of 6 months. The chief complaints that had prompted patients to consult their doctor were: epigastric discomfort (18.7 per cent); dizziness (12.2 per cent); headache (9.8 per cent); insomnia (8.4 per cent); general malaise (7.5 per cent); feverishness (4.7 per cent); cough (4.7 per cent); menstrual disturbances (3.3 per cent); and low back pain (3.3 per cent). Somatic symptoms were complained of initially by 96 per cent of the sample. Practically no depressed patient mentioned emotional distress initially as the chief complaint. Many of the sample had pain as the sole or coexisting complaint – 85 per cent in all had pains or aches of some description. Headaches, for example, were present in 85.4 per cent of the sample. The authors thus warn of the dangers of missing the diagnosis of depression because of the possible facade of somatic symptoms.

Case study: Psychosomatic symptoms in Nanjing, Peoples Republic of China

Ots[49] studied 243 patients, many of whom had 'psychosomatic disorders', attending a traditional Chinese medicine (TCM) clinic in Nanjing. He points out that in China, as in Taiwan and Hong Kong, the open expression of emotion is not encouraged. Instead, the main 'medical care-seeking behaviour' of people suffering from severe unhappiness or psychosocial stress is the presentation of physical complaints, mostly of the 'liver' and 'heart'.

Unlike Western medicine, TCM is not dualistic and does not strictly separate emotions and physical functions; both are seen as part of the same phenomenon. That is, 'specific emotional changes and specific somatic dysfunctions are viewed as corresponding with each other and often as identical'. Although TCM ostensibly focuses on the abnormalities of a particular organ, such as those of the 'liver', 'heart' or

continued

'kidney', these diagnoses must be understood as not referring (in most cases) to an actual physical disease, but to *metaphors* for certain emotional states. Each diagnosis (such as 'liver disease') is really 'a metaphor whose primary referent is not a particular organ but an emotion diagnosed via the patterns of somatic symptoms'. Thus although TCM emphasizes *physical* symptoms (and treatments) rather than psychological ones, the practitioners are able to 'read' these somatic symptoms as essentially an emotional message, and thus identify the underlying psychological problem. In the nosology of traditional Chinese medicine, 'liver' is a metaphor for anger, 'heart' for anxiety, 'spleen' for depression and 'kidney' for a decline in reproductive powers. In the clinic, about 80 per cent of the liver-related diagnoses given did *not* relate to actual physical diseases of the liver (such as hepatitis), but rather to aspects of *anger*. For example, a diagnosis of 'liver-*yang* flaring up' meant that the individuals were suppressing their anger, and this had affected their body, particularly their liver. If not treated, it might even lead to 'liver attacking spleen' – a disorder of the spleen. In other words, anger turned inwards might eventually cause depression.

Therefore, Ots points out that although traditional Chinese practitioners focus mainly on somatic symptoms, they do *not* ignore emotional states, whatever their cause; to them 'emotions are merely understood as pathogenic factors which cause disturbances of the organs and their functions'. Treatment here would consist not of psychotherapy or catharsis (which cultural norms would not permit), but would aim instead 'to harmonize the emotions by harmonizing bodily functions'. In the case of 'liver-anger', it is the liver itself that is treated, usually by a combination of 10–15 herbal medicines.

Ots suggested therefore that Western models of psychosomatic disorders may not be easily applied to China, since the culture there gives both patients and practitioners a different body awareness, and the Chinese 'are culturally trained to "listen" with their body' in a way unfamiliar to Western medicine.

Cultural somatization

Somatization often takes the form of vague, generalized symptoms, such as tiredness, weakness, fever or 'pains everywhere'. However, in some cultural or social groups a special form of somatization takes place; the selection of one particular organ as the main focus of all symptoms and anxiety. This phenomenon could be termed *cultural somatization*, and the organ chosen often has a symbolic or metaphoric significance for the group concerned – such as the liver, spleen, kidney or heart in Ots's study in China. Other examples include the heart in Iran (*narahatiye qalb* or 'heart distress') and in the Punjab (*dil ghirda hai* or 'sinking heart'), the liver in France (*crise de foie*), the bowels in the UK[50] (and other countries), and the penis in some Chinese groups (*koro*). In each case, not only do individuals suffer from a particular symptom but they also become the 'embodiment'[51] of core cultural themes of the society in which they live.

This shared focus on a particular organ or body part must be differentiated from the more personal, idiosyncratic forms of somatization described by Western psychoanalysts. For example, Freud and Breuer's[52] model of hysteria suggests that certain localized physical symptoms (such as pain or paralysis in a limb or body part) could be the expression of a particular intrapsychic conflict, unique to that individual. In this case, the selected body part had a special, symbolic significance for the person concerned. Researchers of psychosomatic disorders have adopted a similar approach in trying to understand the reasons for 'organ choice' – that is, why one organ in an individual is selected as a target organ while another is not[50]. In many individual cases, though, and irrespective of the cultural context, the choice of target organ is likely to be based on both cultural *and* individual criteria.

Mumford[53] proposed a useful model for understanding how somatization relates to cultural background. He suggests that there are three levels at which culture may shape the evolution of somatic symptoms, from first awareness to actual clinical presentation. They are:

1. *Language and idiom*, without which the sensation cannot be expressed
2. *Concepts of health and disease*, without which the symptom cannot be interpreted
3. *Culturally sanctioned illness behaviour*, without which the symptom cannot be presented to other people in order to obtain treatment of relief.

In most communities, all three of these levels are necessary in order for cultural somatization to take place and to be recognized as such by all concerned.

The concept of 'psychosomatic'

Although first used in 1818[54], the term psychosomatic has been most widely applied since World War Two. It refers to conditions that have both a psychological *and* a physical component, often with some causal connection between the two. Generally it is used to describe conditions whose origin is entirely psychological and where no physical abnormality can be found (such as tension headaches or irritable bowel syndrome), or those where there *is* a physical disorder, but it is precipitated or worsened by psychological factors (such as asthma attacks precipitated by family conflict). However, both anthropologists and medical researchers have criticized this term for the mind–body dualism that it implies. As Lipowski[55] puts it, 'psychosomatic connotes an assumption that there exist two classes of phenomena, i.e. psychic (mental) and somatic, which require separate methods of observation and distinct languages for their description'. That is, the term imposes a 'methodological and semantic dualism' onto the nature of human suffering. Despite its attempts to combine the 'disease' and 'illness' perspectives, the essential dualism of the concept still remains. Furthermore, psychosomatic disorders are an anomalous category within biomedicine. Unlike many 'real' diseases in the medical textbooks, they often include conditions that are difficult to diagnose, explain, predict, treat or prevent, and there is often no definite physical abnormality to be found. In some cases, therefore, this may lead to 'victim-blaming'; putting the responsibility for therapeutic failure on patients and supposed defects in their psyche.

A further problem is the linear, *causal* relationship that the term implies between certain psychological factors (such as personality, character, traits, conflicts or emotions) and specific symptoms or physical changes. Earlier this century, this 'psychogenicity' hypothesis suggested that certain personality types or people with certain character traits suffered from certain types of physical diseases – for example, asthmatics were often said to be 'passive and dependent people'[56]. Each psychosomatic disorder, therefore, was said to be associated with its own specific form of psychopathology. Some of the psychoanalytic literature has further implied a spatial model of body and mind, whereby an inner (psychic) reality somehow acts upon an outer (physical) one to cause psychosomatic symptoms. As one psychoanalyst, McDougall[57], puts it: 'such somatic phenomena arise in response to messages from the psyche'. This image of active psyche and passive body ('the mind is making use of the body in order to communicate something, to tell a story'[57]) is now common in much of the psychosomatic literature, including discussions of somatization. It sometimes includes the notion of an inherited or acquired 'weakness' of the part of the body where these mental forces have their greatest effect.

Other authors have tried to widen the definition of psychosomatic to include social and contextual factors, and to develop more *multicausal* models. Engel[58], for example, proposed a 'biopsychosocial model', which would be less dualistic and would integrate mental and physical factors with social ones – especially the events surrounding the origin of the disorder. Other multicausal models included that of Alexander and colleagues[59], who proposed that these disorders were due to three factors:

1. The individual's 'characteristic psychodynamic conflict pattern', present from childhood
2. A specific 'onset situation', which involved activation of this conflict pattern
3. 'Factor X', defined as a specific organ vulnerability or weakness.

From a family therapy perspective, Minuchin and colleagues[60] developed the 'family systems theory', whereby the family is seen as a system of inter-relationships that strives to maintain equilibrium – even at the cost of causing a psychosomatic disorder (such as anorexia nervosa) in one of its members (see below).

More recently, psychosomatic research has concentrated on sophisticated *physiological* models, which seek to connect certain psychological states with specific physiological changes in the body, especially in the immune, endocrine and neural systems. The new field of psychoneuroimmunology (PNI)[61], for example, has shown how sensitive the immune system is to changes in psychological state, such as depression. Other work has focused on how physical factors – such as chromosomal, metabolic or endocrine abnormalities – can in turn influence the emotional and intellectual state, as well as behaviour. Like earlier models of psychosomatic disorders, many of these contemporary physiological models are also dualistic, since they often ignore the role of social and cultural factors in the origin, interpretation and management of the condition.

In recent years, the term 'psychosomatic' has increasingly become a part of Western folk culture – just as it is in the discourse of biomedicine. Anthropology can help in understanding how this concept has diffused into the population, and how it is now understood. In English-speaking countries particularly, the word often suggests that the condition is somehow not as 'real' as physical illness, and that its origin and chronic course is somehow the patient's 'fault'. In some cases, prolonged contact with health professionals may contribute to this process. People may learn from them, and from other sources, the moral implications of these disorders, and of their failure to recover from them despite medical treatment. As one woman with ulcerative colitis in the Massachusetts study[45] stated: 'What I heard from all the doctors was that it was my fault, and if only you did what they said, everything would be OK', while a medical student, also with ulcerative colitis, remarked: 'I searched very hard and for a reason – why me? Everyone told me it *must* be psychological, there must be a large psychological component – it's in the medical textbooks'.

From an anthropological perspective, therefore, many of the current psychosomatic theories – whether dualistic, multicausal, systemic or physiological – are useful but often insufficient. For a fuller picture, they also need to include the role of *context*, whether cultural, social, political or economic, in the origin, presentation and understanding of the disorder. In this respect, some of the anthropological theories outlined in this book are particularly useful. They include concepts of the cultural constructions of body and self (Chapter 2), 'illness' (Chapter 5), pain (Chapter 7), placebos and nocebos (Chapter 8), ritual (Chapter 9) and stress (Chapter 11), as well as of cultural and symbolic healing (see below). Only in this way can a fuller, more holistic understanding of the subtle ways in which certain phenomena – physical, psychological, social and cultural – all blend together in certain situations of human suffering, and in certain individuals, be obtained. In this sense, it is proposed that this field of study should be more accurately called the study of *psychosociosomatic* disorders.

This approach is best described in the case of the culture-bound disorders.

Culture-bound psychological disorders

The 'culture-bound disorders' are a group of folk illnesses, each of which is unique to a particular group of people, culture or geographical area. Each is a specific cluster of symptoms, signs or behavioural changes recognized by members of those cultural groups and responded to in a standardized way (see Chapter 5). They usually have a range of symbolic meanings, moral, social or psychological, for both the victims and those around them. They often link an individual case of illness with wider concerns, including the sufferers' relationship with their community, with supernatural forces and with the natural environment. In many cases they play an important role in expressing and resolving both anti-social emotions and social conflicts in a culturally patterned way. Because they tend to occur in certain types of social, personal and cultural contexts, they could also be termed '*context*-bound disorders. The conditions in this group range from purely behavioural or emotional disorders to those with a large somatic component. Among the dozens that have been described[62] are: *amok*, a spree of sudden violent attacks on people, animals and inanimate objects, which afflicts males in Malaysia; *Hsieh-ping*, a trance state among Chinese, where patients believe themselves possessed by dead relatives or friends whom they had offended; *koro*, a delusion among Chinese males that the penis will retract into the abdomen and ultimately cause death; *mal deojo* or evil eye among Latin Americans (and other groups), where illness is blamed on the 'strong glance' of an envious person; *latah*, a syndrome of hyper-suggestibility and imitative behaviour found in South East Asia; *voodoo death* in the Caribbean and elsewhere, where death follows a curse from a powerful sorcerer; *Shinkeishitsu*, a form of anxiety and obsessional neurosis among young Japanese; *windigo*, a compulsive desire to eat human flesh among the Algonkian-speaking Indians of central and north-eastern Canada; *susto* (or 'fright') in most of Latin America, a belief in 'loss of soul'; and the *narahtiye qalb* ('heart distress') and *dil ghirda hai* ('sinking heart') described in Chapter 5.

Culture-bound syndromes are by no means all as 'exotic' as this list suggests. Elsewhere in this book it has been suggested that a number of common behaviours, idioms of distress, perceptions of bodily states and also certain diagnostic categories can all, in certain contexts, be regarded as Western culture-bound disorders. These include obesity, anorexia nervosa, premenstrual syndrome and the Type A coronary-prone behaviour pattern. In a review of this subject, Littlewood and Lipsedge[63] added to this list a number of other conditions common in the contemporary UK, including: *parasuicide*, an overdose with medically prescribed drugs; *agoraphobia*, 'The Housewives' Disease'; *shoplifting* by well-off, middle-aged women; *exhibitionism* (or 'flashing'); and *domestic sieges*, where a divorced man denied access to his children, for example, holds the family hostage in their home. In each of these the authors saw certain recurrent patterns of public behaviour, each of which encapsulate some of today's core cultural themes and values. Like the conditions mentioned earlier, they can therefore be regarded as *culture-bound*. Housewives' agoraphobia, for example, can be seen as both a ritual display of – and a protest against – the cultural pressures and injunctions on women, especially those that state that 'a woman's place is in the home'. By 'over-conforming' to this stereotype, the woman is able to dramatize the situation, mobilize a caring family around herself, and at the same time also restrict her husband's movements by forcing him to stay at home and look after her.

New culture-bound syndromes

In addition to these, a number of new syndromes have recently appeared in the industrialized world. Although many are created mostly by the media and are not yet fully-fledged culture-bound syndromes, they have begun to penetrate widely into popular culture and discourse. Some have a more medical origin, and have even found their way into psychiatric textbooks. In an increasingly secular age, many of them represent medicalized images of antisocial or nonconformist behaviour (see Chapter 5) and often lie on the border between 'mad' and 'bad' behaviour. In Britain, these emerging culture-bound syndromes include:

- aggressive behaviour or 'rage' syndromes, such as *road rage* (conflict between motorists), *air rage* (violent behaviour on an air flight) and *trolley rage* (conflict between customers in a supermarket)
- violent, repetitive behaviour syndromes, such as *serial killing, child abuse, 'granny bashing'* (abuse of the elderly), *bullying* (among schoolchildren) or the *battered wife syndrome*
- addiction or dependency syndromes, such as *workaholism* (addiction to overworking), *shopaholism* (addiction to shopping), *chocoholism* (addiction to chocolate), *lottomania* (addiction to buying lottery tickets), *sex addiction*, and addiction to computer games
- energy-loss syndromes, such as *burnout* (especially among those in the caring professions), *stress* (see Chapter 11) and *yuppie 'flu* (myalgic encephalopathy or ME)
- miscellaneous syndromes, such as *school refusal syndrome, attention deficit hyperactivity disorder* (ADHD) and *false memory syndrome.*

Even when there is some proven physical or psychiatric basis for them (as there is, for some on this list), these syndromes often condense wider social and cultural and concerns into a single diagnostic image or metaphor, and often this is seen as the perverse product of modern life. Over the years, several of these syndromes have become more popular, while for various reasons others have gradually declined. As an example, Acocella[64] has detailed the rise and fall of the *multiple personality disorder* (MPD) in the USA over the past 20 years, and relates it clearly to certain social trends and intellectual fashions that have also ebbed and flowed within that same period.

In addition to the more specific and standardized culture-bound syndromes, both non-Western and Western, a more diffuse cultural patterning determines the language of distress in which certain types of psychological or social disorder are expressed in each society. Here, the mode of presentation is culture-bound, though not the exact pattern of symptomatology. Examples of this, quoted above, are the largely somatic presentation of depression among Chinese in Taiwan, Hong Kong and the People's Republic of China, Asian immigrants in the UK, and working-class Americans. However, in other cases a particular pattern of symptoms and how people interpret them can be described as 'culture-bound', even though they do not form as standardized a syndrome as those listed above. Bose[65], for example, has described a culture-specific idiom of distress among some British Bangladeshis in London. Here, a wide range of expressions of extreme personal distress are interpreted by the patients, their families and religious healers as evidence of *upridosh*, or possession by malign spirits (*jinns*). These displays of distress, both emotional and behavioural, may include refusing to eat, muteness, crying, shouting, swearing, 'disrespectful behaviour' and visual hallucinations or visionary experiences. Bose points out how this idiom of distress has no exact equivalent in psychiatric nosology, and can only be fully understood from within the specific cultural frame of reference, and the life circumstances, of the individual patient concerned.

It could be argued that *all* syndromes, whether physical, psychological or social, are to some extent 'culture-bound'. That is, there is always some unique, local cultural perspective on the condition, even if it is a standard biomedical disease. However, with their dramatic changes in behaviour and mental state, the absence of clear physical changes, and the many symbolic meanings attached to them, the conditions mentioned above do constitute a specific class of phenomena of great interest to medical anthropologists.

The following three case studies describe: an example of a well-known and widely spread culture-bound disorder from Latin America; another syndrome afflicting some Latino immigrants to the USA; and two inter-related syndromes found in South Africa.

Case study: *Susto* in Latin America

Rubel[16] described the characteristics of *susto* (or 'magical fright'), which is also known as *pasmo*, *jani*, *espanto*, and *pédida de la sombra*. It is found throughout Latin America in both rural and urban areas, among both men and women, and among both Indians and non-Indians. It is also found among Hispanic Americans, especially those in California, Colorado, New Mexico and Texas. It is based on the belief that an individual is composed of a physical body and of one or more immaterial souls or spirits which, under some circumstances, may become detached from the body and wander freely. This may occur during sleep or dreaming, or as the consequence of an unsettling experience. Among Indians, it is believed to be caused by the soul being 'captured' because, wittingly or not, the patient disturbed the spirit guardians of the earth, rivers, ponds, forests or animals. The soul is believed to be held captive 'until the affront has been expiated'. Among non-Indians, this 'soul loss' is usually blamed on a sudden fright or unnerving experience. Its clinical picture consists of:

- becoming restless during sleep
- during waking hours, complaining of depression, listlessness, loss of appetite and lack of interest in dress and personal hygiene.

The healing rites, carried out usually by a folk healer or *curandero*, consist of an initial diagnostic session where the cause of the specific episode is identified and agreed, and then a healing session whereby the soul is 'coaxed and entreated to rejoin the patient's body'. The patient is massaged, rubbed and sweated to remove the illness from the body and to encourage the soul to return. Rubel relates the incidence of the condition to a number of epidemiological factors (see Chapter 12), including stressful social situations, especially where the individual cannot meet the social expectations of his own family and cultural milieu.

Case study: *Ataques de nervios* among Latinos in the USA

De La Cancela and colleagues[66] have described *ataques de nervios* (attacks of nerves) among Puerto Ricans and other Latino immigrants in the USA. These attacks are a specific and 'culturally meaningful way to express powerful emotion'. They usually have an acute onset, with a variety of physical symptoms including shaking, feelings of heat or pressure in the chest, difficulty in moving limbs, numbness or tingling of hands or face, a feeling of the mind 'going blank', and sometimes a loss of consciousness, or abusive behaviour. These acute episodes usually follow the gradual build-up of *nervios* (nerves) from the general problems of life, especially with family relationships, housing or money. An 'attack' is then usually precipitated by some specific stressful event. The authors point out that for most Latinos it is not seen as an 'illness' needing medical attention, but rather as an expression of upset, anger, frustration or sadness at the stressful event, as well as a temporary escape from it and a way of getting sympathy and help from other people. However, they suggested that this disorder cannot only be understood at the micro-level; the social, political and economic status of Latinos in the USA, and 'the sense of hopelessness, helpless, and lack of control' many of them experience, need to be examined. Stressful experiences in the countries of origin (especially in Central America), coupled with the effects of migration – such as the disruption of family life, unemployment, discrimination, overcrowded housing and changes in gender roles – are all part of this wider context. Added to the sense of social and political helplessness are the constant 'demands to submerge cultural identity and assimilate to the United States culture', and the lack of respect accorded to their cultures of origin. The authors suggested, therefore, that as well as treating individuals with this condition, and their families, attention must also be paid to wider socio-economic realities, because 'in the long run *ataques* may be more effectively dealt with in the sociopolitical arena'. Therefore health providers 'need to engage in social action and advocacy focusing on the social problems and material conditions that give rise to *ataques de nervios*'.

Case study: *Amafufunyana* and *ukuthwasa* in South Africa

Swartz[67] described two common culture-bound disorders among Xhosa- and Zulu-speaking African people in South Africa. Both are forms of spirit possession, though one is considered negative, the other positive. *Amafufunyana* is a form of hysteria, with agitated and uncontrolled behaviour and sometimes suicide attempts. It is believed to be caused by possession by malign spirits, sometimes sent by sorcery. Among the Zulu, according to Ngubane[68], possession is sometimes by 'a horde of spirits' from different ethnic groups. It can occur in individuals, or in larger outbreaks – such as in a girls' school. Like *nervios* or 'nerves' (see Chapter 11), it afflicts mainly people (especially women) who are in a relatively powerless social and economic position, especially at times of major social change and disruption. As such, it helps to draw attention to their suffering and to mobilize a caring network around them. Treatment is usually a ritual of exorcism by a traditional healer. By contrast, *ukuthwasa* – a similar form of spirit possession – has a more positive outcome. It is 'the state of emotional turmoil a person goes through on the path to becoming an indigenous healer'. Here possession is a necessary sign of the victim's 'calling' to be a healer. It signals a positive relationship to the ancestors, who will one day help them in their healing task. However, as Swartz points out, neither of these conditions forms a discrete or standardized entity. While the labels *amafufunyana* and *ukuthwasa* do have meaning, 'these meanings shift in different circumstances', and in different contexts. Like 'nerves', they can cover a variety of conditions and human situations. *Amafufunyana*, particularly, offers victims a way of explaining *post hoc* what has happened to them, as well as placing blame for it elsewhere. Similarly, the definition of *ukuthwasa* 'lies partly in the experience of the person undergoing it, and partly in the way these are handled by existing healers'. However, where somebody with this condition fails to become a healer, they may be rediagnosed by the community as having *ukuphambana*, or madness.

As the examples above illustrate, culture-bound disorders can only be fully understood by looking at the wider context in which they appear. In some cases, this context may include many of the political, economic, social and gender issues of the wider society.

Cultural and symbolic healing of psychological disorders

In many non-Western societies, particularly in rural or small-scale communities, mental illness is often considered to be more of a *social* event, one that intimately involves the patient's family, friends and community. In many cases, both mental and physical ill health are interpreted as indicating conflicts or tensions in the social fabric. Kleinman[69] uses the term *cultural healing* for when healing rituals attempt to repair these social tears and 'reassert threatened values and arbitrate social tensions'. Healing takes place at many levels; not only is the patient restored to health, but so is the community in which he or she lives. The aim of the healer, like the Ndembu *chimbuki* described in Chapter 9, is to resolve the conflicts causing the patient's illness, restore group cohesion and integrate the patient back into normal society. Unlike in the Western world, emotional disorders are often seen as *useful* to the community. For example, Waxler[15] notes how in many small-scale societies mental illness can be useful, even necessary; it incurs obligations between people (such as the obligations of family, friends and neighbours to attend and pay for a public healing ritual), and this has an *integrating* function, strengthening the ties within and between groups. In these societies, few other specialized institutions (such as a centralized legal, political and bureaucratic organization) exist to promote integration, and deviance (such as mental illness) can play this role. This usually occurs within a shared cognitive system, where everyone shares similar views of the aetiology of misfortune and ill health. If mental illness in one individual is ascribed to sorcery or witchcraft from someone in another group (family, clan or tribe), the offender's group has incurred obligations to the victim's group, which must be repaid in a public ceremony. This helps recreate the ties between groups and also reasserts the boundaries between them, and in the process the mentally ill person is reintegrated into society. According to Waxler, this process, and the key role of the family in caring for the patient, means that in traditional non-Western societies mental illness seems to be more easily cured and much more short-lived. She contrasts this with the West, where psychiatric treatment does not have this integrating function (which is fulfilled by the political, bureaucratic system and so on), and mental illness serves to *alienate* the sick individual even further from society. It establishes boundaries around the patient, and does not create or re-establish social ties between kin and other groups (except perhaps within the nuclear family) or make clear the boundaries between groups. The Western schizophrenic is assumed to have a chronic, relapsing disease process that may always recur, and is 'a schizophrenic in remission' rather than 'a person who had schizophrenia'. She therefore relates this lack of an integrating function with the long illness careers and poor prognosis of Western psychotics.

However, Kleinman[69] points out that 'cultural healing' may heal social stresses 'independently of the effects they have on the sick person who provides the occasion for their use'. In some cultures, the resolution of social conflicts may not be as beneficial to mentally ill patients as Waxler suggests; it may involve imprisoning, killing or driving them from the community. For example, in the past those 'possessed' by evil spirits in the New Hebrides and Fiji were routinely buried alive. However, in many non-industrialized societies the mentally ill are usually well cared for within their families or communities.

In more traditional societies, mental illness is usually dealt with by folk healers such as the Taiwanese *tang-ki*, the Ndembu *chimbuki*, the Latin American *curandero*, the Moroccan *fqih*, the Malaysian *bomoh* or the Zulu *isangoma*. Some of the practices and psychotherapeutic functions of these ritual healers have already been described. Perhaps the most famous is the *shaman*, who appears in many different cultures, from Alaska to Africa, and whose Western equivalents are mediums, clairvoyants and 'channellers'. Like the mentally ill person who is 'possessed' by spirits, the shaman also allows himself to become temporarily possessed by certain spirits. Lewis[70] points out that, by contrast with the patient, his possession is 'controlled' during the healing seance and thus occurs when and where he chooses. In this condition of controlled abnormality, the fact that he is able to master or neutralize the spirits is of great reassurance to the community. He is also able to identify and exorcise malign spirits possessing the ill person, and in the process alleviate anxiety, fears, guilt and conflicts. Murphy[71] has described some of the psychotherapeutic aspects of shamanism as part of his ritual of cultural healing. These include:

- working within the shared beliefs of the group, and thus reinforcing them
- involving the individual as well as the community in the ritual, during which time the patient remains surrounded by familiar friends and relatives
- by becoming 'possessed', illustrating his mastery over the other spirits causing ill health.

In his seance, the shaman identifies the cause of mental illness (such as breach of a taboo) and prescribes the appropriate expiatory acts, which are believed to effect the cure, and then demonstrates that the patient has indeed recovered. That is, 'through suggestion and the patient's personal involvement in the cure, these visible acts further promote in the patient a psychological realization that he is returning to a state of health'. According to Lewis, by the wide role that he plays in the religious and social life of his community, 'the shaman is not less than a psychiatrist, he is more'[70].

Symbolic healing

'Cultural healing', with its focus mainly on the social dimensions of healing, is really only a special form of what anthropologists have called *symbolic healing* – that is, healing that does not rely on any physical or pharmacological treatments for its efficacy, but rather on language, ritual and the manipulation of powerful cultural symbols. As well as the more traditional folk or religious healing described above, it also includes the various types of 'talk therapy' common in the West – such as psychoanalysis, psychotherapy and counselling.

This section examines a number of key questions raised by symbolic healing. How does it work? What are its effects on mental illness? Does it have common features in whatever society it occurs?

In understanding this phenomenon, the previous discussions of the placebo effect (Chapter 8), ritual healing (Chapter 9), folk healers (Chapter 4), illness narratives (Chapter 5) and even the 'total drug effect' (Chapter 8) are all relevant. In addition, the innovative work of Dow[72], Kleinman[73], Csordas[74], Moerman[75] and others are particularly useful in helping to identify certain basic themes that seem to underlie virtually *all* forms of symbolic healing, whether sacred or secular, and wherever they occur.

Before this type of healing can take place – involving a particular healer, client and community – a number of conditions must be fulfilled. These conditions apply both to secular healing such as the Western 'talk therapies' and to the more religious forms of healing, and include the following.

1. The healer must have a coherent system of explanation, or frame of reference, for the origin and nature of the problem, and how it can be dealt with. Dow[72] called this the *mythic world* – 'a model of experiential reality', whose elements 'represent solutions to personal human problems', and which is composed of culturally specific beliefs, metaphors and idioms. It may consist, for example, of a belief that malign 'spirits' (or 'intrapsychic conflicts') are responsible for all mental illness and extreme emotional states. In many cases – especially in small-scale societies – the mythic world is common to most members of the group: but it may also be created *de novo* by some charismatic healer or cult leader, or be shared by only a tiny group of adherents, as in the new cults, religions, lifestyles, talk therapies and healing systems that are now proliferating in Europe and the USA[76]. The mythic world may exist only in an oral form or be standardized in certain texts (or textbooks). It may take many forms, sacred or secular – for example, as a religious cosmology (Ayurveda), a folk tradition (spirit possession), a theory of personality (Freudian psychoanalysis) or a scientific model of the body (biomedicine).
2. The mythic world must include what Kleinman[73] describes as a *symbolic bridge* between personal experience, social relations, and cultural meanings. That is, suffering individuals in that society must be able to understand their own situation and its resolution in terms of its imagery and symbols (such as spirit possession, or intrapsychic conflict). In many cases these symbols are already familiar to these individuals since, as Finkler[77] puts it, they 'emerge from the depths of their cultural experience and ... reach the bearers of that culture at the most profound levels of their existence'. They represent 'the deep cultural grammar governing how the person orients himself to the world around him and to his inner world'[61], and serve to link the individual to the social world – and often to the supernatural world as well.
3. When a suffering individual consults a healer, the healer aims to activate this 'symbolic bridge' by *convincing* the clients (if they require convincing) that their own particular problem *is* explicable in terms of the symbols of the mythic world. That is, the patients have to be persuaded that their suffering can be redefined or 'reframed' as, for example, evidence of spirit possession, neurosis or evil eye affliction. Thus the healer's aim at this stage is to get 'the patient to accept a particularization of the general mythic world as a valid model of the patient's experiences'[71], and to achieve this they may use many different theatrical or rhetorical techniques.

4. Once patient and healer have reached this consensus, the healer needs to get the patient *emotionally* (as well as intellectually) 'attached' to the symbols of their mythic world. That is, before therapeutic change can take place, patients must first become more self-aware, feel emotionally involved in the healing process, and see these symbols (whether they are spirits or intrapsychic conflicts) as relating to them personally and to their situation. This is done, for example, by interpreting a patient's excess rage as evidence of 'possession' by an angry evil spirit, or of severe inner 'conflicts' dating from childhood, or by interpreting feelings of depression as being due to 'soul loss' (as in *susto*). In each case, the aim is not only to relate the patients' emotions (including their hopes and fears) to the symbols of the healer's mythic world, but also to link the individual patients thereby to wider social, cultural and cosmological concerns.
5. The healer now begins to guide *therapeutic change* by manipulating the symbols of their mythic world. For example, having identified the spirit possessing the patient, he goes through a complex ritual of exorcism, at the end of which the anxious patients are reassured that the spirit has left them and that they can now resume their normal life. Or, they may be reassured by a psychotherapist that they have at last 'worked through' certain archaic, inner conflicts. Or, as in the case of *susto*, they may be told after a ritual that their soul has, at last, been safely returned to their body. In each case, Kleinman[72] points out that the 'healing, as a sacred or secular ritual, achieves its efficacy through the transformation of experience'. The patients learn to re-evaluate and 'reframe' their past and present experiences. Furthermore, Kleinman[73] saw this process, and the symbols used within it, as a way of linking the patient's 'self' (both psychological and physical) to the social relations and cultural concerns of the wider society. Thus a successful transformation will affect not only their emotional state, but also their physiology, their relationships with other people and their relationship to the culture at large. In many cases the symbols that achieve this are not only the conceptual symbols of the mythic world, but also the more tangible ritual symbols described in Chapter 9.
6. The 'healed' patients have acquired a new way of conceptualizing their experiences in symbolic terms, and a new way of functioning – both of them confirmed by the healer. In the process, they have also acquired a newly fashioned *narrative* of their past and present, and of their likely future. Whether this narrative is short (as in spirit exorcisms) or lengthy (as in psychoanalysis), it summarizes *post hoc* what happened to them and why, and how the healer was able to restore them to happiness or health.

Symbolic healing thus often takes place at many levels simultaneously; psychological, physical, social, cultural and spiritual. As with the placebo effect, the exact mechanisms of its effects on physiology (for example, relieving muscular tension, reducing pain sensation or lowering blood pressure) are not clearly understood; nor whether they are mediated by the autonomic nervous system, the endocrine system, the immune system or the neuropeptide (endorphin) system.

Secular symbolic healing: the 'talk therapies'

In the Western world most forms of 'talk therapy', with the exception of family therapy, focus mainly on the individual patient, as do many of the alternative/complementary therapies described in Chapter 4. Whatever their ideology, the majority of talk therapists will see their individual clients as the main 'problem', and their emotional state, behaviour, insights and delusions as the main areas of concern. Most of the clients' treatments will take place in specialized settings, such as a psychotherapist's office, far removed from their social milieu and characterized by both privacy and confidentiality. Where patient and therapist come from similar backgrounds, they may share many assumptions about the likely origin, nature and treatment of psychological disorders. However, the proliferation of new talk therapies has meant that, in many cases, the patients may have to *learn* this world view gradually, acquiring with each session a further understanding of the concepts, symbols and vocabulary that comprise it. This can be seen as a form of 'acculturation' whereby they acquire a new mythic world couched, for example, in terms of the Freudian, Jungian, Kleinian, Laingian or other psychological models. This mythic world, shared eventually by patient and therapist, is often inaccessible to the patient's family or community, who in any case are excluded from the consultation.

Psychoanalysis

Psychoanalysis is a special and influential form of symbolic healing, found almost exclusively in the Western world and providing the basis for many of the other 'talk therapies'. To Dow[72], it is 'probably the most significant psychotherapy in Western culture'. Stein[78] has argued further that its concepts provide a useful way of understanding the universal characteristics of the human condition, whatever the cultural or social context. As a form of therapy, though, it has specific features very different from most forms of cultural healing. Its focus is only on the individual, irrespective of home environment and socio-cultural background, and healing sessions involve only a solitary analyst and a solitary client. The sessions take place in a specified place (the analyst's office) and at a specified time, and in most cases they last exactly 50 minutes. Lying on a couch in this office, with the analyst out of sight and sitting silently behind them, the clients are encouraged to 'free associate', to 'say anything that comes into your head'. As a form of healing, its emphasis is on phenomena believed to originate *within* the individual psyche as they emerge during the analytic session – especially the meanings given by the client to their past experiences. In the session, as Dow[72] puts it, 'transactional symbols are developed by the analyst from the content of the mythic world constructed by the patient', and these will form the basis of the therapeutic stages outlined above. Above all, the emphasis of psychoanalysis is on the treatment of the individual rather than of the social domain. As one analyst[79] puts it, 'the wish for further insight in order to discover the unconscious meaning of unsatisfactory life situations or incomprehensible symptoms implies acceptance of the fact that ultimately the causes of psychological symptoms *lie within oneself*'.

Anthropologists have argued that, whatever the reasons for its efficacy, the practice of psychoanalysis can also be understood as the expression of certain core Western cultural values[80] – especially those of the educated middle-classes. Included here could be the emphasis on self-awareness, insight, 'personal growth', individualism, privacy and confidentiality; the high value placed on language and the ability to verbalize one's distress; and the location of conflicts (especially sexual ones) deep within the psyche, rather than in the social world outside. Its metaphors of the psyche are often spatial (as well as dualistic); an 'inner' psyche hidden within an 'outer' body, and the consequent need for 'insight'. Its view of time is, to some extent, paradoxical; on the one hand, a rigid adherence to Western monochronic 'clock time', strictly enforcing the 50-minute consultation, on the other hand, an open-ended period of therapy, sometimes lasting for many years. As in some other forms of symbolic healing, analyst and client share in the creation of a personalized *narrative* of misfortune, and one embellished and refashioned over many years.

By contrast, more traditional forms of symbolic healing tend to be less structured, last a shorter time, take place in the presence of other people and be linked more to the social or supernatural aspects of daily life. They do not seek insight from the patient, or aim at their individuation or 'personal growth'. These differences, as Kleinman[81] points out, 'illumine the radical differences between egocentric Western culture and sociocentric non-Western cultures, and disclose that culture exerts a powerful effect on care'.

The setting of symbolic healing

Symbolic healing usually takes place at specified times and in specified places. As described in Chapter 9, the *setting* itself plays a crucial role in the healing process; setting the stage, creating a mood of expectation, and giving information to the clients about the healers – especially their interests, background, the source of their power and what they believe in. For example, patients entering Sigmund Freud's consulting rooms in Vienna or London would find the desk and shelves filled with artefacts from ancient Greece, Rome and Egypt, reflecting his interest in his clients' early, hidden childhood experiences, and his remark that the analyst's work 'resembles to a great extent an archaeologist's excavation of some dwelling-place that has been destroyed and buried'[82].

In religious healing, the setting may be a church, a temple, a shrine, a tomb, the home of a religious leader or a sacred place of pilgrimage. For example, El-Islam[83] describes how, in many

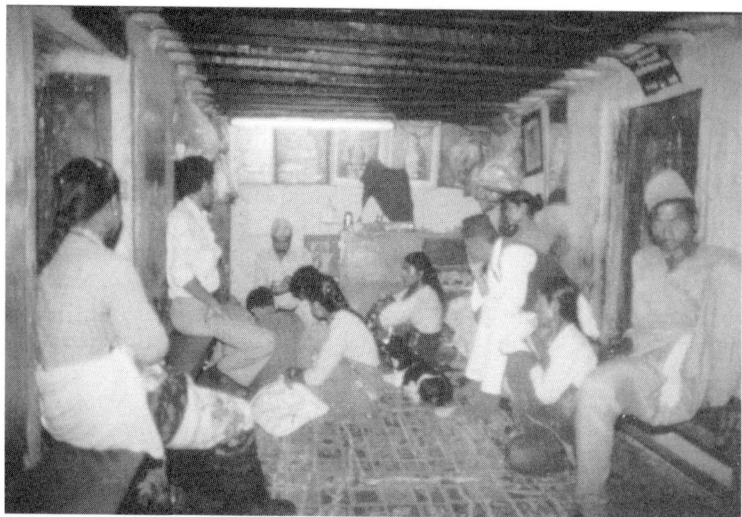

Figure 10.2 A *jhārphuke vaidya*, or Hindu Tantric healer, and his clients in the Kathmandu Valley, Nepal. He offers healing for a variety of ailments, including physical disease, social problems, and mental illness – especially when due to witchcraft or other supernataural causes (Source: David Gellner).

Arab countries, the families of people with severe mental problems (frequently blamed on the evil eye, sorcery or possession by *jinns*) often turn first to forms of ritual healing. These may include visits to the tombs of famous *sheikhs*, consultations with a respected *sheikh* or master (*Al-Asyaad*), the use of amulets containing holy verses, and purification rituals (*Mahuw* or *Mahaya*) that involve drinking or washing in water that has been washed off Koranic verses written on a plate. In *Umbanda*[84], a popular Brazilian religion that has incorporated elements of Catholicism, Afro-Brazilian beliefs and European Spiritism, consultations and healing take place during public religious rituals (*sessões*). They are usually held in special centres (*terreiros*) decorated with brightly-painted images and murals of the various deities. During the service, Umbanda initiates can become possessed by these deities – such as the *orixas* (African deities or their Catholic equivalents), *caboclos* (Indian deities) or *Pretos Velhos* (spirits of old African slaves). In this altered state of consciousness they are able to act as 'spirit consultants' to other members of the congregation, divining the causes of their illness or misfortune with the aid of their spirits and then healing it, often by exorcism.

Whether symbolic healing is sacred or secular, the setting in which it occurs and the ritual symbols used within it are crucial parts of the healing process. Both play an essential, though non-verbal, role in the creation of the mythic world, in terms of which healing will take place.

The efficacy of symbolic healing

It is difficult to evaluate the efficacy of different forms of symbolic healing, since definitions of therapeutic success vary among them. Some seem to relieve one type of psychological distress, but not another. For example, in a detailed study of healing in a spiritualist temple in rural Mexico, Finkler[85] found that it was ineffective for the psychoses but useful for 'neurotic disorders, psychophysiological problems and somatized syndromes'. It enabled patients to abandon their sick roles, return to normal behaviour, and eliminate the feeling of 'being sick'. Similarly, in a study of therapeutic outcomes from a Taiwanese healer or *tang-ki*, Kleinman[86] found that symbolic healing was mainly effective for episodes of neurosis and somatization, and its value more in healing the 'illness' than in curing the 'disease'. It was effective in fitting the illness episode into a wider context – explaining it in familiar terms, mobilizing social support about the victim and reaffirming basic values and group cohesion – and thus reducing anxiety in both the victims and their families. In a study in Tamil Nadu, southern India, Campion and Bhugra[87] found that of 198 psychiatric patients attending hospital, 45 per cent had earlier sought help from a Hindu, Muslim or Christian religious healer. Of these, 30 per cent felt that they had got some benefit from the consultation, although the majority (90 per cent) had discontinued this treatment by the time of hospitalization. Overall, most anthropologists would agree therefore that – for whatever reason

– many people *are* helped by symbolic healing, whether religious or secular.

'Healing', however, is not identical to 'curing', especially in the case of severe psychosis or physical disability. Individuals and their families may feel that they have been 'healed', even though they have not yet been 'cured' in conventional psychiatric or medical terms. This distinction is clearer in some forms of religious healing, such as faith healing. As Csordas[88] points out, there are crucial differences between secular healing (with its mind–body dualism), such as medicine or psychotherapy, and religious healing (with its tripartite division of mind–body–spirit). In his study of Catholic Charismatic healing in the USA[89], he described their four distinct types of healing: *physical healing* of bodily illness; *inner healing* of emotional scars or mental illness; *deliverance* from the adverse effects of demons or evil spirits; and *spiritual healing* of the soul injured by sin, primarily by means of the Sacrament of Reconciliation (confession). Even if the first three fail in a particular case, and the person remains mentally or physically ill, spiritual healing is still possible as what Csordas calls 'a hedge against the failure of healing prayer'.

It should be pointed out that, as described in previous chapters, *all* forms of healing, including medical and surgical treatments[90], have some symbolic component to them. Both Western medicine and psychiatry are symbolic systems as well as technical ones. With the gradual diffusion of their concepts and techniques worldwide, there is an increasing likelihood of complex interactions or conflicts between the different mythic worlds of traditional and psychiatric approaches to mental illness, as illustrated in the following case studies.

Case study: A case of 'fox possession' in Sapporo, Japan

Etsuko[91] described the case of Michiko, a 43-year-old single woman complaining of possession by a fox spirit (*kitsune-tsuki*), a common idiom of mental disorder in Japan. Her illness began after her parents died, when she became distressed and 'strange voices and noises came to my ears. I felt very uneasy'. She was seen by psychiatrists but 'the medicine was no help, but it's natural that spirits can't be cured by medicine. And doctors would never understand spirit possession'. To get relief, and an explanation for her symptoms, she consulted in turn seven different shamans. At the seventh one, a shaman of the Shugendo sect of Buddhism, a series of seances confirmed that she was possessed by an evil fox spirit because – among other reasons – she and her ancestors had killed many foxes in their previous lives. After several rituals, Michiko claimed that the fox spirit had told her important facts; in particular, that she was really of noble birth, and that her misfortune was not her fault but the result of her being born under an unlucky star. Gradually the fox evolved from a possessing spirit to be her personal deity; at the same time, she became transformed from being a client into being a shaman in her own right. Her psychological state improved markedly, as 'the illness of possession was replaced by a shamanistic ability brought about by her steady effort in religious practice'. At the same time as this improvement was taking place, the psychiatrists judged her condition to have deteriorated, to have gone from auditory hallucinations and possession state to delusional perceptions, grandiose beliefs and signs of chronic schizophrenia. This case illustrates, therefore, the discrepancy between being 'healed' and being 'cured' – at least from a psychiatric perspective.

Case study: Psychiatric and religious healing in Jerusalem, Israel

Bilu and colleagues[92] described how secular (psychotherapy) and sacred (Jewish mysticism) forms of healing can intersect in a medical milieu in Jerusalem, Israel. By using hypnosis, guided imagery and conventional psychotherapy, the therapists were able to treat Avraham, a religious psychotic patient, by working within his own mythic world and its complex metaphors and symbolism – drawn largely from Jewish mysticism. By encouraging him, under hypnosis, to confront the black 'demon' that was persecuting him, and chase it away ('Go, go, go away because you do not belong to our world!'), they were able to greatly improve his emotional state and social functioning. During the therapy sessions Avraham was symbolically led through a desert until finally he found peace in a quiet green oasis – a manifestation of Paradise and the Garden of Eden – filled with 'pure springs, sweet odors, beautiful gardens, and particularly

continued

pious inhabitants'. His personal cure was thus linked to the wider cultural themes of Exodus and redemption in Jewish tradition and theology, already familiar to the patient.

Case study: Spiritist healing in Porto Alegre, Brazil

Greenfield[93] examined the healing practices of a new syncretic religion, a Spiritist group known as *Casa do Jardim*, in Porto Alegre, southern Brazil. Its imagery is an unusual fusion of Afro-Brazilian folk religion and ideas drawn from medical science; several of its healers are themselves physicians. They believe in two parallel worlds, one material and the other spiritual, with communication possible between the two. Each human being has a spirit as well as a body, and under some circumstances that spirit can also get ill. In that case, the healers will 'uncouple' it from the body and send if off to the spirit or astral world, where teams of 'spirit doctors' will diagnose and treat it in a 'spirit hospital' called the *Amor e Caridade* before returning it, healed, to its body. Mental illness is believed to be due to disincarnate evil spirits from the astral plane imposing themselves on the living. Its treatment is by 'disobsession' – the healer 'incarnating' the offending spirit, lecturing it on the error of its ways and then sending it back to the astral plane. Like other healing groups, the *Casa do Jardim* provides social support, practical help and psychotherapy, especially for 'unaffiliated individuals who face the increasing uncertainty and insecurity of life in disorganized, anomic, urban Brazil'.

Anthropology and family therapy

Anthropology is essentially the study of groups rather than of individuals, though sometimes individuals are studied within the context of certain groups. In all human societies, the primary social group is always the *family*. The composition of the family varies greatly between cultures, as does the role that it plays in the lives of its members. Outside the urban areas of the industrialized world, where the nuclear family (a couple and their children) is often the norm, the extended multigenerational family (usually a couple, together with one or more married children and their children and spouses) is one of the commonest kinship patterns found worldwide. In poorer parts of the world, this larger family unit, though linked to the wider society, often acts as a miniature and self-contained community or self-help group, whose members share many of their resources and many of the tasks and responsibilities of everyday life. In whatever form it takes, and in whatever culture it appears, the family is always a *social* as well as a biological unit, and it always includes members who are not biologically related to it. As well as marriage partners and their families of origin, it may also include honorary relatives or 'fictive kin', such as close friends or neighbours, or even health professionals.

In recent years there has been an increasing overlap in interest between medical anthropologists, family therapists and some psychiatrists. All three are interested in widening the definition of 'patient' beyond the individual, to include their family and, where relevant, their community as well. For many clinicians, like some of the folk healers described in Chapter 4, the family and not the individual has become the main focus for both diagnosis and treatment.

One obvious problem is that the definition of 'family' is not universal. There is wide cross-cultural variation in patterns of kinship, and anthropologists have described many different types of family structure. Children in different parts of the world may be the result of different forms of marriage: monogamy (one wife, one husband), polygyny (one husband, several wives) or – more rarely – polyandry (one wife, several husbands)[94]. As well as extended families and nuclear families, there are joint families (a household composed of married siblings, spouses and children) and one-parent families (usually mother and child). In recent years a number of *new* types of family structure have also appeared, especially in Western countries. These include adoptive or fostering families, childless marriages by choice, communes (organized like large extended families), lesbian and gay couples, and the complex combinations of step-children, step-parents and in-laws that have resulted from high rates of divorce and remarriage. Certain other social groupings can also function as quasi-families for some of their members. These include clubs, self-help groups, youth gangs, military regiments, cults, corporations, voluntary organizations, and even the personnel of a hospital ward.

In many parts of the world, the concept of 'family' also includes the dead. In an emotional sense, therefore, as mentioned in Chapter 9, the dead never die. In much of Asia and Africa and in parts of Latin America the ancestors are still regarded as part of the family, and even though invisible they continue to play important roles in daily life. They are often consulted or worshipped, or shrines are erected to them. In many parts of Africa they are also the guardians of the social order, and punish transgressions among their descendants by causing them to suffer misfortune or fall ill. Contact with the ancestors is usually maintained by regular rituals, attended by most of the family. In the annual Mexican 'Day of the Dead' (*El Día de los Muertos*), for example, the family gathers at the graveside of their relative, decorates it with photos and mementos, and then 'shares' a communal meal with them[95]. This ritual also serves to remind the living that the dead are still very much part of their lives. In some cultures, the links between living and dead are more pervasive and constraining. Widows, for example, may be forbidden ever to remarry, since they are considered permanently married to their dead husbands.

However it is constituted, it is useful to view the family as a small-scale society, or even as a small 'tribe', with its own distinctive organization and culture. In many ways, what may be termed this *family culture*[96] is very similar to that of the wider society, but it also has certain unique and distinctive features of its own. As described at the beginning of this book, a culture includes a set of implicit and explicit guidelines telling people how to view the world, how to experience it emotionally and how to behave in it – especially in relation to other people, the natural world and supernatural entities or gods. Families, like larger cultural groups, also have their own particular view of the world, their own codes of behaviour, gender roles, concepts of time and space, private slang and language, history and myths and rituals. They also have ways of communicating psychological distress to one another and to the outside world.

This family culture can be either protective or pathogenic to health, depending on the context. For example, certain types of family structure may contribute to the development of alcohol abuse among the children later in life (see Chapter 8), while others may protect against this. The family can also be seen as a 'system', in which the pattern of inter-relationships can have important influences on both health and disease[97]. This *systems theory* or cybernetic model suggests that family dynamics are often aimed at maintaining a state of equilibrium between these various relationships, even at the cost of psychologically 'scapegoating' one of its members. For example, Minuchin and colleagues[60] have shown how certain types of family structure are more likely to cause psychosomatic disorders such as anorexia nervosa in some of its members. These 'psychosomatic families' maintain their cohesion, continuity and sense of equilibrium, not only by producing this disorder in one of its members, but also by helping to maintain it. The recovery of the 'identified patient' (in this case, the anorexic young girl) may well cause the break-up of such a pathological family. In this case, as in others, focusing only on the individual and not on their family makes a fuller understanding of the problem difficult to achieve.

Byng-Hall[98] has described the concept of *family script*, which is transmitted from generation to generation. These scripts are ways of behaving, of viewing the world and of reacting emotionally to it. As with culture in general, most of these scripts are outside of conscious awareness. Their role is to provide a sense of stability and continuity, and a set of guidelines for performing the daily drama of a family's life. They often function to avoid potentially dangerous conflicts within the family. Each generation of the family knows its allocated role within this continuing drama, and sometimes this role may determine when and how they get ill, or even die. The script may also influence the clustering of certain symptoms within a particular family, and how these symptoms are passed on from parents to children[99]. Family scripts can be maintained by the family's own myths and folklore, which are passed on from generation to generation; in some cases, these myths may have originated centuries before the birth of its present members[98]. Many years later, these *family myths* may still be exerting a negative effect on both the mental and physical health of its members.

The relation of *culture* to family dynamics is complex, and to some extent controversial. McGoldrick and colleagues[100] have provided a comprehensive selection of mini-ethnographies of the family cultures of different ethnic groups in the USA – such as the 'Irish family', 'the

Italian family' and the 'British American family' – and the problems that family therapists face when dealing with each of them. Although it is certainly possible, and useful, to make some generalizations about, say, Italian families, and the cultural themes they have in common, the danger of stereotyping *all* Italian families still applies. Furthermore, listing the supposed cultural traits of families from different ethnic groups often ignores major differences between families (based on region, economic position, social class, education etc.), even if they come from the same ethnic group. Maranhao[101], in his critique of McGoldrick's book, has also argued that 'family oriented ethnic groups' are sometimes described in it as if their differences from the Anglo-Saxon family type (with its emphasis on individual rather than family goals) were 'pathological' by definition. Overall, in his view, knowledge of the cultural background of a family is useful but not essential for therapy to take place – 'the interviewer does not have to know anthropology, but just be a sensitive family therapist'.

DiNicola[102] has suggested two alternative ways of describing the relationship between a family's mental health and its culture of origin. *Cultural costume* is 'the particular set of recipes the individuals or families of a community have to give meaning and shape to their experiences and to communicate these experiences through shared ceremonies, rituals and symbols'. It is therefore the repertoire of cultural beliefs and behaviours of which each family culture is a particular (and sometimes unique) expression. The cultural costume becomes *cultural camouflage* 'when culture is invoked as a smokescreen to obscure individual states of mind or patterns of interaction in the family'. That is, the family claims that pathological behaviour patterns within it are only normal expressions of its cultural background. DiNicola quotes, as examples of this: 'My husband drinks very hard, he's Irish,' or 'My son had a breakdown because he stopped going to the Orthodox church and lost the Greek way'.

Lau[103], like Maranhao, points out how west European or North American family therapists may misdiagnose family patterns from other cultures as pathological or deviant. This is especially likely where the family structure is less familiar to them, as in one-parent families (among some West Indians) or in multigenerational extended families (among Asians, Chinese and Greek Cypriots) who are living in the same household. She points out that in many cultures outside the Western world, 'breaks are not expected between the generations and continuity in the group depends on the presence of three generations'. Notions of individual autonomy and differentiation therefore have a different meaning in these groups from the Western nuclear family model. In dealing with families from ethnic minorities, Barot[104] has further suggested that a focus on their culture may be insufficient because a wider analysis of the institutional and structural factors (such as unemployment, racial discrimination, poor housing, inadequate social and health care facilities and the effects of migration) that may also adversely affect their lives is required as well. Furthermore, these external factors may act to weaken the traditional culture and cohesion of those families, so that 'culture' is no longer a viable explanation for many of the pathological breakdowns in family life.

From an international perspective, several detailed studies have shown fundamental variations in family culture between different parts of the world – though, as noted above, these broad generalizations do not take into account variations *within* each country or community. Tamura and Lau[105], for example, have contrasted Japanese and Western (particularly British) family structures. In Japan, the culture stresses the *interconnectedness* of relationships, especially within the family. A high value is placed on the unity and wellbeing of the group, and the 'family self' – the 'basic, inner psychological organization' of the Japanese – 'involves intensely emotional intimacy relationships, high levels of receptivity to others, strong identification with the reputation and honour of the family and others'. The individual is thus seen as part of a 'web of interconnectedness', rather than as merely a 'skin-encapsulated ego'. The core of a Japanese family is the mother–child dyad, rather than the husband–wife dyad in the West; because children are firmly in the woman's domain, many Japanese men may be reluctant to accompany their wives to a therapist if their children have problems.

By contrast, family structure in North America and north-western Europe stresses the *separateness* of individuals – their degree of autonomy and individuation from one another – rather than their interconnectedness. Westerners are expected to see themselves as autonomous, independent, individual units, with sharp boundaries between themselves and others. Human growth and emotional development in the family life cycle is seen as a process of individuation, while in Japan it involves the transition from one form of integration to another. Tamura and Lau thus warn against imposing the Western notion of 'hyper-individualism' on Japanese families, or misinterpreting connectedness as 'enmeshment' or inadequate individuation. Japanese therapists tend to see family problems as resulting from *too little* connectedness rather than too much, and therefore aim to strengthen integration of the family unit rather than fragment it. In carrying this out, their clients expect them to be authoritative, directive and also 'connected' – almost as if they were senior family members. Finally, Japanese families may avoid seeing a therapist because of feelings of shame and guilt for their inability to deal with the problem within the privacy of the family.

In India, Shankar and Menon[106] stress that the traditional extended or joint family is a key resource in the care of people with serious mental illness, such as schizophrenia. Given the widespread poverty and unemployment – as well as the paucity of psychiatric hospitals, trained mental health professionals and social welfare benefits – therapists planning interventions with families of schizophrenics therefore 'need to take into account the complex matrix of social, economic, cultural, and infrastructural factors that exist in the country'. Thus the majority of the seriously mentally ill are managed by their families, who represent 'the cornerstone of client care in the community'. Because these families (unlike many of their Western equivalents) 'have at no time received the label of being aetiological agents of the illness', they do not feel any sense of guilt if asked to participate in their relative's therapeutic programme. In dealing with Indian schizophrenics, Shankar and Menon therefore suggest that no attempt should be made to blame the family either for causing the illness or for any relapses. Instead, they should be treated as an ally in treatment and not as a potential enemy. The therapist should be sensitive to their needs, as well as those of their ill relative, and should aim to strengthen their positive role in the care of the patient. They should be given ample information on schizophrenia, and encouraged to supervise the patient's medication and to identify any early signs of relapse.

El-Islam[83] has listed 'certain widely shared features of general relevance to psychiatry' in the Arab world, while also emphasizing the enormous cultural diversity within those communities. He describes the strong extended family structure, which favours 'affiliative behaviour' at the expense of 'differentiating behaviour'; that is, 'traditional child rearing instils behaviour oriented towards accommodation, conformity, cooperation, affection, and interdependence rather than behaviour oriented towards individuation, intellectualisation, independence and compartmentalisation'. Also, in more traditional communities, women 'are at a socio-cultural disadvantage in relation to men'; polygyny is still practised, arranged marriages are common, and divorce is more easily obtained by men than by women. In this setting, conflicts may arise between older family members and a more Westernized younger generation, especially over attitudes to sexual behaviour, education and the choice of marriage partner. However, El-Islam notes that, for those of its members who have a mental illness (such as schizophrenia), the extended family provides a more therapeutic setting, and with a better prognosis, than would institutionalization.

Therefore, as this section illustrates, family therapy provides one of the most fruitful areas of co-operation between psychology, psychiatry and medical anthropology – especially in understanding the family's role in both the cause and cure of mental illness – and research in this area is likely to increase in the future.

Migration and mental illness

Studies carried out in various countries have indicated that immigrants often have a higher rate of mental illness than either the native-born population or the population in their countries of origin. This is indicated by higher rates of admission to mental hospitals, and higher indices of alcoholism, drug addiction and attempted suicide. Some of these studies on immigrants to the UK, such as Asians, West Indians, Africans, Irish, Poles and Russians, are described in Chapter 11. Some immigrant groups appear to be more vulnerable to certain illnesses than to others; for example, Irish immigrants to the UK have significantly higher rates of alcoholism, while West Indians have the highest rate of schizophrenia of all the immigrant groups. In his study of mental illness among immigrants to Australia, carried out in Victoria, Krupinski[107] found that depressive states were particularly common among British and East European migrants, and the latter group also had the highest rate of schizophrenia. Overall, immigrants showed a much higher rate of psychological instability than exists in the Australian-born population.

Cox[108] has summarized the three hypotheses that seek to explain this high rate of mental illness associated with migration:

1. Certain mental disorders incite their victims to migrate (the *selection* hypothesis)
2. The process of migration creates mental stress, which may precipitate mental illness in susceptible individuals (the *stress* hypothesis)
3. There is a non-essential association between migration and certain other variables, such as age, class and culture conflict.

In the first group, restless and unstable people are believed to migrate more often, in an attempt to solve their personal problems. In another study in Australia, for example, Schaechter[109] found that 45.5 per cent of non-British female immigrants admitted to a psychiatric hospital within 3 years of migration had suffered an established mental illness prior to migration. If 'suspected cases' of mental illness prior to arrival were added, the figure rose to 68.2 per cent. Other studies, from different parts of the world, have shown that a certain percentage of immigrants *do* have a history of previous mental disorders in their countries of origin.

The 'stress' hypothesis, described in Chapter 11, emphasizes the role of changes in the migrants' 'life space', where the basic assumptions on which their world is founded can no longer be taken for granted. Littlewood and Lipsedge[110], in their study of mental illness among immigrants to the UK, point out that these disorders result from the complex interplay of many factors, including both 'selection' and 'stress'. These include material and environmental deprivation such as overcrowding, shared dwellings, lack of amenities, high unemployment and low family incomes, as well as racial discrimination, and conflict between immigrants and their local-born children. Language difficulties also play an important part, especially among female immigrants who arrive later in the country than their menfolk and who are often confined within the home and family. For example, a study in Newcastle[111] found that 58 per cent of Pakistani women spoke little or no English, and 15 per cent of men and 66 per cent of the women had received little or no schooling and were entirely illiterate. These socio-economic factors, coupled with the stress of culture change and the influence of selection, explain much of the increased rates of mental illness among first-generation immigrants. A further factor, mentioned earlier, is that diagnostic and admission rates in psychiatry may reflect political, racial or moral prejudices, and misinterpret the immigrants' cultural beliefs and reactions to their plight as evidence of 'madness' or 'badness'.

Within both immigrant populations and ethnic minorities, certain groups seem to have different rates and forms of mental illness. According to Littlewood and Lipsedge[110], 'there appear to be no simple explanations for the different rates of mental illness applicable to all minority groups'. Some factors seem more significant in some groups than in others, and the best way to compare groups would be to add up all these negative factors – selection, stress, multiple deprivations, language difficulties, loss of status (both social and professional), clash between old and new cultural values and so on – to find a 'score' indicating the risk factors for that community. For example, they note how West African students seem particularly vulnerable to mental illness due to dissatisfaction with British food and weather, to discrimination, economic and legal difficulties, experience of the 'typical British personality', sexual isolation, more mature age, middle-class aspirations and fear of withdrawal of their grants if they fail their examinations. Those with the lowest rates of mental illness – the Chinese, Italians and Indians – have in common a great determination to migrate, migration for economic reasons, an intention to return home, little attempt at assimilation, and a high degree of entrepreneurial activity. Immigrants who were forced to leave their countries as refugees and who cannot return are by contrast likely to have a higher rate of mental illness. Krupinski[107] has examined some of these variables among immigrant groups in Australia; he relates their high rates of mental illness to the fact that many are single young men migrating from the UK and western Europe, among whom there is a proportion of already unstable persons (including some chronic alcoholics arriving from the UK). The stresses of migration seem to affect migrants from southern and eastern Europe especially, particularly those in the latter group who had suffered traumatic experiences in the war or loss in occupational status in Australia. Seventy per cent of East European migrants with university degrees now belonged to a lower socio-economic class, compared with only 20 per cent of British graduates. Krupinski also found that schizophrenia occurred most frequently among male immigrants 1–2 years after arrival, while in females the peak was found after 7–15 years. The late onset among females was ascribed to the onset of menopause, and the ending of the maternal role with the departure of grown-up children. In addition, a high proportion of female non-British immigrants could not speak English even after many years in the country, especially those from southern Europe. As with the Pakistani women in Newcastle, their social and linguistic isolation was believed to contribute to their high rate of mental breakdown.

Looked at in perspective, migration (both between countries and within a country) seems to carry with it the increased risk of mental illness, although the reasons for this are complex and not fully understood. However, as some authors[112] have pointed out, studies of the mental health of immigrants are difficult to interpret unless controls for such factors as age, social class, occupational status and ethnic group on one hand, and culturally biased diagnostic methods on the other, are used. Unless this is done, it cannot be demonstrated clearly that there is a significant association between migration and the rates of mental illness among migrants.

While most of the studies of this problem have concentrated on the immigrants and their response to their condition, the cultural attributes of the *host* community are just as important. Such factors as xenophobia, discrimination, racial prejudice[113] (both individual and institutionalized) and racial harassment are all likely to contribute towards the immigrant's mental and physical ill health, as are the economic and political conditions prevailing in the host community.

Within many immigrant and ethnic minority communities, certain cultural traits (such as family cohesion and religion) may protect against mental illness, while others are likely to contribute to an increase. These may include a rigid division among the sexes, the social isolation of women, multiple religious taboos and prescriptions, residential patterns which encourage several generations of a family to live in the same house, intergenerational conflicts and pressure on children to succeed financially or academically. Some of these examples of 'culturogenic stress' will be reviewed in Chapter 11.

Cross-cultural psychiatric diagnosis

This chapter has illustrated some of the complexities in making cross-cultural psychiatric diagnoses, and especially the problems of defining 'normality' and 'abnormality' in the members of other cultures. A further problem is that clinicians may *over*emphasize culture as an explanation for patients' behaviour, and thus ignore any underlying psychopathology[114]. In making cross-cultural diagnoses, therefore, the clinician should always be aware of:

- the extent to which cultural factors affect some of the diagnostic categories and techniques of Western psychiatry
- the role of the patients' culture in helping them understand and communicate their psychological distress
- how the patients' beliefs and behaviour are viewed by other members of their cultural group, and whether their abnormality is viewed as beneficial to the group or not
- whether the specific cluster of symptoms, signs and behavioural changes shown by the patients are interpreted by them, and by their community, as evidence of a 'culture-bound' psychological disorder
- whether the patient's condition is indicative not of mental illness, but rather of the social, political and economic pressures upon them[114].

Recommended reading

Dow, J. (1986). Universal aspects of symbolic healing: a theoretical synthesis. *Am. Anthropol.*, **88**, 56–69.

Kirmayer, L. J. and Young, A. (1998). Culture and somatization: clinical, epidemiological, and ethnographic perspectives. *Psychosom. Med.*, **60**, 420–30.

Kleinman, A. (1988). *Rethinking Psychiatry*. Free Press.

Littlewood, R. and Lipsedge, M. (1989). *Aliens and Alienists*, 2nd edn. Unwin Hyman.

Simons, R. C. and Hughes, C. C. (1985). *The Culture-Bound Syndromes*. Reidel.

Swartz, L. (1998). *Culture and Mental Health: A Southern African View*. Oxford University Press.

11 Cultural aspects of stress

The nature of stress

The concept of 'stress' was first described by Hans Selye in 1936[1], and since then more than 110 000 papers have been published on it in the academic literature[2]. On the level of popular culture, however, 'stress' has also become one of the most pervasive metaphors for personal and collective suffering in the late twentieth century.

In Selye's original model, stress represents the generalized response of the organism to environmental demands. It is an inherent physiological mechanism which prepares the organism for action, and which comes into play when demands are placed on it. Not all stress is harmful to the organism; at a moderate level ('eustress') it has a protective and adaptive function. However, at a higher level ('dystress') the stress response can cause pathological changes and even death. The actual environmental influence – whether physical, psychological or socio-cultural – that produces stress is termed a *stressor.* Selye has described the sequence of events whereby an organism responds to a stressor as the General Adaptation Syndrome (GAS). This usually has three stages:

1. The *alarm* reaction, whereby the organism becomes aware of a specific noxious stimulus
2. The stage of resistance or *adaptation*, in which the organism recovers to a functional level superior to that before it was stressed
3. The stage of *exhaustion*, where the recovery processes, under the continuing assault of stressors, are no longer able to cope and to restore homeostasis.

In this final stage, the physiological changes that have taken place in the organism now become pathological to it, and disease or death results. From a physiological point of view, the GAS is said to be mediated via the adrenal medulla and the hypothalamic–pituitary–adrenocortical axis, and involves a wide range of physical changes[3].

Critiques of Selye's model

Selye's early model, although widely accepted as basic for all stress research, has been criticized on several counts – in particular, for its rather mechanistic approach and its overemphasis on the physiological dimensions of the stress response. Psychologists such as Weinman[4] have pointed out the importance of the *psychological* responses or coping strategies of the individual confronted by a stressor. These range from an initial 'alarm and shock state', with feelings of anxiety or of being threatened, through attempts to cope with the subjectively unpleasant situation, to a range of more extreme psychological reactions such as depression, withdrawal, suicide or resort to 'chemical comforters'. These responses, as well as the *meanings* people give to their stressful experiences, are all influenced by the individual's personality, education, social environment, economic situation and cultural background. As such, they are of more interest to the social scientist than the purely physiological stress responses.

A further salient critique of Selye's model, and of much of the subsequent literature on stress, comes from the anthropologist Allan Young[5]. He argues that 'stressors' are often described in the stress literature as if they were abstract 'things', separated from a particular social and political context, and a particular time and place. Sometimes they are described almost as if they were invisible pathogens or forces that cause illness or unhappiness to certain individuals. Furthermore, the focus on these decontextualized stressors and their physiological effects may lead to ignoring the larger economic and social forces acting upon the individual, which may also have an adverse effect on health.

Pollock[6], too, has criticized Selye's approach, pointing out that his original model of how stress acts physiologically was a mechanical one, taken from physics and engineering. However, since then stress theory has become heavily 'psychologized', with an increasing emphasis on the pathogenic role of emotions and perceptions, but 'it still relies for its validation on the physiological models with which it is fundamentally non-compatible'. In addition, the key link in stress theory – the postulated process by which stress is actually transformed into illness – 'remains unclear and unproven', and many of the studies carried out on this link have produced 'inconsistent, contradictory or inconclusive results'.

Another critique of the model is that it overemphasizes the *external* origin of stress, so that the individual often appears in the stress literature as a passive victim of circumstances. However, from a psychological point of view, many sources of stress may originate *within* the individual. Whatever their origin in early development, these intrapsychic factors – such as exaggerated fears, chronic anxiety, aggressiveness, insecurity, over-sensitivity or false expectations of life – may all contribute towards one individual having a much more stressful life than another.

Finally, the assumption that stress is always negative in its effect on the individual can also be challenged. McElroy and Townsend[7], for example, point out that in many cultures certain rituals can actually induce physical and emotional stress as part of a healing process. These rituals may include painful stimuli (such as fire-walking), physical exhaustion, sleep deprivation, extreme heat or cold, hyperventilation or altered states of consciousness – sometimes with the aid of hallucinogenic drugs (see Chapter 8). To members of these cultural groups, these stressful processes are an essential prerequisite to being healed. Furthermore, on a physical level, some of these culturally-induced stressors may cause the release of endorphins, or endogenous opiates, which induce feelings of wellbeing, reduce pain perception and have a variety of other positive physiological effects[7].

Despite these and many other criticisms, Selye's model of stressors and stress responses is useful as a starting point in understanding how human beings cope with the adversities of life. It can be used as an analytical tool, provided there is an awareness of its limitations and that the role of *context* – psychological, social, cultural and economic – is always included when trying to understand why one individual or group finds some situations stressful, while others do not.

Relation of stressors to stress response

By definition, a 'stressor', according to Selye, is an environmental influence or agent that produces a stress response in the organism. The range of possible stressors is therefore extremely wide, and a list could include such events as severe illness or trauma, natural disasters, bereavement, divorce, marital conflict, unemployment, retirement, interpersonal tensions at work, religious or other persecution, financial difficulties, changes in occupation, migration, wartime combat, and excessive exposure to heat, cold, damp or noise. However, the relationship between stressors and their response is more complex than this list suggests. For example, the same event might cause stress in one individual but not in another. Also, as Parkes[8] points out, stress can arise from usually positive experiences such as promotion, engagement, the birth of a child or winning a great deal of money, all of which involve a change in lifestyle. Individuals vary in how they cope with and adapt to these life changes, and to more adverse circumstances such as bereavement. In both cases, as the World Health Organization[9] pointed out, stress (and the diseases that result from it) represents an unsuccessful attempt on the part of the body to deal with adverse factors in the environment'. Thus 'disease is the body's failure to become adapted to these adverse factors rather than the effect of the factors themselves'. There are many reasons for this failure of adaptation, including the physical, psychological and sociocultural characteristics of the individual. For example, elderly frail people are more likely to experience cold or very humid weather as 'stressful' than younger, more robust people. Also, some situations (such as retirement) may cause a stress response in one person but not in another. Weinman notes that 'specific situations or objects are threatening to the individual because they are perceived as such rather than because of some inherent characteristic'[4]. Some of the social or cultural factors that apparently predispose to, or protect against, the stress response will be described later in the chapter.

According to Selye[2], the relationship between particular stressors and the response they elicit is marked by *non-specificity*. That is, it cannot be predicted what specific stress-related disease (such as peptic ulceration, psychiatric disorders, hypertension or coronary thrombosis) will result from a specific stressor (such as marital conflict, frustration at work, combat fatigue or burns). A stressor such as marital conflict may result in peptic ulceration in one individual, and bronchial asthma in another. In psychosomatic research (see Chapter 10) this is known as the problem of *organ choice*, and many theories have been put forward to explain why one organ is 'chosen' and not another[10]. In practical terms, therefore, a stressor and its effect can only be linked circumstantially, and to some extent only *post hoc*, though more experimental evidence is accumulating on the nature and prevalence of this link.

Stress can also be viewed either as a causal factor in disease or as a contributory one, by reducing the individual's 'resistance' to disease processes such as viral infections[11] or rheumatoid arthritis[12]. The relatively new field of *psychoneuroimmunology* (PNI) (see Chapter 10) has tried to examine the relationships between psychological state, the endocrine system and the body's defences or immune system[13]. Although still characterized by non-specificity, there is evidence that depression and anxiety may adversely affect the immune system and thus increase susceptibility to infections and other illnesses[13]. In other cases, an individual with a pre-existing organic disease might have a relapse in response to stress, as described by Trimble and Wilson-Barnet[14] in the case of epileptic seizures. Finally, the physical disease itself may be a stressful experience which can delay recovery or cause other forms of ill health, especially if it involves loss of income or of job security or a change in personal relationships.

Stress and life changes

Many of the stressors mentioned above, such as bereavement, migration or the birth of a child, involve prolonged, major *changes* in the patterns of people's lives. In recent years, more attention has been paid to the possible negative effects of these changes on both mental and physical health. From this point of view, stress represents an inadequate adaptation to change, an unsuccessful attempt on the part of the individual to cope with and adapt to the changed circumstances of their lives – whether promotion at work or the loneliness of widowhood. Parkes[8] provides a useful way of viewing these changes or psychosocial transitions. He points out that the change is likely to take place in that part of the world which impinges upon the self – the 'life space'. This consists of 'those parts of the environment with which the self interacts and in relation to which behaviour is organized; other persons, material possessions, the familiar world of home and place of work, and the individual's body and mind in so far as he can view these as separate from his self'. They also involve changes in the basic assumptions that people have made about their worlds, for these can no longer be taken for granted. In Parkes' view, the psychosocial transitions most likely to cause stress are those that are lasting in their effects, take place over a relatively short period of time and affect many of the assumptions that people make about their worlds. In that sense, the sudden unexpected loss of a spouse or job is likely to be more stressful than other slower transitions, such as those involved in growth and maturation. Changes such as bereavement, losing a job, or migration will involve many aspects of an individual's life space, such as social relationships, occupational status, financial security and living arrangements, and are more likely to provoke a stress response.

The effects of these changes on both mental and physical health have been studied by several investigators. In their study of bereavement, for example, Parkes and colleagues[15] examined the death rates of 4486 widowers aged 55 years or older for 9 years following the death of their wives. Of these, 213 died in the first 6 months of bereavement – 40 per cent above the expected death rate for married men of the same ages. The death rate from degenerative heart disease was 67 per cent higher than expected. The mortality rate dropped to that of married men after the first year. The authors ascribed the increased death rate to 'the emotional effects of bereavement with the concomitant changes in psychoendocrine function'. Other studies have reached similar conclusions; in a significant number of cases ill health is preceded by a high level of psychosocial transitions or 'life events', especially if these events are perceived as negative.

The precise causal link between these life changes and the occurrence of ill health remains unclear, though various hypotheses have been advanced. Murphy and Brown[16], in examining the question 'whether stressful situations bring about episodes of illness associated with pathological structural changes occurring in a tissue, system or area of the body', point out that in most cases illness will *not* follow from an experience of stress, but where it does the link is likely to be a psychiatric disturbance. They cite evidence that individuals with psychiatric disorders have a significantly higher rate of organic illness, and hypothesize that 'stressful circumstances lead to organic illness by first producing a psychiatric disturbance'. In their study of 111 women in London, 81 had developed a new organic disease (from which they had previously not suffered) in the previous 6 months. Of this latter group, 30 per cent (24) had had at least one severe life event before the onset of ill health, compared with 17 per cent of a matched comparison group. However, this association applied only to women aged between 18 and 50 years, where 38 per cent had had at least one severe event compared with 15 per cent of a control group. In this age group, 30 per cent had experienced the onset of psychiatric disturbance in an average period of 7 weeks before the start of their illness, compared with an expected 2 per cent in the control group. The authors conclude that 'it is the onset of psychiatric disturbance rather than a severe event that is the immediate cause of organic disorder for those [women] under 50'. The events most likely to cause psychiatric disorders are those involving long-term threat to the 'life space', such as an unplanned pregnancy, or terminal illness in a relative. However, the exact physiological mechanism whereby life events, psychiatric disorder and organic illness are interlinked remains unclear. Engel[17] has also pointed out how sometimes illness and even death can be preceded by a period of psychological disturbance, during which the person feels 'unable to cope'. He termed this the 'giving-up–given-up complex', and suggests that this state 'plays some significant role in modifying the capacity of the organism to cope with concurrent pathogenic factors'. It is characterized by: a feeling of psychological impotence or helplessness ('giving-up'); a lowered self-image as one who is no longer competent, in control or functioning in the usual manner; a loss of gratification from human relationships and social roles; a disruption of the sense of continuity between past, present and future; and reactivation of earlier memories of helplessness or giving-up. In this state, the person is less likely to deal with pathological processes, though the complex itself does not 'cause disease directly but rather contributes towards its emergence'. Once again, the precise physiological mechanism by which this occurs remains unclear. However, the three perspectives mentioned above – 'psychosocial transitions', 'life events' and the 'giving-up–given-up' complex – all provide useful ways of viewing the effects on health and illness of such dramatic changes in life space as migration, urbanization, conquest, refugee status, rapid social or technological change and voodoo death.

Factors influencing the stress response

In Selye's original model, stress represented a pathological physical response to environmental demands. However, as noted earlier, this response is mediated by a number of other factors, including:

1. The characteristics of the individuals concerned
2. Their physical environment
3. The social support available to them
4. Their economic status
5. Their cultural background.

Individual characteristics

The individual's characteristics that influence response to stress are partly physical (such as age, weight, build, genetic make-up, state of nutrition and previous health) and partly psychological. Weinman[4] points out how differences in personality affect response to stress, from phlegmatic types to those whose response is primarily somatic –

such as the 'gastric responders' or 'cardiovascular responders'. Infantile and childhood experiences also play some part, as do the individuals' perception of whether they have control over their lives or not. In the work situation, for example, Karasek and colleagues[18] have related a low sense of personal control to high levels of stress response. To a variable degree, the individual's outlook on life, including his or her hopes, fears and ambitions, is conditioned by socio-cultural background as well as by early upbringing.

Physical environment

Physical sources of stress include extreme heat, cold, dryness and damp, and sources of tissue damage such as pathogenic organisms, burns or trauma. In all these cases, the nature and extent of the environmental stressor will influence the severity of the stress response.

Social support

Social and cultural factors tend to overlap in practice, but will be considered separately. Several authors have noted the importance of social support, at all stages of life, in protecting against stress. Weinman[4] notes how 'insufficient early support can give rise to physical and behavioural abnormalities, including a reduced ability to withstand stress' later in life. Brown and Harris[19] have demonstrated that women who lost their mothers before the age of 11 years are more vulnerable to depression in adulthood, and a close and confiding relationship with another person helps protect against stress and psychiatric disorder. Kiritz and Moos[20] also pointed out the relationships of social environment to stress. In their view, social support and a sense of group cohesion protect against stress, while a sense of personal responsibility for others increases the physiological stress response. It is also increased by work pressure (to complete a large number of transactions per unit time), uncertainty (about the possibility of physical or psychological harm) and change in their psychosocial environments (such as job relocation or redundancy). Some social factors, such as violence – whether domestic, crime-related or political – can be important stressors, with a major impact on the mental and physical health of the individual.

Economic status

Economic factors are especially relevant to the stress response. Unemployment, deprivation and poverty (and the associated poor housing, diet, sanitation, clothing and exposure to crime and violence) are potent stressors in any community, as is loss of income and financial insecurity resulting from either physical or mental ill health. The competitiveness, high expectations, long hours and lack of job security associated with so many careers in the industrialized world today also leads to a heightening of the stress response.

Cultural background

Cultural factors play a complex role in the response to stress. In general, this role might considered to be either protective or pathogenic. Culture also helps to shape the *form* of the stress response into a recognizable language of distress. That is, different cultural groups exposed to similar stressors may display different types of stress response, as may men and women within the same cultural group. In their study of French, American, Filipino and Haitian college students, Guthrie and colleagues[21] found clustering of the different symptoms of stress in the four groups. The Americans, for example, reported more gastrointestinal symptoms, while the French reported more changes in mood or thought content. The Filipinos, especially the women, tended to emphasize cardiovascular symptoms, such as a rapid heartbeat and shortness of breath. Symptoms such as dizziness, headaches, nightmares and muscle twitches were more often mentioned by women in all four groups, and the authors suggest that 'in certain societies it may be less socially acceptable for males to admit and experience this constellation of symptoms'. The cultural values of a group may also *protect* against stress – for example, by strengthening social and family cohesion and mutual support, which enable the individual to cope better with the vicissitudes of life. A culture's world-view can also have this effect, by placing individual suffering in the wider context of misfortune in general. This is characteristic of religious world-views, especially those with a fatalistic view of misfortune as being an expression of divine will or fate. Membership of a group with such a shared conceptual system also helps give

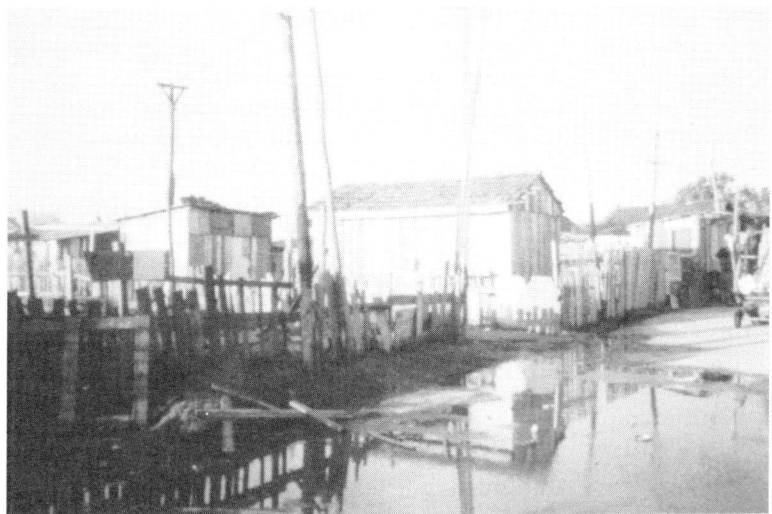

Figure 11.1 A *favela* or shanty town in Porto Alegre, Brazil. Poverty, unemployment, poor housing, and inadequate sanitation are all major sources of stress in many parts of the world (Source: Cecil Helman).

meaning and coherence to daily life, and reduces the stress of uncertainty. Cultures that value meditation and contemplation rather than competitiveness and material achievement are probably less stressful overall to their members. A further factor is that in many societies the rearing of children (and the stress that goes with it) is shared among several adults of an extended family as well as the parents, and this may also have a protective function. In looking at non-Western or pre-industrial societies, however, care should be taken to avoid what has been termed 'the myth of the stress-free "primitive" existence'[22]. Contrary to the WHO's contention[9] that stress as 'a traditional method of adaptation has become inadequate in the psychological, social and economic circumstances of modem society', the evidence is that traditional societies, too, have their full share of damaging stressors.

'Culturogenic' stress: the nocebo effect

While culture can protect against stress, it can also make it more likely. That is, certain cultural beliefs, values, expectations and practices are likely to *increase* the number of stressors that the individual is exposed to. For example, each culture defines what constitutes 'success' (as opposed to 'failure'), prestige (as opposed to loss of face), 'good' behaviour (as opposed to 'bad') and good news (as opposed to bad tidings), and there is considerable variation between these in different societies. In part of New Guinea, for example, failure to have enough pigs or yams to exchange with other tribal members on certain occasions may lead to a stressful loss of face; in the Western world, failure to 'keep up with the Joneses' in terms of consumer objects may also result in subjective stress. In each society, individuals try to reach the defined goals, levels of prestige and standards of behaviour that the cultural group expects of its members. Failure to reach these goals, even if the goals seem absurd to members of another society, may result in frustration, anxiety, depression and even the 'giving-up–given-up' complex described below. Some beliefs can be directly stressful, such as the belief that one has been 'cursed' or 'hexed' by a powerful person against whom there is little defence. In some cases, as in 'voodoo death', this may result in the victim's death after a short period of time. Other cultural values that may induce stress are an emphasis on warlike activities, or intense competition for marriage partners, money, goods or prestige. The unequal distribution of wealth in a society, based on its economic culture, is usually stressful to its poorer members, whose lives are a daily struggle for survival; however, economic privileges also sometimes involve high levels of stress, due to competitiveness and fear of the poor.

In its effect upon the health of the individual, therefore, there are both negative and positive sides to belief. As Hahn and Kleinman[23] put it, 'belief kills; belief heals'. Those beliefs and behaviours that contribute to stress, and are acquired by growing up within a particular society, can therefore be regarded as a form of culturally induced or 'culturogenic' stress.

This type of stress is also an example of the nocebo phenomenon (from the Latin root *noceo*, I hurt), which is the negative effect on health of beliefs and expectations – and therefore the exact reverse of the placebo phenomenon (see Chapter 8).

Culturogenic stress: some examples

The most extreme form of culturogenic stress and the nocebo effect described by anthropologists is known as 'voodoo death', 'hex death' or 'magical death', which Landy[24] prefers to term *socio-cultural death*. This phenomenon has been reported from various parts of the world, including Latin America, Africa, the Caribbean and Australia, and is usually found in traditional, pre-industrial societies. In magical death, people who believe they have been marked out for death by sorcery sicken and die within a short period, apparently of natural causes. Once victims and those around them believe that a fatal curse has been placed upon them, then all concerned regard them as doomed. As Landy puts it, a 'process is set in motion, usually by a supposed religious or social transgression that results in the transgressor being marked out for death by a sorcerer acting on behalf of society through a ritual of accusation and condemnation; then death occurs within a brief span, usually 24 to 48 hours'. The anthropologist Claude Levi-Strauss[25] has provided a graphic account of this process, beginning with the individual's awareness that he is doomed, according to the traditions of his culture. His family and friends share this belief, and gradually the community withdraws from him. Often they remind the unfortunate victim that he is doomed, and virtually dead. Then:

> Shortly thereafter, sacred rites are held to dispatch him to the realm of shadows. First brutally torn from all of his family and social ties and excluded from all functions and activities through which he experienced self-awareness, then banished by the same forces from the world of the living, the victim yields to the combined terror, the sudden total withdrawal of the multiple reference systems provided by the support of the group, and, finally, to the group's decisive reversal in proclaiming him – once a living man, with rights and obligations – dead and an object of fear, ritual, and taboo'.

This situation is a classic example of Engel's 'giving-up–given-up' complex, which he sees as a life setting conducive both to illness and to sudden death. He has analysed the reports of 170 cases of sudden death[26], and finds certain common themes in most of them:

- they involve events that are impossible for the victim to ignore
- the individual experiences or is threatened with overwhelming emotional excitation
- the person believes he or she no longer has control over the situation.

Ten of the cases involved sudden death during loss of status or self-esteem; for example, two men who were confidently expecting promotion to important positions dropped dead when their expectations were unexpectedly dashed. Various hypotheses have been advanced to explain the mechanism of culturogenic sudden death. Cannon[27] believed it was due to overactivity of the sympathetic nervous system – the 'fight or flight' response – in a situation where the victim is (culturally) immobilized and can do neither. According to Engel[28], it is due to vasovagal syncope and cardiac arrhythmias in a patient with pre-existing cardiovascular disease. This occurs in cases of emotional arousal and psychological uncertainty, where both the sympathetic ('fight–flight') and parasympathetic ('conservation–withdrawal') systems are simultaneously activated. In Lex's[29] view this simultaneous activation takes place in the settings characteristic of magical death. In this state the nervous system is 'tuned' or over-sensitized, and the individual is more vulnerable to suggestions that he will die by magical means; he is also vulnerable to acute parasympathetic hyper-reactivity, or vagal death.

'Magical death' is an extreme and dramatic form of the culturogenic stress response. It represents the reverse of Hertz's[30] model of bereavement (see Chapter 9), for here social death *precedes* biological death by a variable period of time. In a Western setting, long-term admission to a psychiatric institution, old age home, geriatric ward or prison can also be seen (in some circumstances) as a form of socio-cultural death. It involves a major change in life space, and a new set of stressors for the inmates of these institutions, and has been well described by Erving Goffman[31] in his work on the impact of these 'total environments' on their inmates.

A modern form of social death was commonly seen among the victims of the acquired immunodeficiency syndrome (AIDS), especially in the first years of the epidemic. Cassens[32] described the many stressful social consequences that occurred for homosexual men who had been diagnosed as having this condition. As well as the physical illness itself, they had to cope with guilt, anxiety and the fear of certain death, and the prejudices of other people (see Chapter 5). There was also a loss of privacy about their sexuality, possible loss of employment and rejection by family and friends, and constant exposure to lurid stories in the media with their 'tones of sin and retribution' – which could only enhance their sense of social isolation and rejection.

Another, though much less extreme, example of culturogenic stress is the damaging effect on health and behaviour of certain *diagnostic labels* – for example, patients told by their doctor 'you've got cancer', 'you've got a weak heart' or 'you've got hypertension'. In Waxler's[33] view, certain diagnostic labels can affect patients' symptoms, behaviour, social relationships, prognosis and self-perception, as well as the attitudes of others towards them. This may even occur in the absence of physical disease. In this case, the nocebo phenomenon results from lay beliefs about the origin, significance, severity and prognosis of 'a weak heart' or 'hypertension', and about the behaviour appropriate to sufferers from that condition. Patients may see themselves as ill or disabled, while family and friends may begin treating them in a particular way – encouraging them to change their diet or behaviour, or to take special precautions. Like the patient, the relatives' attitudes are shaped by cultural beliefs about the significance of certain diseases. In the case of children, this might have lifelong effects; parents of a child labelled 'asthmatic' may, based on their own childhood memories of what asthma entailed, prohibit the child from a wide range of social or sporting activities. A diagnostic label can thus become a form of self-fulfilling prophecy. Some individuals who are labelled as 'ill' may become enmeshed within certain institutions that sustain the label rather than encourage its disappearance. Waxler notes how organizations such as Alcoholics Anonymous, for example, may inadvertently prolong an individual's label of 'illness' because 'a large percentage of AA members' social lives centers on the organization and other members, thus isolating them from normal relationships and further strengthening their role as "alcoholics"'. She quotes another study of a group of American farmers who had no evidence of cardiac disease, but who labelled themselves as having 'heart disease', due to misunderstanding their doctors' diagnosis. As a result they took more heart-related precautions, and generally acted like cardiac invalids. As Waxler points out, the label itself – what the farmer or his family *believed* to be the case – had an important effect upon his behaviour, even when he had no symptoms and no disease. Another example of how labelling can affect everyday behaviour is described by Haynes and colleagues[34], who screened factory workers for hypertension. In those (asymptomatic) patients who were told they had 'hypertension', absenteeism from work rose by 80 per cent, greatly exceeding the 9 per cent rise in absenteeism in the general employee population during the same period. Certain diagnostic labels, therefore, if they provoke anxiety and foreboding (such as 'cancer'), are likely to act as additional stressors, especially if the person is already physically ill.

Similarly, certain settings (such as a hospital clinic or doctor's office) can also induce so much anxiety that it causes a physiological response, which can be misdiagnosed as disease. The two best-known examples of this phenomenon are 'white coat hypertension'[35] and 'white coat hyperglycaemia'[36]. In the former, higher blood pressure readings are found when taken in a medical setting, compared to measurements taken in the patient's home. In the latter, it is the blood glucose level that is higher when measured in the clinic, compared with a similar test carried out in the home.

A final example of how the cultural values of a society may contribute towards stress and disease in its members is seen in the case of coronary heart disease (CHD). This condition is believed to have a multifactorial aetiology, and a number of risk factors that predispose to its development have been described. These include a high dietary intake of saturated fats, lack of exercise, cigarette smoking, raised serum cholesterol and hypertension. However, the work of Friedman and Rosenman[37] suggests that psychosocial patterns, especially behaviour patterns and personality type, also play a role in its aetiology, particularly in susceptible individuals. They have described the characteristics of what they term the *Type A behaviour pattern* (TABP) – in particular, the chronic struggle to achieve an unlimited number of goals in as short a time as possible. Those individuals displaying the TABP show marked aggressiveness, ambition and competitive drive; they are work-orientated and 'workaholic' people, preoccupied with deadlines and chronically impatient[37]. Their personal lives are emotionally parched and incomplete, and both family and leisure are less important to them than work and ambition. Long-term follow-up studies have shown that individuals with this behaviour pattern are about twice as likely to develop CHD as other adults of similar age without these traits (known as the *Type B* behaviour pattern)[38]. According to Friedman and Rosenman, modern Western industrial society encourages the development of Type A traits, and rewards them. Those who exhibit them often become successful executives, professionals, politicians, managers, technocrats and salesmen. However, these rewards often involve constant anxiety about failure, demotion or loss of control. Appels[39] saw this type of personality as one who cannot manage or handle the pressures of the industrialized, fast-moving and achievement-orientated society and who, by this very failure, shows the characteristics of this society in an excessive way. In his study of 22 societies he found that the mortality rate from CHD was positively correlated with a cultural emphasis in the societies on the need for achievement. Waldron[40] has examined the relationship of Type A behaviour and gender within the USA, where the risk of CHD is twice as great in men as in women. She suggests that while men's excess vulnerability may be partly due to hormonal factors, cultural factors also play a part. In particular, Type A behaviour can contribute to success in traditional male roles and professions, but not in the traditional female role in society. Accordingly, parents and other socializing institutions may promote Type A characteristics in boys but not in girls, and later in life this may protect a higher proportion of the women from the risk of CHD.

It is possible therefore to view the Type A behaviour pattern as a Western culture-bound syndrome (see Chapter 10), embodying many of the cultural values of an industrial, capitalist society, where competition, ambition, materialism and the time-urgency of rush hours and deadlines are all part of daily life. Furthermore, this model of stressful behaviour also encompasses some of the *contradictions* within the cultural values of Western society, and the Type A individual is the living embodiment of those contradictions. On the one hand, for example, he conforms to the social values of his society – to what Weber[41] terms its 'philosophy of avarice' – and is rewarded for doing so, but on the other hand his hostile, competitive behaviour is also *anti*social, damaging to himself, his family, his friends and those he works with. It can be argued that this paradox of values – that some forms of antisocial behaviour are being constantly rewarded by society – is symbolically resolved (at least for a while) when he is 'punished' by suffering a heart attack, and emerges from the hospital as a chastened, fragile and less aggressive Type B[42].

Chapter 12 will include discussion of how some immigrants to the USA, such as the Japanese, seem to be partly protected by their cultural background against the risk of both Type A behaviour and CHD, provided they retain many of their traditional cultural values.

Stress and migration

Migration from one culture to another (or from one part of a country to another) is often a traumatic experience, involving major disruptions in the individual's 'life space'. As Eitinger[43] noted, new immigrants have to deal with isolation, helplessness and a feeling of insecurity in their surroundings, coupled with a flood of incomprehensible stimuli. Not only have they left family, friends and a familiar locality, but many of their assumptions about their world are no longer valid. They are often faced with language difficulties, with hostility or indifference from the host population, and with new cultural practices that may be at variance with their religious beliefs. Also, migration is often not only between cultures but also from a small village community to a big metropolis; from the life of a peasant on his own little plot of land to that of an unskilled labourer in the big city. While some of the migrant's cultural values, such as an emphasis on family cohesion, may be protective against stress, the experience of migration is usually a profound psychosocial transition – analogous in some ways to bereavement or disablement. Eisenbruch[44] has coined the term *cultural bereavement* for those groups of people who have suffered a permanent traumatic loss of their familiar land and culture. This applies especially to unwilling migrants such as exiles and refugees, suddenly uprooted during war or persecution. The stressful changes that such a group may undergo in its collective grief are analogous to those suffered by individual mourners, and may include pathological and atypical grief reactions.

Actual physical migration is not the only cause of stress. One can also 'migrate' socially and economically, from one social class to another, without actually changing locality. For example, a person who was born poor but who then makes money (or wins a lottery or other prize) and rises rapidly in the social scale, even without actually leaving the home village, town, or neighbourhood, can be considered a type of social migrant. Often this rise in social status can be a major psychosocial transition, involving considerable stress; new insecurities, anxieties and pressures, possible alienation from family and friends, the fracturing of old relationships and so on. For example, Dressler[45] has described the types of stress response (such as a rise in blood pressure, or psychosomatic symptoms) that are often associated with modernization, economic development, social change and upward social mobility in some communities in the Caribbean and the USA. In many cases economic development raises expectations, fuels competitiveness, increases dissatisfaction and widens the gap between rich and poor. In this situation, both those who rise socially and those who fail to do so can suffer from considerable stress, although for different reasons and in very different ways.

Some of the stress responses (both physical and psychological) of immigrants to the UK and the USA have been examined in a number of studies outlined below, though the exact mechanism by which these relate to migration is complex and not yet fully understood.

Case study: Effects of migration on blood pressure

Cassell[46] has reviewed the research done on the effects of migration on blood pressure. In one study, the blood pressure of black migrants from the Southern USA to Chicago was compared with that of Chicago-born blacks. It was found that the longer the period of city life, the higher their blood pressure. In another study, the blood pressures of inhabitants of the Cape Verde Islands (off West Africa) were compared with those of Cape Verdeans who had migrated to the eastern USA. The immigrants showed higher pressures at each age, and a sharper difference between young and old than did the islanders. Other studies showed higher rates of hypertension among Irish immigrants to the USA (32 per cent) when compared with their brothers living in Ireland (21 per cent). In Cassell's view, the findings of these studies are unlikely to be due to genetic differences between those who emigrate and those who stay behind, but possibly to genetic differences in the susceptibility to environmental influences among individual migrants. These influences include such physical factors as caloric intake, physical activity and salt intake, and the absence of certain parasites and diseases in the host country which, in the country of origin, usually cause wasting, anaemia and a fall in blood pressure. However, psychosocial factors also play a part, particularly the disappearance of a coherent value system and its replacement by different values and different situations, where the migrant's traditional way of coping with life is no longer effective.

Case study: Mental illness among immigrants in Manchester, UK

Carpenter and Brockington[47] examined the incidence of mental illness among Asian, West Indian and African immigrants living in Manchester. It was found that the migrant populations had about twice the first admission rate to mental hospitals that British-born subjects had, especially those migrants aged 35–44 years, and also Asian women. Schizophrenia was particularly common among the immigrants, especially with delusions of persecution, a phenomenon noted in many other studies of migrants. The authors hypothesized that 'social and lingual isolation ... insecurity and the attitudes of the milieu are the explanations for the development of persecutory delusions'.

Case study: Psychiatric admissions to hospitals of foreign-born people in Bradford, UK

Hitch and Rack[48] studied the rates of first admission to psychiatric hospitals in Bradford, and found that foreign-born people had substantially higher mental illness rates than British-

continued

born people. The rates of psychiatric breakdown of a sample of Polish and Russian refugees in Bradford were measured 25 years after they had settled in the UK. While both had higher rates of mental illness (especially schizophrenia and paranoia) than the UK-born population, the Poles had a higher rate than the Russians. The most vulnerable group was the Polish females. The authors suggest that the difference between the immigrant groups was due partly to minimal cohesion among the Poles, and also to a strong sense of national, ethnic identity among the Russians (many of whom were Ukrainians). This ethnic social support not only afforded a protection against environmental stress, it also bestowed identity, though the Russians appeared to have maintained this identity more than the Poles. Many years after migration, though, both immigrant groups were especially vulnerable to first-time mental illness. The authors suggested that 'the combination of wartime experiences and culture shock may have been met with adequate coping mechanisms, but nevertheless rendered the personality vulnerable to later stress'. In middle age, when children have moved away from home and spouses or relatives have died, an immigrant who still speaks broken English and has no English friends will become particularly vulnerable to environmental stressors, with the consequent danger of mental or physical illness.

Case study: Attempted suicide among immigrants in Birmingham, UK

Burke, in three studies published in 1976, examined the rate of attempted suicide among Irish[49], Asian[50] and West Indian[51] immigrants in Birmingham. His findings indicate that immigrants have a higher rate of attempted suicide than the populations in their countries of origin, and this applies particularly to female immigrants. In Birmingham, those born in Northern Ireland or the Irish Republic had about a 30 per cent higher rate than the native population (as measured in Edinburgh), and higher rates than both Belfast and Dublin. Other indices of stress, such as the rates of alcoholism, drug addiction or mental illness, were also raised in this immigrant group. Asian immigrants (from India, Pakistan and Bangladesh) had a lower rate of attempted suicide than the native-born population, but their rate was higher than that of their countries of origin, especially among females. Burke points out that language difficulties for women may play a major part in this, since Asian men have usually migrated several years earlier, and have had a greater opportunity to learn the language and familiarize themselves with English culture. Female immigrants are often expected to remain at home, and there is also some culture conflict for younger Asian women and girls between the values of home and those of school or workplace. Among West Indians, too, attempted suicide was less common than in the native-born population, but West Indian women had a higher rate than women in the Caribbean; that is, the 'stresses that follow immigration and contribute to attempted suicide are more likely to affect women than men'. Part of the stress on young West Indians arises from the insecurity of low paid jobs, fear of not being able to cope financially and emotionally, housing difficulties, and the absence of the extended family in an urban setting. All of these 'may effectively reduce the tolerance of immigrants in withstanding these stresses'.

Case study: Suicide levels among immigrants in England and Wales

Raleigh and Balarajan[52] analysed national suicide rates among 17 immigrant groups in England and Wales for the years 1979–1983. Using mortality data on male and female immigrants aged 20–69 years, they found that many immigrant groups, especially Poles, Russians, French, Germans, South Africans, Scots and Irish, had much higher rates of suicide than the native population of England and Wales. The rates among Scottish and Irish immigrants aged between 20 and 29 years were particularly high. Other groups, such as migrants from the Caribbean, the Indian subcontinent, Italy, Spain and Portugal, had much lower rates than the national average. However, when the suicide rates of these various communities were compared to those of their countries of origin, they were found to be very similar. This was particularly true of male immigrants, but less true of females, especially from Ireland and Poland. The authors thus concluded that, as suicide levels in the immigrant groups differed less from levels in their home countries than from levels in England and Wales, 'the findings do not suggest that migration increases the risk of suicide'. Although they agreed that 'the economic and social changes associated with migration can often be stressful', they suggested that 'reaction to such stress is conditioned by the social and cultural attitudes inculcated in the country of origin'.

It should be emphasized that these four studies dealt predominantly with the *first* generation of immigrants to the UK, people who were born outside the country. They do not necessarily apply to those born and raised in the UK, whose experiences and degree of acculturation are likely to be different from those of their parents. Some of the evidence of stress among the second generation, born in Britain, has already been described in Chapter 10. In addition, while all the studies seem to indicate higher levels of certain physical, emotional and social problems ('stress responses') among first-generation immigrants, there are some inconsistencies among them. Burke's studies[49,50,51], for example, indicate higher levels of *attempted* suicides among immigrants to the UK, while Raleigh and Balarajan[52] found *actual* suicide levels no higher among the immigrant population – although they did note that from 1970 to 1983 in England and Wales, suicide rates did significantly increase among some immigrant groups, especially those born in Russia, Ireland and South Africa. Furthermore, there are apparently wide variations in how different groups respond to the experience of migration. While these studies are useful in illustrating the high level of stress among immigrants, they do not provide enough data on *how* the cultural practices and world-view of immigrants – and of the host community itself – interact in the migrant situation. For example, which cultural traits in immigrant communities protect them from stress or predispose towards it? Do some cultural groups migrate less 'stressfully' than others? Is the status of temporary migrants (such as *gastarbeiters*) less or more stressful than that of permanent migrants, exiles or refugees? What are the effects of racial discrimination and racial prejudice, both individual and institutional, on immigrants' mental and physical health? Are some host cultures more 'stressful' to immigrants than others?

Another factor, mentioned in Chapter 10, is that the medical and other authorities in the host community determine whether deviant behaviour among immigrants is regarded as 'mad' or 'bad', and this can significantly affect the morbidity statistics among immigrant populations.

Collective stress and social suffering

Under some conditions, an entire population may be said to be 'under stress'. This form of social suffering is particularly common in conditions of war, civil unrest, natural disasters, population movements, political oppression, economic insecurity and extreme poverty. In some cases, several of these factors may operate at the same time and in the same place.

In the sense of collective suffering, the twentieth century may be seen as one of the most stressful in human history. In addition to two world wars, there have been numerous civil wars, interethnic strife and widespread political repression. There has been genocide and ethnic cleansing, including the Armenian massacres of World War One, the Nazi holocaust of World War Two, the genocides of Cambodia and Rwanda, and the mass killings in Bosnia, Kosovo and elsewhere. In addition, Desjarlais and colleagues[53], in the *World Mental Health* report, cited the numerous low-intensity wars – such as those that have ravaged parts of Africa, Latin America, and Asia for many years – as a particular cause of considerable stress and tension at the population level. In these conflicts the aim is usually control over populations rather than territory and, as a result, violence often takes take place anywhere within the country, and can affect civilians as well as soldiers. As with other conflicts this century, these low-intensity wars have left large numbers of people with the *post-traumatic stress disorder* (PTSD) – suffering long-term symptoms of anxiety, depression, psychosomatic disorders and social dysfunction, and 'flashbacks' to traumatic events – even long after the conflict is over and the 'stress' of it has receded[53,54]. Because many of these conflicts have taken place in poorer countries, at the margins of the world economy, the access of millions of victims to medical and mental health facilities is often very limited.

In circumstances where a similar level of stress is shared by many others in the population, what is the effect of this on the individual? Does it help make their own experience less stressful in some way, or more so? And how can communities who have collectively suffered social stress heal themselves in a collective way?

According to Desjarlais and colleagues[53], a collective healing process almost always involves people talking openly about their pain and suffering. Often the authorities have imposed a 'wall of silence' that has to be breached before healing can take place. Expressing these narratives or trauma stories, either in public or to a therapist, is one way that people can give meaning to their experience, enabling them to leave the past behind them (see Chapter 5). In South Africa, for example, Swartz[54] has described the situation of the many millions of non-white people who lived under the oppressive racist system of *apartheid*. Over almost 50 years, many of them were subject to constant humiliation, social and economic discrimination, the break-up of families, arbitrary arrest, forced relocation, and sometimes torture, extra-judicial killings and 'disappearances'. Although the effects of this system on the health of the population are difficult to quantify, it has left behind a considerable legacy of social, psychological and economic problems, including poverty, violence, crime and substance abuse. In order to heal itself on a collective level, post-*apartheid* South Africa has tried to achieve a shared 'national healing' of this stressful period by setting up a Truth and Reconciliation Commission (TRC). Its main slogan is: 'Truth: The Road to Freedom'. To a large extent, this model is based on psychoanalytic approaches to individual psychotherapy – 'finding the truth as a basis for healing'. The TRC has encouraged both perpetrators and victims to describe publicly the traumatic events that actually occurred under *apartheid*, and their role in it, in order to get either amnesty or compensation. However, Swartz points out that national healing, although essential, may not necessarily heal individual victims. In some cases the revelations at the TRC may prove cathartic to those who partake in them, but in others they have the opposite effect – reminding people of distressing events, and making them feel even worse as a result. In either case, an individual's response both to suffering ('stress') and to national healing, even if it is part of a more collective experience, is often idiosyncratic, difficult to predict and, like other forms of stress response, marked by non-specificity.

Refugees and stress

Today, the most common form of collective stress is probably to be found among *refugees*. In 1993 it was estimated that there were between 15 million and 50 million of them world-wide, from wars, civil unrest and natural disasters[55]. Another estimate in 1995[56] assessed that there were 20 million 'official' refugees world-wide, and another 20 million people internally displaced within their own countries. The United Nations High Commission for Refugees has estimated that about 80 per cent of refugees are women and children[56]. Many refugees will have witnessed or personally experienced acts of extreme violence, sometimes including sexual abuse. As well as loss of home, property and possibly loved ones, they will also have experienced a major psychosocial transition. Many of them will be suffering from what Eisenbruch terms 'cultural bereavement'; grieving for the loss of all the familiar cultural reference points that defined who they were and how they were to live their lives. They will also have lost their livelihood, their sense of security and continuity, and even their sense of self. Many will encounter hostility among their host populations. Others will experience outbreaks of infectious diseases and other health problems. There may also be alcohol or drug abuse, or different forms of antisocial behaviour – especially among the youth. Overall, flight from one's home under these circumstances is likely to lead to major physical, emotional and cognitive distress, and often long-term PTSD[54], among refugee populations. To a certain extent, some protection for the refugees may arise from the social support available to them, especially if this comes from family, friends, people from their own community or voluntary workers. Religious figures and traditional healers may also play a positive role. In some cases, religious faith or ideological conviction can also help ameliorate the stress of their situation. Given the vast scale of many refugee situations today, both individual and collective healing may only be possible on a relatively small scale. For many individual refugees, true healing can only begin when they return home safely or when they become reconciled to a new life, in a new country.

Lay models of stress and suffering

In the past few decades the concept of 'stress' outlined above has increasingly entered popular discourse, and is now commonly used in books, magazines, radio and television programmes. Lay concepts of stress are often those of a diffuse and invisible force, somehow mediating between individuals (and their mental and physical state) and the social environment in which they live and work.

The lay concept of stress can be regarded as one of the most pervasive and multidimensional folk illnesses of contemporary Western society. More importantly, in the modern age it is also one of the most widely used *metaphors* for human suffering, and especially one that places responsibility for that suffering outside the individual. Like 'heart distress' and 'sinking heart' (see Chapter 5), lay notions of stress blend together into a single image, a cluster of negative feelings, emotions and physical sensations, as well as certain social, cultural and economic circumstances. In doing so, it has absorbed older, more traditional models of misfortune and unhappiness, especially where they originate outside the individual. It has become a secularized version of more supernatural concepts, such as witchcraft, sorcery and other forms of interpersonal malevolence, as well as of fate, divine punishment and possession by malign spirits. Modern images of stress provide a fascinating illustration of how Selye's original concept has entered popular culture and blended with older models of misfortune, becoming a point of overlap between popular, medical and religious explanations for human suffering.

In the author's study[10] performed in Massachusetts, USA, 95 per cent of a sample of patients with psychosomatic disorders blamed their condition and personal suffering on 'stress', though they varied widely on what they meant by this term. It was variously described as:

- an invisible force in the environment, pressing down on the individual (to be 'under acute stress')
- an invisible and malevolent force, usually produced by other people, that enters your body and then causes disease ('stress can cause my bronchi to spasm', 'stress goes to the weakest organ. I let it get to me and eat me away')
- something that 'builds up' inside you unless you can get it out ('a good relationship can make you stay healthy, because you can ventilate a lot of stress').

'Stress' explanations are just as common in Britain, too. In one study[57] of 406 patients in an English general practice, 53 per cent of them blamed their illnesses on different types of stress – which they thought could be relieved by medical explanations of their condition and by discussion of their symptoms.

In English-speaking countries, a number of recurrent images or metaphors associated with the word 'stress' can therefore be identified. Each is a metaphor for a sense of personal suffering, and often of helplessness. Many of them overlap with lay concepts of 'nerves' (see below). Most of these metaphors, though not all, are drawn from the artefacts and technology of everyday life; heavy objects, machines, cars, batteries, electrical wires, strings, rubber bands, kettles, crockery and pottery. Some of them refer to the stress itself, others to reactions to the stress. Among the most common of these metaphors are the following:

1. Stress as a heavy *weight*. In this image, stress is conceived of as a heavy invisible weight, burden or force that somehow 'presses down' on the individuals from above – especially onto their chest, head or shoulders – and which they have difficulty in carrying. Examples include 'to be under a lot of stress', 'to be under pressure', 'to be under tension', to 'have things piling up on top of me', 'to have a lot on one's mind' (or 'on one's plate').
2. Stress as a *wire* or line. In this image, the nerves are described as if they were a series of wires, lines, rubber bands, or strings (similar to violin or guitar strings). For example, some people are 'highly strung', 'taut', 'tense', 'tightly wired' or 'at the end of their tether', while others have nerves that 'snap', or have become 'frayed' or 'jangled'.
3. Stress as *internal chaos*. Here the image is of some uncontrollable internal disorder, chaos, change or movement within the body. Examples include 'to be churned up', 'to be all mixed up', 'to be all shook up' or to have 'butterflies in the stomach'.
4. Stress as *fragmentation*. Here the image is of an object that fragments under stress, almost as if it were a plate or earthenware pot. Examples include 'to crack up', 'to fall apart', 'to break', 'to feel shattered' or 'to go to pieces'.
5. Stress as a *malfunctioning of a machine*. In this image, the body and self are seen as a machine or engine that can no longer

function. Examples include to 'have a nervous breakdown', 'to be burnt out', 'to grind to a halt', 'to crash' or to 'need one's batteries recharged'.

6. Stress as *depletion of a vital liquid*. Here the image is of the depleted level of some vital fluid, such as blood or breast milk, or – in an overlap with point (5) – of fuel or steam. Examples include 'to feel drained' or 'empty', to feel 'sucked dry', to 'run out of gas', to be 'running on empty', to 'run out of steam' to be 'at a low energy level'.
7. Stress as *inner explosion*. This image, drawn largely from the Age of Steam, conveys the idea of the build up of an internal force or pressure which, in the absence of some safety valve, suddenly and dramatically explodes. Examples include 'to get it off one's chest', 'to burst a boiler', 'to blow one's top' or 'to blow a gasket'.
8. Stress as *interpersonal force*. This image is similar to (1) above, but includes the idea of one person somehow causing (consciously or unconsciously) another person to feel stressed or to get ill. Examples include 'my boss gives me a lot of stress', 'I get a lot of stress from living with her', 'she gave him a nervous breakdown' or 'he broke his mother's heart'.

The frequent use of mechanical or machine metaphors to describe ideas of stress is also linked to another common contemporary image in both stress literature and popular discourse; the dangerous, disease-producing nature of 'modernity' itself. This idea of modernity as being pathogenic is not, in itself, modern. In 1897, for example, the famous physician Sir William Osler described 'arterial degeneration' as resulting from 'the worry and strain of modern life', and from 'the high pressure at which men live, and the habit of working the machine to its maximum capacity'[58]. Much of the contemporary New Age and other metaphysical movements also see modern life, modern diets and urban living as inherently stressful[59]. As one American woman put it to McGuire[60], stress 'has to do with some kind of thing that's very much a part of our Western culture – accomplishment-oriented, striving, being seen, having a big voice ... Making it, striving, getting ahead, that kind of thing. Really makes us crazy and makes us sick'. Often these ideas are associated with a sense of nostalgia for some more 'natural' way of living – for a pre-industrial, more communal, non-competitive and notionally stress-free Garden of Eden.

'Nerves'

One of the commonest folk images of suffering, found in many different forms and in many different cultures, is the idea of 'nerves'. It seems to be particularly common among women, especially in Europe, North and South America and all the English-speaking countries, and usually overlaps with lay concepts of stress. Like stress, it incorporates physical, psychological and social experience into a single image. It also places the emphasis on an ostensibly physical phenomenon; the malfunctioning of a diffuse part of the body vaguely described as 'the nerves'. As illustrated earlier, these can be conceptualized in many different ways. However, unlike in the stress model there seems to be more emphasis on *internal reasons*, within the individual, for their emotional suffering or illness and their vulnerability to the stress of daily life. Thus some people are just born with 'weak nerves' or 'bad nerves', some inherit them from their parents, while others acquire them in childhood or adulthood – when their nerves were 'frayed', 'shattered', 'broken', or 'shot to ribbons' by some traumatic event. In each case, 'nerves' are blamed for predisposing the individual to ill health. As one 72-year-old asthmatic woman put it: 'A nervous person gets asthma. All through my life I never thought I was a nervous person, but I must have been. Behind it all there must have been a case of nerves'[10].

Anthropological studies of 'nerves' reveal that it is not a single image, folk category or culture-bound syndrome. Nor is there a clear and consistent set of symptoms associated with it. Rather, the concept of 'nerves' can only be understood in terms of the specific and local social *context* in which the word is used; as a way of explaining an individual's personality, for example, or their emotional, physical or social reactions to certain events. One problem is that physicians often misinterpret the significance of 'nerves' and the vague symptoms associated with it. As Finkler[61] points out, they often 'objectify and separate the disorder from the patient's experience in which the disorder is embedded', and assume that it is due to physiological malfunction. By concentrating on the 'disease' rather than the 'illness' dimension of

Case study: *Nervios* in San Jose, Costa Rica

Low[62], in her study in San José, Costa Rica, found that both men and women, of all ages and from all social classes, could be afflicted by 'nerves' (*nervios*). In a culture where family links and the *tranquilidad* (tranquillity) of family life are very important, it is often a symptom of family discord or disruption of the family structure. For example, a crisis of *nervios* may be precipitated when a son marries an undesirable woman, when a child is born illegitimately, or when a sudden bereavement occurs. People also blame their own *nervios* on a poverty-stricken childhood, an alcoholic father or a mother who was unwed when she gave birth to them. It can manifest by a variety of vague physical and emotional symptoms, including headache, insomnia, vomiting, lack of appetite, fatigue, anger, fear and disorientation. All of these indicate that the individual feels out of control, or separated from body or self. It is thus a culturally sanctioned way of signalling to others that something has gone wrong with family relationships, and that they need sympa thy and attention. Overall, the belief in *nervios* is a way of 'encouraging culturally appropriate behaviour and an adherence to cultural norms', especially those that reinforce family relationships and thereby enhance family cohesion.

Case study: *Nevra* among Greek immigrants in Montreal, Canada

Dunk[63] described 'nerves' (*nevra*) among Greek immigrants in Montreal, a form of somatization found mainly among women. An attack of *nevra* manifests as a feeling of loss of control, of 'being grabbed by your nerves', which then 'burst' or 'break out'. At the same time there is often screaming, shouting, throwing things and hitting one's children. Often there are vague physical symptoms, such as headaches, neck pain, shoulder pain and dizziness. Sufferers from the condition commonly use the expression 'my nerves are broken!'. Its cause can be related to the specific conditions of the immigrants' lives, including: economic pressures, crowded living conditions, the effects of migration upon the family, gender-role conflicts and the women's double burden of running a home and going out to work. It is thus a culturally constituted metaphor for distress, and a cry for help; it can be viewed as a realistic way of coping when responded to positively by family members and others.

'nerves', they may therefore miss its true significance and how it can be treated.

As these examples indicate, lay models of stress and 'nerves' are highly variable. They cannot be fully understood without taking into account the context in which these terms are used. Part of this context involves those traditional explanations for misfortune that have been absorbed into these modern models of stress or 'nerves'. In other cases – as with the *Ataques de nervios* of Latino immigrants, described in the previous chapter – the wider picture must be taken into account, especially the social, political and economic context in which these immigrants find themselves. Overall, the concept of 'stress', although based originally on a limited, mechanistic model, has become one of the most pervasive images of human suffering of the modern world.

Recommended reading

Ader, R. A., Cohen, N. and Felten, D. (1995). Psychoneuroimmunology: interactions between the nervous system and the immune system. *Lancet*, **345**, 99–103.

Hahn, R. A. (1997). The nocebo phenomenon: concept, evidence, and influence on public health. *Prev. Med.*, **26**, 607–11.

McElroy, A. and Townsend, P. K. (1989). *Medical Anthropology in Ecological Perspective*, 3rd edn, Chapter 7. Westview.

Helman, C. G. (1987). Heart disease and the cultural construction of time: the Type A behaviour pattern as a Western culture-bound syndrome. *Soc. Sci. Med.*, **25**, 969–79.

Pollock, K. (1988). On the nature of social stress: production of a modern mythology. *Soc. Sci. Med.*, **26**, 381–92.

Young, A. (1980). The discourse on stress and the reproduction of conventional knowledge. *Soc. Sci. Med.*, **14B**, 133–46.

12 Cultural factors in epidemiology

Epidemiology is the study of the distribution and determinants of the various forms of disease in human populations. Its focus is not on the individual case of ill health, but rather on groups of people, both healthy and diseased. When investigating a particular disease (such as lung cancer), epidemiologists try to relate its occurrence and distribution to a variety of factors associated with most victims of that condition (such as smoking behaviour) in order to discover its probable aetiology. The factors most commonly examined are the age, sex, marital status, occupation, socio-economic position, diet, environment (both natural and man-made) and behaviour of the victims. Their aim is to uncover a causal link between one or more of these factors and the development of the disease.

Hahn[1] has compared the ways that epidemiology and anthropology approach the study of health phenomena, and how each discipline can contribute towards the other. Despite obvious differences – 'anthropologists deploy universals to arrive at particulars, epidemiologists tolerate particulars in their quest for universals' – he sees much in common between the two. Both deal with the study of *populations* rather than individuals. Both seek to understand the role of social (and other) variables in the lives of individuals, and how they impact upon them. Each can offer a unique, if complementary, perspective on human health and the reasons for human disease. Although medical anthropology is more concerned with cultural variables (such as health-related beliefs and behaviours), many epidemiological concepts (such as those of probability, or 'risk factors') are increasingly of relevance to it.

Most epidemiological surveys utilize one of two approaches; sometimes a combination of the two. The *case–control* method examines a sample of the population suffering from a particular disease. If it is possible to demonstrate a statistically significant correlation between certain factors and the occurrence of the disease, such as a long history of cigarette smoking in those suffering from lung cancer, then a causal link can be postulated. In the *cohort study* approach, a healthy population (some of whom are associated with hypothetical risk factors such as smoking) is followed up over time, waiting for a particular disease to occur. If those associated with a particular risk factor are found to be more likely to develop the disease subsequently, then a causal link between the risk factor and the disease can be postulated. In many of these epidemiological studies, though, the precise nature of this link cannot be explained, and must remain presumptive until further evidence is accumulated. In other cases, such as lung cancer and smoking, or congenital birth defects and thalidomide use during pregnancy, the aetiological link is much clearer, and can also be explained in physiological terms.

On an individual level, however, the notion of 'risk factors' has only a limited predictive value. For example, not all heavy smokers will develop lung cancer; not all immigrants will suffer a suicidal depression; and nor will all 'Type A personalities' develop coronary heart disease. In understanding why a particular individual gets a particular disease, at a particular time, a much wider range of factors – genetic, physical, psychological and socio-cultural – must all be taken into account, as well as the inter-relationships between them. This multifactorial explanation of ill health is often more useful than postulating a simple cause–effect relationship between one risk factor and one type of disease. As Kendell[2] has pointed out: 'In medicine, as in physics, specific causes have given way to complex chains of event sequences in constant interplay with one another. The very idea of "cause" has become meaningless, other than as a convenient designation for the point in these chain of event sequences at which intervention is most practicable'.

Both anthropologists and sociologists have made important contributions to the understanding of how these complex factors are related to disease. They have pointed out how such variables as social class, economic position, gender, life events, and cultural beliefs and practices can be correlated with the incidence and distribution of certain diseases. Sociologists Murphy and Brown[3], for example, in their study of 111 women in London, demonstrated how both psychological and physical ill health was preceded by one or more severe life events in the previous 6 months (see Chapter 11). On a more macro level, the Black Report[4] in 1982 showed how in the UK there is a relationship between social class and health, and how members of the lower socio-economic classes have poorer health and a higher mortality than their fellow citizens in the more affluent classes. In the developing world, too, there is a clear relationship between health and income. In many of these countries much of the population, already weakened by poor nutrition, will suffer from infectious and other communicable diseases. These diseases are often transmitted with the help of polluted water and food supplies, poor sanitation and inadequate housing, all of which can be improved by an adequate income[5]. In most cases economic inequality, both within and between countries, is likely to make this situation much worse. Therefore, at a macro level, these types of economic and social factors – as well as the political organization of the particular society – must always be taken into account before considering the exact role of cultural factors in health and illness.

In the developing world, anthropological insights have been especially useful in unravelling the causes of more exotic diseases such as *kuru* (a progressive degenerative disease of the brain), which epidemiological studies in the 1950s found to be confined to women and children in a small area of the Eastern Highlands of New Guinea. The disease was virtually unknown among men. Various theories were advanced to explain this, but it was eventually found to be caused by a 'slow virus' infection in the brain, which was transmitted by the ritual cannibalism of dead relatives practised only by some women and children in that area[6]. Other anthropological research has shed light on why people smoke, drink, take narcotic drugs, mutilate their bodies, avoid nutritious diets, reject contraceptive advice, have dangerous pastimes and follow stressful occupations or lifestyles. Marmot[7] points out how cultural factors (as well as social and psychological ones) may influence much of this risk-related behaviour. He notes how in most medical epidemiological studies the risks associated with such factors as smoking, intake of certain foods or obesity are examined, but often scant attention is paid to cultural influences shaping dietary patterns, obesity or smoking. Those studies that have looked at these cultural dimensions point out that cultural beliefs and practices are only part of the multifactorial aetiology of disease. In the case of *kuru*, for example, the virus, the social division between the sexes, and the practice of cannibalism all share in its aetiology and explain its distribution.

Throughout the world, anthropological insights are of particular relevance in community-oriented primary care (COPC)[8], which focuses on the primary health care of individuals and families, but also on the health needs and health problems of their local community. Part of the continuing surveillance of the community's health involves an awareness of the role of *cultural* beliefs and behaviours in either improving health or causing disease.

These cultural factors, where they can be identified, are often difficult to quantify and are therefore less attractive to medical epidemiologists and statisticians. Nor is there a neat, measurable 'dose–response' relationship between a particular cultural factor and a particular disease, as there might be between a pathogenic organism (or chemical) and the disease that it causes. Nevertheless, despite this difficulty in quantifying cultural factors, there *is* sufficient evidence available to confirm their role in the development of disease, even if this role is contributory rather than directly causative. It should also be noted that, in some cases, cultural factors may *protect* against ill health. In the studies by Marmot and colleagues[9,10] quoted below, the rates of coronary heart disease (CHD) were compared between samples of Japanese men living in Japan, Hawaii and California. The degree of their adherence to traditional Japanese culture and world-view correlated with their incidence of CHD; it was found that the rate of CHD among the Japanese-Americans was the highest of the three groups, and this matched their increasing distance from their traditional culture.

This type of study also has the value of pointing out the relative importance of genetic and environmental factors – of 'nature' and 'nurture' – in the causation of disease. If three groups of Japanese with similar backgrounds have different rates of CHD, then environmental influences must somehow be implicated.

Culture and the identification of disease

The cultural and social background of the epidemiologist and of the populations studied may affect the validity of the epidemiological data gathered. First, there are still differences in the diagnostic criteria used to define particular diseases, between epidemiologists in different countries. These differences in labelling policy may give an inaccurate picture of the incidence of certain diseases in different countries. For example, Fletcher and colleagues[11] examined the apparent predominance of 'chronic bronchitis' in England, and of 'emphysema' in North America. It was found that this was largely due to the fact that the *same* constellation of symptoms was diagnosed as chronic bronchitis in the UK but as 'emphysema' in the USA. Other studies among British and American psychiatrists (see Chapter 10) have shown differences in diagnostic criteria between the two groups, with American psychiatrists diagnosing schizophrenia more readily than their British counterparts. A similar study[12] showed apparent sharp differences in the incidence of schizophrenia in France and England. First admission rates to psychiatric hospitals for this condition, for patients below the age of 45 years, were much higher in France; however, they were much lower after that age. The study suggests that the different incidence of the disorder in the two countries is more apparent than real, and due largely to diagnostic bias. French psychiatrists are reluctant to diagnose schizophrenia after 45 years of age, while more likely to diagnose it under 45 years – when 'the French concept of schizophrenia ... seems to encompass a variety of chronic states that would be excluded in the United Kingdom for lack of symptoms'.

Another study[13] also showed marked differences in the rates of diagnosis of various diseases by doctors in five European countries. These differences, it was suggested, may either be the result of actual variations in disease morbidity in the five countries, or they may be due to differences in the ways doctors in those countries actually *interpret* and diagnose certain symptoms and signs.

Zola[14] points out how the perceived incidence of a disease in a particular community depends on its actual incidence, and the degree of its recognition (by patients or doctors) as being something 'abnormal'. In the latter case this depends on the social context in which the disease occurs, and whether there is a 'fit' between the symptoms and signs and the society's definition of what constitutes 'abnormality'. He quotes studies illustrating how Arapesh women report no pain during menstruation, though quite the contrary is reported in the USA. Other studies, quoted by Fox[15], have shown how congenital dislocation of the hip is considered 'normal' (though not necessarily good) among the Navaho Indians of the southwestern USA, and how in 'Regionville' backache was considered 'abnormal' by the higher socioeconomic groups, but not by the lower socioeconomic class. Lay definitions of abnormality or disease determine, to some extent, whether these conditions find their way to doctors, and thus into the morbidity statistics. In Zola's words, 'a selective process might well be operating in what symptoms are brought to the doctor ... it might be this selective process and not an aetiological one which accounts for the many unexplained or overexplained epidemiological differences observed between and within societies'.

Epidemiology is directed more towards the study of 'disease' rather than that of 'illness'. Its scientific approach leads to an emphasis on 'hard' or objectively verifiable data, such as abnormal blood pressure readings, graphs, blood tests or other measurable changes in the body's structure or function. However, this excludes the many forms of illness, particularly the culture-bound folk illnesses described in Chapters 5 and

10, where physiological data are often absent. Anthropologists like Rubel[16] have suggested that epidemiological techniques used to study such diseases as tuberculosis or syphilis can also be applied to folk illnesses such as *susto* in Latin America. These folk illnesses are perceived as 'real' by members of these societies, just as medical epidemiologists see tuberculosis as 'real'. They can also have marked effects on people's behaviour, and on their mental and physical health. In Rubel's view, the unique constellation of cultural beliefs, symptoms and behavioural changes that characterize *susto* recur with remarkable constancy among many Hispanic-American groups, Indian and non-Indian alike. By studying ethnographic case histories of those suffering from the condition, Rubel was able to isolate certain variables usually associated with each occurrence of the illness. He suggests that *susto* and other folk illnesses can be thought of as having multifactorial aetiology; that is, they result from the complex interplay of the victim's previous state of health, personality (including self-perception of success or failure in the performance of social expectations) and the social system in which he or she lives (particularly its role expectations). *Susto* occurs in social situations that the individual finds stressful, such as an inability to meet the expectations of family, friends or employers, and is 'the vehicle by means of which people of Hispanic-American peasant and urban societies manifest their reactions to some forms of self-perceived stressful situations'. While its identification rests mainly on folk perceptions and the observations of anthropologists, the techniques of epidemiology should be valuable in relating its occurrence to social, cultural or psychological variables.

Cultural factors in the epidemiology of disease

As mentioned above, cultural factors can be causal, contributory or protective in their relation to ill health. In this section a number of these cultural factors are listed, many of which have already been described in more detail in previous chapters. The list is not meant to be exhaustive, but rather a selection of those factors most commonly examined by anthropologists and epidemiologists. Their relevance is illustrated later in the chapter by a number of case histories.

Economic situation

This includes:

- whether wealth is evenly distributed throughout the society
- whether the sample group is poor or wealthy relative to other members of the society
- whether income is sufficient for adequate housing, nutrition and clothing
- the cultural values associated with wealth, poverty, employment and unemployment
- whether the basic economic unit (of earning, accumulating and sharing wealth) is the individual, the family or a larger collectivity.

Family structure

This includes:

- whether nuclear, extended, joint or one-parent families are the rule
- the degree of interaction, cohesion and mutual support among family members
- whether the emphasis is on familial rather than on individual achievements
- whether responsibility for child-rearing, the provision of food, and care of the elderly, sick or dying is shared among family members.

Gender roles

This includes:

- the division of labour between the sexes, especially who works, who remains at home, who prepares the food, and who cares for the children
- the social rights, obligations and expectations associated with the two gender roles
- cultural beliefs about the behaviour appropriate to each gender (such as alcohol consumption, smoking and competitive behaviour being regarded as 'natural' for men but not for women)
- the threshold for consultation with a doctor for each of the genders
- the degree of 'medicalization' of the female life-cycle.

Marriage patterns

This includes:

- whether monogamy, polygyny or polyandry are encouraged

- whether the *levirate* or *sororate* are practised (see Chapter 13)
- whether marriage is *endogamous* (where individuals must marry within their family, kin-group, clan or tribe) or *exogamous* (where they must choose a partner from outside these groups).

In the case of endogamy there is a greater likelihood of the 'pooling' of recessive genes, with a higher incidence of such inherited diseases as haemophilia, thalassaemia major, cystic fibrosis and Tay-Sachs disease.

Sexual behaviour

This includes:

- the age of first sexual relationships
- whether promiscuity, pre- or extramarital sexual relations are encouraged or forbidden
- whether these sexual norms apply to men, to women or to both
- whether special sexual norms (such as celibacy or promiscuity) are applied to restricted groups within the society (such as nuns or prostitutes)
- whether recourse to prostitutes is socially acceptable or not
- whether homosexuality, both male and female, is tolerated or forbidden
- whether certain sexual practices (such as anal intercourse) are regarded as acceptable or not
- whether there are taboos on sexual intercourse during pregnancy, menstruation, lactation or puerperium.

Contraceptive patterns

This includes cultural attitudes towards contraception and abortion. A taboo on both of these enlarges family size, and in some cases may have a negative effect on maternal health. Certain forms of contraception or abortion may also be dangerous to maternal health. Attitudes to the use of condoms and other forms of barrier contraception may influence the spread of sexually transmitted diseases such as chlamydia, gonorrhoea, syphilis, hepatitis B and AIDS.

Population policy

This includes cultural beliefs about the optimal size of the family (such as the 'one child' policy in China) and the gender of its children – the incidence of infanticide and illegal or self-induced abortion may be related to these beliefs. Wagley[17] described a Brazilian Indian tribe, the Tenetehara, who believe a woman should have no more than three children and that these should not be all of the same sex. If a woman with two daughters gives birth to a third, the third daughter is killed. Over time, such beliefs can affect the size and composition of local communities. It also includes whether having many children is seen as a sign of full adulthood, masculinity or femininity.

Pregnancy and childbirth practices

This includes:

- changes in diet, dress or behaviour during pregnancy
- the techniques used in childbirth and the nature of the birth attendants
- the position of the mother during labour
- care of the umbilical cord (in some cultures, neonatal tetanus can result from the practice of applying dung as a dressing to the newly cut umbilical cord[18])
- customs relating to the puerperium, such as social isolation or the observance of special taboos
- whether breast or artificial infant foods (such as powdered milk) are preferred.

Child-rearing practices

This includes:

- the emotional climate of child-rearing – whether permissive or authoritarian
- the degree of competitiveness encouraged among children (which may be related to mental illness, suicide attempts and development of the 'Type A' coronary-prone behaviour pattern in later life)
- the degree of physical or emotional abuse regarded as 'normal' by the society[19]
- initiation rituals carried out after birth and at puberty (such as circumcision and scarification).

Body image alterations

This includes:

- culturally sanctioned bodily mutilations or alterations, such as male or female circumcision, scarification, tattooing, ear and lip

- piercing, foot binding and forms of cosmetic surgery (like augmentation mammoplasty operations)
- cultural values supporting or discouraging certain body shapes, such as slimness, tallness or obesity, especially among women.

Diet

This includes:

- how food is prepared, stored and preserved
- whether there is any gender bias in how portions of food are allocated
- the utensils used in cooking and storing food
- whether food routinely contains contaminants (such as aflatoxins)
- whether food is symbolically classified into 'food' and 'non-food', 'sacred' or 'profane' food, or 'hot' and 'cold', irrespective of nutritional value
- whether vegetarianism or meat-eating is the rule
- whether special diets are followed during pregnancy, lactation, menstruation and ill health
- whether dietary fads and fashions are common
- the use of Western foodstuffs (with high salt, fat and refined carbohydrate levels) in non-Western communities as a sign of 'modernization'.

Dress

This includes:

- cultural prescriptions about forms of dress appropriate for men and women, and for special occasions
- fashions of dress, such as tight dresses or corsets, high-heeled or platform-heeled shoes – which may relate to the incidence of certain diseases or injuries
- body adornments, such as cosmetics, jewellery, perfume and hair dyes, which may cause skin diseases.

Long dresses that cover much of the body may predispose to certain conditions; for example, the Underwoods'[20] related the long dress and veil worn by women in Yemen, as well as their confinement to 'harems', to their increased rate of osteomalacia, tuberculosis and anaemia. In the UK, lack of sunlight combined with a vegetarian diet, confinement to home and long dresses are believed to contribute to high rates of osteomalacia in Asian females[21].

Personal hygiene

This includes:

- whether personal hygiene is neglected or encouraged
- whether, and how often, hair is washed or cut
- how often clothing is changed
- whether rituals of washing and purification are carried out on a regular basis
- whether bathing arrangements are private or communal.

Housing arrangements

This includes:

- the construction, siting and internal division of living space
- whether this space is occupied by members of the same family, clan or tribe
- the number of occupants per room, house or hut (which may influence the spread of infectious diseases)
- how indoor space is allocated by age, gender or marital status
- how the living space is heated or cooled in different seasons of the year
- whether anti-mosquito screens are integrated into the construction of windows and doors, or used to divide up internal living space.

Sanitation arrangements

This especially concerns:

- the modes of disposal of human wastes
- who carries out the disposal
- whether wastes are routinely buried or not
- whether wastes are disposed of near residences, food supplies, bathing areas or water sources.

Occupations

This includes:

- whether men and women follow similar or different occupations
- whether certain occupations are reserved for particular individuals, families or groups within the society – as in the traditional caste system in India, or the former *apartheid* system in South Africa

- whether certain occupations have a higher prestige and get higher rewards in some societies (such as the Type A executive in Western society)
- the use of certain techniques, such as traditional methods of hunting, fishing, agriculture or mining, which are associated with a high incidence of accidental death, trauma or infectious diseases
- some modern industrial occupations that are also associated with certain diseases (such as pneumoconiosis in coal miners, bladder cancer in dye workers, silicosis in metal grinders or mesotheliomas in asbestos workers).

Religion

This includes:

- whether a religion is characterized by a coherent, reassuring world-view
- whether it requires such religious practices as fasts, food taboos, ritual immersions, communal feasts, circumcision, self-mutilations or flagellation, fire-walking, or mass pilgrimages, all of which may be associated with the incidence of certain diseases.

Mass pilgrimages, for example, may be linked to the outbreak of infectious diseases such as meningitis or viral hepatitis.

Funerary customs

This concerns especially:

- how and when the dead are disposed of, and by whom
- whether the corpse is buried or cremated immediately or displayed in public for some time (which may aid the spread of infectious diseases)
- the sites of burial, cremation or display of the corpse, and whether these are near to residences, food or water supplies.

Culturogenic stress

This includes:

- whether culturogenic stress (and the nocebo effect) is induced, or aggravated, or sustained by the culture's values, goals, hierarchies of prestige, norms, taboos or expectations
- whether the culture fosters 'workaholism', or more relaxed attitudes to daily life
- whether there is conflict between the social expectations of one generation and those of the next.

Migrant status

This includes:

- whether the immigration was voluntary ('pull'), as with economic migrants, or involuntary ('push'), as with refugees
- whether migrants have adapted to their new culture in terms of behaviour, diet, language and dress
- whether they are subject to discrimination, racism or persecution by the host community
- whether their familial structure and religious world-view remain intact after migration
- whether they have access to their familiar religious figures or traditional healers
- the culture of the host community, especially its attitude to immigrant populations.

Seasonal travel

This includes regular, seasonal patterns of mass migration, whether of tourists, pilgrims, nomads or migrant workers. While nomads usually migrate as a community, tourists and migrant workers often migrate as individuals or in small social units. In both cases, absence from community, family and home may sometimes predispose to high rates of alcoholism and/or sexually transmitted diseases (such as AIDS and hepatitis B).

Use of 'chemical comforters'

This especially includes:

- cultural values associated with smoking, alcohol, tea, coffee, snuff, prescribed and non-prescribed drugs, and the use of hallucinogens as sacramental drugs
- the use of intravenous 'hard' drugs by an addict sub-culture and the prevalence of needle-sharing among those groups (relevant to the spread of both hepatitis B and AIDS)
- the use of more contemporary 'designer' drugs, such as 'Ecstasy'.

Leisure pursuits

This includes:

- the various forms of sport, recreation and tourism

- whether these involve physical exercise or not
- whether they are competitive or not
- whether they are associated with the risks of injury or disease
- whether they involve prolonged exposure to sunlight (and ultraviolet radiation).

Domestic animals and birds

This includes:

- the nature and number of pets and domestic livestock
- whether they are kept within the home or outside it
- the degree of direct physical contact between individuals and these animals.

Various viral illnesses have been linked to domestic pets, such as benign lymphoreticulosis ('cat-scratch fever') and psittacosis ('parrot fever'), and also protozoal diseases such as toxoplasmosis, transmitted by cat faeces.

Self-treatment strategies and lay therapies

This includes all the treatment used within the popular and folk sectors described in Chapter 4, such as the use of herbal remedies by traditional healers, patent medicines, special diets, bodily manipulations, injections and cupping. Lay healing that takes place in a public ritual, rather than a private consultation, may predispose to the spread of infectious diseases. Certain alternative therapies, such as acupuncture, may be implicated in the spread of hepatitis B and other infections. It also includes cultural attitudes to medical treatments and preventive strategies, such as antibiotics, oral rehydration therapy and immunizations.

Summary

This section summarizes some of the cultural factors that may be of relevance to epidemiologists. Many of them have already been discussed in more detail earlier in this book. It should be noted, however, that in many cases of disease, *several* cultural factors actually coincide – such as occupation, use of 'chemical comforters', and dietary preferences – some of which may be pathogenic to individuals, others protective. For example, a case–control study of laryngeal cancer in Shanghai, China[22], found that cigarette smoking was a major risk factor in both sexes (86 per cent of the male cases and 54 per cent of the females), as was the intake of salt-preserved meat and fish, while for men, occupational exposure to asbestos and coal dust was a definite risk factor. By contrast, a high intake of garlic, fruits (particularly oranges and tangerines) and certain dark green/yellow vegetables protected all groups against getting laryngeal cancer.

The importance of some of these cultural factors to the study of the origin and distribution of disease is illustrated in the following case studies.

Case study: Cervical cancer in Latin America

Cervical cancer is a well-documented example of the role of cultural factors – in this case, sexual norms and practices – in the distribution of a disease. Various studies have shown it to be rare in nuns and common in prostitutes. It is extremely uncommon among Jewish, Mormon and Seventh Day Adventist women. Women with cervical cancer are more likely to have experienced early commencement of coitus, early marriage, multiple sexual partners and multiple marriages. Although the exact cause of cervical cancer is still unknown, it is believed to be multifactorial in origin, and there is a strong suspicion that a viral infection (human papilloma virus, HPV) may be implicated[23].

It was originally thought that a woman's sexual behaviour alone could determine her risk of cervical cancer. However, Skegg and colleagues[24] have pointed out that its incidence is very high in Latin America, where women are expected to have only one sexual partner in their lives, and strong cultural sanctions exist against their having pre- or extramarital sexual relationships. They suggest that, *if* the hypothesis of the infective origin of cervical cancer is correct, then in some communities a woman's risk of getting the disease will depend less on her sexual behaviour than on that of her husband or male partner. One should therefore look at the patterns of sexual behaviour in a society as a whole, especially the sexual habits of the *men*. On this basis, they postulate three types of society:

1. 'Type A', where both men and women are strongly discouraged from pre- or extramarital relations (for example, Mormons or Seventh Day Adventists)
2. 'Type B', where only women are strongly discouraged from extramarital sexual

continued

relations but men are expected to have many (especially with prostitutes), as in many Latin American societies and in Europe last century
3. 'Type C', where both men and women have several sexual partners during their lives (as in modern Western 'permissive society').

The incidence of cervical cancer is lowest in Type A and highest in Type B societies. In Type A groups, such as Jews, Seventh Day Adventists and Mormons, the low incidence could be due to endogamous marriage and monogamous patterns of sexual behaviour, as well as to low recourse to prostitutes. In Latin America, by contrast, recourse to prostitutes is common. In one study quoted by Skegg and colleagues, 91 per cent of male Colombian students reported premarital intercourse, and 92 per cent of these men had experienced intercourse with prostitutes. The authors suggest that this might account for the high incidence of cervical cancer in Latin America, as the prostitutes could act as a reservoir of infection. Similarly, the decline in mortality from the disease in the UK and USA (Type C societies) may be due to changing patterns of sexual behaviour among men, with less recourse to prostitutes in a more 'permissive' society.

Case study: Cultural practices and hepatitis B

Brabin and Brabin[25] reviewed the role of cultural factors in the transmission of the hepatitis B virus. The level of infection by the virus varies widely between countries, ethnic groups, tribes and even neighbouring villages. Part of the reason for this is a number of cultural factors, including sexual behaviour patterns, family and marriage patterns, and cultural changes affecting women and their childbearing age. For example, the risk of infection with the virus varies with the level of promiscuity, and the spouses of promiscuous partners are therefore at greater risk from infection, which is particularly important in the case of pregnant women. They point out that marriage patterns that permit extramarital relations, polygamy, frequent divorces or the exchange of partners may all contribute to spread of the virus, as may widespread recourse to prostitution, especially in tropical countries. Family patterns involving frequent adoption of children and their movement between households, and the movement of women in marriage between villages, may also provide channels for the spread of infection. By contrast, marital patterns that forbid marriage between different communities or segments of a community may confine the infection to certain geographical or ethnic pockets; for example, Chinese immigrants in the UK and USA and Fijian Indians all have low levels of HBsAG, characteristic of their homelands. Finally, social changes such as war, migrations and social upheaval may break down barriers that contained the virus in a local environment, and spread it further afield. Since the prevalence of hepatitis B antigen (which correlates with the rate of vertical transmission of the virus) declines with age, most vertical transmission occurs when women bear children at a younger age. Cultural changes that produce a later age of marriage and childbearing will therefore reduce this transmission, and the spread of infection. The authors conclude that, especially in the case of hepatitis, 'interpretation of epidemiologic data in non-Western societies demands a cultural perspective if modes of transmission are to be correctly defined and intervention planned'.

Case study: Coronary heart disease among Japanese in Japan, Hawaii and Cahfornia

In a number of studies, Marmot and colleagues[9,10] examined the epidemiology of coronary heart disease, hypertension and stroke among 11 900 men of Japanese ancestry living in California, Hawaii and Japan itself. The aim was to identify the influence of *non*-genetic factors on these three groups, by comparing disease rates of the two migrant groups and those of Japanese who had not emigrated. They found that there is a gradient in the occurrence of coronary heart disease (CHD) between the three groups, with the lowest rate in Japan, intermediate in Hawaii and highest in California. The influence of other risk factors commonly associated with high CHD rates, such as hypertension, diet, smoking, weight, blood sugar and serum cholesterol levels, was examined. It was found that the gradient in the incidence of CHD could not be explained only by the presence of these risk factors (for example, those who smoked similar amounts in the three groups still showed a gradient in the incidence of CHD). However, the incidence of CHD *was* found to be related to the degree of adherence to the traditional Japanese culture they were all brought up in. The closer their adherence to these traditional values, the lower was their incidence of CHD. Within California, those Japanese-Americans who had become most westernized in outlook had higher rates than those immigrants who followed their more traditional lifestyle. Marmot and Syme[9] point out that 'these results support the hypothesis that the culture in which an individual is raised affects his likelihood of manifesting coronary heart disease in adult life', and that this relationship of culture of upbringing to CHD 'appears to be independent of the established coronary risk factors'. In the case of the Japanese, the cultural emphasis is on group cohesion, group achievement and social stability. In this cultural group, as in other traditional societies, it is suggested that 'a stable society whose members enjoy the support of their fellows in closely knit groups may protect against the forms of social stress that may lead to CHD'.

Case study: Cultural practices and parasitic diseases

Alland[26] examined the relationships between certain cultural practices and the incidence, distribution and spread of parasitic diseases. Many of his findings apply also to infectious diseases. He notes how the arrangement of living space, the type and arrangement of houses and the numbers of people per room or house may all influence the spread or containment of disease. The social isolation of certain sub-groups, such as within a rigid caste system, may affect the spread of epidemics into certain communities. Population movements, such as a nomadic lifestyle, also help to spread parasitic and other infections, sometimes through the wider distribution of their human wastes. Certain cultural practices that separate man from the extra-human environment of some parasitic organisms also help reduce infections. For example, the practice of digging deep latrines (as opposed to discharging waste products into rivers or streams) offers protection against those parasitic infections that are spread by urine or faeces. Contamination of water supplies is also prevented by its location far from domestic animals or human habitations, and by the separation of drinking sources from water used for bathing or laundering. Other cultural practices, such as frequent spitting, may increase the spread of viral and other infections through the community. Patterns of visiting the sick, or attending large public rites or festivals, may also be related to the spread of epidemics. Certain agricultural techniques, such as the cultivation of rice paddies, may increase the danger of schistosomiasis and other parasitic infestations. Certain forms of dress, such as tailored clothing, apparently provide a better environment for lice or fleas to live in than do loose togas, while the sharing of clothing within a family may also spread these infections. These and other cultural practices may influence the distribution of a wide range of parasitic, bacterial, viral and fungal infections.

Case study: AIDS and sexual practices in urban Brazil

Parker[27] studied sexual attitudes and practices in urban areas of Brazil, in relation to the growing incidence of AIDS in that country. Based on his fieldwork, he criticized the assumption that 'sexual practices are constant cross-culturally – that sexual behaviour is largely unaffected by its specific social and cultural context'. He pointed out that models of AIDS transmission (and therefore of prevention) developed in the USA and Western Europe may be inappropriate to the Brazilian cultural context. The assumption that there are just three types of sexual behaviour – heterosexuality, homosexuality and bisexuality – with clear boundaries between these groups does not reflect Brazil's complex cultural reality. For example, not all homosexuals are regarded as being really 'homosexual'. Brazilian culture differentiates between the active, penetrating partner (the *homem* or 'man'), and the passive 'woman' (known as the *viado* or *bicha*). Social stigma attaches mainly to the latter, while the *homem* can have sexual relations with either women or men, 'without sacrificing his masculine identity'. The same distinction applies also to the more active male prostitutes (the *miche*), as opposed to the more passive transvestites or *travesti*. In popular thought, therefore, 'the category of *homossexuais* or "homosexuals" has generally been reserved for "passive" partners, while the classification of "active" partners in same-sex interactions has remained rather unclear and ambiguous'. This ambiguity can in turn undermine preventive strategies and health education that are directed only against the more obvious *viados*.

Another significant feature in Brazil is the widespread practice of anal intercourse, both

continued

between men and men, and between men and women. It is also common between male clients and female prostitutes. In adolescence, too, anal intercourse is common, mainly in order to avoid both unwanted pregnancy and rupture of the hymen – still an important sign of a young woman's sexual purity. The apparently frequent incidence of anal intercourse among different groups in Brazil thus 'makes the epidemiological picture of AIDS there quite distinct from the picture in Europe and the United States'; these patterns 'significantly change the definition of "high-risk" groups in Brazil and may well further the spread of AIDS to the population at large'. Thus Parker concluded that epidemiological research on AIDS should recognize the disease as 'simultaneously a socio-cultural and biological phenomenon', and that preventive strategies should always take this into account.

In addition to the conditions just described, one other set of cultural factors is becoming increasingly important in the contemporary world; the effects on health of *migration*. There is now a considerable body of research that links migration and refugee status to an increased incidence of certain illnesses, both mental and physical, though the exact link between migration and illness is not clear. These studies (some of which were quoted in Chapters 10 and 11) indicate, for example, a higher incidence of mental illness, attempted suicide and hypertension among some immigrants, compared to the incidence of these conditions in the host countries and in their countries of origin. As with coronary heart disease among Japanese-Americans, it appears that the cultural lifestyles of both immigrant and host communities as well as the fit (or lack of fit) between the two, coupled with the economic situation of the country and its attitudes towards newcomers, may all contribute towards the increased incidence of these stress-related conditions.

Variations in medical treatment and diagnosis

Epidemiological techniques can also be used in the study of differences in the diagnostic and treatment behaviour of doctors from various countries. Some of the differences between British and American and between British and French psychiatrists in the frequency with which they diagnose schizophrenia and affective disorders have already been described in Chapter 10. In the case of medical treatments, the rate of a particular treatment (such as tonsillectomy) in two countries can be compared with the actual prevalence (in both countries) of the condition (in this case recurrent tonsillitis) for which the treatment is usually prescribed. If the rate of tonsillectomies is much higher in one country, in the absence of a proportionately higher rate of tonsillitis, then it can be inferred that cultural influences on both doctor and patient are responsible for this. Obviously both economic and technological factors, as well as the supply of both medical manpower and hospital facilities, play a part in this phenomenon, and such a study is more valid if carried out between countries with similar levels of social and industrial development.

Case study: Comparison of surgical rates in the USA, Canada and England and Wales

Vayda and colleagues[28] compared overall surgical rates in Canada, England and Wales, and the USA between 1966 and 1976. In particular, they examined the *relationship* between:

1. Operative rates per 100 000 population in each of the three countries
2. Selected resources (surgical manpower and hospital beds)
3. National priorities, as measured by percentage of gross national product (GNP) spent on health care
4. Disease prevalence, as measured by mortalities for selected diseases for which surgery is one form of treatment.

The rates of 10 common operations were computed in the three countries and compared. These operations were: lens extraction; tonsil surgery; prostatectomy; excision of knee cartilage; inguinal herniorraphy; cholecystectomy; colectomy; gastrectomy; hysterectomy; and Caesarean section. During the 10 years studied, overall surgical rates in England and Wales were found to have remained constant, while Canadian rates were also relatively constant, but US rates increased by about 25 per cent. Canadian rates, though, continued to be 60 per cent higher than the British rates, and the US rates, which were 80 per cent greater than those in Britain in 1966, were 125 per cent greater than England and Wales in 1976. Caesarean sections increased in all three countries from 53 per cent to 126 per cent. In 1976 about 12 per cent of all Canadian and American births were delivered in this way, but only 7 per cent in England and Wales. Hysterectomy rates were twice as high in Canada and the US as in the British sample. In comparing the availability of hospital beds, the British sample had the lowest number (and the lowest number of operations) of the three in 1976, and while Canada had 30 per cent more hospital beds than the US, overall US operative rates were 40 per cent higher than Canada's rate. In the decade under study, England and Wales spent about 5 per cent of their GNP on health care, Canada spent about 7 per cent and the US about 9 per cent. The study could find no clear correlation between operative rates in the three countries and the availability of either hospital beds or medical manpower; nor were they related to differing mortality rates (as a measure of prevalence) of the selected diseases between the countries. Instead, the differences were due to 'differing treatment styles and philosophies of patient management', the different value systems of these countries, the priority they assign to health care (as reflected in the percentage of GNP allocated to health care), and changes in technology (especially the increase in cardiac, vascular and thoracic surgery in the US and Canada). The authors note that 'differing operative rates are more a reflection of consumer and provider preferences; consequently, outcomes must be measured in terms of quality of life and postoperative morbidity rather than by mortality'. This is because most operations done are elective or discretionary, and not done for any potentially fatal condition; this explains why the differences in operative rates were not related to differing mortalities from the selected conditions. The study demonstrated, therefore, that 'at least three industrialized Western countries have tolerated substantial differences in their frequencies of surgery without consistent unfavourable outcomes'. To some extent, therefore, the *cultural* values of the surgeon, the patient and the society in which they live play a part in determining the frequency with which surgery is used as a treatment for certain conditions.

Recommended reading

Brabin, L. and Brabin, B. J. (1985). Cultural factors and transmission of hepatitis B virus. *Am. J. Epidemiol.*, **122**, 725–30.

Hahn, R. A. (1995). *Sickness and Healing: An Anthropological Perspective*, pp. 99–128. Yale University Press.

Marmot, M. (1981). Culture and illness: epidemiological evidence. In: *Foundations of Psychosomatics* (M. J. Christie and P. G. McIlett, eds), pp. 323–40. Wiley.

Marmot, M. G. and Syme, S. L. (1976). Acculturation and coronary heart disease in Japanese Americans. *Am. J. Epidemiol.*, **104**, 225–47.

Parker, R. (1987). Acquired immunodeficiency syndrome in urban Brazil. *Med. Anthropol. Q.* (new series), **1**, 155–75.

13 Medical anthropology and global health

Traditionally, most anthropologists have studied small-scale societies, or relatively small groups of people within a wider society. They have usually aimed at a *holistic* view of a particular culture or community, including how its different aspects are connected with one another – to understand, as Mars[1] puts it, 'the articulation of family and kinship organization with grass-root political power and authority, the relation of these to religious beliefs and practices, and the place taken in all these affairs by the way goods and services are produced and distributed'.

Medical anthropologists, too, have concentrated mainly on health problems at the local (and occasionally national) level. However, in recent years many of the major threats to human health – such as overpopulation, pollution, global warming, drug abuse and the AIDS epidemic – can no longer be confined, or dealt with solely behind local or national boundaries. In an increasingly mobile and interdependent world, they are truly *global* in both their origins and their effects. Furthermore, information about these problems has also become global as more areas of the world are connected with one another by telecommunications, the Internet, radio, television, jet travel and mass tourism.

For these reasons, future research in medical anthropology is likely to focus not only on how certain cultural and social factors can damage individual health, but also on the health of the human species as a whole. This will involve adopting a much more global perspective – a holistic view of the complex interactions between the cultures, economic systems, political organizations and ecology of the planet itself.

Medical anthropology, as a *biocultural* discipline integrating both medical science and biology with the social and behavioural sciences, brings a unique perspective to the study of these global health problems. Its comparative, cross-cultural approach coupled with the collection of physical and psychological data gives it an overview of the diversity of beliefs and behaviours found world-wide, and the relation of these to health and disease.

It can also help explain the effects and causes of these global problems at the *local* level. To take one example, the acquired immunodeficiency syndrome (AIDS) now poses a threat to health on a global level. Faced with this situation, detailed in-depth ethnographic studies can provide information regarding:

- how an increase in AIDS can affect the social, economic and cultural life of a particular community
- how beliefs and behaviours within that community change (or do not change) to meet this threat
- what explanations are given (in terms of local beliefs) for the origins of the disease and why some people are afflicted by it and others not
- whether sufferers from it can mobilize social support or find themselves stigmatized and rejected
- how sexual relationships, marriage patterns, family structures and religious rituals are altered by the disease
- whether changes occur in the way that different genders and generations relate to one another
- the strategies of prevention and self-care used by the community, and how these articulate with local and national medical systems

- the shifts that take place in the patterns of work, migration and residence.

All these anthropological approaches to health problems, however, have to take place against the background of one key issue in global health: *poverty*. According to the World Health Organization[2], extreme poverty is the greatest killer and cause of ill health and suffering across the globe. Together with economic inequality, it is responsible for more physical and mental ill health than any other cause.

To illustrate the relevance of medical anthropology to certain global health problems, a few key areas have been selected for further discussion. They are:

1. Overpopulation
2. Urbanization
3. AIDS
4. Primary health care
5. Malaria
6. Pollution and global warming
7. Deforestation and species extinction.

Overpopulation

Overpopulation is one of the most serious global problems, and the situation is worsening every year. Despite attempts to slow it down, the world's population is still growing exponentially. It has been estimated that by the year 2025 it will have increased from 5.5 billion to at least 8 billion, or even more[3]. As well as this massive population increase (which is mostly confined to the poorer countries), energy consumption by the richer countries is increasing at an even faster rate. Overall, world energy consumption has grown from an estimated 1 terawatt in 1890 to 3.3 in 1950 and 13.7 in 1990 – and on average, poor people use one-tenth of the energy of rich people[3]. Overpopulation, plus the overuse of energy sources (such as fossil fuels), is potentially a dangerous combination, with deadly results for global health. These include widespread starvation, disease, poverty and civil unrest; the depletion of valuable fossil fuel reserves; and environmental dangers such as climatic changes and global warming (due to the 'greenhouse effect'), the rise of sea-levels with flooding of coastal plains, increased heat waves and droughts, and natural disasters such as hurricanes and cyclones[2].

Family planning programmes

Various strategies have been put forward to deal with the growing problem of overpopulation, including international programmes such as those of the WHO or of the International Planned Parenthood Federation, and national ones such as the 'one child' policy in the People's Republic of China. Most of these family planning programmes have been targeted on women, and have aimed at increasing their awareness of the benefits of reducing family size, allowing longer gaps between pregnancies and using the various forms of artificial contraception now available.

At present, an estimated 43 per cent of married couples world-wide are using some form of modern contraception. This includes 52 per cent of couples in the richer, developed world, and 27 per cent in the developing world (although in China the figure is 73 per cent)[4]. Also, an estimated 30 million legal abortions were carried out world-wide in 1987, as well as 10–22 million illegal ones[4]. As a form of population control and family planning, abortion can pose many dangers to health, including haemorrhage, infection and perforation of the uterus, especially in the hands of untrained personnel. It has been estimated that between 100 000 and 200 000 women die each year in developing countries from the complications of illegal abortions[4].

Despite their good intentions, family planning programmes have often been unsuccessful in reducing population growth. In many parts of the world, the idea of limiting one's fertility has either been rejected outright or accepted only very reluctantly. It is thus important to recognize, as Warwick[5] points out, that the demand for family planning is *not* universal, and it is not accepted by many different cultures. There are many reasons for this.

In most cases, the meaning of family planning is closely related to the value given to children. In many cultures, having a child is the visible sign of adult status; also, for many men, the birth of a son is the ultimate proof of their virility. In those communities where starvation, poverty, insecurity and a high infant mortality rate are common, fertility is given a very high social value. Having many children is one of the few ways that people can ensure their future, especially where the state is weak, has few resources and cannot provide comprehensive care for its citizens. The traditional extended family provides its members with a small-scale society of their own. It functions as a social and economic unit, sharing in the creation and distribution of resources, providing its members with a miniature social security system and helping them with the care of children, the elderly and the infirm.

A further salient reason for the rejection of family planning is that some world religions disapprove of *all* artificial forms of birth control, preferring instead more 'natural' (rhythm) methods. However, at both national and local levels there are many other reasons why family planning programmes are not successful. Warwick[5] notes that 'in every country, at least one group is opposed to organized family planning for some reason', and the opposition may be based on religious, cultural, economic or political criteria. In some developing countries, for example, family planning programmes originating in the West may be seen as just another form of colonialism, imposing itself on the local culture and population and weakening them in the process. Also, in those multi-ethnic countries where there have been conflicts between different communities, such as Sri Lanka, Lebanon, Malaysia, Fiji, South Africa and India, these conflicts 'may create feelings that a large population is vital to communal survival and that family planning helps one's enemies'[5].

Another factor influencing the acceptability of contraceptive techniques is cultural beliefs about the *body*, particularly the female reproductive system. These include ideas, such as those described among some low-income groups in the USA[6], of the uterus being a hollow organ, closed throughout the month and only 'open' during menstruation. Becoming pregnant is therefore only possible just before, or just after the period when it is still 'open' (during the period itself intercourse is strictly forbidden), and therefore there is no need to take contraceptive precautions during the rest of the month.

In addition, women in many cultures see menstrual blood as 'polluting' or 'poisonous', and fear the effects of a decreased menstrual flow, when more of the 'poison' will remain within their bodies (see Chapters 2 and 6). This is one of the reasons why the contraceptive pill, which may cause lighter menses or even their cessation, has been rejected by many women world-wide. For example, Good[7] describes how, in Maragheh, Iran, lighter periods due to the pill are blamed for causing women to have the folk illness 'heart distress' (see Chapter 5), and are therefore avoided. In Scott's study[8] in Miami, Florida, many of the women interviewed saw the pill as dangerous for this same reason, fearing that the accumulated blood would cause them to have 'blood pressure', mental illness, or to be nervous or depressed. In those groups that see menstrual blood as polluting and dangerous to other people, the intermenstrual 'spotting' sometimes caused by the pill may also lead to its rejection: it might also prevent them from taking part in certain religious rituals and festivals due to their temporary state of 'pollution'.

Similarly, cultural attitudes can influence whether the intrauterine contraceptive device (IUCD) is acceptable or not. Some may welcome the IUCD, which often causes heavier periods, as a way of increasing the monthly loss of their 'poisonous' blood. Others may reject it, based on folk models of female anatomy. For example, in Jamaica, MacCormack[9] found that some women believed the uterus and vagina to be a single tube, open at both ends, and feared that the IUCD might therefore move and get lost somewhere within the body. Snow[10], in her study of low-income African-Americans, found similar beliefs about IUCDs. Because menstrual blood was seen as polluting and shameful, the idea of exposing oneself to a strange physician for the IUCD to be inserted *during* a period (which it usually is) was met with revulsion.

In Japan, there has been widespread public and official rejection of oral contraception. Sobo and Russell[11] ascribed this to traditional Japanese beliefs about how the human body should always be in accordance with nature – unlike the Western desire to always conquer nature. By making the fertile female body infertile, artificial contraceptives (including the pill, surgical sterilization or the IUCD) violate this relationship. The pill particularly is seen changing the body's natural ecology, depriving the body 'of the opportunity to follow its natural, self-determined rhythm'.

As well as these cultural beliefs, family planning methods can also be rejected for more practical reasons such as availability or cost – especially in areas of extreme poverty. Also, since *all* forms of artificial contraception (including sterilization) carry with them certain risks and side effects, knowledge and experience of these within a community will obviously influence whether women are willing to accept them or not.

As mentioned above, most family planning programmes have been targeted on women. As

McCally[4] put it: 'The control of population growth appears to be in women's hands. The empowerment of women, meaning access to education, health services, employment and public health, is coming to be understood as a major determinant of fertility'. Reproductive decision-making may not, however, be only the prerogative of women. Decisions on fertility also depend on local cultural conditions, patterns of marriage and residence, and the ways that individual women are embedded in family and kinship networks. Dyson and Moore[12], for example, point out differences in the power of women to make decisions about fertility between north and south India. According to their research, women in the north tend to marry younger than those in the south, to be more controlled by their husband's family, and to be under stronger pressure from them to produce many children, especially sons.

Family planning programmes also need to target *men*. At present, many of the programmes aimed at men seem mainly to emphasize the use of condoms for AIDS prevention rather than as a regular form of contraception within a relationship. Arguably, by emphasizing only the female link to fertility, some men may even be led to conclude that if fertility is solely a female issue, then so is responsibility for infertility as well (see Chapter 6). Getting the co-operation of men (as well as women) is especially important in male-dominated societies, where they make most of the fertility decisions. Among the Hausa of northern Nigeria, for example, Renne[13] describes how married women are often kept secluded within their homes. This *auren kulle* ('marriage lock') means that they have little access to contraception without their husband's permission. They have few financial resources, so cannot afford to buy contraceptives, and in any case are discouraged from visiting chemist's shops or clinics unless accompanied by their husband or an older female relative.

Because of the diversity of populations, many anthropologists have therefore concluded that there cannot be a universal model of family planning that is applicable to *all* parts of the world. Within many countries, different regions, religions, ethnic groups, social classes and local communities may all have very different attitudes towards family planning, and each may require a different type of programme. In some cases, especially where the population is culturally, ethnically or socially diverse, this may make a national family planning strategy difficult, if not impossible.

Thus Warwick[5] suggests that, as well as programmes at the national and international levels, *local* communities should also be involved in family planning programmes. This will involve regular consultations with the community, being sensitive to their cultural needs, expectations and concerns (for example, having female staff conduct interviews and examinations), and enlisting the opinions and co-operation of local religious and political leaders. It also means recognizing that 'in some regions socio-cultural conditions may not be ripe for any kind of family planning program. Life may be too precarious, the value of children too high, the politics too polarized, or the issue of fertility control too remote to make such an investment worthwhile'.

Finally, like all other forms of health aid and intervention, family planning programmes cannot take place in a vacuum. They should always be part of a more holistic approach that also involves social and economic development, such as the reduction of poverty, improved health care, better nutrition, higher levels of literacy and employment, and the reduction of maternal and infant mortality. From a global perspective, this will also involve a more equitable distribution of resources between the poorer and richer parts of the world, and a reduction of energy consumption by the latter.

Urbanization

A parallel phenomenon to overpopulation has been the massive increase in *urbanization*. At the beginning of the nineteenth century the world's urban population totalled less than 50 million; in 1988 it was estimated that by the year 2000 it would be 3.1 billion[14]. Many parts of the world have seen the development of huge 'mega-cities' such as Cairo, Calcutta, Mexico City, Sao Paolo, Bombay, Jakarta and Manila, due mainly to natural increase, but also to migration of people from the countryside in search of a better life. In 1988 it was estimated that by the year 2000 there will be 60 cities with a population of over 5 million – 61 per cent of the increase from natural growth, the rest from migration. Most of these will be in the developing world, where an estimated 44 per cent of the population will be living in these huge cities.

The rapid growth of the *urban poor*, often living in shanty towns, slums or squatter settlements 'in the shadow of the city', has accompanied the rise of urbanization. The percentage of urban dwellers living in these slums and shanty towns varies from 79 per cent in Addis Ababa, 67 per cent in Calcutta and 60 per cent in Kinshasa to 30 per cent in Rio de Janeiro, 23 per cent in Karachi and 20 per cent in Bangkok[14].

The urban poor face numerous health problems, often worse than those of their rural counterparts. Many of these are a combination of the problems of underdevelopment (such as malnutrition and infectious diseases) and those of development (pollution, noise, traffic accidents etc.). Harpham and colleauges[15] described how these problems have three main sources:

1. *Direct problems of poverty*, such as unemployment, low income, limited education and literacy, inadequate diet, lack of breast-feeding, and prostitution
2. *Environmental problems*, due to poor housing, overcrowding, inadequate sanitation and water supplies, lack of waste disposal, air pollution, traffic accidents, the siting of hazardous industries nearby and lack of land to grow food on
3. *Psychosocial problems*, such as stress (see Chapter 11), insecurity, marital breakdown, depression, alcoholism, smoking, domestic violence and drug addiction.

These health problems are rarely confined to the slum communities themselves. In Mexico City, for example, there are so many people without proper sanitation that a 'faecal snow' often falls on the city as the wind sweeps up dried human waste[4]. As illustrated below, these overcrowded urban environments can also become breeding grounds for several infectious diseases – some spread by humans, other by vectors such as mosquitoes.

Case study: Dengue and urbanization in Mérida, Mexico and El Progresso, Honduras

Kendall and colleagues'[16] study of Mérida and El Progresso indicates how an increasing urban population, and especially the growth of slums and shanty towns, is creating new ecologies of disease. In many urban areas of Central and South America and the Caribbean, overcrowding, population mobility, pollution, poor sanitation and the accumulation of garbage are all helping the rapid spread of certain diseases. These include insect-borne diseases such as dengue, and its variant dengue haemorrhagic fever (DHF), malaria, yellow fever, elephantiasis and Japanese encephalitis. DHF is caused by a virus and transmitted by mosquitoes, especially *Aedes aegypti* (which can also transmit yellow fever). It can cause bleeding disorders and death, and there is no specific treatment or vaccine for it at present. In urban areas, the mosquitoes breed in collections of stagnant water such as in rainwater pools, barrels, bottles, discarded tyres, flowerpots, vases and animal drinking troughs. However, many people are still unaware of the dangers posed by mosquitoes in an urban environment and of the need to take precautions against them. In Mérida, although most of the population knew about dengue from public health education programmes, some confused it with other fever-producing illnesses such as *derengue* (a disease of cattle), *deshidratación* (dehydration) and 'flu; they were also unaware that insects were its vectors, blaming instead certain 'winds' for carrying it and other febrile illnesses. In El Progresso, too, most people knew of dengue, but many confused it with 'flu, and also believed that it came from the 'winds' or from garbage rather than from mosquito bites. The authors concluded, therefore, that given the growth of urbanization and of these 'new' urban diseases, their control 'will require theoretical knowledge about the organization of urban environments and its relationship to disease, new methodologies to encourage participation and social activism in health, and increased knowledge about influencing health behaviour'.

Anthropological research in the new mega-cities, especially among the urban poor, can contribute to the provision of community-oriented primary care (COPC) – a form of health care that emphasizes the importance of relating health care provision to local needs and conditions[17]. Here, its role is to assess the specific health needs and problems of a particular community, to raise awareness of the role of cultural beliefs and behaviours in their health (and health care), and to act as their advocates to the medical and other authorities where necessary. Ethnographic research can also be relevant to the planning, application and evaluation of a variety of primary health care programmes at both national and international levels, as illustrated later in this chapter.

The acquired immunodeficiency disease (AIDS)

AIDS is one of the deadliest diseases of the modern age, and a major threat to global health. The World Health Organization estimated that, by 1995, some 6000 people were being infected by the virus every day[2]. According to a comprehensive review by Mann and colleagues[18], 164 countries had reported cases of AIDS to the WHO by 1992. Nearly 2.5 million people, including more than 550 000 children, had died from the disease; 75 per cent of these deaths had occurred in Africa, including 90 per cent of all children dying from the disease. In the Americas, where 268 477 cases had been reported, the USA alone accounted for 80 per cent of them (44 per cent of the global total), while most of the remainder occurred in Canada, Brazil and Mexico. In many industrialized countries, AIDS is now among the 10 leading causes of death for men aged 35–44 years; in New York City in 1988–1989, it was also the leading cause of death among women aged 25–39 years. As well as actual cases of AIDS, about 12 875 450 people had been infected by the HIV virus by 1992, and it was estimated that this would have risen to nearly 20 million (2.3 million of them children) by 1995, and that 90 per cent of all HIV infections would have occurred in the developing world. Since 1985 there have been some changes in the virus's pattern of transmission – mainly a fall in the rates of homosexual transmission, but an increase by heterosexual sex and injection drug use. Overall, it was estimated that by the year 2000, between 5.9 million and 20.4 million adults would have died from this deadly disease.

AIDS is not only unique from a biological point of view. Because its spread is so clearly linked to certain patterns of human behaviour, especially sexual behaviour, it is truly both a biological *and* a socio-cultural phenomenon. As such, any attempt to control its spread cannot focus only on the search for a vaccine or a pharmacological cure. It must also take into account the complex social, cultural and economic environments in which the disease is embedded, and which may either help or hinder its spread.

The following section outlines some of the many ways that research in medical anthropology (and other social sciences) can, and already has, contributed towards an understanding of these various socio-cultural factors.

Metaphors of AIDS in the Western world

Many of the metaphors associated with the very word 'AIDS' in contemporary Western society have already been described in Chapter 5. Mention has also been made of how its use in the media, and in both medical and popular discourses, may play a political role, stigmatizing and alienating even further those groups (such as homosexuals, drug addicts or immigrants) said to be most at risk of the disease[19]. Thus Frankenberg[20], in his analysis of the portrayal of AIDS in modern literature, points out that 'the paradox that AIDS is popularly seen both as a disease of the few and other, and as the ultimate threat to the many and same'.

These prejudices and the fears associated with them can undermine attempts to identify, treat and control the disease, and to offer its victims the care and compassion they deserve. Thus the moral and ideological attitudes of a society towards AIDS are just as relevant to its control as is the search for an effective vaccine. As Clatts and Mutchler[21] note, it is therefore important to examine 'what society does to people with words and the images the words evoke'. They note that a culture's metaphors play a prominent role in defining the identity of self, us and others, and how these relate to one another. In the USA, the discourse on AIDS defines the victim as the ultimate 'other' – 'alien, antisocial, unnatural, dangerous and threatening'. They describe how, gradually, the images of illness and evil have merged, until to say someone 'has AIDS' is also to say that they are 'dangerous and untouchable', and their disease a manifestation of their inner 'moral evil and/or mental illness'. Stigmatized groups such as homosexuals and drug addicts are often associated with images of a personality type –'compulsive, out of control, and maladjusted'. Clatts and Mutchler point out that this identification of AIDS only with the deviant 'other', as well as over-confidence in the powers of medicine to cure the disease, may be dangerous, since it 'has lulled the American public into believing that they are "safe" so long as they adhere to the virtuous venting of desire'.

Cultural representations of AIDS

AIDS is a global disease, but different human groups differ widely in their understanding of its origins, significance and modes of spread, as well as in the *meanings* they ascribe to it. This is a further example of the split between 'disease' and 'illness' described in Chapter 5. In many ways AIDS has become the pre-eminent folk illness of the modern age, absorbing, in each local context, a variety of indigenous images, metaphors and cultural themes. As in all forms of human misfortune, these provide answers to questions that people ask themselves, such as 'why me?' and 'why now?'.

In many countries now, widespread publicity about AIDS has led some anxious or depressed individuals to develop what may be termed *folk AIDS* . This is a type of illness without disease that has also been termed 'pseudo-AIDS'[22] or 'AIDS neurosis'[23], and in which people become convinced that they have the disease, even though there is no medical evidence for this. One reason for this, as Miller and colleagues[22] point out, may be that the early symptoms of AIDS – such as lethargy, loss of appetite and weight, and excessive sweating – are similar to those of anxiety and depression, and some individuals may thus misinterpret them. In Japan, Miller[23] has reported the widespread incidence of 'AIDS neurosis' – the first case being reported back in 1985 – with many officials convinced that it is 'a distinctly Japanese illness'. She quotes one AIDS counsellor as saying: 'Japanese are at much greater risk for developing AIDS neurosis, than they are of getting AIDS'. The syndrome is usually characterized by somatic complaints, depression, sleep disturbances, suicidal ideas and the delusion, despite evidence to the contrary, that they are HIV seropositive.

In other contexts, cultural representations of AIDS may be a blend of medical and indigenous beliefs – as a physical disease, but also as a punishment for sinful behaviour. For example, Ingstad[24] described how, in Botswana, traditional healers knew of AIDS, but saw it as just a new form of *meila*, a folk illness caused by the breaking of certain sexual taboos (see below). In the USA, Flaskerud and Rush[25] found similar beliefs among some African-Americans, with AIDS being seen as 'punishment for sin'; a result of breaking religious and moral laws, especially those against homosexuality or extramarital sex. These cultural representations are not static, however. Anthropologists have shown how they can change over time as new information (often from health education programmes) is received and then blended with older, more traditional beliefs, as illustrated in the following case history.

Case study: Changing concepts of AIDS in Do Kay, Haiti

Farmer[26] described how concepts of AIDS (*syndrome d'immunodéfiecence acquise*, or *sida*) gradually changed during the period 1983–1989, in the rural village of Do Kay, Haiti. In 1983–1984, the village had heard only vague rumours of a 'city disease' (*maladi lavil*); very few knew how it was transmitted, or how serious it was. By 1985–1986, and drawing on folk models of illness causation, the idea had become common that *sida* was a 'sickness of the blood', something that 'spoils your blood, and makes you have so little blood that you become pale and dry'. Partly due to public health programmes, these beliefs gradually became linked to vague understandings of *sida* as due to an irreversible pollution caused by blood transfusions or same-sex relations, as well as by weakness from overwork in the city, or by travel to the USA. In 1987, a consensus about the symptoms of *sida* had begun to develop, especially its association with diarrhoea and tuberculosis. That same year, the first resident of Do Kay fell ill with the disease; this was widely blamed on a 'sent sickness', or sorcery, due to envy. The victim's family consulted a voodoo priest, who confirmed this, and identified certain individuals responsible for it. When another villager fell ill with the disease, though, most did not believe that she actually had *sida*, as she was considered 'too innocent' to be the victim of envy. By 1988–1989, after both villagers had died and a third had fallen ill, a consensus about the disease had developed in Do Kay. *Sida* was seen as two entities, both caused by a microbe; a 'natural' illness, caused by sexual contact with someone who 'carries the germ', and an 'unnatural' illness sent by sorcery from a malicious person. Condoms were helpful against the former, but useless against the latter. The 'unnatural' *sida* could only be prevented by using charms that could 'protect you against any kind of sickness that a person would send you'.

Thus, as Farmer pointed out, over the 6-year period 'the term *sida* and the syndrome with which it is associated came to be embedded in a series of distinctly Haitian ideas about illness'. These in turn link the sudden appearance of the disease to wider social and political issues, which he described as 'the endless suffering of the Haitian people, divine punishment, the corruption of the ruling class, and the ills of North American imperialism'.

Public and professional knowledge of AIDS

In many parts of the world, increasing numbers of education programmes have tried to disseminate knowledge about AIDS to the public. However, for a variety of reasons, large numbers of people are still unaware of how it is transmitted and how it can be prevented. In a study in Walsall, England, for example, Smithson[27] found good general knowledge of AIDS (90 per cent had got their information from television, and 80 per cent from newspaper articles), but also some significant misconceptions about how it could be spread. Twenty-six per cent, for example, thought they could get it from giving a blood donation, 16.1 per cent from sharing crockery or cutlery, and 15.6 per cent by using a toilet previously used by an AIDS patient. As part of the same study, health personnel (such as nurses and laboratory technicians) were asked the same questions: 17.8 per cent of them also believed AIDS could be caught by donating blood, and over half were fearful that they could catch AIDS from patients. In another study of 399 individuals in San Francisco, New York and London, Temoshok and colleagues[28] found that a general fear of AIDS, as well as anti-gay prejudice, was associated with a low knowledge of AIDS; there was a lower level of knowledge and higher level of general fear of the disease in London, compared to San Francisco, with New York intermediate between the two. From this study, however, it was 'not clear whether fear and ... prejudice promote ignorance, or whether ignorance increases fear and prejudice'. In either case, knowledge of the disease is not enough; the role of irrational fears and prejudices is also important in determining whether people change their behaviour or not.

Snow[29] described how, in some poor neighbourhoods, African-American folk beliefs also ascribe AIDS to 'toilets', 'filth', 'touching', 'kissing' and 'mosquitoes'. Some see it as evidence of 'bad blood' ('So many things can go wrong with your blood; like AIDS, a lot of things will give you impure blood'), others as the result of 'lowered resistance to impurities, poor health habits, exposure to cold, improper nutrition, or 'a body weakened by menstruation'. The belief that mosquitoes can transmit the disease has also been found in Namibia, as has the notion that asymptomatic carriers are not infectious[30].

Knowledge about how to prevent AIDS is particularly important among the young, though it may not necessarily be translated into action. In Brazil, for example, the largest and most populous nation in South America, 26 per cent of its population is under the age of 20 years, and AIDS is an increasing health problem[31]. In a large study of a student population (aged 13–22 years) in Porto Alegre, southern Brazil, De Souza and colleagues[31] found that while 95 per cent had high levels of knowledge about the physiology of reproduction, this did not always translate into safer sex precautions. While 42 per cent of the sample had already had a sexual relationship, and 35 per cent had sex at least once weekly, 52 per cent of them did *not* take any systematic or regular contraceptive precautions. Whatever the reasons for this, the authors conclude that this situation places many Brazilian teenagers at a high risk for unwanted pregnancies, as well as for sexually transmitted diseases such as AIDS.

Although such studies of beliefs about AIDS and its prevention may be useful in providing a baseline for future health education, anthropologists have often warned that beliefs and behaviours are not necessarily identical; people may not actually do what they say they do (see Chapter 14). Research indicates that knowledge of risk does not, in itself, always result in a change of behaviour – as shown by the many people who continue to smoke, drink and drive under the influence of alcohol, despite knowledge of the many risks involved[27]. The psychological reasons for this 'split' are complex, and often ill understood. On an individual level, they may include a belief that one is 'lucky' or 'blessed' (and thus immune to danger), a subconscious desire to be damaged or killed, or even a craving for the excitement of risk-taking. As one study of the sexual behaviour of young men in a Thai village put it, 'HIV provides another opportunity to test their invulnerability; to display a badge of courage to their friends'[32]. Thus, studies of beliefs and behaviours often require further anthropological investigation in order to understand why people behave (or do not behave) in a particular way, despite the health education messages that they have been exposed to.

Social dimensions of AIDS

People diagnosed as having AIDS (or as being HIV positive) often become the victims of discrimination and prejudice, even of violence. In extreme cases, this social rejection may lead to the 'social death' described in Chapter 9. Anthropological studies can provide baseline data on the attitudes, prejudices and stereotypes about AIDS held by the rest of the population, and the degree of stigma attached to it. Katz and colleagues[33], for example, interviewed a group of 433 adults – mainly nurses, medical students and chiropractic students – in New York City about how they perceived sufferers from serious diseases, including AIDS. The study revealed that AIDS is a 'severely stigmatizing condition', and for all groups in the sample the status of AIDS sufferers was as 'social deviants who are seen as themselves responsible for having this disease'. In Owambo, Namibia, Webb[30] also found that AIDS was a highly stigmatized disease, and that many believed that 'those who are infected will knowingly infect others, either deliberately through some malicious motive, or as a result of their inability to remain abstinent'. As Temoshok and colleagues[28] note, there are 'cultural differences in the degree of interaction with and prejudice against the higher risk groups based on fear of the disease'. Data on these differences, therefore, can be used to design public education programmes that aim at decreasing ignorance of the disease, and irrational fear of it. However, stigma does not attach only to the so-called high-risk groups and individuals in society. Stanley[34], in her study of white middle-class women with HIV, has shown how in the USA (as elsewhere) stigma extends also to all parts of the population who are HIV positive, irrespective of their sexual orientation, gender, economic status or ethnicity.

One growing area of research is into the *social networks* of those with HIV. Not only is this useful in tracking the spread of the virus, but it enables understanding of the social context of at-risk behaviours, such as syringe-sharing or unprotected sex. Thus Parker and colleagues[35] have investigated the sexual networks of HIV-positive men in London, in order to identify how at-risk behaviours help spread the virus. Certain situations, such as sex between older and younger men, or between male prostitutes and their clients, were identified as particularly likely to spread the infection throughout a much wider network of people. In New York City, Neaigus and colleagues[36] have shown how the 'risk networks' of intravenous drug users often overlap with their social networks – that is, people shared syringes mainly with those with whom they were already closely involved. Thus 70 per cent injected or shared syringes with a spouse or sex partner, a close friend or someone that they knew fairly well. This implies that changing risk networks can be very difficult, since these networks are an important part of addicts' daily lives (see Chapter 8). However, these same social ties with other drug-users can be a useful route – in the form of peer pressure and emotional support – through which to spread messages about the ways to reduce high-risk behaviours. For example, these ties can be used to develop a collective self-organization of drug injectors, 'in order to make HIV risk reduction a permanent feature of drug injectors' subculture'.

Anthropologists can therefore often help identify the social networks, self-help groups and other community resources that can be mobilized to help those with AIDS, and which can then be integrated into their long-term treatment. This is particularly important in cities since, in Western countries particularly, AIDS is predominantly an *urban* disease. By the end of 1991, for example, nearly 20 per cent (37 436) of all AIDS cases identified in the USA were reported in New York City, which was second only to San Francisco in the cumulative numbers of cases per 10 000 population[37]. Despite their anomie, urban environments offer some advantages over rural ones for people with AIDS: greater concentration of medical resources; more developed support networks and self-help groups; and a greater tolerance of diverse lifestyles. Health education programmes therefore need to take into account both the social and cultural diversity of urban populations, and the many different kinds of community support available for those with the disease.

Sexual practices and behaviour

The spread of AIDS is closely linked to sexual behaviours, but this intimate area of human relationships has always been notoriously difficult to study. In recent years, however, a number of anthropological studies have begun to remedy this situation, and have provided useful data for public health programmes. These studies reveal that patterns of 'normal' and 'abnormal' sexual behaviour (heterosexual and homosexual) differ widely between, and within, different societies. For example, anal intercourse has been reported as being relatively common among both heterosexuals and homosexuals in Brazil[38], compared to some other countries. Another example is the significant variation found world-wide in the incidence of extramarital sex, and the fact that in most societies it is commoner among men than among women (see Chapter 6) – a crucial fact, because in many parts of the world AIDS is increasingly becoming a heterosexual disease[32]. Furthermore, where such double standards of sexual morality exist, with women (but not men) expected to be chaste, faithful and virginal at marriage, women may be put at risk from their husband's behaviour, especially their recourse to prostitutes[39].

In Mexico, Carrier[40] describes the significance for AIDS prevention of the cultural values of urban (and mainly *mestizo*) males. These include the importance of family, manliness (*machismo*), strict gender roles, the dichotomization of women as being either 'good' or 'bad', and the shame attached to homosexuality. As in Brazil[38], the sharp division of gender roles means that there are two distinct groups of homosexual men; those that play the active, insertive 'masculine' (*activo*) role, and those that are passive (*pasivo*) and penetrable. Only the second group is considered to be truly homosexual, as well as 'feminine'. The *activo* group is not stigmatized as homosexual – 'the masculine self-image of Mexican males is thus not threatened by their homosexual behaviour as long as the appropriate role is played and they also have sexual relations with women'. That is, 'although involved in bisexual behaviour, they consider themselves to be heterosexual'. The emphasis on *machismo* encourages males to have 'multiple, uncommitted sexual contacts which start in adolescence' as a sign of manliness. By contrast, the dichotomization of women into 'good' (virginal, faithful, respectable) and 'bad' (those who have already acquired a 'spoiled identity') is accompanied by constraints on female sexual behaviour that can last 10–12 years, from adolescence to young adulthood. During this period it is the 'bad' women who are sought after; they may play the role of prostitute (*puta*), lover (*amante*) or common-law wife. In some cases, homosexual partners may offer 'a free or certainly a lower-cost alternative to whatever female partners are available'. Carrier also points out that after marriage, 'male extramarital relationships may be only with females, but they may also include or be only with males'. Overall, he concludes that 'more sexually active single males in Mexico have had sexual intercourse with both genders than have Anglo-American males'. In terms of preventive strategies, he suggests that, as most bisexual and homosexual men live with their families, a national health education campaign should focus on the family rather than individuals, educating the family about the importance of safer sex practices by their members. Another useful strategy, given widespread poverty in some areas, would be increased availability of free or low-cost condoms, as well as of spermicidal lubricants (for those playing the *pasivo* role).

Attitudes to condom use

Despite decades of advice about the need for 'safe sex', and the value of condoms in preventing HIV infection, many people in high-risk groups still continue to reject them. In some cases this is due to the condoms being unavailable or unaffordable. In others it may be due to certain cultural attitudes towards them. As Whitehead[41] notes, condoms often have a 'symbolic power' or sociocultural meaning in different communities, which can affect people's response to them. Schoepf[42] described some of the widespread folk beliefs about condom use, and their supposed dangers for women, in parts of Central and East Africa. These include infections, permanent sterility and even death, should a condom break and remain inside the vagina. In Uganda, Obbo[43] described how these fears have had a major effect, since some women see condoms as threatening to their reproductive health. In a society where there is social pressure on them (as on men) to prove their fertility, where barren women are pitied and mothers are respected, and where women gain access to social status and resources by marriage and child-bearing, the

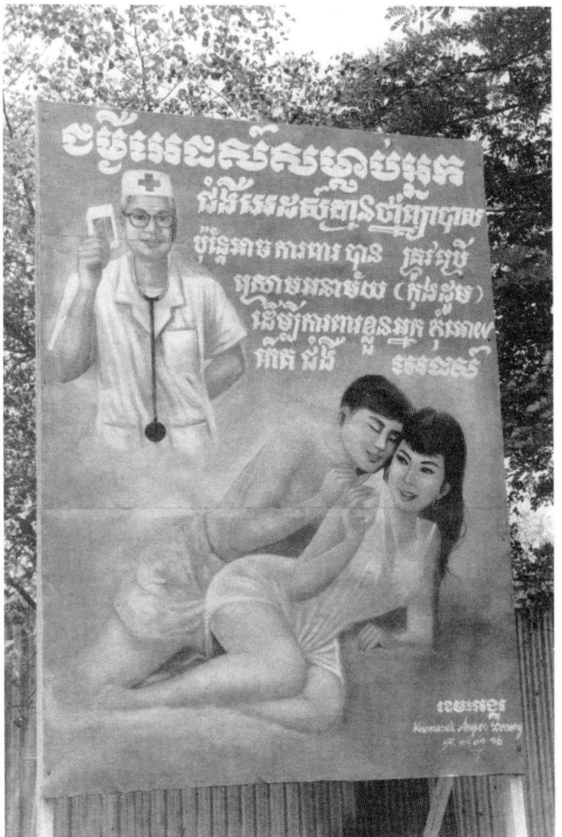

Figure 13.1 Street poster in Cambodia promoting safe sex and the use of condoms to prevent AIDS (Source: Sean Sprague/Panos Pictures, No. Cam: 439).

risks of condom use seemed high. Added to this was the opposition of some Ugandan churches, and the authorities' belief that easy availability of condoms promotes promiscuity. Elsewhere, Preston-Whyte[44] has described other folk beliefs, in South Africa, about how the condom itself may cause AIDS, or that because it holds bodily fluids these may be mis-used by sorcerers.

Men in many countries reject condom use for a number of reasons, often related to beliefs about its effect on reducing sexual sensation ('taking a shower in a raincoat'). In other cases, these beliefs may be related to other aspects of masculine identity. In a study of urban, low-income African-American men in Baltimore, Whitehead[41] found that barriers to condom use may be linked to:

- ideas about the importance of fathering children, as part of male identity
- sexual prowess, and conquests, as evidence of masculine attractiveness
- economic capability, as an attribute of masculine status and power.

In this community, as in many others worldwide, men's core identity and sense of self-esteem (especially that of younger men) may lead them to take many risks in their daily lives. Not using a condom is just another form of risk-taking behaviour, among many others.

Women are often reluctant to initiate condom use, in case they are seen as being too sexually experienced and too 'forward' in their behaviour[45]. Others may feel that to suggest a condom may threaten the survival of their relationship, damaging intimacy by suggesting that they don't trust their sexual partner. But another major issue here is the differential in *power* – physical, social and economic – between women and men in many societies. Often younger or poorer women feel unable to resist the pressure from men not to use a condom[32]. This is particularly the case with prostitutes, who in any case may use condoms with clients, but prefer not to use them with in their more intimate relationships with boyfriends (see below).

Patterns of female and male prostitution

In many parts of the world, prostitution, both male and female, is an important source of HIV infection[46] – as it is of other sexually transmitted diseases. Like other forms of human behaviour, prostitution can only be fully understood in terms of the specific cultural and social *context* in which it appears. For example, the Western model of 'career' (or full-time) prostitution, tacitly tolerated by the authorities within a red light district, may not be applicable elsewhere. In many poorer countries, prostitution is a more complex phenomenon. It may involve, for example, what may be termed 'episodic prostitution', where – for economic reasons – women (and less commonly men) sell sex before or during marriage, or after being widowed or divorced. Their prostitution career may last only a few months or years, interspersed with marriage and/or childbearing. Thus, prostitutes are not a homogeneous group, and within the same city or region several *different* types of prostitution may be found. Carrier[40] notes how a study in Mexico identified nine different types of prostitutes selling their services to male clientele from all social classes: 'street walkers; itinerant travellers; dance hostesses and barmaids; taxi girls; professionals living in brothels; semi-professionals; lovers (*amantes*); call girls; and companions for parties or vacations'. Each of these types of commercial sexual activity offers different types of risk of AIDS transmission, and may well require a different form of intervention.

In most settings, *poverty* and the economic dependence of women are major causes of female prostitution, especially in its 'episodic' form. They may be widowed, divorced or abandoned by husbands, and forced into it to feed their families, or their husband may be too sick or elderly to work. In some parts of Africa they may have to repay the 'bridewealth' paid for them by their husband, after getting divorced, or if they do not wish to be 'inherited' by their dead husband's brother (see below). In their personal lives they may thus be wives, mothers or grandmothers, and have other sexual relationships that are not in any way commercial. In other cases, as described by Webb[30] in northern Namibia, 'transactional sex' may be a much more informal arrangement between adolescent boys and girls, or between a girl and an older man. However, prostitution is *not* the only economic strategy available to women in poorer regions; as Pickering and Wilkins[47] found in the Gambia, West Africa, there are other ways that divorced or widowed women can make a living, which do not involve selling sex – such as working as a laundress, hairdresser or cook, or selling groundnuts, fruit or alcohol.

Lyttleton[32] described how in Thailand urban dwellers earn nine times the income of rural people, and many 'commercial sex workers' from these poor villages will spend several years in Bangkok building up capital before returning to their villages to raise a family. In the rural areas themselves, commercial sex, though less common, also exists, and a more permissive attitude to sex has spread from city to countryside. In some cities, too, young female students occasionally sell sex at discos or in their dormitories.

Even if prostitutes are willing to adopt 'safe sex' practices, their clients (who have the ultimate economic control in the situation) may object. For example, Leonard's study[46] of 50 male clients of female prostitutes in Camden, New Jersey, showed that 29 had refused to use a condom. Despite being aware of the dangers involved, they tried to 'minimize' this risk by various strategies, including choosing a woman who looked 'clean', 'well-groomed', relatively inexperienced, or free of drugs. Others preferred oral to vaginal sex, believing it to be safer. Thus, because 'condom use is one of the most important points of negotiation for disease prevention between sex partners', AIDS prevention programmes should target not only prostitutes but their clients as well. However, as Waddell's study[45] in Perth, Australia suggests, even if prostitutes are willing to use condoms with clients, they may still refuse to use them in their more intimate relationships with boyfriends or husbands.

As well as female prostitution, male and bisexual commercial sex are a feature of several societies. These include different forms of male prostitution, such as the 'masculine' (*miche*) and more 'feminine' transvestites (*travesti*) in Brazil[38], and the *activo* and *pasivo* in Mexico[31]. In societies with a sexual double standard (as in many parts of Latin America[40] and elsewhere), where adolescent and young adult males are encouraged to have sex but their female counterparts are not, the risk of prostitute use may be increased. Similarly, in several parts of Africa[48] a late marriage age for men, often combined with the need to accumulate a large 'bridewealth' to pay a prospective wife's father, may also increase this risk.

Thus, interventions to reduce HIV transmission in prostitution need to take into account the economic, social and cultural context in which this type of behaviour takes place. They also need to consider the intimate emotional relationships in which prostitutes are involved, and their possible role in the transmission of the disease.

Intravenous drug use and needle-sharing

In the USA, intravenous drug users (IVDUs) are the second largest at risk group for AIDS[49]. In many other industrialized countries, the situation is similar; in Edinburgh, Scotland, for example, an estimated 60 per cent of the injecting drug users in the city are now HIV positive. In Spain, the spread of intravenous drug use in the population since 1978 has also lead to a wider diffusion of the AIDS virus throughout the country[50]. Increasingly, IVDUs have become an important source of HIV exposure for the heterosexual population.

Detailed ethnographic studies indicate that IVDUs, and the addict sub-cultures that they form, are *not* homogeneous; they vary in motivations, attitudes, sexual behaviours, social networks, the actual drugs they use and the techniques of injection that they employ. In most cases, however, the sharing of needles is a major source of HIV infection, though it sometimes overlaps with other at risk behaviours. Page and colleagues[49] studied 230 injecting drug users, most of them African-American, living in poor neighbourhoods in Miami, Florida. Of the sample, 104 were found to be HIV positive, and this was clearly correlated with their practice of needle sharing. In preparing for injection, not only were needles often shared among them, but many also cleaned their syringes in the same jar of water or drew their drugs from the same receptacle. In addition, 136 of the sample had, at one time or another in their lives, traded sex for money; of these people, 45 (33 women and 12 men) had worked as prostitutes for periods ranging from a few months to several years before the study began.

In another study of 438 IVDUs in San Francisco, Newmeyer and colleagues[51] found that more than 90 per cent of them admitted to recent sharing of needles and syringes (though only 9 per cent of the sample were HIV positive). While 86 per cent said they cleaned their needles between sharing episodes, this was not done consistently, and much of this cleaning consisted of only a simple water rinse. Part of the reason for needle sharing was that at that stage (1985–1986) there was a chronic shortage of needles, as public policy made it illegal to possess them (unless for certain 'medically arranged circumstances'). Newmeyer and colleagues suggest therefore that IVDUs could prevent the spread of AIDS in four ways: by stopping drug use completely; failing that, by not injecting the drugs; if injecting, by not sharing needles and other equipment; and by disinfecting the injecting equipment that is being shared. Their research indicated that only the last option would be acceptable to most IVDUs, and that it could be done effectively by cleaning equipment with household bleach. They also concluded, however, that because 'changing sexual practices of IVDUs will be more difficult than changing their needle-using behaviour', the focus of interventions should be mainly on the latter.

Sibthorpe[52], in a study in Oregon, examined the reasons why so many IVDUs refused to use condoms and practise 'safe sex'. Of the 161 drug users interviewed, the vast majority did *not* use condoms regularly (but 58 per cent of the sample saw their risk of contracting HIV as zero or slight). The use of condoms correlated with the types of sexual relationships they were involved in; the greater the social (and emotional) distance between partners (such as that between prostitute and client), the more likely they were to use them. In more intimate *relationships*, though, there was resistance to them; not using a condom was equated with love and trust – the very basis and proof of intimacy. Thus some prostitutes would use condoms with clients, but not with their husbands or boyfriends ('that's my man, that's the difference'). Sibthorpe points out that in the USA, AIDS prevention has focused on the 'personal responsibility model' of risky behaviours, rather than on the *relationships* in which they occur. Because sex within an intimate relationship is 'one of the bases of human social relations', condom use in these close relationships can be deeply threatening to both partners, signifying either guilt or suspicion and calling into question 'the commitment, attachment, and exclusivity' of the relationship. She therefore concludes that the 'greatest gains in safer sex practices can be expected in those relationships that only minimally affirm social bonds', while in more intimate relationships, changing to condom use may be much more difficult.

Thus, as Page and colleagues[49] warn, 'inter-community variations in self-injection practices are potentially infinite, and each variant may be accompanied by different kinds of risks of HIV infection'. For this reason, strategies developed for one country, region, city or community may not be completely appropriate for another, and *local* conditions must always be taken into account.

Traditional and alternative healers and AIDS

Studies of health care pluralism (see Chapter 4) in both richer and poorer parts of the world are also relevant to AIDS research. As in other serious diseases, such as cancer, chronic pain or disability[53], for which medicine can offer no 'quick fix', many AIDS patients may choose to use different types of self-treatment or to consult with traditional or alternative practitioners. Self-treatment is especially common in the industrialized world (see below). In a study in gay men with AIDS in West Hollywood, California[54], for example, while 92 per cent were currently using biomedical treatments, 69.2 per cent were also using one or more alternative therapies at the same time, and a further 19.3 per cent had used them in the past. Thus, only 11.5 per cent had never made use of any form of alternative therapy.

In some cases, communities may consult traditional or religious healers in an attempt to prevent the disease striking in the first place, and these healers may become useful allies in controlling the spread of the disease. In Botswana, Ingstad[24] describes how the various traditional Tswana healers – such as the *ngaka ya diatola* ('doctor of the bones'), *ngaka ya dishotswa* ('doctor of herbs') and *profiti* (a 'prophet' of the Independent African Churches) – often have different attitudes to the origins and treatment of AIDS. Some see it as a 'modern disease', which traditional medicine is unable to help. Others see it as a 'Tswana disease', a version of *meila* (an indigenous folk illness) that they could treat by traditional methods. In this condition, disease and misfortune are ascribed to the breaking of sexual taboos, which forbid intercourse within certain periods of time – such as during menstruation or shortly after childbirth. This makes men vulnerable to 'pollution' originating within the female body (in her blood), which the man can then transmit to any other women with whom he has intercourse. As with AIDS, blood and semen are seen as the vehicles for transmission of the 'pollution'. Ingstad suggests that in the future Tswana traditional healers may have an important role to play in AIDS prevention by, for example, encouraging the use of condoms: 'Advocating condoms as a way to prevent *meila* probably carries more incentive than advocating them to prevent pregnancy or other sexually transmitted diseases'.

In terms of the *treatments* for AIDS offered by non-medical healers in different cultures, further studies are urgently needed on their efficacy (or lack of efficacy). It should be noted, however, that in some cases folk definitions of efficacy may be different from those of biomedicine. For example, both religious and secular forms of symbolic healing (see Chapter 10) may be very helpful to sufferers and their families, for they may be able to 'heal' the individual, even if they cannot 'cure' the disease. On the other hand, other forms of folk and alternative healing may have a more negative effect on health. Injectionists, acupuncturists and those who practise ritual scarifications, bleeding or 'cupping' may all inadvertently help the spread of the disease. In either case, anthropology can contribute towards an understanding of the social, psychological and physical effects (on the immune system, for example) not only of secular folk remedies such as herbs, massage, moxibustion, but also of the different forms of symbolic healing practised world-wide.

Finally, it is possible that some IVDUs regard themselves, however perversely, as 'healer's in their own right, seeing the drugs that they ritually inject into themselves and others as a form of medicine for the physical and psychological symptoms of withdrawal. In that sense, they are acting as what may be termed 'auto-injectionists'.

Case study: Alternative approaches to HIV and AIDS in the USA

O'Connor[55] has described the many forms of self-treatment and alternative strategies now being used in the USA, especially by gay men in the PWA (people with AIDS) community. Since the mid-1980s there has been a well-organized grass-roots response to the epidemic, with the proliferation of self-help organizations and networks of information. They aim not only to help those with the disease, but also to promote further research and different forms of treatment, especially as conventional medicine seems to offer little but palliation. She describes dozens of alternative or complementary forms of self-treatment, including:

- nutritional approaches, such as macrobiotic and yeast-free diets, the 'Immune Power Diet', food supplements, antioxidants, and mega-doses of vitamins or minerals
- herbal treatments, such as echinacea, ginseng, garlic, St John's wort, aloe vera, astragalus or Bach flower essences
- homeopathic treatments, such as nux vomica for severe nausea, or arnica for muscular pains)

continued

- traditional Chinese medicine, both herbal preparations and acupuncture
- New Age holistic approaches, such as guided imagery, visualization, therapeutic touch, *reiki*, *Qi Dong* or crystal healing
- psychological and metaphysical approaches, such as religious healing services, prayer, and positive thinking to increase 'psycho-immunity'
- conventional pharmaceuticals used in 'unofficial' ways, or before being given official approval (such as 'underground drugs' obtained from 'guerrilla clinics', treatment study groups or from abroad). O'Connor points out that most of these treatments are intended to *supplement* rather than supplant conventional medical treatment. For the PWAs, they are ways of taking personal responsibility for their health, and asserting their rights and expertise in their own condition and its treatment.

Bodily mutilations and alterations

As described in Chapter 2, many of the forms of bodily mutilations practised world-wide can involve risks to health. Among those that may help spread the HIV virus are tattooing, scarification, circumcisions, ear and lip piercing, and the sharing of blood in ceremonies marking membership of a cult or 'blood brotherhood'. Rituals where blood is regularly spilt – by self-flagellation or piercing of the skin – may also sometimes be implicated. *All* forms of bodily mutilation should therefore be taken into account when planning an AIDS prevention programme. Where a particular cultural group is unwilling to abandon these practices, aid workers may be able to convince them to use sterile needles and instruments and disinfectants (for circumcision or scarification, for example), and to supply these free of charge where necessary.

Patterns of migration and the spread of AIDS

Studies of regular patterns of population movement, such as those of migrant labourers, seasonal farm workers, truck drivers, travelling businessmen or tourists, are relevant to an understanding of how AIDS spreads within and between different countries. Where people (usually men) migrate as individuals rather than as part of an established family unit, there is a greater risk of acquiring sexually transmitted diseases, including AIDS. For example, Webb's study[30] of the Owambo region of Namibia indicated a number of transmission routes of HIV infection linked to population movements. These included:

- migrant labourers working in mines and urban areas in the south of the country, who had sexual relations there during their absence from home
- traders and truck drivers who travelled regularly along the main trunk road from the south (HIV infection tended to cluster in areas closest to the roadside, where traffic densities were greatest)
- military personnel stationed at various bases in the area (many of whom had previously lived in Zambia and Angola, during the war for independence).

In Thailand, too, Lyttleton[32] described how large numbers of seasonally migrating workers (including prostitutes) as well as about 200 000 truck drivers 'many of whom ply the length and breadth of the country, stopping at the many truck-stop brothels', may also aid the spread of the disease. As well as these more regular population movements, the creation of refugees – especially the mass uprooting of people by war or civil unrest – may also be related to an increased incidence of certain diseases, including AIDS.

Finally, the process of migration into cities is also important since, in some cases, social constraints on behaviour may be less powerful than they would be in small rural communities. Overcrowding, contact with people from different backgrounds and exposure to advertising and the media may all weaken these social constraints in an urban environment, and increase the incidence of alcoholism, drug abuse, teenage pregnancies and sexually transmitted diseases – especially AIDS. In other cases, population movements to the city may follow a more circular pattern, with newly urbanized people maintaining close links with their rural roots and traditional values, and returning there regularly to visit their families, and *vice versa*.

Marriage and kinship patterns

In different cultures, certain patterns of kinship and marriage may sometimes increase the risk of the HIV virus spreading within a community. These include polygyny and polyandry (see Chapter 10), 'ghost marriage' and 'women marriage' (see Chapter 6). Polygyny is particularly important, since the Embers[56] estimate that it is still practised in some form in about 70 per cent of human societies. In this situation, a husband who has contracted the HIV virus may thus pass it on to several women, and then on to their children. In addition, some societies which practise the *levirate* (or 'widow inheritance'), where a man is obliged to marry his brother's widow, or the *sororate*, where a woman is obliged to marry her deceased sister's husband[56], may also be more at risk of the spread of AIDS. In the industrialized world, where the rates of separation, divorce and remarriage are greatly increasing, the effect may sometimes be similar.

Evaluation of preventive strategies

Anthropology is useful in the follow-up or *evaluation* of preventive strategies. Because of the diversity of at-risk groups, local interventions are usually also necessary in addition to national (or international) public health campaigns[30,32]. In many communities, outreach programmes have been successful in bringing information about AIDS prevention (as well as condoms and other items) to different communities, and to particular groups of people within them. Daly and Horton[57] point out that 'the best workers are often recruited from the target group itself', whatever that is. Thus some outreach programmes have recruited prostitutes as, in effect, 'community health workers', encouraging them to distribute condoms, spread information about AIDS and refuse to have unprotected sex with their clients.

In San Francisco, community health outreach workers (CHOWs) were used to convince IVDUs of the value of sterilizing their injecting equipment with household bleach, and together with educational literature they handed out thousands of 1-oz bottles of bleach to them. In London and other European cities, 'needle exchanges' have been set up to supply sterile needles and syringes to addicts, free of charge and with no questions asked.

In Thailand, Lyttleton[32] has described how the comprehensive National AIDS Program, begun in 1989, provides considerable information about AIDS prevention to the population, especially via the media and in schools, clinics and hospitals. At the level of the rural village, however, local custom and belief may make this information less effective in altering behaviour. In one north-eastern village, for example, the people saw some of the at-risk behaviours, including visiting prostitutes, as 'something belonging to city lifestyles' rather than their own. The overemphasis on prostitution as a source of AIDS meant that for some men, sleeping with several different village women is not 'promiscuous', unlike a single visit to a CSW' (commercial health worker). Others avoided cheaper prostitutes, whom they perceived as more likely carriers, but instead used 'good girls', such as students. So many men disliked using condoms that some prostitutes did not insist on their use on every occasion, especially if the clients were 'local government officials who pull rank', young men claiming to be virgins who wanted their first experience to be 'natural', and men regarded as 'respectable' or who were regular clients. Thus Lyttleton emphasizes that, in addition to national campaigns about avoiding at risk behaviours, 'to understand the spread of HIV, both real and potential, the local meaning attached to these acts is essential knowledge'.

Some AIDS prevention programmes may also fail because they assume, quite erroneously, a high level of literacy in their target population, or even access to radio or television. Others may neglect to take into account *economic* influences on behaviour, such as widowed, divorced or abandoned women being forced to work as prostitutes in order to feed their families, or poor village girls in Thailand having to work for several years in the city in order to accumulate money for their future[32]. Other economic constraints include the inability to afford basic medical treatment, including drugs, tests, hospitalization and rehabilitation, and a lack of money to buy condoms or bleach (in the case of IVDUs) or to travel to a clinic to get them. For example, prostitutes who have many clients in a single night may be unable to afford to supply each with a condom, even if these are available. In poorer countries the economic *impact* of AIDS is substantial, especially in terms of health care costs and reduction in the labour force, and any programme must take these facts into account.

A further aspect of programme evaluation is an assessment of the role of national and international *bureaucracies* in education, research and the provision of medical care (see below). As well as their institutional sub-cultures (which may either help, or reduce their effectiveness), the economic, political[58] and religious influences on AIDS prevention programmes also need to be assessed, as do the human rights of those who have the disease[59]. The attitudes of health professionals may also have a negative effect on AIDS surveillance and treatment. Some studies have shown how many AIDS victims still distrust the medical system to provide them with effective and non-judgmental health care. For example, a study of 632 homosexual men in England[60] found that 44 per cent of them had never informed their general practitioners of their sexual orientation, and that of the 77 who were HIV positive, 44 per cent had not told them of this fact.

Overall, the medical system's tendency towards 'cure' rather than 'care', and its emphasis on the physical rather than the psychological, social and cultural aspects of ill health (see Chapter 5), means that input from anthropologists and other social scientists is urgently needed in both the planning and evaluation of AIDS prevention programmes. Furthermore, the success of a programme should always be monitored not only from the perspective of the medical authorities but also from that of the at-risk community themselves, and where possible they should assist in helping to design more effective interventions in the future.

Primary health care

In 1978, the World Health Organization issued its famous declaration in Alma-Ata of 'Health for All by the Year 2000'[61]. This ambitious plan aimed to develop, throughout the world, a *comprehensive* system of primary health care (PHC). The programme was to consist, as Mull[62] puts it, of 'essential health care made universally accessible to individuals and families by means acceptable to them, with their full participation, and at a cost that they, their community and the country as a whole could afford'. As part of the comprehensive approach, health care was to be accompanied by improved health education, nutrition, sanitation, immunizations, family planning, maternal and child health, and the supply of essential drugs (see Chapter 8). Above all, it represented a move away from the curative, 'quick fix', centralized medical model towards a more preventive, decentralized and *community*-based strategy[62].

This comprehensive approach was seen as crucial in tackling global health problems, especially in Third World countries. In these poorer countries, infant and child mortality rates are many times higher than those in the industrialized world. It has been estimated that 12 million children die of poverty every year[3], many of them from preventable or treatable diseases. These deaths occur mainly from infectious diseases such as respiratory illnesses, neonatal tetanus, diarrhoeal diseases, polio, diphtheria, pertussis, measles, rubella, tuberculosis, cholera, typhoid and yellow fever[63]. Others die from parasitic diseases such as malaria, bilharzia, leishmaniasis and, increasingly, from AIDS and hepatitis B. Most of these causes of early death are associated, directly or indirectly, with *poverty*, and can be either prevented or treated – as they have been in most industrialized countries.

Critics of the plan for world-wide comprehensive PHC pointed out its considerable cost, the shortage of available health care personnel and the practical difficulties of community participation. Some health planners suggested instead a more *selective* form of PHC that would focus on specific health problems (such as diarrhoeal diseases), especially those of infants and children. The policy of 'child survival' became paramount, and has now been adopted in some form by most organizations involved in international health. Its strategies have been summarized by UNICEF as 'GOBI-FF'[61–63], that is:

*G*rowth monitoring
*O*ral rehydration
*B*reast-feeding
*I*mmunization
*F*amily planning
*F*ood supplements.

A further '*F*' was added, for '*F*emale literacy'[64], since there is evidence that higher levels of maternal literacy are associated with a decrease in both the birth rate and in infant mortality rates[63]. This is due, among other reasons, to women being able to read health-related pamphlets or information, and the instructions on containers of medicines.

Mull[62] has criticized selective PHC for its narrower approach, instead of Alma-Ata's more comprehensive strategy, and its emphasis on community participation and empowerment: it advocates 'dealing with measurable disease entities so that quantifiable results could be produced at the lowest possible cost'. He also points out that GOBI-FFF targets mainly children and younger women, while ignoring the rest of the community. Men, too, need to be involved in health care interventions, since many may not necessarily follow their wives' or mothers' health advice. To prevent them drinking, smoking, being too competitive or adopting at-risk sexual behaviours, health interventions may have to be brought to them in the workplace or via (male) community leaders. Also, as Green[65] found in Bangladesh, although women provided the main care for children, it was the men who decided which medicine to buy if the children were ill.

Despite the conceptual split between the 'comprehensive' and 'selective' approaches to PHC, Mull[62] points out that in many international aid programmes a pragmatic fusion of the two has actually taken place; for example, a 'top-down' and selective focus on a particular health problem (such as diarrhoeal illnesses) combined with interventions that improve nutrition, sanitation, water supplies, female literacy and popular participation at the community level.

Problems of GOBI-FFF

Some of the specific problems associated with applying each aspect of the GOBI-FFF strategy have been described in more detail earlier in this book. They include oral rehydration therapy (Chapter 1), breast-feeding and food supplements (Chapter 3), and family planning (above). In many cases, both organizational and local cultural factors may make them difficult to apply. For example, although paediatricians agree on the value of growth monitoring (mainly height and weight) as a way of identifying malnutrition or other developmental problems, it can also be seen as a Western, culture-bound way of defining 'health'. As described in Chapter 5, the numerical definitions used to define 'normality' may not match indigenous beliefs about whether a child is healthy or not. Parents may see a child as 'healthy' if he or she can smile, play, talk, respond affectionately, or perform certain domestic or ritual tasks, irrespective of its height and weight. Furthermore, some mothers may fear the envy of others if, at the clinic, their own child is found to be more 'normal' than other children, or they may fear being accused of witchcraft or 'evil eye' if the situation is reversed. The next section will concentrate mainly on immunizations and on the prevention and treatment of diarrhoeal and respiratory diseases, including tuberculosis.

Immunizations

An estimated 5 million children die each year from diseases preventable by immunizations[62]. Heggenhougen and Clements[66] point out two key problems faced in trying to immunize a large proportion of the world's population:

1. The technical and organizational problems of making vaccines available to those who need them (this includes the need for a 'cold chain', whereby vaccines remain at a constant low temperature from the place of production to the site of immunization)
2. The need to increase acceptability of vaccines, even when they are available.

The technical issues include the cost, production and efficacy of the vaccines, and how they are distributed. Organizational problems include: when and how immunization campaigns are to be put into practice; whether they should target particularly vulnerable groups or the entire population; whether they should be separate, or integrated with the rest of PHC; how communication with the community can be effectively organized; and whether local healers, such as traditional birth attendants, should be involved in the campaign. However, they point out that immunizations alone often do not reduce overall mortality rates unless *other* issues, such as malnutrition, are also dealt with. Overall, there is thus 'a need to be aware that immunizations do not represent a magic, or universal protection against all ill'. In terms of acceptability, they link low levels of acceptability with a number of factors, including: low socio-economic status; large families; low educational level of mothers; social isolation; and migrant status (including nomadic lifestyles). Coverage for handicapped or otherwise disadvantaged children has also been shown to be low, as has been that for girls in comparison to boys. By contrast, those 'predisposed to immunization' tend to believe that their susceptibility to a disease is high, that the consequences of getting it would be serious, that immunization is the most effective way of preventing it, and that there are no serious barriers to immunization.

Certain indigenous beliefs may either help or impede immunization campaigns; in general, in order for these to be successful they should somehow 'make sense' in terms of people's own perceptions of ill health. Nichter[67] points out that limited information combined with some local beliefs may lead to fears or false expectations of a particular immunization campaign. In his study in south India, he found that only 11 per cent of the households in North Kanara district, and 28 per cent in South Kanara, had a family member who had been informed as to the illness prevented by the immunization they had received. In most cases, health workers had merely told them that 'vaccinations are good for health and they prevent disease'. Some pregnant women thought that vaccinations were 'tonic injections' that would cause them to have big babies, and thus difficult deliveries. Told by health workers that the vaccines were powerful 'health injections', other people thought that they were too strong for a body in a 'weakened' state, such as a child who was weak or ill, especially with fever, productive cough or diarrhoea. Others thought that vaccines, like ear piercing or ritual scarification, 'shocked' the body back to health. Other beliefs about vaccines included that they removed 'toxins' from the body, protected against *all* serious infectious diseases as well as mystical illnesses such as *krimi*, were 'long-lasting doses of antibiotic' that travelled all over the body to reduce illness, and reduced children's future fertility. Furthermore, many people did not trust the competence of the PHC staff administering the injections, especially if they were outsiders and not accountable to the community. On the other hand, health workers in those target communities might sometimes be reluctant to give immunizations, for fear of being blamed if they fail to work or if they cause side effects. Where side effects to a particular vaccine do occur, mothers often reject all other forms of vaccination on the assumption that they are all 'similar', and therefore have similar bad reactions.

Nichter further points out that while there are advantages in health workers' identifying a vaccine by the name of an illness with which people are familiar (such as whooping cough), this may be more difficult where the disease to be prevented has a vaguer, more diffuse clinical picture (such as a rash or fever). Also, in many cases people believe that a vaccine may protect against a specific disease or a range of diseases that they fear, even if this is not the case. For example, in his research in south Kanara[68], Nichter found that while 50 per cent of mothers surveyed thought that vaccinations protected their children against specific illnesses (such as polio, or TB), 28 per cent thought that they protected them against all 'big' or serious illnesses found in that community. He points out therefore that these false expectations may contribute to the perception among many people that vaccinations are not very effective.

Finally, the members of a community may not understand why only children, and sometimes women, are the main targets of vaccination campaigns, while men and older children are ignored. They might advance a whole range of conspiracy and political theories to explain why they, too, are not being given the powerful 'government injections' said to enhance health and protect against disease[68].

Overall, an understanding of indigenous ideas about both diseases and vaccines is therefore crucial to the success of any immunization programme. As Heggenhougen and Clements[66] put it, 'messages which contradict beliefs, habits and action which people have invested with time, effort and resources and around which people have based their lives, will require considerably more force, ingenuity, and/or repetition in order to impress than messages which agree with their way of doing things'.

Diarrhoeal diseases

Some of the issues related to diarrhoeal diseases, and the acceptance of oral rehydration solution (ORS), have already been discussed in Chapter 1. These diseases, which kill about 5–7 million people every year, are largely linked to *poverty*, with the resultant poor nutrition, water supplies, housing, sanitation and garbage disposal. Before diarrhoeal illnesses can be permanently reduced, or eliminated, these socio-economic issues will have to be addressed[69]. In addition, Weiss[70] has described the many *cultural* explanations found world-wide about the origin, significance or treatment of diarrhoeal illnesses. For example, in many cultural groups (including in Latin America and South Asia) they are blamed on an imbalance of 'heat' and 'cold' either within the body or in the environment. In other groups, 'bad breast milk', heavy foods, dirt or pollution may be blamed. Supernatural causes (see Chapter 5) of diarrhoeal illnesses include the evil eye, witch-craft, sorcery, malign spirits, divine punishment, contact with a menstruating woman, parental sexual infidelity, or having sex during pregnancy or lactation. Indigenous treatments may involve herbal remedies, patent medicines, religious rituals, changes in diet or breast-feeding, and even 'cleansing the gastrointestinal tract with enemas, purgatives, and emetics'.

Nichter[71] stresses the importance of understanding whether communities differentiate between ordinary (usually viral) diarrhoea and the more dangerous *dysentery* (due to bacteria such as *shigella*). As well as ORS, the latter may require antibiotic treatment, and often hospitalization. He points out that in some communities the bloody diarrhoea associated with dysentery may be considered more serious than the more watery, secretory diarrhoea, but in others the situation may be reversed. In Mindoro, in the Philippines, for example, he found that the emphasis by health workers on the dangers of dehydration meant that villagers feared the (less severe) form of watery diarrhoea more than dysentery. Fever and pain, not blood in the stools *per se*, were seen as reasons for going to the clinic. In Sri Lanka, bloody diarrhoea is associated with 'heat' trapped in the body, and is treated by ingesting 'cooling substances', as well as medicines and ORS. Some people refuse antibiotics, though, which they see as 'dangerous heating agents for bloody diarrhoea'. By contrast, others refuse ORS for watery diarrhoea, 'because cultural common sense dictates drying up watery stool'.

Both community health workers and traditional healers have been used to promote the use of ORT within their communities. However, these healers are not a homogeneous group, and often vary in their knowledge of ORT and in their willingness to use it. In Montrouis, Haiti, for example, Coreil[72] found that while 74 per cent of mothers had heard of ORT, only 51 per cent of healers had. Of all the healers, 32 per cent had taught mothers about ORT, and 2 per cent had used it themselves. Midwives and 'injectionists' were more knowledgeable about ORT, and more willing to use it, than were both herbalists and shamans. Of all the traditional healers, traditional birth attendants – because of their close involvement in maternal and infant care – are probably best placed for advising mothers on the benefits of ORT.

Respiratory infections: acute and chronic

In most of the Third World, *acute respiratory infections* (ARIs) are one of the major causes of death in infants and young children under 5 years of age. In India, for example, an estimated 500 000–750 000 children die of these infections every year[73]. The ARIs most commonly implicated are pneumonia, bronchitis, bronchiolitis and tuberculosis. Like diarrhoeal diseases, they are often associated with poverty and deprivation, and sometimes complicate other childhood infections such as measles and pertussis.

As with diarrhoeal illnesses, anthropological studies of ARIs have examined indigenous beliefs and practices, forms of traditional healing, and attitudes to medical treatments[73]. Local perceptions of these conditions are particularly important, since they may influence the point at which parents define them as potentially dangerous (and seek further help), and also whether this occurs before or after the infection has had a chance to spread to the rest of the family or community. These indigenous beliefs may include, for example, notions of 'normal' and 'abnormal' ways of breathing, the significance of different types of cough, wheeze, phlegm or fever, and so on. In terms of explaining the origin and significance of ARIs, many of the lay theories of illness aetiology described in Chapter 5 also apply. Another important issue is the use of Western pharmaceuticals (such as antibiotics) bought over-the-counter from local pharmacies or medicine vendors (see Chapter 8), since these may lead to the development of resistant strains of bacteria responsible for ARIs. The important role of anthropological insights in developing preventive and treatment strategies for these illnesses has been recognized by WHO, with its Programme for the Control of Acute Respiratory Infections[74].

Among more chronic respiratory diseases, *tuberculosis* (TB) is the most serious. Globally, about 1700 million people are or have been afflicted by the disease[75]. Every year, an estimated 8 million cases of TB occur worldwide, as well as about 3 million deaths from the disease; 95–99 per cent of these deaths occur in developing countries[75]. The WHO's *World Health Report 1995*[76] estimated that the disease was responsible for about 7000 deaths every day, and that in 1995 there would be 8.8 million new cases of the disease. Usually it is a disease of poverty, associated with poor nutrition, overcrowding and inadequate health care. Recently, however, cases of TB in the Western world have been increasing, often in poor inner-city neighbourhoods, and sometimes in association with AIDS or other diseases. One estimate was that, by the year 2000, some 1.4 million cases of tuberculosis (14 per cent of the global total) will be associated with HIV infection[77]. Attempts to treat it and control its spread have encountered a number of social and cultural problems. According to a review by Rubel and Garro[78], the two main barriers to successful control are a delay in seeking treatment and the abandonment of treatment before it becomes effective. Cultural beliefs about the significance of early symptoms of the disease play a particularly important part. For example, a study they carried out among Mexican migrant workers in southern California found considerable delays (8½ months on average) between the onset of symptoms and the decision to consult a doctor. Many of them misinterpreted their early symptoms – such as cough, fatigue, loss of weight, headaches, back pains or running nose – as evidence of less serious conditions, such as *gripe* (grippe) or *bronquitis* (bronchitis), or even *susto* (see Chapter 5). Many attributed their fatigue and weight loss to hard work and lack of sleep, and initially treated themselves by smoking and drinking less, going to sleep earlier, using patent medicines and leading what they perceived to be a healthier lifestyle. A further reason for treatment delay (as well as its early abandonment) is the marked *stigma* associated with the disease in many parts of the world. The authors quote a study among Zulu in South Africa, which found that to suggest that sufferers from TB were infectious was tantamount to identifying them as witches or sorcerers, since these were the only people in that community with the power to cause illness to other people. A study in Mexico City showed that 52 per cent of patients discharged from hospital after treatment for TB were not allowed to go home due to the hostility of their families; another showed that many patients had abandoned their treatment early due to the costs of transport to the clinic, a dread of family disintegration, and fear of rejection by their families (25 per cent of the defaulters had not told their families of their true diagnosis). Since successful completion of treatment is associated with good social support from the family, the stigma associated with the disease may be one reason why attempts to control it can fail. Other reasons for failure relate to the health care system itself, and the ways that TB clinics are organized. For example, arranging appointments at inconvenient times, repeating registration of patients at every visit, seating people in overcrowded and poorly ventilated waiting rooms, seeing them rigidly in order of registration (and ignoring any extenuating circumstances), and physicians using technical jargon when talking to patients, may all contribute to people's reluctance to come to a clinic for treatment or follow-up. Thus, there are many reasons for the persistence of TB and the failure of treatment, including its cost and availability. In designing more effective interventions, Rubel and Garrow suggest that it is necessary to assess 'how people use knowledge to interpret symptoms of this chronic, debilitating disease at the time that they seek help and how their help-seeking decision is influenced by financial, transport and other considerations'.

Case study: Folk models of tuberculosis in Dongora, southern Ethiopia

Vecchiato[79] described folk beliefs about tuberculosis, and self-treatments, in a farming community of the Sidama people in southern Ethiopia. Despite a high prevalence of tuberculosis in that area, and despite the fact that no social stigma was attached to it, only a fraction of the cases presented themselves to the local clinic. However, most Sidama did recognize the symptoms of the disease, which they blamed either on over-work or on poor nutrition (though some accepted that it spread by contagion, or by 'inhaling dust particles'). However, 52.1 per cent believed that traditional remedies (*Sidama taghiccho*) were much more effective in treating tuberculosis than modern ones, while only 37.8 per cent preferred the latter. Traditional treatments included eating a nutritious diet (especially meat, milk and *ensete* porridge), ingesting several types of herbal remedies (mostly used as emetics, to vomit out the 'bad blood' that accumulates internally), or getting a traditional healer (*oghessa*) to apply smouldering wooden rods to 'cauterize' the diseased parts of the body, especially the chest. Vecchiato noted that one reason that anti-tuberculosis drugs such as streptomycin were often rejected was that they have no emetic effect, and suggests that future anti-TB programmes take into account these indigenous beliefs, and work with them where possible. As a starting point, they should acknowledge that the Sindama *can* accurately diagnose pulmonary TB, that they do have a sense of diseases being contagious, and that they do see the value of a highly nutritious diet when ill. He also suggests that attempts be made to discover whether traditional herbal remedies are effective in treating TB, or not.

Community resources in PHC

The emphasis in the Alma-Ata declaration on *community participation* in PHC has meant that a number of community resources have been used to facilitate PHC at the local level. These include:

1. Community health workers
2. Community health groups
3. Traditional healers
4. Community leaders.

Community health workers (CHWs) are generally members of a particular community whose task is to improve the health of that community, often in co-operation with the health care system or with national or international aid agencies. They may be selected by their communities, though sometimes this is done by local leaders or by outside agencies. They advise the community on preventive strategies and give advice on child care, healthy nutrition, immunizations and hygiene, as well as providing some limited curative and first-aid services; in addition, many become more general agents for change in the community, in areas outside the health field. Since Alma-Ata, many thousands have been selected and trained, in 62 many different countries, and in both rural and urban areas[80]. They include the 'barefoot doctors' in China, the 'family welfare educators' in Botswana, the 'village health development workers' in Indonesia, the 'village health volunteers' in Thailand and the 'community health agents' in Egypt. In most cases, CHWs are given a short course of training – usually a few weeks to a few months – and a small amount of equipment, such as a few basic drugs, some dressings, disinfectants, thermometer, and scales and charts for measuring the weights and heights of children. In some countries, the training of CHWs has been much more extensive – such as that of the *feldsher*[81], or physician's assistants, in rural parts of Russia and the former USSR, who have provided some basic PHC at the village level since Peter the Great founded them in the eighteenth century, and whose training currently lasts up to 2½ years[81].

However, the use of CHWs is still controversial. For one thing, their selection and training raises the problems of how 'community', 'health' and 'worker' are each defined. The definition of a 'community', for example, may be a bureaucratic fiction, imposed on a disparate group of people by some distant official or aid agency with little local knowledge. For one thing, these communities are not static; many are in a constant state of flux, as some people migrate in from rural areas while others leave in search of work. Nor are they homogeneous. Slums and shanty towns, especially those with a high proportion of rural migrants, often have many different communities within them – formed by people from the same village or region, or based on different religious, ethnic or social backgrounds. Each micro-community, and often each gender, may have very different attitudes to health and illness, and utilize a different range of traditional cures and healers (see Chapter 4).

Definitions of 'health' are also problematic since, as illustrated throughout this book, medical and lay definitions of health are often very different. Which definition, then, is the CHW meant to promote? If these workers are seen to be merely the agents of the health service, can this reduce their credibility in the eyes of their community? Finally, many of these CHWs are not 'workers' in the formal sense; most are unpaid volunteers, or receive very little money for their time and effort.

Another argument against CHWs is that, with their limited period of training, they are not 'real' health practitioners, and can only provide 'second-class health care for second-class citizens'. In many cases, ill people prefer consulting a 'real' doctor, whatever the cost, effort or travel involved. A follow-up study of Tanzanian CHWs[82], for example, found that although the community was generally in favour of them, they (and the CHWs themselves) were primarily interested in them providing *curative* rather than preventive services. Also, 53 per cent of the 344 CHWs interviewed had had no supervisory visit from any health agency in the previous 3 months. The combination of inadequate diagnostic and treatment skills, infrequent supervision and shortage of drugs undermined the acceptance of CHWs by their communities; despite this, they were seen as a valuable resource, and 88 per cent of those trained since 1983 were still active 5 years later.

Other local resources may be *community health groups*, which are organized to share information about health issues (such as the importance of family planning, breast-feeding or immunizations) and to give help to their members. Many are women's groups, especially antenatal and mother-and-baby groups, and are often facilitated

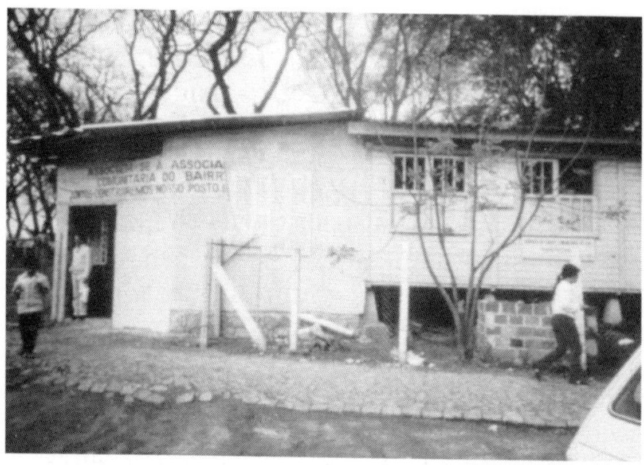

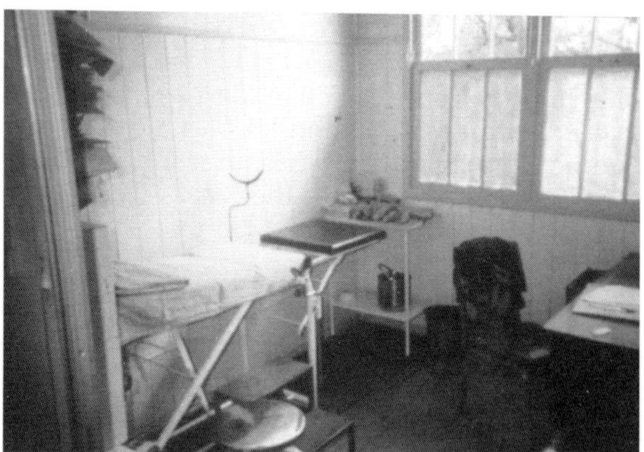

Figure 13.2 A primary health care clinic in a *favela* or shanty town in Porto Alegre, southern Brazil, built and run in co-operation with the local community (Source: Cecil Helman).

by local CHWs. *Traditional healers* have also been promoted as an intrinsic part of PHC, and some of the arguments for and against them have been summarized in Chapter 4. In some cases the roles of CHW and traditional healer may overlap, either directly or indirectly due to familial links. In the author's study in Porto Alegre, southern Brazil, for example, the majority of the 150 community health workers (*agente de saúde*) recruited to work in the shanty towns (*favelas*) had at least one traditional healer in their family tree. The intention of WHO has been to involve traditional healers in PHC, for example in the Essential Drugs Programme (see Chapter 8), but without causing too much disruption to local cultural patterns[83]. That is:

> the establishment of primary health care services in developing countries should not result in abrupt disruption of prevailing cultural patterns in rural communities. The work of traditional healers, for example, should be adapted and supplemented so as to ensure that innovation is successfully integrated into existing systems of care.

A final resource used in PHC are *community leaders*, or people of influence – such as local schoolteachers, religious figures or political leaders – since their co-operation might be vital for the success of any health care initiative. In many systems of PHC, these community resources are often combined with local clinics or 'health posts' situated in villages or urban shanty towns and staffed by doctors, nurses or other health professionals, often in co-operation with CHWs. More serious cases would then be referred to regional district hospitals, or sometimes to more specialized hospitals elsewhere. To some extent, this shift towards a community-based PHC also means a shift away from a medical model that has become increasingly expensive, over-specialized and over-dependent on technology. It also implies the development of a new kind of doctor, who sees successful PHC as not only an applied medical science, but as an applied social science as well.

The role of anthropologists in PHC

Since Alma-Ata, many anthropologists have been involved in the planning, application and evaluation of PHC programmes[62–64], and in increasing community participation in health care. As well as their expertise in local cultures, health beliefs and practices and traditional forms of healing, Donahue[84] sees their role as 'culture brokers', mediating between the needs of local communities and those of the health care system: 'Anthropologists can provide direct feedback to the community which they have studied. Their knowledge of the structural–cognitive systems of both the traditional and the modern medical systems allows them to find points of articulation between the two'. Mars[1] suggests that 'in an attempt to link social reality to social planning', medical aid programmes should develop a network of 'barefoot anthropologists' – and one trained anthropologist could, with the aid of locally recruited assistants, monitor up to 10 small-scale communities and facilitate a two-way communication in order to modify and influence more centralized policy decisions.

It should be stressed, however, that 'anthropologist' is not necessarily synonymous with 'Western anthropologist'. In many different contexts, especially in non-Western countries, it is those anthropologists and other social scientists that come from those countries (or even from those communities) who may be the best people to act as consultants and researchers. These people, who understand the subtleties of local custom and belief and are native speakers of the language, may be better able to avoid the 'cultural imprint of the West' inherent in many PHC programmes (see below). This type of input is crucial in community-based PHC, since these programmes have often been developed by a distant international bureaucracy in Europe or North America, or by a national urban elite with little knowledge of local conditions in rural areas or in the poorer neighbourhoods of their own cities.

PHC and cultural concepts of time

One important reason for the failure of health education and preventive strategies, in PHC and elsewhere, is a difference in the perception of *time* between health planners and local communities. Many of these programmes are designed by middle-class individuals and targeted on people much poorer than themselves, and much of the health education is based on what may be termed a 'middle-class investment model'. That is, 'invest' in yourself now (by education, savings, a nutritious diet, avoiding smoking, using a condom, and 'deferring gratification'), and this behaviour will result in your reaping a 'profit' (or 'interest' on your 'investment') many years in the future. In terms of health, this profit will be in the form of better physical health, a better quality of life and increased life expectancy. However, this approach ignores the daily reality of people living precarious, poverty-stricken lives. The daily, sometimes hourly, struggle for survival – for food, shelter, money and safety – of many people living in slum or shanty town communities, especially where there is no social welfare system, means that they live in a very short time span. People living this precarious existence may not be able to plan more than a day or two ahead; to expect them, for example, to avoid smoking so that in 15 or 20 years time they will not develop lung cancer or heart disease is simply impractical, especially with adolescents and younger people – who also have a very different sense of time. As well as changing the socio-economic realities in which they are embedded, programmes in health education need to stress the short-term benefits of a change in behaviour. They may also need to break down long-term health interventions into much shorter time units (such as the 'day at a time' approach of Alcoholics Anonymous) in order to reflect the way different people experience time in their daily lives.

Socio-economic considerations and PHC

As mentioned earlier, many of the health problems addressed by comprehensive PHC are the result, direct or indirect, of poverty – especially the inability to afford adequate food, housing, clothing, sanitation, garbage removal, transport and health care[85].

For the rural poor of Third World countries, another major obstacle to health and health care is not their cultural belief systems, but the lack of any physical *infrastructure*, especially of roads, railways, bridges, electrical power, street lights, telephones, hospitals and clinics[86]. Poor-quality roads, infrequent or expensive public transport and long distances to travel to a clinic may all influence their ability and willingness to seek medical care. Also, within a particular country, wealthier regions may be better able to afford the infrastructure of health than poorer ones. In India, for example, the richer states of Maharashtra and Gujarat have 1.5 and 1.1 hospital beds respectively per 1000 population, while the rates for the poorer states of Bihar and Madhya Pradesh are only 0.3 and 0.4 respectively[86]. There is also a significant shortage of doctors, nurses and other health professionals in many poorer countries, and an urban bias in their distribution (see Chapter 4).

However, all attempts at improving health and preventing disease will be pointless unless larger social, economic and ecological issues are also addressed. These include the overpopulation, pollution and global warming mentioned above, but also the transnational marketing of 'chemical comforters' such as tobacco[87], pharmaceuticals (see Chapter 8) and addictive drugs. Another issue is the enormous *inequality* in wealth and resources between different parts of the world; it has been estimated that the world's richest 20 per cent are 150 times richer than the world's poorest 20 per cent, and that the gap between the two is steadily widening[2]. Finally, it is also pointless to save children from infectious diseases if they are going to be killed by crime, war or other forms of violence. The *British Medical Journal*[3] estimates that developing countries spend about $38 on arms for each person, but only $12 on health, and that the entire annual budget of the WHO amounts to just 3 hours of world expenditure on arms. As well as using up scarce resources, these arms are a major threat to human life. The *New York Times*[88] estimates that about 100 million landmines now threaten civilians in more than 60 countries, and have caused tens of thousands of deaths and injuries, especially in Afghanistan and in South-East Asia (about 30 000 people in Cambodia have lost limbs, mostly from mines). At the same time, the market for these mines is worth $200 million per year, and they are produced by some 100 companies and government agencies in 48 countries. A related issue is that war, civil unrest and ecological disasters usually result in *refugees* – currently estimated as between 15 million and 50 million world-wide[3], but mostly located in poorer countries. Some of the many physical and psychological effects of refugee and migrant status have been described in Chapter 11.

The evidence, therefore, is that the organization of any system of PHC, whatever its ideology or origin, must always take these wider socio-economic and ecological issues into consideration. That is, in order to be truly effective, it must always have some 'comprehensive' element in it[62].

Health care bureaucracies and PHC

To understand any form of PHC fully, the role played in it by the culture of medicine itself must be examined (see Chapter 5), as well as that of its various institutions, such as hospitals, medical schools, government departments and the bureaucracies of international aid agencies. Each of these has its own institutional sub-culture, hierarchy, ideology (whether political, religious or secular) and view of health, illness and the nature of medical care. In examining PHC, therefore, medical anthropology is not just about the health beliefs and behaviours of different cultures and communities; an essential part of its perspective is an understanding of how these institutional factors can either help or hinder the successful delivery of health care.

Foster[89] points out that health professionals easily accept the premise that the principal barriers to health care lie within the target community. The assumption is that 'effective health care can be achieved only when members of traditional communities change their health behaviour. Rarely if ever is the question asked, "How can anthropologists help to change bureaucratic behaviour that inhibits the design and operation of the best possible health care systems?"'[89]. Furthermore, 'among health personnel there is a hopeful assumption that there is a right "key" which, if only anthropologists can discover it, will unlock the door to wholehearted community co-operation in primary health care activities'[71]. Similarly, Coreil[90] warns that 'studies are commissioned with the hope that social science can pinpoint a simple key element that can be manipulated in such a way to make the whole system work as desired'. The assumption is that 'if changing behaviour will result in effective primary health care, it must be community, not bureaucratic, behaviour that changes'.

Foster[91] emphasizes the enormous strides that international health agencies (such as WHO) have made in meeting the world's health needs, especially in developing countries. However, he sees many of them, although international in ideology, as bearing 'the cultural imprint of the West'. He describes three premises that underlie many international medical aid programmes:

1. That the developed world possesses both the talent and the capital for helping 'backward' countries to develop
2. If some people have 'know-how', and others do not, those with the 'know-how' are the proper ones to plan and execute the transfer
3. Particular institutions and modes of operation that have met the needs of the developed world are the appropriate templates for the developing world, i.e. 'the health strategies that have served the West are universal, equally suited to Boston or Bombay'.

This section illustrates, however, that *local* realities – social, cultural and economic – and the needs and desires of local communities also need to be taken into account when designing any system of PHC. For this reason, many of the insights of medical anthropology, usually based on detailed micro studies in local communities, can be useful to those who plan, administer and evaluate primary health care programmes. They can help design systems of PHC at the local, national and international levels, which are humane, culturally appropriate and cost-effective, and which meet the needs not only of medical bureaucracies but also of the local communities themselves and the individuals within them.

Malaria

Malaria is one of the world's most dangerous and widespread parasitic diseases. More than half the population of the world is estimated to live in areas where malaria transmission occurs to some degree[92]. The majority of cases occur in tropical Africa, but they also occur in parts of Asia and Latin America. It is especially common in poor, deprived and undeveloped regions, where it has an enormous effect on public health. World-wide, 300–500 million suffer from the disease each year, often severely[92]. It kills between 1.5 and 2.7 million people annually[92], and over a million of these deaths are in children below the age of 5 years although they also include many older children, pregnant women and non-immune travellers[92]. Overall, it is responsible for 10–30 per cent of all hospital admissions world-wide[93]. Malaria is often associated with other conditions, such as malnutrition, respiratory infections, AIDS or tuberculosis.

Like other global diseases, high rates of malaria are a feature of poverty and inadequate health services. Urbanization, the growth of shanty towns, overcrowding, poor nutrition, economic inequality, civil disorder, patterns of migration and the movement of refugees, as well as the high cost of anti-malarial drugs, all make the situation much more difficult to control. However, like AIDS, malaria can also help to *cause* poverty, and can be a major brake on economic development[93]. Improving the living standards of ordinary people in poorer countries through economic advancement can be almost impossible without a sound malaria control policy and the allocation of appropriate funds. As well as the growing costs of treatment and prevention, adults with the disease are often too exhausted to work, and children feel too tired or unwell to study in school[94].

To deal with this situation, the World Health Organization, together with other United Nations agencies, launched the Global Malaria Control Strategy (GMCS) in 1995. Its aim was to ensure that 90 per cent of the world's malaria-endemic countries would implement national malaria control programmes as soon as possible. By mid-1997 this target had been met, with 47 of the 49 malaria-endemic countries in Africa completing their national plans of action, while outside Africa 57 other countries had also reoriented their malaria control programmes in accordance with the GMCS[92]. However, these national policies are not enough. For their success, they also need economic development – in order to afford better housing, improved sewerage, more swamp drainage and more effective drug therapies – as well as community participation in all prevention and treatment strategies.

Despite all these initiatives, malaria remains one of the worst of global health problems. This is due partly to widespread economic underdevelopment and to the emergence of species of mosquito resistant both to pesticides and to the drugs that prevent and treat the disease[95]. However, in certain communities, a variety of *cultural* beliefs and practices are also part of the problem.

Folk beliefs about malaria

Several anthropological studies have shown how folk beliefs can influence whether a community co-operates with a malaria control programme, whether it recognizes the early symptoms of the disease, and whether or not it accepts medical treatment for it. These beliefs also influence how people explain the origin and nature of the disease itself. Two key issues, in all of these anthropological studies, are:

- whether people connect mosquito bites to the origin of the disease
- how people interpret the significance of fever, and whether or not they relate it to malaria.

In south-eastern Tanzania, for example, Muela and colleagues[96] found that while 98 per cent of people interviewed believed that mosquito bites did cause malaria, many also believed in *other* modes of transmission – such as drinking or wading through dirty water, or being exposed to 'intensive sun'. At the same time, the symptom of malaria most frequently reported was *homa*, or fever. However, *homa* had a broader meaning, since it could also express a general malaise or diffuse body pains. In the rainy season, when the wetness and heat favour mosquito breeding, people tended to identify *homa* with malaria. However, in the dry season, they were more likely to attribute the same fevers to hard work, exposure to the cold, or to 'intensive sun'. Furthermore, people often differentiated between two types of *homa* – one due to malaria, a 'natural' disease that was easily treated, and another 'unnatural' form caused by spirits or witchcraft (*uchawi*), which was more difficult to treat. In the latter form, witchcraft was said to cause an illness that exactly mimics malaria, but is *not* the same disease. Seventy-three per cent of mothers in the study believed that this 'fake malaria' could be produced by witchcraft, and 62 per cent that witches could make the parasites invisible. That is the reason, they believed, why hospital tests sometimes could not detect the disease, and why medical treatments sometimes failed to cure it. Where the 'hospital people' could not help, a traditional healer (*mganga*) was often called in. Even when people felt that they had the 'real' malaria, and had accepted medical treatment, they might blame witchcraft if the treatment failed or if the condition recurred or suddenly worsened. Furthermore, people with 'real malaria' often asked the question *why* – 'why did the mosquito sting my child and not someone else's?', 'why did it happen to me?', 'why now?' – questions that can only be answered by a traditional healer. In the case of children, virtually all their mothers in the study who suspected malaria would go first to a hospital, but if there was no relief for their children, 60.6 per cent would then turn to a traditional healer. During the *mganga*'s treatment of witchcraft, anti-malarials would not be taken, since they were considered ineffective or even dangerous at that time.

Another study[97] carried out in a different region of Tanzania also found that people differentiated between several types of fever or *homa*. 'Malaria fever' (*homa ya malaria*) was only one of a group of mild conditions, regarded as not very dangerous, especially as the fever often came and went. It was recognized as occurring when mosquitoes were very numerous, in the rainy season between April and May. More severe fevers, known as 'fevers which do not respond to hospital treatment' (*homa zisizokubali tiba za hospitali*), were blamed on spirits, witchcraft, sorcery or other causes. They included serious childhood illnesses known as *degedege*, characterized by a sudden onset, high fever, trembling, delirium, stiffness of limbs, convulsions and a high mortality rate. People were not clear about their cause; sometimes they were blamed on spirits, but only occasionally were they ascribed to malaria. It was also believed that a child with *degedege* should not have a needle inserted into the skin; this might cause malevolent spirits to enter the body, and cause rapid death. In this region, therefore, many people did not give malaria control a high priority, as it was only seen as a mild fever. Often they did not associate their *homa ya malaria* with more serious complications such as cerebral malaria, severe anaemia or malaria in pregnancy.

In India, a study by Lobo and Kazi[98] in Surat district, Gujurat state, also found different folk models of fever, and of the causes of malaria. As in the Tanzanian examples, fever was regarded as a disease in itself, as well as a symptom. In the three villages they studied, people recognized 30 *different* types of fever (or *tav*). However, the situation was complicated by the fact that there was a wide variation, even within the same village, in how people described these fevers, their possible cause and how they should be treated. In different villages, people described similar fevers but gave them different names – or they gave them the same name, but were referring to different types of fever. In general, though, to most people in the district, malaria was seen as one particular type of fever, of which two forms were recognized; *sado* or simple (mild) malaria, and *zeri* or 'poisonous' (severe) malaria. Lobo and Kazi point out that these two categories of folk malaria were not necessarily synonymous with biomedical malaria, and may even not overlap with it. There was wide variation in beliefs about other symptoms associated with these types of malaria (especially the *sado* form) in the three villages. For example, in one village *sado* malaria was associated with loss of appetite, lethargy, bitter taste in the mouth, drowsiness and sweating, while in another village it was associated mainly with cold, body aches, headache, 'loosening' of the body, pain below the knee, waist pain and fluctuating fever. *Zeri* malaria was usually associated with symptoms such as a longer-lasting fever, acute shivering, weakness, severe pains, vomiting and, sometimes, convulsions. In terms of the aetiology of these malarial fevers, 59.5 per cent were not sure what caused malarial fevers, while only 34.1 per cent of the sample blamed them on mosquito bites.

These examples indicate, therefore, that folk beliefs about fevers in general, and malaria in particular, often vary widely within the same country, the same region, and even within the same village. Furthermore, in many communities there is no universal agreement that malaria is caused by insect bites; nor is there agreement on the types of fever characteristic of the disease, or the treatment appropriate for it. Therefore, any malaria control programme needs to take into account local beliefs about the disease, and how it may be prevented or treated.

Case study: Beliefs about malaria in a farming community in southern Ghana

Agyepong[99] has described beliefs about fevers, including malaria, in a farming community of the Ga-Adangbe tribe in southern Ghana. She describes *asra* – a symptom complex which can include fever, but also some or all of the following: chills, headaches, bodily pains, yellow eyes, a bitter taste in the mouth, deeply coloured urine, loss of appetite, weakness, vomiting, pallor of palms and soles, and cold sores around the mouth. A more serious, less common, version was *asraku*, where the person has high fever, confusion, and 'acts like a madman'. Only a small minority believed that mosquitoes could cause *asra*. Almost all members of the community agreed that *asra* was caused by contact with excessive external heat, especially from sunlight, but also from cooking, burning charcoal or standing too close to a fire. This heat causes *asra* by accumulating in the body, and upsetting the body balance by an effect on the blood. The prevailing view was that *asra* could not be prevented. It was an unavoidable fact of life, and of having to work outdoors in the harsh sunlight. Treatment for the condition mostly took place at home, and only rarely at medical facilities. Home remedies included herbs to 'wash the blood of the illness', so that it was sweated out through the skin or else passed out in the urine. Only if these remedies failed did they resort to pharmaceuticals bought over-the-counter, such as analgesics or, occasionally, low doses of chloroquine.

Attitudes to malaria treatment

People diagnose malaria, in themselves and in others, by a number of methods. These include the clinical presentation, the season of the year when it occurs, and the personal circumstances that preceded the illness. Where malaria is endemic in a community, some form of *self-treatment* is usually common; either the use of traditional home remedies, or of pharmaceutical drugs bought from a retail outlet[100]. This approach is partly due to the high cost of medically prescribed drugs[101], but also to folk beliefs about the origin and nature of the disease itself. Depending on these beliefs, the ill person may be first treated at home[100] or else be taken straight to a hospital[97] or sometimes to a traditional healer[97]. In most cases people move back and forth between biomedical and traditional systems, depending on their condition. The process usually begins with self-treatment, but later this is often carried out in parallel with medical treatment. Self-treatment strategies sometimes replace medical care, especially if the drugs fail to work and the patient deteriorates. In that case, a traditional healer may be consulted. In the study by Muela and colleagues[96], for example, when a patient failed to recover or relapsed, a *mganga* would be consulted – first to diagnose witchcraft or evil spirits, then to neutralize them by rituals or herbal treatment. This in turn might pose serious problems for successful treatment, since 96 per cent of the sample believed that once herbal medicines were begun, anti-malarials should not be given. Taking them at the same time as chloroquine was dangerous, as the effect on the patient might be too strong, and their blood 'start boiling'.

Mwenesi and colleagues[100], in the Kilifi coastal district of Kenya, also found that most mothers who diagnosed malaria in their children first turned to over-the-counter drugs bought from a retail outlet. Twenty-nine per cent of mothers had given their children anti-malarial drugs, and 30 per cent antipyretics or other medications (including antibiotics). Only 25 per cent had taken the child to a clinic; 9 per cent had given them no treatment at all; and 7 per cent had given them a home remedy such as a herbal preparation of the *neem* tree (*Azadirachta indica*). The most popular choice was a combination of antipyretics and anti-malarial drugs. Similarly, in southern Ghana, Agyepong[99] found that *asra* was first treated at home by a complex mixture of herbs or pharmaceuticals. The herbs were given to 'wash the blood of the illness', the drugs to treat the specific disease. Among the Mende people of Sierra Leone, Bledsoe and Goubaud[102] found that malaria was treated by certain foods or condiments (especially pepper), by certain herbs, by rubbing white chalk into the skin, and sometimes by Western pharmaceuticals. They found that many people chose these drugs on the basis of *colour*, choosing white medicines to relieve fever because they were seen as analogous to the traditional white chalk and its assumed 'bitterness', which is said to produce warmth and reduce fever. For that reason, people would accept medicines such as chloroquine, provided that it was white, or if its bitterness was not disguised by sugar coatings. But this also meant that other white or bitter medicines, such as aspirin, heart drugs, anti-diarrhoeals and anti-hypertensives, would also be considered as acceptable treatment for malaria.

These studies indicate, therefore, some of the reasons why medically prescribed anti-malarials may be accepted or rejected by a particular community. They also suggest why these drugs are often combined with other forms of treatment, either self-administered or from a traditional healer, in ways that 'make sense' to the community in terms of their local cultural beliefs.

Attitudes to malaria prevention

In many communities, malaria is so common that it is sometimes regarded as a normal (if undesirable) part of everyday life, and not as something that doctors can ever prevent. Similarly, mosquitoes and their bites are such a common part of life that people may believe that nothing can be done to eradicate them[96–99]. Furthermore, preventive strategies for malaria have to take into account the fact that many people do not connect mosquito bites to the disease. If, as in Agypong's study[99], people believe that malarial fever (*asra*) is caused by external heat, then, as one informant put it: 'There is nothing that we can do [to prevent it]. Unless you can provide us with other jobs so we do not work too hard in the sun'. Modern methods of prevention on a community level – such as better housing, screens erected across windows and doorways, drainage of stagnant water, spraying of potential reservoirs of the parasite, use of insect repellents, and bed nets impregnated with pesticide – often do not make sense in terms of indigenous folk beliefs. They may also be unaffordable, especially the high cost of pesticides and anti-malarial drugs produced by the Western pharmaceutical industry[101].

In many communities there are well-tried traditional ways of repelling mosquitoes, to prevent their bites or the diseases that they might carry. In Gujurat, for example, Lobo and Kazi[98] have described how these methods include covering the body with sheets to protect it, or using the smoke of burning cow dung or *neem* leaves. However, they found considerable resistance to the use of mosquito bed nets. Of the

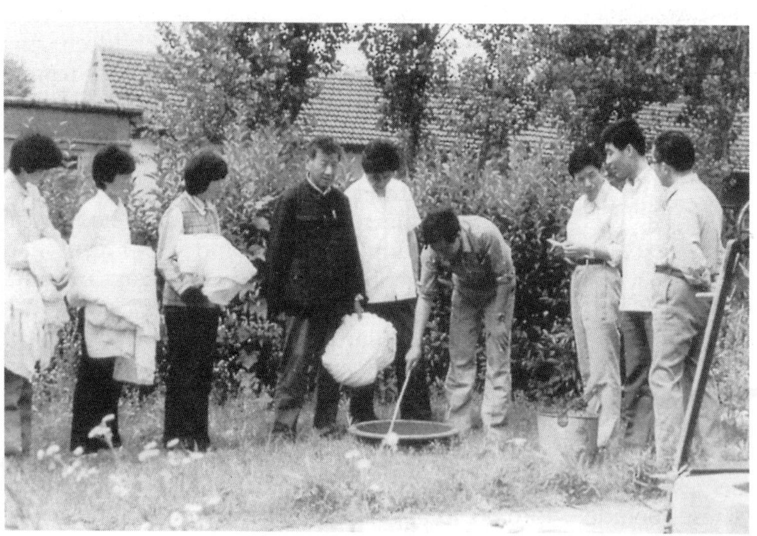

Figure 13.3 Community participation in malaria prevention. Householders in a Chinese village dip their mosquito bed nets in an insecticide (deltamethrin) to protect themselves against mosquito bites (Source: WHO/TDR/Y. Zhao, *World Health*, No. 3, May–June, 1998, page 10).

only 30 per cent who owned one, only 53.7 per cent used them regularly. People described them as very expensive, and as uncomfortable or suffocating, and there were often difficulties in finding a place to suspend them over the sleeping area. Also, some people (13.3 per cent) preferred sleeping out in the open, especially in very hot weather. In addition, cultural concepts of *personal space*, including who should sleep where, based on age, gender and status, made their use problematic. For example, elderly members of the family usually slept out on the verandah. This was partly because they were closer to toilet facilities, but also because of a cultural need to keep a physical distance from grown-up daughters and daughters-in-law and their children. In many households children slept in the kitchen, as it was believed that kitchen smoke repels mosquitoes. In some households, a young couple without children would sleep in the kitchen, but older couples in the sitting room. Within the houses, families slept in beds or cots, or sometimes on the floor – especially in the poorer social castes. All these variations in the location and allocation of sleeping spaces make the universal use of bed nets very difficult. As well as requiring a place to hang them from, these nets impose individual 'bubbles' of space (see Chapter 2) on communities and families who value communality and a greater sharing of personal space than is common in the industrialized world.

Thus, any attempt to get community participation in malaria prevention needs to take these cultural beliefs and concerns into account. The role of economic factors must also be considered, since many people simply cannot afford bed nets[103], anti-malarial tablets, different types of dress, and more protective housing arrangements. Nor can they afford to change traditional ways of agriculture, even if this bring them into regular contact with reservoirs of mosquitoes.

Malaria and migration

Outbreaks of malaria are often linked to massive movements of human populations. In some parts of the world, the disease is extremely common among refugees. It is one of the main killers of people fleeing from armed conflict, especially civil wars and social unrest, in developing countries[104]. Often these people are displaced from an area where malaria is uncommon to areas of high transmission. Having no natural immunity, they succumb quickly to the disease and its complications. This has particularly been the case in Africa, in regions where malaria is endemic and where large number of refugees have resulted from conflicts in Rwanda, Burundi, the Democratic Republic of the Congo, Somalia, eastern Sudan, Ethiopia, Kenya and Malawi[104]. In Asia, a similar problem has occurred among Cambodian refugees on the Thai-Cambodian border, and among refugees from Afghanistan in Pakistan and elsewhere. In these cases, medical interventions have to focus not only on bringing health care quickly to the refugee camps, but also on finding out the cultural beliefs and practices of the refugees themselves. This type of rapid research (Rapid Assessment Procedures) in emergency relief situations is listed in Chapter 14, and has been described in more detail by Slim and Mitchell[105].

Other population movements that can contribute to the spread of the disease include tourist air travel[105] – either of sick people or of mosquitoes themselves, carried in clothing and baggage – or migrant labour. In poorer counties particularly, where there is often marked economic inequality between regions, patterns of migrant labour can expose more people to the disease. Liese[93], for example, has described how, in Brazil, the relative poverty of the countryside leads people to seek work in towns and cities as migrant labourers. Each year, thousands of young men are being attracted to the gold rush in the Amazon basin. Many of these would-be miners or *garimpeiros* live in poor conditions, in houses without proper walls, and have poor nutrition. Many suffer from malaria. Coming from the south of the country, they have never before been exposed to the disease and, having little natural immunity, it affects them severely. They transport malaria with them when they return back home to visit relatives or friends. When they have spent their savings, they trek back to the Amazon, and the process starts all over again.

The examples outlined above illustrate, therefore, that the effective prevention and treatment of malaria requires a holistic approach. This includes economic development, alleviation of poverty, better housing and work conditions, and access to affordable anti-malarial drugs, insect repellents and impregnated bed nets. It also requires an understanding of folk beliefs about the origin, nature, recognition and treatment of the disease. As well as malaria, this holistic approach is also important for the control of other mosquito-borne diseases such as yellow fever, dengue, and filariasis.

Pollution and global warming

In 1944, the anthropologist Malinowski differentiated between the 'basic' human needs necessary for biological survival (such as metabolism, movement, growth, health and reproduction) and 'secondary' (or derived) needs (necessary for social life)[106]. These man-made 'derived needs' included systems of laws, values, religion, art, ritual, language and symbolism, but they also included material objects, artefacts and technology. With socio-economic development, 'new needs appear and new imperatives or determinants are imposed on human behaviour'. The problem is that these new culturally derived needs, such as the 'need' in Western society always to eat food with a knife and fork or to own a motor car and a refrigerator, often become seen as if they were as 'basic' or biological as the need for food or shelter, and become difficult to do without. In looking at ecological issues, therefore, anthropological studies of these culturally derived, quasi-basic needs are important, since their constant production by advertising and industry can outstrip the planet's resources, create inequality and dissatisfaction, and be dangerous to the environment.

To take one small example, the widespread use of chlorofluorocarbons (CFCs) in both refrigerators and aerosols has been found to contribute towards the thinning of the ozone layer, as well as to global warming (the 'greenhouse effect'), both of which can seriously damage human health[107]. Although economic factors (such as the profits involved in producing, promoting and selling these products) play a major role in their popularity, so do culturally influenced beliefs and behaviours. For example, where aerosols are used as deodorants, air cleaners, hair lacquers and furniture polish, their use is clearly influenced by certain cultural values, which are constantly reinforced by advertising. In Western countries, particularly, these stress the importance of living in an odour free environment, with an absence of both natural body odour and extraneous smells within the home. They also promote certain hair styles and colours (particularly those suggesting a youthful appearance), and emphasize shiny, reflecting surfaces on furniture within the home as a sign of order, affluence and social respectability.

Another more pervasive example is the *motor car*, an invention that has had a profound effect on human life, transforming societies, cultures, economies, landscapes and human relationships all over the world. However, the cost of this invention has been high. As well as the many millions killed or maimed in traffic accidents since cars appeared early this century (approximately 200 000 people died in traffic accidents in 1985 world-wide[108]), they have been responsible for enormous damage to both human health and the environment. The best-known example of this is air pollution from car exhaust fumes – mainly carbon monoxide, ozone, nitrous dioxide and hydrocarbons. In overcrowded cities with high traffic densities, air pollution can have serious and permanent effects on health, particularly on the respiratory system. In addition, the combustion of leaded gasoline (banned in the USA, but still common elsewhere) can lead to the fallout of lead oxide in dust, which may then contaminate food, the soil, crops and the feed of livestock, and cause serious health problems – especially in children[109].

The car, however, is not only a form of transport. It is also a symbolic object that has different *meanings* for different people, depending on their culture and socio-economic background, their gender and age group. It often symbolizes values of prestige, power, autonomy, individualism and mobility (both social and geographical); images often created, or sustained, by the motor industry.

As with population control, attempts to reduce air pollution from car exhausts need to take some of these socio-cultural issues into account. National traffic policies (such as enforcing lowered speed limits, subsidizing unleaded gasoline, checking car exhausts, increasing car tax and banning cars from city centres) may not be the only solution. Before people can be converted from private to public and less polluting forms of transport, such as railways, not only must these be easily accessible and affordable, but it is also important to understand why so many people seek to own cars in the first place. Here, anthropological studies of the cultural roles of car ownership can be useful, as part of a national transport policy.

For example, Miller[110] has described how in Chaguanas, Trinidad, the car is 'a vehicle not only for transporting people spatially but also conceptually from one set of values to another'. These new values include notions of *individuality*, since in contemporary Trinidad 'the car is probably the artefact which outweighs even clothing in its ability to incorporate and express the concept of the individual'. In conversation, people are sometimes identified not by name, but by the make or number plate of their cars. For young males, particularly, cars have become the means of realizing their inner fantasies of independence from family, successful seduction and sexual attraction (street wisdom insists that 'women will not look at men who don't have cars'). As a public way of expressing individuality, cars can be 'customized' by special decorations to their upholstery or exteriors, clearly marking the status and character of the owner. One result of this is 'an unwillingness to walk, once in possession of a car'; huge traffic jams are commonplace as people drive to work or school, even when it is very near to home. Thus in Trinidad, as elsewhere, the car has become 'as well-established a vehicle for expressive identity, as it is a vehicle for transport'. Public health measures to reduce air pollution need to take these cultural factors into account. As with advertisements for tobacco and alcohol, the constant creation of 'derived needs' – and the emphasis on meeting these only by the consumption and public display of a material object, such as a car – will have to be dealt with, before the damage to the environment becomes irreversible.

As this section briefly illustrates, there is often a connection, direct or indirect, between the ecology of the planet, the health of its inhabitants and certain cultural beliefs and behaviours. As well as human practices that cause environmental pollution, they include deforestation, the use of nuclear power and weaponry, the extinction of many species of wildlife and the emphasis on short-term profits and political power over the long-term interests of humanity. All need to be considered by the medical anthropologist of the future, since human culture influences how those problems are produced, whether they are recognized and whether or not they are dealt with.

Deforestation and species extinction

One of the major threats to global health is *deforestation*, especially of the rainforests. Less than 50 per cent of the area covered by prehistoric tropical rainforests still remains, but it is currently being cut down or burned at a rate of about 142 000 square kilometres per year (approximately 1.8 per cent of the total area still standing)[111]. Forests – 'the Earth's lungs' – play a crucial role in stabilizing global gases, thus reducing the greenhouse effect, and in maintaining global rainfall patterns. Their destruction can result in a reduced rainfall in adjacent areas and irreversible soil erosion, causing crop failures and a fall in food production. As well as its effects on the planet's ecology, there are three other serious problems associated with deforestation:

1. *Destruction of indigenous peoples* living in forest areas, both physically and culturally, by direct violence from loggers, ranchers, miners or government officials, or by the actual destruction of their habitat and hunting grounds
2. *Species extinction* of animals, birds, plants and microbes, including many that could be used in the development of medicines
3. *Infectious diseases* resulting from destruction of the natural habitats and ecological niches of certain viruses or their vectors, and their release into human populations.

In many cases, anthropologists have been able to contribute a more detailed understanding of the problem. For example, they have provided considerable data on indigenous tribal groups, especially within the Third World (such as Brazilian Indians), and on how many are dying as a result of destruction of the forests in which they live and hunt or by diseases brought in from the outside world[112]. Many have acted as advocates on their behalf to government and other bureaucracies, in an attempt to stop what may amount to genocide. Frequently, they have pointed out to those living in industrialized countries that they could learn valuable lessons from these indigenous peoples; especially their respect and reverence for the natural environment and its limited resources.

The destruction of natural species, especially plant, bird, animal and microbial, poses a special threat to global health. Within the next 50 years, an estimated one-quarter of all species will become extinct, particularly those lost by the rapid tropical deforestation[111]. At the current rate, this would mean an estimated 27 000 species lost every year – or more than 74 per day. An important result of this would be the loss of many thousands of potential medicines, of use in treating many different diseases. At present, Chivian[111] estimates that about 80 per cent of all people living in developing countries (about two-thirds of the world's population) rely almost exclusively on traditional medicines using natural substances, mostly derived from plants; even in the USA, 25 per cent of all prescriptions dispensed from community pharmacies between 1959 and 1980 contained active ingredients extracted from plants. Many of these plants have been used by indigenous healers for centuries before the development of modem pharmaceuticals, and are still being used. Among the better-known medicines derived from plants are quinine and quinidine (from cinchona bark), D-tubocurarine (from the *Chondrodendron* vine), aspirin (from willow bark), digitalis (from foxglove), morphine (from the opium poppy), and the cancer drugs taxol (from the Pacific yew tree) and vinblastine and vincristine (from *Vinca rosa*, the periwinkle plant)[111]. Over the years, anthropological studies of traditional healing and indigenous pharmacopoeias have been a useful source of information about many other plant-based medicines, their advantages and disadvantages, and how they are used by human groups in different parts of the world[113].

Another danger of deforestation is the release of new infectious diseases into human populations due to the destruction of natural habitats and the disruption of delicate local ecologies. For example, the cutting down of tropical rainforests (as in the Amazon area) displaces forest rodents, who were the usual reservoir hosts of sandflies (which carry protozoa of the genus *Leishmania*). As a result, the sandflies turn temporarily to biting humans, and thereby increase the incidence of *Leishmaniasis* – a serious disease said to affect over 12 million people world-wide[111]. Similarly, ticks, tsetse flies (carriers of African sleeping sickness) and kissing bugs (carriers of Chagas disease, common in Central and South America, and affecting 15–20 million people) may all be released by the destruction of their usual habitats. Several viral illnesses have also recently 'emerged' from forest regions as a result of deforestation. Among them is *Kyasanur forest disease* (KFD), carried by *Haemophysalis spinigera* ticks, which usually feed on small forest animals in the tropical forests of southern India. With the introduction of sheep and cattle into previously forested areas, they become reservoirs of the disease, as do the humans who tend them[111,114]. As with other 'new' viral diseases, anthropologists have studied the impact of these epidemics on particular communities.

Case study: Community reactions to Kyasanur forest disease (KFD) in South Kanara district, southern India

Nichter[114] described KFD in South Kanara District as essentially a 'disease of development' – the result of deforestation and the rearing of cattle in the cleared scrublands between villages and forest. Many of those afflicted were poor agricultural workers, who tended these tick-bearing cattle. In the area, the local cosmology divides the universe into three realms; that of humans, that of the wild (forest), and the realm of spirits mediating between the two. Danger is inherent in any meeting between the human and spirit realms, and when the spirits are not controlled the results may be 'crop failures, epidemics, and the violent death of humans and domestic animals'. Faced with the outbreak of KFD, the villagers in the area assumed that the spirits were punishing some moral transgressions on their part, and tried to placate them by various rituals; their belief in KFD's supernatural causation was reinforced by the failure of doctors to cure it. During the epidemic, many victims refused to go to hospital, for both cultural and economic reasons, preferring instead to be treated at home by a private Ayurvedic practitioner. They feared that to die in hospital would be to have a 'bad death', and their unsatisfied spirit (*preyta*) would cause problems to their surviving kinsfolk. To appease such a spirit would then entail expensive rituals that they could not afford. Hospitalization also meant the loss of another healthy wage earner, who would be forced to help nurse the patient in hospital. By contrast, the private practitioner, although less (medically) effective, was more sensitive to popular health beliefs than the hospitals, prescribed special diets in keeping with those beliefs and was quite liberal in his administration of diazepam (Valium) to patients having a wide variety of illnesses. By treating them at home, he also helped avoid the expense of a 'bad death'. Nichter points out that, at first, government officials played down the link between KFD and deforestation, and did not sufficiently tap community self-help as a resource in dealing with the epidemic. Despite their belief in the mystical origin of the disease, the villagers' 'effort to appease this spiritual cause of KFD did not preclude an interest in controlling ticks as an instrumental cause of disease'.

As well as deforestation, many species of wildlife have been hunted almost to extinction, not as a source of food but rather for more cultural reasons. These include:

- whales hunted early in the century to provide whalebone for women's corsets
- thousands of animals shot annually on safaris in Africa to provide trophies for wealthy hunters
- sharks killed as a source of 'shark fin' soup, popular in the Far East
- foxes, mink and rabbits killed to provide fur coats for fashionable women
- rhino horns used, in a powdered form, as an aphrodisiac in parts of Africa
- elephant tusks, to provide ivory for ornaments
- tigers killed for their organs, used in traditional medicaments in India and China
- bears, hunted in parts of Asia for their gallbladders, reputed to have a medicinal value.

In each of these cases of environmental destruction, Cortese[115] points out that human belief systems are part of the problem, especially the anthropocentric view of the world that 'man is the most important of all the species and should have dominion over nature', and that the world's resources are 'free and inexhaustible'. One of the consequences of this belief, and the economic and political systems that go with it, is the present ecological crisis, and its growing threat to global health.

The roles of anthropology in a global health strategy

This chapter has outlined not only some of the global health problems that we face today, but also the inherent tension between national (and international) solutions to them on one hand, and local social and cultural conditions on the other. In other words, there is a basic *paradox* at the core of almost all global health strategies, whether they are for population control, improvement in nutrition, prevention of AIDS, promotion of breast-feeding, or any other form of health promotion. This paradox can be expressed as:

1. Global health problems require a global health strategy
2. No global health strategy can be universally applicable to *all* parts of the world, due to the wide diversity of human population groups – especially at the local level.

Given this situation, some of the possible roles of medical anthropology in a global health policy can summarized as follows:

1. To carry out detailed research in local communities and social groups into the social and cultural dimensions of specific health problems and diseases
2. To provide a comprehensive database on the social and cultural composition of different communities world-wide, based on prior research by other anthropologists
3. To study the relationship between health beliefs and behaviours in particular contexts or communities; i.e. to explore the differences between what people *say* they believe or do and what they actually *do* in practice, and explain the reasons for these discrepancies
4. To mediate between health interventions at the local level and policy makers at the national or international levels in order to adapt the programme to specific local conditions
5. To aid in these interventions at the *local* level by:
   a. ensuring that the programme 'makes sense' to the community, in terms of their local social, cultural, and economic realities
   b. identifying community resources useful for health education or health care, as part of a national or international programme
   c. monitoring the impact of these programmes on the local community
   d. developing a network of locally recruited 'barefoot anthropologists'[1] (research assistants) or social scientists, to assist in the planning, application and evaluation of the programme
   e. providing feedback for policy makers on the progress and impact of the programme
   f. adapting health education programmes to disseminate information through culturally appropriate channels within the community (such as teachers, religious leaders or traditional healers)
   g. acting as advocates, or cultural interpreters, for the community to health bureaucracies and policy makers at the national or international levels

6. To organize educational programmes on the social and cultural dimensions of health and disease for policy makers, and for other researchers
7. To monitor the institutional cultures of national and international medical aid agencies, to improve their efficiency and help reduce ethnocentric bias
8. To develop and test new research instruments (such as rapid assessment procedures) to study particular health problems in specific local and national contexts (see Chapter 14).

Recommended reading

Baer, H., Singer, M., and Susser, I. (1997). *Medical Anthropology and the World System*. Bergin and Garvey.

Chivian, E., McCally, M., Hu, H. and Haines, A. (eds). (1993). *Critical Condition: Human Health and the Environment*. Massachusetts Institute of Technology Press.

Coreil, J. and Mull, D. J. (eds). (1990). *Anthropology and Primary Health Care*. Westview Press.

Harpham, T., Lusty, T. and Vaughan P. (eds). (1988). *In the Shadow of the City: Community Health and the Urban Poor*. Oxford University Press.

Nichter, M. and Nichter, M. (1996). *Anthropology and International Health: Asian Case Studies*, pp. 329–65. Gordon and Breach.

ten Brummelhuis, H. and Herdt, G. (eds). (1995). *Culture and Sexual Risk: Anthropological Perspectives on AIDS*. Gordon and Breach.

Warwick, D. P. (1988). Culture and the management of family planning programs. *Stud. Fam. Plan.*, **19**, 1–18.

World Health Organization. (1995). *The World Health Report 1995 – Bridging the Gaps*. WHO.

World Health Organization (1998). United against malaria *World Health*, **3** (special issue).

14 New research methods in medical anthropology

To meet the challenges of both international and local health problems – many in need of urgent intervention – a number of new research techniques have been developed in medical anthropology, as well as in psychology and sociology. All of them aim to provide a new understanding of health and illness, especially of health-related beliefs and behaviours. Many of these take the form of *qualitative* techniques, though they are often now combined with more quantitative (or measurement-based) techniques within the same project[1]. These may include large-scale population surveys of morbidity and mortality, and of the prevalence and incidence of certain diseases. These days, furthermore, a problem is frequently researched using several different qualitative techniques at the same time, and as part of the same study[2]. They are drawn from a 'toolbox' of several of the data collection methods mentioned below. Often these are combined with the more traditional participant-observation technique of ethnography[3], described in Chapter 1. Using several different techniques to examine the same research question has an important advantage. When analysing the data, a strong *agreement* between the findings from two or more of these different techniques is then usually seen as an indication (and a way of confirming) the validity of those data – a process known as triangulation[4] (see below).

While quantitative studies often try to discover *what* has happened in particular situation, most research projects in medical anthropology try to answer the question *why*?[5] Why, for example, do some people prefer traditional or alternative healers for some conditions, but not for others? Why do some people change their diet during illness, pregnancy or lactation in ways harmful to their health? Why do some groups reject one form of medical treatment, but accept another? Why are some conditions regarded as diseases in one group, but not in another? Why are behaviours thought of as 'bad' in one group, regarded as 'mad' in another? Why is contraception accepted by one community, but not by another? Why are levels of alcohol or drug abuse high in one cultural group, but not in another?

Types of data

To examine any of the problems described in this book – particularly the role of health beliefs and behaviours – requires a more holistic and multi-dimensional approach. The researchers have to be sure that they have understood, as far as this is possible, *all* aspects of the situation being studied. To achieve this, researchers should ideally aim to examine, and then to integrate, four different types or levels of data[6], each one collected and analysed in a very different way.

The four levels of data are:

1. What people *say* they believe, think or do
2. What people actually *do*
3. What people *really* think or believe
4. The *context* of the above three points.

Examining only one form of data, such as using a questionnaire to collect statements about stated health beliefs (level 1 data), may often give a very different picture from what is actually observed in their daily lives (level 2 data). The latter data are often collected by the process of participant observation, described in Chapter 1. Discrepancies between levels 1 and 2 data – that is, between what people say they do and what they actually do in practice – have often been reported by anthropologists. They may need to be explained by deeper, more hidden beliefs (level 3 data) – what people *really* believe at the level of their inner 'cultural grammar' (what Hall[7] terms 'primary' or 'secondary' level culture; see Chapter 1) or at the level of the personal unconscious. At this personal level, for example, doctors who advise patients of the dangers of smoking but continue to smoke heavily themselves may possibly do so because:

- they genuinely believe that smoking is harmless
- they assume that they are 'lucky', and will not get ill from smoking, even if other people do
- they actually likes the sense of danger and risk involved in smoking
- they actually want, on some level, to get ill from smoking.

Data at this level may therefore have to be inferred from levels 1 and 2, or revealed by more in-depth and more detailed studies. Although more difficult to discover, data at this level should never be ignored, since many failures of health promotion or disease prevention programmes are due to these types of phenomena. Finally, data at levels 1, 2 and 3 can also be heavily influenced by the *context* in which those data were gathered, and information on this context (i.e. level 4 data) needs to be explicitly noted in any description of the research findings[6].

Influences on data collection

Unlike the traditional quantitative or 'positivist' approach to research, especially in the social sciences, *qualitative research* recognizes that certain factors inherent in the research project itself can influence the phenomena under study, and thus the types of data that can be obtained. This is particularly true in studies of human populations and their culture or social organization. In these settings, this recognition of the subjective and contextual aspects of qualitative research is a major strength of its approach, and not a weakness. This is because it provides readers of the research with much more information on which to base their evaluation of its findings and their opinion of its validity. This differs from quantitative scientific research (in the social sciences), which still commonly promotes the myth of the 'invisible researcher' (and research technique) whose presence supposedly has no influence whatsoever on the people being studied.

The major influences on data collection recognized by qualitative research are:

1. The attributes of the *researcher*
2. The attributes of the *research technique*
3. The *context* in which the research takes place.

The implications of this are that, in some cases, different researchers, even when using the identical questionnaires, may produce very different data from the same population. Often this is due to some subtle influence of their personal attributes, such as age, gender, ethnicity, dress, body language, tone of voice, religious or political background, and so on, on the people being interviewed. In addition, each research technique also imposes its own specific influence on the people being studied, particularly on what they say and do during the study, the questions that they answer, and the ones they do not. At its simplest level, this includes research techniques such as self-administered questionnaires, which require high degrees of literacy or numeracy in the study population, or familiarity with such culture-bound approaches as the multiple-choice questionnaire. More subtly, however, it refers to the influence of, say, the visible presence of a tape-recorder or video camera in the interview, and how this may cause either self-consciousness and withdrawal in the people being interviewed, or a tendency to over-dramatize answers. Finally, the *context* in which the research is carried out – the setting, and circumstances where the data are actually gathered – may also influence the data obtained. People behave differently in different contexts, and the same questionnaire administered in a hospital ward, police cell, supermarket or at the subject's home may all give very different results.

Qualitative research methods

In recent years, an increasing focus has been on research methods that can collect ethnographic data in a relatively short period of time compared to the lengthy periods of traditional ethnography. These techniques are becoming more popular and sophisticated. They are regarded as particularly useful in the planning, design and evaluation of health education, disease prevention and international aid programmes. They are particularly relevant in situations where research (and policy decisions to be based on that research) need to be fairly close together in terms of time. This is the case in situations of emergency (such as refugee crises or natural disasters) or in outbreaks of infectious diseases, where rapid control can save many lives, especially among the young, elderly and vulnerable. Traditional fieldwork or *ethnography*[3], which can take up to 2–3 years to complete, write-up and analyse, is simply not useful in this type of situation.

Some of these newer and more rapidly administered research techniques are summarized below.

Open ended questionnaires

These can be structured, or semi-structured. They may be directed at a particular research question (such as dietary taboos during pregnancy), or at a wider issue (such as beliefs about the origin, presentation and treatment of infertility). Open-ended questions are, for example, 'What causes tuberculosis?', 'Why have you become ill?', 'How do you feel about your condition?', 'What causes tuberculosis?'. Often one or more such open-ended questions are included in a more structured or even a multiple-choice questionnaire. Answers to these open questions are either written down by subjects, or recorded and then transcribed. Examples of open-ended questionnaires (clinical questionnaires) relating to the topics in this book are listed in the Appendix.

Rapid assessment procedures

Rapid assessment procedures (RAP)[8] are increasingly popular in international medical aid and health promotion programmes. Among the best known of them are *rapid ethnographic assessment*[9], *focused ethnographic study*[10], *rapid epidemiological assessment*[11] and *rapid rural appraisal*[12]. In each case the research can take between several weeks and several months, and is often carried out by a team of researchers rather than a single researcher. This research is usually carried out in co-operation with the community – in fact, communal participation is necessary for *all* forms of RAPs. During the research, members of the research team each study different aspects of the community's daily life, especially their health-related beliefs and behaviours, with the aid of a booklet of standardized research questions and open-ended questionnaires. These may include their social and economic organization, gender roles, health beliefs, local folk illnesses and culture-bound syndromes, infant-feeding practices, use of traditional healers, self-treatment strategies, diet and nutrition, and housing arrangements. Others researchers will collect demographic and census data, and try to assess the health status of the community by carrying out surveys of morbidity and mortality – often in relation to specific diseases, such as malnutrition, tuberculosis or AIDS. Usually the study will focus on a specific health problem or research question, such as family planning, malaria control or AIDS prevention. In the study of refugee groups, Eisenbruch[13] has also developed another type of rapid assessment procedure; the *cultural bereavement interview*, a way of understanding how refugees have responded to their experiences of displacement – physically, emotionally and socially (see Chapter 11).

In recent years, RAPs have been used to study aspects of: infant feeding practices[14], malnutrition[15], acute respiratory infections[10], women's reproductive health[16], childhood development, HIV and AIDS[17], immunizations, infant mortality[18], attitudes to epilepsy[19], and community health needs[20]. For example, Pelto and Grove[10] described how a focused ethnographic study was developed for the World Health Organization to study acute respiratory infections in children, and some of the useful findings from it. In many cases, these RAPs need to be combined with data gathered from longer-term, more intensive fieldwork, and often with more clinical or epidemiological data as well.

Focus groups

Focus groups[21,22] are intensive interviews with a small group of people (usually 8–12), each of whom shares certain attributes. Ideally, they should not have met each other before. The focus group may be, for example, a group of pregnant teenagers, of male adolescents, drug abusers or

AIDS patients. The aim is to observe and record the health-related beliefs and behaviours of this particular group of people, as revealed in the group discussion – particularly by their answers to key questions and the interactions between group members. The group is run by one or more facilitators, and proceedings are taped and then transcribed. Focus groups are often useful as part of RAPs. Some of the advantages and pitfalls of this technique are summarized by Asbury[22].

Free listing

The aim of this technique is to reveal underlying health beliefs by asking subjects to list as many items as possible on a particular subject[23]. For example, 'Tell me all the types of fevers that children suffer from', 'List all the ways that diarrhoea is treated in your community', 'Tell me all the symptoms of tuberculosis that you know' or 'List all the foods that are bad (or good) for diabetes'.

Pile sorting

This usually follows from free listing. Subjects may be given the list of items gathered above, each of which is written on a separate card. They are then asked to sort them into piles according to certain criteria. For example, 'please put in one pile all the types of childhood fever that you think should be brought to a clinic, on another pile those you would treat yourself at home, and on another all those you think should be treated by a traditional healer'. The subjects are then asked to talk about the piles, and to describe in detail the reasons for their choices[23].

Rank ordering

This is an elaboration of pile sorting, whereby subjects are asked to group the cards (compiled from free listing) into hierarchies in terms of specific criteria. For example, grouping types of childhood fever according to severity in three groups, from 'most severe' to 'moderate' and down to 'mild'[23].

Semantic network analysis

This technique overlaps somewhat with free listing. Its aim is to reveal, often with the aid of 'free association', all the concepts, images, fears, prejudices and assumptions that are linked in people's minds to a particular word or phrase. This can include a particular symptom, disease (such as 'cancer') or diagnostic label. It is useful for the study of folk illnesses and their symbolic associations, as in Blumhagen's study[24] of 'hyper-tension' and Good's[25] description of 'heart distress' in Iran.

Family interviews

These are often based on the concepts and techniques of enquiry of family therapy. These concepts include that of 'family systems theory'[26], which views the family as a system of relationships that always strives for equilibrium. They aim to examine specific aspects of the family culture[27] and its relevance to health, illness and lifestyle. In this type of study, the definition of 'family' may often be quite broad, and include many non-biological members (see Chapter 10) who also play significant roles in family life.

Narrative analysis

This usually includes analysis of autobiographical accounts of ill health, doctor–patient interactions, surgical operations and diagnostic tests; or of significant life events such as childbirth, bereavement or severe illness. It also includes the collection of longer life histories, from some selected informants[28]. All are either written down (by the subject or the researcher), video-taped or tape-recorded.

Collection of medical folklore

This is the study of inherited folklore – within families, communities and wider populations – that relates to health, illness and medical care. It usually includes the collection of traditional remedies, 'old wives' tales' and methods of diagnosis. It is collected either as oral folklore (gathered usually from older members of the community), or from published texts, home-doctor books, pamphlets or advice leaflets. An example of this approach is Snow's in-depth study[29] of traditional African-American health beliefs and folk medicine.

Analysis of written or visual material

This material may include diaries, family photographs, historical records, census reports, maps, newspaper articles, advertisements, self-help pamphlets, shrines, wills and even novels relevant to a particular area, group of people or type of ill health.

Videotapes, audio tapes, and photographs

These techniques are used especially in studying specific events within health care, such as doctor–patient or nurse–patient consultations, behaviour in a clinic waiting room, or the body language of health professionals or their patients. Although useful, this is a 'snapshot' technique, capturing only a moment in time. It tells little about what happened before or after, the recording, or about the inner belief systems of the participants.

Genealogies and genograms

These are collected from informants, and are useful for understanding the patterns of kinship and marriage within a family or community[30], the inheritance of patterns of lifestyle (such as alcoholism, drug abuse and teenage pregnancy) or of symptom patterns within a family (the 'family symptom tree'[31]), and the origins and persistence of hereditary diseases (such as cystic fibrosis or Tay-Sachs disease).

Social network analysis

This involves compiling a chart of the network of the people associated with a particular individual[32]. It may focus on family, friends, neighbours, work associates, sexual partners, members of the same club or church, or any particular combination of these. It is especially useful in contact tracing during outbreaks of infectious diseases (including sexually transmitted diseases), in monitoring the spread of health-related information in a community, and in studies of the social support available to ill individuals. An example of this technique is Parker and colleagues' study[33] of the transmission of HIV in London by analysing the sexual networks of a sample of people who are HIV positive.

Mapping and modelling

In these techniques subjects are asked to portray – by drawings, diagrams, artwork or even sculptures – certain aspects of their daily lives or belief systems. For example, these may include drawing a map of their home, village, or local community, drawing diagrams of the body's interior to show the location of organs, or indicating on a standardized outline of the body (as in Boyle's study[34] of body image among English patients) the location of bodily organs or systems. Most studies of body image have used this approach, such as MacCormack's study[35] of Jamaican women's understanding of their own reproductive systems. A combination of mapping and open-ended questionnaires – the 'drawing-interview' – was used in the COMAC Childhood and Medicines Project on childhood perceptions of illness in nine European countries, carried out in 1990–1993[36]. Here each child in the study was asked to make a drawing of the last time that they were ill, and was then interviewed in depth about the content and meaning of the drawing they had made.

Projective techniques

These are similar to use of Rorschach and other tests in psychology. Groups or individuals are exposed to the same photograph, slide, film, model or written vignette, and are then asked to describe and comment on it. This is useful in revealing hidden assumptions about levels of understanding (level 3 data). For example, a sample of mothers may be shown a set of 10 photographs of children, some of which are visibly suffering from a particular disease, and asked to pick out and talk about which children they see as healthy or unhealthy, and how they would deal with the situation. Another projective technique – observed play with dolls (often made with explicit sexual organs) – has been used in eliciting evidence of sexual abuse from children.

Structured vignettes

This technique, developed by Greenhalgh and colleagues[37], aims to overcome what could be termed *deference bias* – the tendency of some subjects from disadvantaged backgrounds to agree automatically with any question the researcher asks, especially if the researcher comes from a more affluent or educated background. The vignette is a fictional story, in the form of a tape-recording, text or even a cartoon, presented to the subject for comment.

The aim is to reveal a subject's belief system (level 3 data) by noting how much he or she agrees or disagrees with the story. If a tape-recording is played, it may then be played back slowly, sentence by sentence; after each, the subject is asked, for example, 'Do you agree that this person would have acted (or thought) in this way?' Some deliberately incorrect statements may be included, to check for deference bias. Presenting it as a fictional vignette reduces the element of intimidation and the desire to please the investigator.

Ethnography of a medical institution

These use traditional participant-observation techniques to study the institutional culture, norms, rituals, social organization, use of language and division of labour within a medical or nursing environment. Often the researchers work within the institution for a period of time (as, say, hospital porters, nursing assistants or receptionists), in order to carry out their fieldwork. The settings could include a hospital ward, clinic, doctor's office, medical school or nursing college. Examples include Goffman's work[38] on the culture of mental hospitals, Katz's study[39] of surgical rituals in the USA and Barrett's study[40] of how schizophrenia is defined and treated within a state psychiatric hospital in Australia.

Ethnography of a folk, traditional or 'alternative' healer

This is a participant-observation study which usually involves 'sitting in' with one or more healers and observing the ritual setting of their work, the techniques that they employ, and the types of responses that their patients have to them. It often also involves trying to assess the efficacy of these techniques *vis-à-vis* those of conventional Western medicine. Examples of this type of ethnography include Kleinman's study[41] of the work of the *tang-ki* or folk shaman in Taiwan, Finkler's study[42] of spiritual healers in Mexico, and Simon's study[43] of a Xhosa folk healer in Transkei, South Africa.

Computer analyses

The chief value of these software programs lies in their capacity to analyse large bodies of text, to select out certain themes or clusters of themes and to reveal relationships between them, or between them and certain demographic or other variables[44]. Many computer programs are useful in converting qualitative data (in the form of texts or transcripts) to quantitative data (in the form of statistical analyses, models, charts, tables, graphs or diagrams). There are now numerous software programs available that are commonly used to analyse data in medical anthropology. They include: NUDIST, ETHNOGRAPH[45], ANTHROPAC[45,46], TEXTBASE ALPHA[45], EPISTAT, ZYINDEX[45], GOPHER[45], TALLY[45] and AnSWR[47].

Summary

Keesing[48] has remarked that anthropology is more 'concerned with meanings rather than measurement, with the texture of everyday in communities, rather than formal abstraction'. Despite this, most medical anthropology research these days usually includes collection of some *quantitative* data (such as a village census, household survey, household income studies, caloric intake, food production, crop output, infant mortality or disease prevalence) in addition to these qualitative research methods. The Peltos[49] point out that the task of the modern medical anthropologist is increasingly to develop ways of integrating qualitative with quantitative data – of articulating detailed ethnographic studies of health beliefs and behaviours with the work of epidemiologists and other more quantitative researchers.

In cross-cultural psychiatry, a series of more specialized research instruments – both qualitative and quantitative – has been developed. Mumford[50] has reviewed several of these techniques, whose overall aim is to identify, analyse, measure and compare mental disorders across a variety of cultures. For example, the Bradford Somatic Inventory (BSI) was developed 'to meet the need for a multicultural inventory of common somatic symptoms reported by anxious and depressed individuals in Britain and the Indian subcontinent'[50]. Another example is the 'cultural bereavement interview' mentioned above[13].

The question of validity

Qualitative research techniques do have a number of limitations, in medical anthropology and elsewhere. In particular, they are labour-intensive, require special training for researchers, are suitable mainly for studying small groups of people, and are unsuitable for large-scale population surveys or studies of physiological data. There is also the possibility of the sample interviewed not being typical of the population at large, and of observer bias or disagreement among researchers[6].

In order to minimize these possible biases and maximize the validity of the research findings, the following strategies should be followed:

1. During the research, attributes of the following should be *standardized*:
   a. the researcher
   b. the research technique
   c. the context of the research.

   This means that, as far as is possible, the same researcher (or someone of similar attributes) should carry out all the research, using the same research techniques each time, and it should be carried out each time in the same setting (in terms of place, time, and circumstances).
2. During the research, the *same* phenomena should be studied, using *different* research techniques (chosen from the 'toolbox'), since a high degree of agreement among these findings would be significant, and maximize the chances of validity. This process of seeking agreement or overlap among the findings from different research techniques in the same study is known as triangulation[51].
3. When analysing research findings, such as a body of text produced by an open-ended questionnaire, the aim is to get the *agreement* of several researchers when coding the data and identifying underlying themes. That is, several researchers should independently read and analyse the material, then compare notes in order to identify areas of agreement among them.

These new approaches to qualitative research, and the attempts to make them even more valid and reliable, are now an essential part of most social sciences[52]. They are also particularly relevant to the field of clinically applied medical anthropology as it enters the new millennium.

Recommended reading

Bernard, H. R. (1994). *Research Methods in Anthropology: Qualitative and Quantitative Approaches*, 2nd edn. Sage.

Helman, C.G. (1991). Research in primary care: the qualitative approach. In: *Primary Care Research: Traditional and Innovative Approaches* (P. G. Norton, M. Stewart, F. Tudiver *et al.*, eds), pp. 105–1124. Sage Publications.

Helman, C. G. (1996). The application of anthropological methods in general practice research. *Fam. Pract.*, **13**(Suppl. 1), S13–S16.

Hudelson, P. M. (1994). *Qualitative Research for Health Programmes*. Division of Mental Health, World Health Organization.

Morse, J. M. (ed.) (1992). *Qualitative Health Research*. Sage.

Pelto, P. J. and Pelto, G. H. (1990). Field methods in medical anthropology. In: *Medical Anthropology* (T. M. Johnson and C. E. Sargent, eds), pp. 269–97. Praeger.

Scrimshaw, N. S. and Gleason, G. R. (eds) (1992). *Rapid Assessment Procedures*. International Nutrition Foundation for Developing Countries (INFDC).

Appendix

Clinical questionnaires

In this section short questionnaires are included on the topic of each chapter of the book. As described in Chapter 14, these open-ended, qualitative questionnaires can be used in two ways. Faced with a clinical situation where socio-cultural factors might be relevant, health professionals can ask themselves these questions as a way of increasing awareness of these factors and acting accordingly. Each set of questions can also provide the basis for a small research project on a particular topic within the wider field of applied medical anthropology. In this latter case, it is suggested that the books and journals recommended at the end of each chapter be consulted for further theoretical background before the project is attempted.

Chapter 2: Cultural definitions of anatomy and physiology

1. What alterations in the shape, size, clothing and surface of the patient's body can be ascribed to his or her socio-cultural background?
2. How does the patient conceptualize the boundaries of his or her body?
3. How does the patient conceptualize the inner structure (including the location of organs) of his or her body?
4. How does the patient conceptualize the inner workings of his or her body?
5. To what extent do 1, 2, 3 and 4 affect:
   a. the clinical presentation of the patient's condition
   b. the patient's attitude towards the origin, treatment and prognosis of his or her condition?
6. To what extent do 1, 2, 3 and 4 affect the patient's health?
7. To what extent do 1, 2, 3 and 4 affect compliance with medical treatment or advice?
8. Is medical diagnosis, treatment or advice congruent with 1, 2, 3 and 4?
9. In pregnancy/menstruation/lactation, to what extent do 1, 2, 3 and 4 affect:
   a. the behaviour and diet of the woman
   b. the health of the woman
   c. the health of the foetus or newborn?
10. To what extent does the patient's concept of his or her 'body' coincide with that of the 'self'?

Chapter 3: Diet and nutrition

1. Is the patient's diet nutritionally adequate (and is there evidence of malnutrition)?
2. If the diet is inadequate (or if malnutrition is present), are foodstuffs being excluded from the diet because they are not available?
3. Are foodstuffs being excluded from the diet because the patient cannot afford to buy them, even though they are available?
4. Are foodstuffs being excluded from the diet because they are classified as:
   a. non-food
   b. profane food
   c. 'hot' (or 'cold') food
   d. medicine
   e. low social value food (not signalling correct status, caste, ethnicity, region etc.)?

5. Are foodstuffs included in the diet because they are classified as:
   a. food
   b. sacred food
   c. 'hot' (or 'cold') food
   d. medicine
   e. high social value food?
6. What forms of eating are defined as 'meals' and 'snacks'?
7. In 'meals', what social function does the content, order, preparation and timing of the meal perform for those who take part in it? What does it signal to them, and to others, about the types of relationships between those who take part in it?
8. In pregnancy/menstruation/lactation, is the woman's diet nutritionally adequate? If not, is this because of 2, 3, 4, or 5, or combinations of these?
9. In infant feeding, how do socio-cultural factors affect:
   a. the choice of breast or artificial feeding
   b. the length of breast or artificial feeding
   c. the techniques of weaning, and types of weaning foods used
   d. maternal beliefs about the optimal size, shape and weight of their infants?
10. In infant feeding, how do economic factors affect:
   a. the choice of breast or artificial feeding
   b. the length of breast or artificial feeding
   c. the techniques of weaning, and types of weaning food used?

Chapter 4: Caring and curing: the sectors of health care

1. What sectors of health care can be identified in your society?
2. Within these sectors:
   a. who are the patients and who are the healers
   b. how does one become a patient or a healer?
3. How can the health care provided by each sector be compared, considering:
   a. the availability of healers
   b. the cost of consultations
   c. the formality or informality of consultations
   d. the length of consultations
   e. the types of data considered relevant to the consultation
   f. whether the consultation is private or public
   g. how diagnosis and treatment are carried out
   h. who attends the consultation
   i. the effectiveness (or dangers) in treating disease
   j. the effectiveness (or dangers) in treating illness?
4. Which sources of advice has the patient sought before consulting a health professional?
5. If non-professional advice was sought:
   a. why were non-professionals consulted
   b. what do they provide that professional advice cannot (the perceived benefits of the advice)
   c. was the advice effective, or dangerous to health?
6. If advice from health professionals was sought:
   a. why were they consulted
   b. what do they provide that non-professionals cannot (the perceived benefits of the advice)
   c. was the advice effective, or dangerous to health?

Chapter 5: Doctor–patient interactions

1. In what ways are the health professional's perception, diagnosis and treatment of ill health influenced by his or her:
   a. individual attributes (age, gender, personality, experience, prejudices)
   b. education or sub-culture (ethnic, religious or professional)
   c. cultural background
   d. socio-economic status?
2. Can the cause (or presentation) of the patient's ill health be related to his or her:
   a. individual attributes (age, gender, personality, experience, prejudices)
   b. education or sub-culture (ethnic, religious or professional)
   c. cultural background
   d. socio-economic status?
3. How does the patient view the meaning and significance of his or her ill health?
4. What Explanatory Model does the patient use? What are the patient's answers to the following questions:

   a. What has happened (labelling the condition)?
   b. Why has it happened (aetiology)?
   c. Why to me (relation to diet, behaviour, personality, heredity)?
   d. Why now (timing, mode of onset)?
   e. What would happen to me if nothing was done about it (its likely course, outcome, prognosis and dangers)?
   f. What are its likely effects on other people (family, friends, neighbours, employers etc.)?
   g. What should I do about it – or to whom should I turn for further help (self-treatment, consultations with lay advisers, folk healers, or health professionals)?
5. Does the patient believe that he or she is suffering from a folk illness?
6. How do family and friends view the patient's ill health? What Explanatory Models do they use?

In the consultation:

7. Does the patient have illness as well as disease?
8. Does the patient have illness but no disease?
9. Does the patient have disease but no illness?
10. Is the patient's illness being treated, as well as the disease?
11. Is the diagnosis/treatment/prognosis given to the patient congruent with his or her Explanatory Model? Is consensus between health professional and patient achieved regarding the diagnosis/treatment/prognosis of the patient's ill health?
12. What is the role of context (social, cultural, economic, political) in the origin, presentation, diagnosis and treatment of the patient's condition?

After the consultation:

13. Is there compliance with the health professional's advice or treatment? If not, why not?
14. Is there satisfaction with the health professional's advice or treatment? If not, why not?
15. What is the impact of the medical diagnoses/medical tests/medical treatments on the individual patient's:
   a. physical state
   b. psychological state
   c. behaviour
   d. social relationships
   e. employment
   f. economic status?

Chapter 6: Gender and reproduction

Gender:

1. What elements define the patients' gender as either 'male' or 'female'? Their:
   a. genetic gender
   b. somatic gender
   c. psychological gender
   d. social gender?
2. How does the patient's own gender culture define his or her appropriate:
   a. behaviour
   b. emotions
   c. dress
   d. occupation
   e. leisure activities
   f. use of alcohol, tobacco and drugs?
3. What aspects of the patient's gender culture can be considered either pathogenic or protective of health?
4. Can the origin, presentation or prognosis of the patient's ill health be related to his or her gender culture?
5. What is the relation of the patient's gender to his or her sexual behaviour?
6. To what extent is the patient's sexual behaviour tolerated, or tabooed, by his or her own cultural group?
7. In the patient's own cultural group, is gender defined more by biological criteria (genetic and somatic gender), or by sexual behaviour?
8. Which of the following aspects of the patient's life can be considered to be medicalized:
   a. menstruation
   b. childbirth
   c. menopause
   d. social problems
   e. economic problems?

Reproduction and childbirth:

9. How does the patient's birth culture define the nature and requirements of:
   a. conception
   b. pregnancy
   c. childbirth
   d. puerperium?

10. What rituals and ritual symbols are a feature of the birth cultures of:
    a. the patient
    b. the health professional?
11. What are the advantages and disadvantages for the patient of delivery by:
    a. an obstetrician
    b. a traditional birth attendant?

In males:

12. Are there physical or psychological symptoms suggestive of the couvade syndrome?
13. Are certain beliefs and behaviour prescribed as part of the ritual couvade?

Chapter 7: Pain and culture

1. What is the recognized pattern of pain behaviour (language of distress) in the socio-cultural milieu of:
   a. the health professional
   b. the patient?
2. Is the patient suffering private pain, but not translating it into public pain? If not, why not?
3. Is the patient displaying public pain? If so:
   a. does he or she also have private pain,
   b. what does the patient intend to signal or achieve by the use of pain behaviour?
4. In the patient's socio-cultural background, is pain seen as a 'message' with a religious or healing significance?
5. In the patient's socio-cultural background, is pain behaviour accepted/encouraged/ responded to, or not?
6. In the clinical setting, is pain behaviour accepted/encouraged/ responded to, or not?
7. How does the patient view the origin, significance and prognosis of the pain?
8. How do the patient's family and friends view the origin, significance and prognosis of the pain?
9. Is treatment with analgesics sufficient, or should the illness associated with the pain be treated as well?

Chapter 8: Culture and pharmacology

In drug treatment:

1. What factors are contributing towards the 'total drug effect'? The attributes of:
   a. the drug itself
   b. the patient
   c. the prescriber
   d. the micro-context
   e. the macro-context?

The placebo effect:

2. To what extent is there a placebo element in:
   a. drug treatment
   b. surgical or other treatment
   c. hospital tests
   d. the relationship with the health professional?

Psychological dependence:

3. What symbolic role does the drug or other treatment play in the patient's:
   a. daily activities
   b. self-image
   c. social relationships
   d. relationships with health professionals?
4. Does the patient feel he or she has control over the drug treatment (its dosage, time of ingestion, effects on self or others) or not?
5. Is the drug taken for its effect on:
   a. the patient
   b. relationships with other people?

Physical addiction:

6. Does the patient belong to an addict subculture?
7. If so, what are its values and standards of behaviour?
8. How does the patient view:
   a. other addicts
   b. non-addicts?
9. If there is evidence of stereotyping in 8, how does this affect the treatment of the patient's addiction?
10. In intravenous drug abuse, do the addicts practise 'needle sharing' among themselves?

Alcoholism:

11. In the patient's socio-cultural milieu, what values govern:
    a. normal drinking
    b. abnormal drinking?
12. In normal drinking, what are the rules about:
    a. who is allowed to drink (age, sex, ethnicity, class)

b. in whose company drinking is allowed to take place
c. what can be drunk
d. at what times can drinking take place
e. in what settings can drinking take place
f. the relation of drinking to religious and social festivals?

13. What does the alcohol symbolize to the drinker? What symbolic role does it play in the drinker's:
    a. daily activities
    b. self-image
    c. social relationships
    d. relationships with health professionals?

Tobacco use:

14. What symbolic role does cigarette smoking play in the patient's:
    a. daily activities
    b. self-image
    c. social relationships?

Chapter 9: Ritual and the management of misfortune

1. What rituals (social, religious, personal) exist in the patient's daily life? Do rituals play a central, pervasive role in the patient's life, and do they deal adequately with misfortune, illness and death?

In the consultation:

2. What aspects of the health professional's behaviour, speech, dress, and techniques have a ritual aspect?
3. What ritual symbols are used?
4. What associations do these ritual symbols have for:
    a. the patient
    b. the patient's family or friends
    c. the health professional?
5. Does the ritual, or its absence, positively affect the patient's mental or physical health, or social relationships?
6. Does the ritual serve to integrate the patient back into the community, or to alienate him or her from it?
7. Does the ritual signal a biological and/or social transition in the patient's life?
8. What is the effect of the ritual, or its absence, on the psychological state of the health professional?

In hospital:

9. What aspects of the patient's admission procedure, dress, behaviour, diet, medication and control over time and space have a ritual significance for the patient, and for the professional staff?
10. To what extent do these rituals accelerate or impede the patient's return to health?

In major life changes (pregnancy, birth, bereavement):

11. What rituals are used to symbolize the patient's biological and social transition in:
    a. his or her socio-cultural background
    b. the clinical setting?
12. Is this ritual, or its absence, advantageous (or dangerous) to the patient's mental or physical health, or social relationships?
13. Should more ritual be used, in order to place the transition in a wider social, moral or religious context?

Chapter 10: Cross-cultural psychiatry

In psychiatric diagnosis:

1. Which of the following influences on the diagnostician may affect the validity of psychiatric diagnoses:
    a. cultural factors
    b. social factors
    c. moral attitudes
    d. political pressures?

In cross-cultural diagnosis:

2. In the patient's socio-cultural background, what are the definitions of normal and abnormal social behaviour?
3. Are the patient's beliefs and/or behaviour abnormal by the standards of the community? If they are, is it 'controlled' or 'uncontrolled' abnormality?
4. Do the patient's family and/or friends regard his or her abnormality as beneficial or dangerous to them (or to the wider community)?
5. Are the specific clusters of symptoms and signs interpreted by the patient (or by family

and friends) as evidence of a culture-bound psychological disorder?
6. Is the clinical presentation of the disorder shaped by cultural factors into a culture-bound disorder (such as *susto* or somatization)?
7. What role do cultural factors play in the aetiology of the disorder?

In cross-cultural treatment:

8. Is the illness of the mental disorder being treated, as well as the disease?
9. Should the patient's family and/or friends be asked to take part in the treatment process?
10. Should a folk healer, priest or exorcist be used by the patient (and/or family) as a complementary form of treatment?
11. What could such healers provide that Western psychiatrists cannot?

In symbolic healing:

12. What are its effects on the patient's:
    a. psychological state
    b. physical state
    c. social relationships
    d. socio-economic status?

In family therapy:

13. Are the family dynamics evidence of:
    a. cultural costume
    b. cultural camouflage?
14. In what ways are the structure and dynamics of the family the result of:
    a. psychopathology
    b. cultural background
    c. economic status
    d. external social pressures?

Chapter 11: Cultural aspects of stress

1. Has the patient experienced any major life changes in the past year?
2. Is there any evidence of the 'giving-up–given-up' complex?
3. What cultural factors could have contributed towards the patient's stress response?
4. What cultural factors would protect the patient against the stress response?

In migrant communities:

5. What sources of stress for the migrant can be identified in:
    a. the host community
    b. the migrant community
    c. the changes in life space involved in migration?
6. Is there evidence of cultural bereavement in the migrant or the community?

In lay models of stress:

7. What is meant by the terms 'stress' or 'nerves' when used by:
    a. the patient
    b. their family and friends
    c. the health professional?

Chapter 12: Cultural factors in epidemiology

In studying the origin and distribution of a particular disease:

1. To what extent does the perceived incidence of the disease depend on:
    a. its actual incidence
    b. its recognition by the population as abnormal
    c. its recognition by the researcher as abnormal?
2. What role do cultural factors play in (a), (b) and (c)?
3. What cultural factors can be linked to the occurrence and/or distribution of the disease in a causal way?
4. What cultural factors can be linked to the spread of the disease within the population?
5. What cultural factors may protect some members of the population from the disease?

Chapter 13: Medical anthropology and global health

In family planning programmes:

1. In the patient's socio-cultural milieu, are there taboos (religious, social, cultural) against using artificial contraception?
2. Who makes decisions about reproduction and contraception? Is it:

a. the patient
b. the spouse
c. the family
d. community or religious leaders?

3. Are children seen as proof of:
   a. adulthood
   b. virility
   c. social status?
4. Are there preferences for children of a particular gender?
5. Is menstrual blood seen as 'polluting'? If so, does this affect the acceptance of:
   a. oral contraception
   b. intra-uterine contraceptive devices (IUCDs)?
6. Are beliefs about female anatomy related to the acceptance of IUCDs?

In urbanization:

7. What health problems of the urban poor are due mainly to their:
   a. poverty
   b. physical environment
   c. psychosocial stress
   d. health beliefs and behaviours?

In AIDS:

8. In the patient's socio-cultural milieu, what metaphors for AIDS are common?
9. What is the degree of knowledge of its:
   a. aetiology
   b. modes of spread
   c. treatment?
10. Has the patient experienced prejudice, discrimination or social death?
11. What supportive social networks exist for the patient?
12. Which of the following forms of sexual behaviour are tolerated in the community:
    a. heterosexuality
    b. homosexuality
    c. bisexuality
    d. promiscuity
    e. extramarital sex
    f. recourse to prostitutes
    g. anal intercourse?
13. If there is recourse to prostitutes, is the patient:
    a. heterosexual
    b. homosexual
    c. bisexual?
14. Are the prostitutes:
    a. career prostitutes
    b. episodic prostitutes?
15. Do prostitutes insist on condom use for:
    a. all clients
    b. new clients only
    c. boyfriends or male partners?
16. With intravenous drug users (IVDUs), is there evidence of:
    a. needle sharing
    b. drug sharing
    c. prostitution
    d. unsafe sex practices?
17. If there is recourse to traditional or alternative healers, does their treatment:
    a. cure the disease
    b. heal the disease
    c. transmit the disease
    d. worsen the disease?
18. What bodily mutilations/alterations are commonly used that may transmit the disease?
19. What patterns of population movement may help spread the disease?
20. What marriage patterns may help spread the disease?

In immunizations:

21. Do patients know which disease is being immunized against?
22. Do patients believe that immunizations:
    a. prevent disease
    b. treat disease?

In diarrhoeal diseases:

23. Which types of diarrhoea are regarded as normal?
24. Which types are regarded as abnormal?
25. Which are regarded as more serious:
    a. watery diarrhoea
    b. bloody diarrhoea?
26. Which types are blamed on natural, social or supernatural causes?
27. Which types are treated by home remedies or traditional healers?
28. What are attitudes towards the use of oral rehydration therapy (ORT)?

In acute respiratory infections:

29. What beliefs exist about the significance of different types of:

a. breathing patterns
b. cough
c. wheeze
d. phlegm
e. chest movements
f. fever?

30. What types of home, over-the-counter or medical treatments are thought to be appropriate for each of these?

In malaria:

31. What beliefs exist about the different types of fever?
32. To what extent do people recognize a specific malarial fever?
33. To what extent do they connect malaria with mosquito bites?
34. To what extent do people believe that malaria can be prevented by:
    a. anti-malarial drugs
    b. insect repellents
    c. bed nets
    d. spraying of houses
    e. drainage of stagnant water?
35. To what extent do people believe malaria can be treated by:
    a. Western pharmaceuticals which are self-prescribed, or those medically-prescribed
    b. traditional home remedies
    c. traditional healers?

References

Chapter 1 Introduction: the scope of medical anthropology (pages 1–11)

1. Editorial (1980). More anthropology and less sleep for medical students. *Br. Med. J.*, **281**, 1662.
2. Keesing, R. M. (1981). *Cultural Anthropology: A Contemporary Perspective*, p. 518. Holt, Rinehart & Winston.
3. Leach, E. (1982). *Social Anthropology*, pp. 38–9. Fontana.
4. Keesing, R. M. (1981). *Cultural Anthropology: A Contemporary Perspective*, p. 68. Holt, Rinehart & Winston.
5. Hall, E. T. (1984). *The Dance of Life*, pp. 230–31 Anchor Press.
6. Leach, E. (1982). *Social Anthropology*, pp. 41–3. Fontana.
7. Townsend, P. and Davidson, N. (eds) (1982). *Inequalities in Health: The Black Report*. Penguin.
8. Zaidi, S. A. (1988). Poverty and disease: need for structural change. *Soc. Sci. Med.*, **27**, 119–27.
9. Unterhalter, B. (1982) Inequalities in health and disease: the case of mortality rates for the city of Johannesburg, South Africa, 1910–1979. *Int. J. Hlth. Serv.*, **12**, 617–36.
10. Preston-Whyte, E. M. (1995). Half-way there: anthropology and intervention-oriented AIDS research in Kwazulu/Natal, South Africa. In: *Culture and Sexual Risk: Anthropological Perspectives on AIDS* (H. ten Brummelhuis and G. Herdt, eds), pp. 315–37. Gordon and Breach.
11. Lopez, S. and Hernandez, P. (1986). How culture is considered in evaluation of psychopathology. *J. Nerv. Ment. Dis.*, **176**, 598–606.
12. Weiss, M. G. (1985). The interrelationship of tropical disease and mental disorder: conceptual framework and literature review. Part 1 – Malaria. *Cult. Med. Psychiatry*, **9**, 121–200.
13. Foster, G. M. and Anderson, B. G. (1978). *Medical Anthropology*, pp. 2–3. Wiley.
14. Ember, C.R. and Ember, M. (1985). *Cultural Anthropology*, 4th edn, p. 205. Prentice Hall.
15. Opie, I. and Opie, P. (1977). *The Lore and Language of Schoolchildren*. Oxford University Press.
16. Kaufman, S. (1986). *The Ageless Self*. University of Wisconsin Press.
17. James, A., Jenks, C. and Prout, A. (1998). *Theorizing Childhood*, pp. 22–34. Polity Press.
18. Ember, C. R. and Ember, M. (1985). *Cultural Anthropology*, 4th edn, pp. 169–70. Prentice Hall.
19. James, A., Jenks, C. and Prout, A. (1998). *Theorizing Childhood*, p. 63. Polity Press.
20. Desjarlais, R., Eisenberg, L., Good, B. and Kleinman, A. (1995). *World Mental Health*, pp. 155–78. Oxford University Press.
21. James, A., Jenks, C. and Prout, A. (1998). *Theorizing Childhood*, p. 60. Polity Press.
22. Korbin, J. (1987). Child sexual abuse: implications from the cross-cultural record. In: *Child Survival* (N. Scheper-Hughes, ed.), pp. 247–65. D. Reidel.
23. Desjarlais, R., Eisenberg, L., Good, B. and Kleinman, A. (1995). *World Mental Health*, pp. 207–27. Oxford University Press.
24. Lousteaunau, M. O. and Lobo, E. J. (1997). *The Cultural Context of Health, Illness, and Medicine*, pp. 65–8. Bergin and Garvey.
25. Turkle, S. (1984). *The Second Self: Computers and the Human Spirit*, pp. 281–318. Granada.
26. Johnson, T. M. (1987). Practising medical anthropology: clinical strategies for work in hospital. In: *Applied Anthropology in America* (E. Eddy and W. Partridge, eds), 2nd edn, pp. 316–39. Columbia University Press.
27. Singer, M., Valentin, F., Baer, M. and Jia, Z. (1992). Why does Juan Garcia have a drinking problem? The perspective of critical medical anthropology. *Med. Anthropol.*, **14**, 77–108.
28. Baer, H. A., Singer, M. and Susser, I. (1997). *Medical Anthropology and the World System*. Bergin and Garvey.
29. Foster, G. M. (1987). Bureaucratic aspects of international health agencies. *Soc. Sci. Med.*, **25**, 1039–48.

30. Nakajima, H. and Mayor, F. (1996). Editorial: culture and health. *World Health*, **2**, 3.
31. Agency for International Development (1983). *Proceedings of the International Conference on Oral Rehydration Therapy (ICORT)*, 7–10 June 1983. Agency for International Development.
32. Weiss, M. G. (1988). Cultural models of diarrhoeal illness: conceptual framework and review. *Soc. Sci. Med.*, **27**, 5–16.
33. Mull, J. D. and Mull, D. S. (1988). Mothers' concept of childhood diarrhoea in rural Pakistan: what ORT program planners should know. *Soc. Sci. Med.*, **27**, 53–67.
34. Keesing, R. M. (1981) *Cultural Anthropology: A Contemporary Perspective*, p. 4. Holt, Rinehart & Winston.
35. Pelto, P. J. and Pelto, G. H. (1990). Field methods in medical anthropology. In: *Medical Anthropology* (T. M. Johnson and C. F. Sargent, eds), pp. 269–97. Praeger.

Chapter 2 Cultural definitions of anatomy and physiology (pages 12–31)

1. Fisher, S. (1968). Body image. In: *International Encyclopaedia of the Social Sciences* (D. Sills, ed.), pp. 113–16. Free Press/Macmillan.
2. Polhemus, T. (1978). Body alteration and adornment: a pictorial essay. In: *Social Aspects of the Human Body* (T. Polhemus, ed.), pp. 154–73. Penguin.
3. Warner, E. and Strashin, E. (1981). Benefits and risks of circumcision. *Can. Med. Assoc. J.*, **125**, 967–76.
4. Gordon, D. (1991). Female circumcision and genital operations in Egypt and the Sudan: a dilemma for medical anthropology. *Med. Anthropol. Q.* (new series), 3–14.
5. Ladjali, M., Rattray, T. and Walder, R. J. W. (1993). Female genital mutilation. *Br. Med. J.*, **307**, 460.
6. Jeffcoate, T. N. A. (1962). *Principles of Gynaecology*, 2nd edn, pp. 279–80. Butterworths.
7. Peckham, M., Pinedo, H. and Veronesi, U. (eds) (1995). *Oxford Textbook of Oncology*, Vol. 2, pp. 1325–7. Oxford University Press.
8. MacCormack, C. P. (1982). Personal communication.
9. Garner, D. M. and Garfinkel, P. E. (1980). Sociocultural factors in the development of anorexia nervosa. *Psychol. Med.*, **10**, 647–56.
10. Swartz, L. (1985). Anorexia nervosa as a culture-bound syndrome. *Soc. Sci. Med.*, **20**, 725–30.
11. Rintala, M. and Mutajoki, P. (1992). Could mannequins menstruate? *Br. Med. J.*, **305**, 1575–6.
12. Orbach, S. (1986). *Hunger Strike: The Anorexic's Struggle as a Metaphor for Our Age.* W. W. Norton.
13. Polhemus, T. (1978). Introduction. In: *Social Aspects of the Human Body* (T. Polhemus, ed.), pp. 23–5. Penguin.
14. Gray, B. M. (1982). Enga birth, maturation and survival: physiological characteristics of the life cycle in the New Guinea Highland. In: *Ethnography of Fertility and Birth* (C. P. McCormack, ed.), pp. 75–113. Academic Press.
15. de Garine, I (1995). Sociocultural aspects of the male fattening sessions among the Massa of Northern Cameroon. In: *Social Aspects of Obesity* (I. de Garine and N. J. Pollock, eds), pp. 45–70. Gordon and Breach.
16. Ritenbaugh, C. (1982). Obesity as a culture-bound syndrome. *Cult. Med. Psychiatry*, **6**, 347–61.
17. Helman, C. G. (1978). 'Feed a cold, starve a fever': folk models of infection in an English suburban community, and their relation to medical treatment. *Cult. Med. Psychiatry*, **2**, 107–37.
18. Douglas, M. (1973). *Natural Symbols*, pp. 93–112. Penguin.
19. Scheper-Hughes, N. and Lock, M. M. (1987). The mindful body: a proglomenon to future work in medical anthropology. *Med. Anthropol. Q.* (new series), **1**, 6–41.
20. Gordon, D. R. (1987). Magico-religious dimensions of biomedicine: the case of the artificial heart. Unpublished MS.
21. Csordas, T. J. (1993). Somatic modes of attention. *Cultural Anthropology*, **8(2)**, 135–56.
22. Hall, E. T. (1969). *The Hidden Dimension*, pp. 113–29. Anchor Books.
23. Tamura, T. and Lau, A. (1992). Connectedness versus separateness: application of family therapy to Japanese families. *Fam. Proc.*, **31**, 319–40.
24. Jadhav, S. (1986). *Explanatory Models, Choice of Healers and Help-seeking Behaviour.* Unpublished thesis. National Institute of Mental Health and Neurosciences, Bangalore.
25. Jean, G. (1998). *Signs, Symbols and Ciphers*, pp. 114–6. Thames and Hudson.
26. Levi-Strauss, C. (1967). *Structural Anthropology*, pp. 250–56. Anchor Books.
27. Kaufman, S. R. (1988). Toward a phenomenology of boundaries in medicine: chronic illness experience in the case of stroke. *Med. Anthropol. Q.* (new series), **2**, 338–54.
28. Boyle, C. M. (1970). Difference between patients' and doctors' interpretation of some common medical terms. *Br. Med J.*, **ii**, 286–9.
29. Pearson, J. and Dudley, H. A. F. (1982). Bodily perceptions in surgical patients. *Br. Med. J.*, **284**, 1545–6.
30. Tait, C. D. and Ascher, R. C. (1955). Inside-of-the-body test. *Psychosom. Med.*, **17**, 139–48.
31. Cassell, E. J. (1976). Disease as an 'it': concepts of disease revealed by patients' presentation of symptoms. *Soc. Sci. Med.*, **10**, 143–6.

32. Helman, C. G. (1985). Psyche, soma, and society: the social construction of psychosomatic disorders. *Cult. Med. Psychiatry*, **9**, 1–26.
33. Waddell, G., McCulloch, J. A., Kummel, E. and Venner, R. M. (1980). Nonorganic physical signs in low-back pain. *Spine*, **5**, 117–25.
34. Walters, A. (1961). Psychogenic regional pain alias hysterical pain. *Brain*, **84**, 1–18.
35. Kleinman, A., Eisenberg, L. and Good, B. (1978). Clinical lessons from anthropologic and cross-cultural research. *Ann. Intern. Med.*, **88**, 251–8.
36. Foster, G. M. (1994). *Hippocrates' Latin American Legacy: Humoral Medicine in the New World.* Gordon and Breach.
37. Colson, A. B. and de Armellado, C. (1983). An Amerindian derivation for Latin American Creole illnesses and their treatment. *Soc. Sci. Med.*, **17**, 1229–48.
38. Logan, M. H. (1975). Selected references on the hot–cold theory of disease. *Med. Anthropol. Newsletter*, **6**, 8–14.
39. Snow, L. F. and Johnson, S. M. (1978). Folklore, food, female reproductive cycle. *Ecol. Food Nutr.*, **7**, 41–9.
40. Greenwood, B. (1981). Cold or spirits? Choice and ambiguity in Morocco's pluralistic medical system. *Soc. Sci. Med.*, **15B**, 219–35.
41. Obeyesekere, G. (1977). The theory and practice of Ayurvedic medicine. *Cult. Med. Psychiatry*, **1**, 155–81.
42. Macdonald, A. (1984). *Acupuncture.* Allen and Unwin.
43. Tansley, D. V. (1977). *Subtle Body: Essence and Shadow.* Thames and Hudson.
44. Clifford, T. (1984). *Tibetan Buddhist Medicine and Psychiatry.* Weiser.
45. Helman, C. (1992). *The Body of Frankenstein's Monster*, pp. 19–28. W. W. Norton.
46. Turkle, S. (1984). *The Second Self: Computers and the Human Spirit*, pp. 281–318. Granada.
47. McLuhan, M. (1964). *Understanding Media.* Sphere.
48. Helman, C. (1992). *The Body of Frankenstein's Monster*, pp. 81–93. W. W. Norton.
49. Hall, E. T. (1984). *The Dance of Life: The Other Dimensions of Time.* Anchor Press.
50. World Health Organisation (1980). *International Classification of Impairments, Disabilities, and Handicaps.* WHO.
51. Oliver, M. (1990). *The Politics of Disablement*, p. 12. Macmillan.
52. Oliver, M. (1990). *The Politics of Disablement*, pp. 12–24, 78–94. Macmillan.
53. Susman, J. (1994). Disability, stigma and deviance. *Soc. Sci. Med.*, **38**, 15–22.
54. Reynolds-Whyte, S. and Ingstad, B. (eds) (1995). Disability and culture: an overview. In: *Disability and Culture* (B. Ingstad and S. Reynolds-Whyte, eds), pp. 3–32. University of California Press.
55. Sentumbwe, N. (1995). Sighted lovers and blind husbands: experiences of blind women in Uganda. In: *Disability and Culture* (B. Ingstad and S. Reynolds-Whyte, eds), pp. 159–73. University of California Press.
56. Devlieger, P. (1995). Why disabled? The cultural understanding of physical disability in an African society. In: *Disability and Culture* (B. Ingstad and S. Reynolds-Whyte, eds), pp. 94–106. University of California Press.
57. Ingstad, B. (1995). Mpho ya Modimo – a gift from God: perspectives on 'attitudes' toward disabled persons. In: *Disability and Culture* (B. Ingstad and S. Reynolds-Whyte, eds), pp. 246–263. University of California Press.
58. Levinson, D. and Gaccione, L. (1997). *Health and Illness*, pp. 102–104. ABC-CLIO.
59. Alemayehu, W., Tekle-Haimanot, R., Forsgren, L. and Ekstedt, J. (1986). Perceptions of blindness, *World Health Forum*, **17**, 379–81.
60. Rubinstein, R. (1985). *Take it and Leave It: Aspects of Being Ill.* Marion Boyars.
61. Sacks, O. (1991). *A Leg to Stand On*. Picador.
62. Beecher, H. B., Adams, R. D., Berger, A. C. *et al.* (1968). A definition of irreversible coma: a report of the ad hoc committee of the Harvard Medical School to examine definition of brain death. *JAMA*, **205**, 337–40.
63. Walton, D. N. (1983). *Ethics of Withdrawal of Life Support Systems.* Greenwood Press.
64. McAllister-Williams, R. H. and Young, A. H. (1990). Neuroscience and psychiatry: 'The Decade of the Brain'. *Psychiatry in Practice*, **9**, 12–16.
65. Diamond, N. L. (1993). A brain is a terrible thing to waste. *OMNI*, August, p. 12.
66. Ascherson, N. (1991). Fallen idol. *Independent Magazine*, 16 November, pp. 41–54.
67. Nudeshima, J. (1991). Obstacles to brain death and organ transplantation in Japan. *Lancet*, **338**, 1063–4.
68. Hadfield, P. (1998). No spare parts: cultural qualms are undermining Japan's transplant efforts. *New Scientist*, 31 October, p. 13.
69. Helman, C. (1992). *The Body of Frankenstein's Monster*, pp. 13–18. W. W. Norton.
70. Stacey, M. (ed.) (1991). *Changing Human Reproduction.* Sage Publications.
71. Snowden, R., Mitchell, G. D. and Snowden, E. (1983). *Artificial Reproduction.* George Allen and Unwin.
72. Konrad, M. (1998). Ova donation and symbols of substance: some variations on the theme of sex, gender and the partible body. *J. R. Anthrop. Inst.* (new series), **4**, 643–67.
73. Homans, H. (1982). Pregnancy and birth as rites of passage for two groups of women in Britain. In: *Ethnography of Fertility and Birth* (C. P. McCormack, ed.), pp. 231–68. Academic Press.

74. Snow, L. F., Johnson, S. M. and Mayhew, H. F. (1978). The behavioral implications of some Old Wives Tales. *Obstet. Gynecol.*, **51**, 727–32.
75. Snow, L. F. and Johnson, S. M. (1977). Modern day menstrual folklore. *JAMA*, **237**, 2736–9.
76. Turner, V. W. (1974). *The Ritual Process*, pp. 48–9. Penguin.
77. Skultans, V. (1970). The symbolic significance of menstruation and the menopause. *MAN*, **5**, 639–51.
78. Ngubane, H. (1977). *Body and Mind in Zulu Medicine*, pp. 79, 164. Academic Press.
79. Delaney, J., Lupton, M. J. and Toth, E. (1976). *The Curse: A Cultural History of Menstruation*. Dutton.
80. Snow, L. F. (1976). 'High blood' is not high blood pressure. *Urban Health*, **5**, 5–55.
81. Like, R. and Ellison, J. (1981). Sleeping blood, tremor and paralysis: a transcultural approach to an unusual conversion reaction. *Cult. Med. Psychiatry*, **5**, 49–63.
82. Foster, G. M. and Anderson, B. G. (1978). *Medical Anthropology*, p. 227. Wiley.
83. Bledsoe, C. H. and Goubaud, M. F. (1988). The reinterpretation and distribution of Western pharmaceuticals: an example from the Mende of Sierra Leone. In: Van Der Geest, S. and Whyte, S.R. (eds.) *The Context of Medicines in Developing Countries*, pp.253–276. Kluwer.

Chapter 3 Diet and nutrition (pages 32–49)

1. Levi-Strauss, C. (1970) *The Raw and the Cooked*, pp. 142, 164. Jonathan Cape.
2. Ember, C. R. and Ember, M. (1985). *Cultural Anthropology*, pp. 138–47. Prentice Hall.
3. Jelliffe, D. B. (1967). Parallel food classifications in developing and industrialized countries. *Am. J. Clin. Nutr.*, **20**, 279–81.
4. Foster, G. M. and Anderson, B. G. (1978). *Medical Anthropology*, pp. 263–79. Wiley.
5. Hunt, S. (1976). The food habits of Asian immigrants. In: *Getting the Most Out of Food*, pp. 15–51. Van den Berghs & Jurgens.
6. Littlewood, R. and Lipsedge, M. (1989). *Aliens and Alienists*, 2nd edn, pp. 17–20. Unwin Hyman.
7. Twigg, J. (1979). Food for thought: purity and vegetarianism. *Religion*, **9**, 13–35.
8. Greenwood, B. (1981). Cold or spirits? Choice and ambiguity in Morocco's pluralistic medical system. *Soc. Sci. Med.*, **15B**, 219–35.
9. Harwood, A. (1971). The hot–cold theory of disease: implications for treatment of Puerto Rican patients. *JAMA*, **216**, 1153–8.
10. Tann, S. P. and Wheeler, E. F. (1980). Food intakes and growth of young Chinese children in London. *Community Med.*, **2**, 20–24.
11. Snow, L. F. and Johnson, S. M. (1978). Folklore, food, female reproductive cycle. *Ecol. Food Nutr.*, **7**, 41–9.
12. Etkin, N. L. and Ross, P. J. (1982). Food as medicine and medicine as food: an adaptive framework for the interpretation of plant utilization among the Hausa of Northern Nigeria. *Soc. Sci. Med.*, **16**, 1559–73.
13. Farb, P. and Armelagos, G. (1980). *Consuming Passions: The Anthropology of Eating*, p. 103. Houghton Muffin.
14. Belshaw, C. S. (1965). *Traditional Exchange and Modern Markets*, pp. 12–20. Prentice Hall.
15. Trowell, H. C. and Burkitt, D. P. (eds) (1981). *Western Diseases: their Emergence and Prevention*. Edward Arnold.
16. Jerome, N. W. (1969). Northern urbanization and food consumption patterns of southern-born Negroes. *Am. J. Clin. Nutr.*, **22**, 1667–9.
17. Douglas, M. and Nicod, M. (1974). Taking the biscuit: the structure of British meals. *New Soc.*, **30**, 744–7.
18. Farb, P. and Armelagos, G. (1980). *Consuming Passions: The Anthropology of Eating*, p. 98. Houghton Muffin.
19. Charsley, S. (1987). Interpretation and custom: the case of the wedding cake. *MAN*, **22**, 93–110.
20. Keesing, R. M. (1981). *Cultural Anthropology*, pp. 459–62. Holt, Rinehart & Winston.
21. Lang, T. (1999). Diet, health and globalization: five key questions. *Proc. Nutr. Soc.*, **58**, 335–43.
22. Drewnowski, A. and Popkin, B. M. (1997). The nutrition transition: new trends in the global diet. *Nutr. Rev.*, **55**, 31–43.
23. Dettwyler, K. A. (1992). The biocultural approach in nutritional anthropology: case studies of malnutrition. *Med. Anthropol.*, **15**, 17–39.
24. Artley, A. (1987). Out of sight, out of mind. *Spectator*, **258(8258)**, 8–10.
25. Stroud, C. E. (1971). Nutrition and the immigrant. *Br. J. Hosp. Med.*, **5**, 629–34.
26. Ward, P. S., Drakeford, J. P., Milton, J. and James, J. A. (1982). Nutritional rickets in Rastafarian children. *Br. Med. J.*, **285**, 1242–3.
27. Black, J. (1990). Paediatrics and the Asian child. In: *Health Care for Asians* (B. R. McAvoy and L. J. Donaldson, eds), pp. 210–36. Oxford University Press.
28. Qureshi, B. (1990). Diet and nutrition of British Asians. In: *Health Care for Asians* (B. R. McAvoy and L. J. Donaldson, eds), pp. 117–29. Oxford University Press.
29. Editorial (1981). Asian rickets in Britain. *Lancet*, **2**, 402.
30. Lennon, D. and Fieldhouse, P. (1979). *Community Dietetics*, pp. 78–91. Forbes.
31. MacVicar, J. (1990). Obstetrics: the Asian mother and child. In: *Health Care for Asians* (B. R. McAvoy and L. J. Donaldson, eds), pp. 172–91. Oxford University Press.
32. Mares, P., Henley, A. and Baxter, C. (1985). *Health Care in Multiracial Britain*, p. 49. Health Education Council & National Extension College.

33. Greenhalgh, T., Helman, C. and Chowdhury, A. M. (1998). Health beliefs and folk models of diabetes in British Bangladeshis: a qualitative study. *Br. Med. J.*, **316**, 978–83.
34. International Statistical Institute (1984). *World Fertility Survey: Major Findings and Implications.* International Statistical Institute.
35. Farb, P. and Armelagos, G. (1980). *Consuming Passions: The Anthropology of Eating*, p. 783. Houghton Muffin.
36. Foster, G. M. and Anderson, B. G. (1978). *Medical Anthropology*, pp. 277–8. Wiley.
37. Elliott, L. (1998). Breast is best? *Health Exchange*, Aug 1998, 13–14.
38. Harrison, G. G., Zaghoul, S. S., Galal, O. M. and Gabr, A. (1993). Breastfeeding and weaning in a poor urban neighbourhood in Cairo, Egypt: maternal beliefs and perceptions. *Soc. Sci. Med.*, **36**, 1–10.
39. Goel, K. M., House, F. and Shanks, R. A. (1978). Infant-feeding practices among immigrants in Glasgow. *Br. Med. J.*, **2**, 1181–3.
40. Jones, R. A. K. and Belsey, E. M. (1977). Breast feeding in an inner London borough: a study of cultural factors. *Soc. Sci. Med.*, **11**, 175–9.
41. Tann, S. P. and Wheeler, E. F. (1980). Food intakes and growth of young Chinese children in London. *Community Med.*, **2**, 20–24.
42. Taitz, L. S. (1971). Infantile overnutrition among artificially fed infants in the Sheffield region. *Br. Med. J.*, **1**, 315–16.
43. Burkitt, D. P. (1973). Some diseases characteristic of modern Western civilization. *Br. Med. J.*, **1**, 274–8.
44. Wyngaarden, J. B., Smith, L. H. and Bennett, J. C. (eds) (1992). *Cecil Textbook of Medicine*, 19th edn, pp. 40–41, 667. W. B. Saunders.
45. Fuchs, C. S., Givanucci, L., Colditz, G. A. *et al.* (1999). Dietary fiber and the risk of colorectal cancer and adenoma in women. *New Engl. J. Med.*, **340**, 169–76.
46. Wyngaarden, J. B., Smith, L. H. and Bennett, J. C. (eds) (1992). *Cecil Textbook of Medicine*, 19th edn, p. 1032. W. B. Saunders.
47. Lowenfels, A. B. and Anderson, M. E. (1977). Diet and cancer. *Cancer*, **39**, 1809–14.
48. Newberne, P. M. (1978). Diet and Nutrition. *Bull. NY Acad. Med.*, **54**, 385–96.
49. Kolonel, L. N., Nomura, A. M. Y., Hirohata, T. *et al.* (1981). Association of diet and place of birth with stomach cancer incidence in Hawaii Japanese and Caucasians. *Am. J. Clin. Nutr.*, **34**, 2478–85.
50. Sugimura, T. (1978). Mutagens, carcinogens and tumor promoters in our daily food. *Cancer*, **49**, 1970–84.
51. Seely, S. (1985). Cancer of the digestive tract. In: *Diet-Related Cancer* (S. Seely, D. L. J. Freed, G. A. Silverstone and V. Rippere, eds), pp. 168–79. Croom Helm.
52. Zheing, W., Blot, W. J., Shu, X. *et al.* (1992). Diet and other risk factors for laryngeal cancer in Shanghai, China. *Am. J. Epidemiol.*, **136**, 178–91.
53. Peckham, M., Pinedo, H. and Veronesi, U. (eds) (1995). *Oxford Textbook of Oncology*, Vol. 2, pp. 172–3, 254–8. Oxford University Press.
54. World Cancer Research Fund/American Institute for Cancer Research (1997). *Food, Nutrition and the Prevention of Cancer: A Global Perspective.* WCRF/AICR.

Chapter 4 Caring and curing: the sectors of health care (pages 50–78)

1. Landy, D. (1977). Medical systems in transcultural perspective. In: *Culture, Disease, and Healing: Studies in Medical Anthropology* (D. Landy, ed.), pp. 129–32. Macmillan.
2. Kleinman, A. (1980). *Patients and Healers in the Context of Culture*, pp. 49–70. University of California Press.
3. Chrisman, N. J. (1977). The health seeking process: an approach to the natural history of illness. *Cult. Med. Psychiatry*, **1**, 351–77.
4. Kleinman, A., Eisenberg, L. and Good, B. (1978). Culture, illness, and care: clinical lessons from anthropologic and cross-cultural research. *Ann. Intern. Med.*, **88**, 251–8.
5. McGuire, M. B. (1988). *Ritual Healing in Suburban America.* Rutgers University Press.
6. Levin, J. S. and Coreil, J. (1986). 'New Age' healing in the US. *Soc. Sci. Med.*, **23**, 889–97.
7. Turner, V. W. (1974). *The Ritual Process*, p. 14. Penguin.
8. Lewis, I. M (1971). *Ecstatic Religion.* Penguin.
9. Kleinman, A. (1980). *Patients and Healers in the Context of Culture*, p. 200. University of California Press.
10. Snow, L. F. (1978). Sorcerers, saints and charlatans: black folk healers in urban America. *Cult. Med. Psychiatry*, **2**, 69–106.
11. Ngubane, H. (1981). Aspects of clinical practice and traditional organization of indigenous healers in South Africa. *Soc. Sci. Med.*, **15B**, 361–5.
12. Underwood, P. and Underwood, Z. (1981). New spells for old: expectations and realities of Western medicine in a remote tribal society in Yemen, Arabia. In: *Changing Disease Patterns and Human Behaviour* (N. F. Stanley and R. A. Joshe, eds), pp. 271–97. Academic Press.
13. Reeler, A. V. (1990). Injections: a fatal attraction? *Soc. Sci. Med.*, **31**, 1119–25.
14. Wyatt, H. V. (1984). The popularity of injections in the Third World: origins and consequences for poliomyelitis. *Soc. Sci. Med.*, **19**, 911–15.
15. Kimani, V. N. (1981). The unsystematic alternative: towards plural health care among the

Kikuyu of central Kenya. *Soc. Sci. Med.*, **15B**, 333–40.
16. Karcher, S. (1997). *The Illustrated Encyclopaedia of Divination*. Element Books.
17. Lewis, I. M. (1971). *Ecstatic Religion*, pp. 49–57. Penguin.
18. Martin, M. (1981). Native American healers: thoughts for post-traditional healers. *JAMA*, **245**, 141–3.
19. Fabrega, H. and Silver, D. B. (1973). *Illness and Shamanistic Curing in Zinacantan*, pp. 218–23. Stanford University Press.
20. Finkler, K. (1985). *Spiritualist Healers in Mexico*. Bergin and Garvey.
21. Tessendorf, K. E. and Cunningham, P. W. (1997). One person, two roles: nurse and traditional healer. *World Health Forum*, **18**, 59–62.
22. Lucas, R. H. and Barrett, R. J. (1995). Interpreting culture and psychopathology: primitivist themes in cross-cultural debate. *Cult. Med. Psychiatry*, **19**, 287–326.
23. World Health Organization (1979). *Formulating Strategies for Health for All by the Year 2000: Guiding Principles and Essential Issues*. WHO.
24. World Health Organization (1978). The promotion and development of traditional medicine. *WHO Tech. Rep. Ser.*, **622**.
25. World Health Organization (1979). *Traditional Birth Attendants: An Annotated Bibliography on their Training, Utilization and Evaluation*. WHO.
26. World Health Organization/UNICEF (1992). *Traditional Birth Attendants: A Joint WHO/UNPFA/UNICEF Statement*. WHO.
27. Last, M. (1990). Professionalization of indigenous healers. In: *Medical Anthropology: Contemporary Theory and Method* (T. M. Johnson and C. F. Sargent, eds), pp. 349–66. Praeger.
28. Kossoy, E. and Ohry, A. (1997). The *Feldshers*. Magnes Press.
29. Velimirovic, B. (1990). Is integration of Traditional and Western medicine really possible? In: *Anthropology and Primary Care* (J. Coreil and J. D. Mull, eds), pp. 51–78. Westview Press.
30. Ingstad, B. (1990). The cultural construction of AIDS and its consequences for prevention in Botswana. *Med. Anthropol. Q.* (new series), **4**, 28–40.
31. Warwick, D. P. (1988). Culture and the management of family planning programs. *Stud. Family Planning*, **19**, 1–18.
32. Coreil, J. (1988). Innovation among Haitian healers: the adoption of oral rehydration therapy. *Human Organization*, **47**, 48–57.
33. Razali, M. S. (1995). Psychiatrists and folk healers in Malaysia. *World Health Forum*, **16**, 56–8.
34. Desjarlais, R., Eisenberg, L., Good, B. and Kleinman, A. (1995). *World Mental Health*, p. 110. Oxford University Press.
35. Fulder, S. (1988). *The Handbook of Complementary Medicine*, 2nd edn, pp. 112–13. Oxford University Press.
36. Srinivasan, P. (1995). National health policy for traditional medicine in India. *World Health Forum*, **16**, 190–195.
37. British Medical Association (1993). *Complementary Medicine: New Approaches to Good Practice*, p. 10. British Medical Association.
38. Wirsing, R. L. (1996). The use of conventional and unconventional medicines to treat illnesses of German children. In: *Children, Medicines and Culture* (J. Bush, D. J. Trakas, E. J. Sanz *et al.*, eds), pp. 229–54. Pharmaceutical Products Press (Haworth Press).
39. Eisenberg, D., Kessler, R. C., Foster, C. *et al.* (1993). Unconventional medicine in the United States. *N. Engl. J. Med.*, **328**, 246–52.
40. World Health Organization (1980). Health personnel and hospital establishments. *World Health Statistics Annual*.
41. World Bank (1993). *World Development Report 1993*, pp. 208–9. Oxford University Press.
42. Bennett, S. (1993). Private health care in Third World needs regulating. *Br. Med. J.*, **306**, 673–4.
43. Stacey, M. (1988). *The Sociology of Health and Healing*, pp. 258, 177–93. Unwin Hyman.
44. Littlewood, R. and Lipsedge, M. (1989). *Aliens and Alienists*, 2nd edn. Unwin Hyman.
45. Wing, J. K. (1978). *Reasoning about Madness*. Oxford University Press.
46. Illich, I. (1976). *Limits to Medicine*. Marion Boyars.
47. Stacey, M. (1988). *The Sociology of Health and Healing*, pp. 229–60. Unwin Hyman.
48. Crawford, R. (1977). You are dangerous to your health: the ideology and politics of victim blaming. *Int. J. Hlth Serv.*, **7**, 663–80.
49. O'Brien, B. (1984). *Patterns of European Diagnoses and Prescribing*. Office of Health Economics.
50. Maretzki, T. W. (1989). Cultural variations in biomedicine: the *kur* in West Germany. *Med. Anthropol. Q.* (new series), **3**, 22–35.
51. Payer, L. (1989). *Medicine and Culture*. Henry Holt.
52. Foster, G. M. and Anderson, B. G. (1978). *Medical Anthropology*, pp. 175–86. Wiley.
53. Pfifferling, J. H. (1980). A cultural prescription for medicocentrism. In: *Relevance of Social Science for Medicine* (L. Eisenberg and A. Kleinman, eds), pp. 197–222. Reidel.
54. Goffman, F. (1961). *Asylums*. Penguin.
55. Gamarnikow, E. (1978). Sexual division of labour: the case of nursing. In: *Feminism and Materialism* (A. Kuhn and A. M. Wolpe, eds), pp. 96–123. Routledge and Kegan Paul.
56. Konner, M. (1993). *The Trouble with Medicine*, pp. 22–47. BBC Books.
57. Woolbandler, S., Himmelstein, D. U. and Lewontin, J. P. (1993). Administrative costs in US hospitals. *N. Engl. J. Med.*, **329**, 400–403.
58. World Bank (1993). *World Development Report 1993*, p. 137. Oxford University Press.
59. McLuhan, M. (1964). *Understanding Media*. Sphere.

60. Tenner, E. (1997). *Why Things Bite Back*, pp. 26–70. Fourth Estate.
61. Helman, C. (1992). *The Body of Frankenstein's Monster*, pp. 13–28. W.W. Norton.
62. Kirmayer, L. J. (1992). The body's insistence on meaning: metaphor as presentation and representation in illness experience. *Med. Anthrop. Q.* (new series), **6(4)**, 323–46.
63. Davis-Floyd, R. E. (1992). *Birth as an American Rite of Passage*. University of California Press.
64. Browner, C. H. (1996). The production of authoritative knowledge in American prenatal care. *Med. Anthropol. Q.* (new series), **10(2)**, 141–56.
65. Konner, M. (1993). *The Trouble with Medicine*, pp. 138–60. BBC Books.
66. Barley, S. R. (1988). The social construction of a machine: ritual, superstition, magical thinking and other pragmatic responses to running a CT Scanner. In: *Biomedicine Examined* (M. Lock and D. Gordon, eds), pp. 497–539. Kluwer.
67. Helman, C. G. (1985). Disease and pseudo-disease: a case history of pseudo angina. In: *Physicians of Western Medicine* (R. A. Hahn and A. D. Gaines, eds), pp. 293–331. Reidel.
68. Feinstein, A. R. (1975). Science, clinical medicine, and the spectrum of disease. In: *Textbook of Medicine* (P. B. Beeson and W. McDermott, eds), pp. 4–6. Saunders.
69. Grouse, L. D. (1983). Editorial: Has the machine become the physician? *JAMA*, **250**, 1891.
70. Koenig, B. A.(1988). The technological imperative in medical practice: the social creation of a 'routine' treatment'. In: *Biomedicine Examined* (M. Lock and D. R. Gordon, eds), pp. 465–98. Kluwer.
71. Baer, H., Singer, M. and Susser, I. (1997). *Medical Anthropology and the World System*. Bergin and Garvey.
72. Helman, C. G. (1995). The body image in health and disease: exploring patients' maps of body and self. *Patient Ed. Couns.*, **6**, 169–75.
73. Assal, J. Ph., Golay, A. and Visser, A. P. (eds) (1995). *New Trends in Patient Education: A Transcultural and Inter-disease Approach*. Elsevier.
74. Brennan, A. T., Leape, L. L., Laird, N. M. *et al.* (1991). Incidence of adverse effects and negligence in hospitalized patients. *New Engl. J. Med.*, **324**, 370–76.
75. Brennan, A. T., Leape, L. L., Laird, N. M. *et al.* (1991). The nature of adverse events in hospitalized patients. *New Engl. J. Med.*, **324**, 377–84.
76. Baer, H. A., Singer, M. and Susser, I. (eds) (1997). *Medical Anthropology and the World System*, pp. 220–23. Bergin and Garvey.
77. Haines, A. (1996). The science of perpetual change. *Br. J. Gen. Pract.*, **46**, 115–19.
78. Scott, C. S. (1974). Health and healing practices among five ethnic groups in Miami, Florida. *Public Hlth Rep.*, **89**, 524–32.
79. Brigden, M. L. (1987). Unorthodox therapy and your cancer patient. *Postgrad. Med.*, **81**, 271–80.
80. Stimson, G. V. (1974). Obeying doctor's orders: a view from the other side. *Soc. Sci. Med.*, **8**, 97–104.
81. Stacey, M. (ed.) (1976). *The Sociology of the National Health Service*. Croom Helm.
82. Levitt, R. (1976). *The Reorganized National Health Service*. Croom Helm.
83. Elliott-Binns, C. P. (1973). An analysis of lay medicine. *J. R. Coll. Gen. Pract.*, **23**, 255–64.
84. Elliott-Binns, C. P. (1986). An analysis of lay medicine: fifteen years later. *J. R. Coll. Gen. Pract.*, **36**, 542–4.
85. Dunnell, K. and Cartwright, A. (1972). *Medicine Takers, Prescribers and Hoarders*. Routledge and Kegan Paul.
86. Sharpe, D. (1979). The pattern of over-the-counter 'prescribing'. *MIMS Magazine*, 15 September, 39–45.
87. Jefferys, M., Brotherston, J. F. and Cartwright. A. (1960). Consumption of medicines on a working-class housing estate. *Br. J. Prev. Soc. Med.*, **14**, 64–76.
88. Hindmarch, I. (1981). Too many pills in the cupboard. *New Society*, **55**, 142–3.
89. Warburton, D. M. (1978). Poisoned people: internal pollution. *J. Biosoc. Sci.*, **10**, 309–19.
90. Blaxter, M. and Paterson, E. (1980). Attitudes to health and use of health services in two generations of women in social classes 4 and 5. Report to DHSS/SSRC Joint Working Party on Transmitted Deprivation (unpublished).
91. Pattison, C. J., Drinkwater, C. K. and Downham, M. A. P. S. (1982). Mothers' appreciation of their children's symptoms. *J. R. Coll. Gen. Pract.*, **32**, 149–62.
92. Anonymous (1982). Self-help groups for your patients. *Pulse*, 29 May, 51–2.
93. Levy, L. (1982). Mutual support groups in Great Britain. *Soc. Sci. Med.*, **16**, 1265–75.
94. *Self-help* (undated booklet), p. 25. Leo Laboratories.
95. Robinson, D. and Henry, S. (1977). *Self-help and Health: Mutual Aid for Modern Problems*. Martin Robertson.
96. British Medical Association (1993). *Complementary Medicine: New Approaches to Good Practice*, pp. 28–30. British Medical Association.
97. Fulder, S. and Monro, R. (1981). *The Status of Complementary Medicine in the UK*. Threshold Foundation.
98. National Institute of Medical Herbalists (undated). *Information Leaflet*. NIMH.
99. Community Health Foundation (undated pamphlet). *Your Guide to Healthy Living*. Community Health Foundation.
100. Hyde, F. F. (1978). The origin and practice of herbal medicine. *MIMS Magazine*, 1 February, 127–36.

101. National Federation of Spiritual Healers (undated pamphlet). *About the National Federation of Spiritual Healers.* NFSH.
102. Tod, J. (ed.) (1982). *Someone to Talk To: A Directory of Self-help and Support Services in the Community*, p. 57. Mental Health Foundation.
103. de Jonge, P. (1981). Magical world of Wicca in a Sheffield semi. *Doctor*, 2 July, 30.
104. Royal London Homeopathic Hospital (1978). *One Hundred and Nineteenth Annual Report.* RLHH.
105. Cant, S. L. and Sharma, U. (1996). Professionalization of complementary medicine in the United Kingdom. *Compl. Ther. Med.*, **4**, 157–62.
106. British Acupuncture Association and Register Ltd (1979). Personal Communication, 24 October, Secretary, BAAR.
107. Thomas, K. J., Carr, J., Westlake, L. and Williams, B. T. (1991). Use of non-orthodox and conventional health care in Great Britain. *Br. Med. J.*, **303**, 207–10.
108. *Horoscope* (1981). Advertisement 29, p. 36.
109. British Astrological and Psychic Society (1998). *British Astrological and Psychic Society: Society Information: New Edition – May 1998* (pamphlet). Nutfield.
110. Qureshi, B. (1990). British Asians and alternative medicine. In: *Health Care for Asians* (B. R. McAvoy and L. J. Donaldson, eds), pp. 93–116. Oxford University Press.
111. Council for Complementary and Alternative Medicine (undated pamphlet). CCAM.
112. Research Council for Complementary Medicine (1988). *The First Five Years: 1983–1988.* RCCM.
113. Davies, P. (1984). *Report on Trends in Complementary Medicine.* Institute for Complementary Medicine.
114. Anon (1989). What is the British Holistic Medical Association? *Holistic Health*, **22**, 36.
115. Fulder, S. J. and Monro, R. E. (1985). Complementary medicine in the United Kingdom: patients, practitioners, and consultations. *Lancet*, **2**, 542–5.
116. Institute for Complementary Medicine (1989). Personal communication, 17 July.
117. British Medical Association (1993). *Complementary Medicine: New Approaches to Good Practice*, p. 67. British Medical Association.
118. Office of Health Economics (1981). *OHE Compendium of Health Statistics, 1981*, 4th edn. OHE.
119. Department of Health and Social Security (1982). Personal communication, 24 November.
120. Merry, P. (ed.) (1993). *NHS Handbook*, 8th edn, p. 10. JMH Publishing.
121. Wadsworth, M. F. J., Butterfield, W. J. H. and Blaney, R. (1971). *Health and Sickness: the Choice of Treatment.* Tavistock.
122. Levitt, R. (1976). *The Reorganized National Health Service*, p. 179. Croom Helm.
123. Levitt, R. (1976). *The Reorganized National Health Service*, p. 199. Croom Helm.
124. Fry, J., Brooks, D. and McColl, I. (1984). *NHS Data Book.* MTP Press.
125. Chaplin, N. W. (ed.) (1976). *The Hospital and Health Services Year Book*, pp. 374–7. The Institute of Health Service Administrators.
126. White, A. E. (1978). The vital role of the cottage community hospital. *J. R. Coll. Gen. Pract.*, **28**, 485–91.
127. Levitt, R. (1976). *The Reorganized National Health Service*, p. 94. Croom Helm.
128. Royal College of General Practitioners (1999). *Profile of UK General Practitioners.* RCGP Information Sheet No. 1. RCGP.
129. Harris, C. M. (1980). *Lecture Notes on Medicine in General Practice*, p. 27. Blackwell.
130. Hunt, J. H. (1964). The renaissance of general practice. In: *Trends in the National Health Service* (J. Farndale, ed.), pp. 161–81. Pergamon Press.
131. Levitt, R. (1976). *The Reorganized National Health Service*, pp. 96–7. Croom Helm.
132. Morrell, D. C. (1971). Expressions of morbidity in general practice. *Br. Med. J.*, **2**, 454.
133. Clayson, M. (1993). Primary health care teams. *Practitioner*, **237**, 819–23.
134. Merry, P. (ed.) (1993). *NHS Handbook*, 8th edn, p. 71. JMH Publishing.
135. Morgan, M. (1991). Waiting lists. In: *In the Best of Health?* (F. Beck, S. Lonsdale, S. Newman and D. Patterson, eds), pp. 207–27. Chapman and Hall.
136. Anon (1992). *Private Medical Insurance: Market Update 1992*, p. 3. Laing and Buisson.

Chapter 5 Doctor–patient interactions (pages 79–107)

1. Eisenberg, L. (1977). Disease and illness: distinctions between professional and popular ideas of sickness. *Cult. Med. Psychiatry*, **1**, 9–23.
2. Kleinman, A., Eisenberg, L. and Good, B. (1978). Culture, illness and care: clinical lessons from anthropologic and cross-cultural research. *Ann. Intern. Med.*, **88**, 251–8.
3. Good, B. J. and Good, M. D. (1981). The meaning of symptoms: a cultural hermeneutic model for clinical practice. In: *The Relevance of Social Science for Medicine* (L. Eisenberg and A. Kleinman, eds), pp. 165–96. Reidel.
4. Feinstein, A. R. (1975). Science, clinical medicine, and the spectrum of disease. In: *Textbook of Medicine* (P. B. Beeson and W. McDermott, eds), pp. 4–6. Saunders.
5. Fabrega, H. and Silver, D. B. (1973). *Illness and Shamanistic Curing in Zinacantan: An Enthnomedical Analysis*, pp. 218–23. Stanford University Press.
6. Engel, G. L. (1980). The clinical applications of the biopsychosocial model. *Am. J. Psychiatry*, **137**, 535–44.

7. Cassell, J. (1987). On control, certitude, and the 'paranoia' of surgeons. *Cult. Med. Psychiatry*, **11**, 229–49.
8. Cassell, F. J. (1976). *The Healer's Art: A New Approach to the Doctor–Patient Relationship*, pp. 47–83. Lippincott.
9. World Health Organization (1946). *Constitution of the World Health Organization*. WHO.
10. Fox, R. C. (1968). Illness. In: *International Encyclopedia of the Social Sciences* (D. Sills, ed.), pp. 90–96. Free Press/Macmillan.
11. Blaxter, M. and Paterson, F. (1980). Attitudes to health and use of health services in two generations of women in social classes 4 and 5. Report to DHSS/SSRC Joint Working Party on Transmitted Deprivation (unpublished).
12. Dunnell, K. and Cartwright, A. (1972). *Medicine Takers, Prescribers and Hoarders*, p. 13. Routledge and Kegan Paul.
13. Apple, D. (1960). How laymen define illness. *J. Hlth. Soc. Behav.*, **1**, 219–25.
14. Guttmacher, S. and Elinson, J. (1971). Ethnoreligious variations in perceptions of illness. *Soc. Sci. Med.*, **5**, 117–25.
15. Lewis, G. (1981). Cultural influences on illness behaviour. In: *The Relevance of Social Science for Medicine* (L. Eisenberg and A. Kleinman, eds), pp. 151–62. Reidel.
16. Kleinman, A. (1980). *Patients and Healers in the Context of Culture*, pp. 104–18. University of California Press.
17. Helman, C. G. (1984). The role of context in primary care. *J. R. Coll. Gen. Pract.*, **34**, 547–50.
18. Helman, C. G. (1981). Disease versus illness in general practice. *J. R. Coll. Gen. Pract.*, **31**, 548–52.
19. Rubel, A. J. (1977). The epidemiology of a folk illness: *Susto* in Hispanic America. In: *Culture, Disease and Healing: Studies in Medical Anthropology* (D. Landy, ed.), pp. 119–28. Macmillan.
20. Good, B. (1977). The heart of what's the matter: the semantics of illness in Iran. *Cult. Med. Psychiatry*, **1**, 25–58.
21. Krause, I. B. (1989). Sinking heart: a Punjabi communication of distress. *Soc. Sci. Med.*, **29**, 563–75.
22. Kleinman, A. (1980). *Patients and Healers in the Context of Culture*, pp. 149–58. University of California Press.
23. Frankenberg, R. (1980). Medical anthropology and development: a theoretical perspective. *Soc. Sci. Med.*, **14B**, 197–207.
24. Sontag, S. (1978). *Illness as Metaphor*. Vintage.
25. Kirmayer, L. J. (1992). The body's insistence on meaning: metaphor as presentation and representation in illness experience. *Med. Anthrop. Q.* (new series), **6(4)**, 323–46.
26. Peters-Golden, H. (1982). Breast cancer: varied perceptions of social support in illness experience. *Soc. Sci. Med.*, **16**, 483–91.
27. Herzlich, C. and Pierret, J. (1986). Illness: from cause to meaning. In: *Concepts of Health, Illness and Disease* (C. Currer and M. Stacey, eds), pp. 73–96. Berg.
28. Gordon, D. R. (1990). Embodying illness, embodying cancer. *Cult. Med. Psychiatry*, **14**, 275–97.
29. Hunt, L. M. (1998). Moral reasoning and the meaning of cancer: causal explanations of oncologists and patients in southern Mexico. *Med. Anthropol. Q.* (new series), **12(3)**, 298–318.
30. Weiss, M. (1997). Signifying the pandemics: metaphors of AIDS, cancer, and heart disease. *Med. Anthropol. Q.* (new series), **11**, 456–76.
31. Becker, G. (1997). *Disrupted Lives*, pp. 59–98. University of California Press.
32. Hahn, R.A. (1997). The nocebo phenomenon: concept, evidence, and influence on public health. *Prev. Med.*, **26**, 607–11.
33. Mann, I. M., Tarantola, D. J. M. and Netter, T. W. (eds) (1992). *AIDS in the World*. Harvard University Press.
34. Cassens, B. J. (1985). Social consequences of the acquired immunodeficiency syndrome. *Ann. Intern. Med.*, **103**, 768–71.
35. Warwick, I., Aggleton, P. and Homans, H. (1988). Young people's health beliefs and AIDS. In: *Social Aspects of AIDS* (P. Aggleton and H. Homans, eds), pp. 106–25. Falmer Press.
36. Wellings, K. (1988). Perceptions of risk – media treatment of AIDS. In: *Social Aspects of AIDS* (P. Aggleton and H. Homans, eds), pp. 65–82. Falmer Press.
37. Watney, S. (1988). AIDS, 'moral panic' theory and homophobia. In: *Social Aspects of AIDS* (P. Aggleton and H. Homans, eds), pp. 52–64. Falmer Press.
38. Cominos, E. D., Gottschang, S. K. and Scrimshaw, S. C. M. (1989). Kurn, AIDS and unfamiliar social behaviour – biocultural consideration in the current epidemic: discussion paper. *J. R. Soc. Med.*, **82**, 95–8.
39. Chrisman, N. I. (1981). Analytical scheme for health relief research (unpublished).
40. Gordon, D. R. (1988). Tenacious assumptions in Western medicine. In: *Biomedicine Examined* (M. Lock and D. R. Gordon, eds), pp. 19–56. Kluwer.
41. Snow, L. F. (1976). 'High blood' is not high blood pressure. *Urban Health*, **5**, 54–5.
42. Snow, L. F. and Johnson, S. M. (1978). Folklore, food, female reproductive cycle. *Ecol. Food Nutr.*, **7**, 41–9.
43. Pill, R. and Stott, N. C. H. (1982). Concepts of illness causation and responsibility: some preliminary data from a sample of working class mothers. *Soc. Sci. Med.*, **16**, 43–52.
44. Greenwood, B. (1981). Cold or spirits? Choice and ambiguity in Morocco's pluralistic medical system. *Soc. Sci. Med.*, **15B**, 219–35.

45. Landy, D. (1977). Malign and benign methods of causing and curing illness. In: *Culture, Disease, and Healing: Studies in Medical Anthropology* (D. Landy, ed.), pp. 195–7. Macmillan.
46. Snow, L. F. (1978). Sorcerers, saints and charlatans: black folk healers in urban America. *Cult. Med. Psychiatry*, **2**, 69–106.
47. Spooner, B. (1970). The evil eye in the Middle East. In: *Witchcraft Confessions and Accusations* (M. Douglas, ed.), pp. 311–19. Tavistock.
48. Underwood, P. and Underwood, Z. (1981). New spells for old: expectations and realities of Western medicine in a remote tribal society in Yemen, Arabia. In: *Changing Disease Patterns and Human Behaviour* (N. F. Stanley and R. A. Joshe, eds), pp. 271–97. Academic Press.
49. Lewis, I. M. (1971). *Ecstatic Religion*. Penguin.
50. McGuire, M. B. (1988). *Ritual Healing in Suburban America*, p. 83. Rutgers University Press.
51. Blaxter, M. (1979). Concepts of causality; lay and medical models. In: *Research in Psychology and Medicine* (D. J. Osborne, ed.), Vol. 2, pp. 54–61. Academic Press.
52. Foster, G. M. and Anderson, B. G. (1978). *Medical Anthropology*, pp. 53–70. Wiley.
53. Young, A. (1983). The relevance of traditional medical cultures to modern primary health care. *Soc. Sci. Med.*, **17**, 1205–11.
54. Kleinman, A. (1988). *The Illness Narratives*. Basic Books.
55. Brody, H. (1987). *Stories of Sickness*. Yale University Press.
56. Becker, G (1997). *Disrupted Lives*, pp. 25–58. University of California Press.
57. Blumhagen, D. (1980). Hyper-tension: a folk illness with a medical name. *Cult. Med. Psychiatry*, **4**, 197–227.
58. Helman, C. G. (1978). 'Feed a cold, starve a fever': folk models of infection in an English suburban community, and their relation to medical treatment. *Cult. Med. Psychiatry*, **2**, 107–37.
59. Trakas, D. J. and Sanz, E. (eds) (1996). *Childhood and Medicine Use in a Cross-cultural Perspective: A European Concerted Action*. European Commission.
60. Bush, P. J., Trakas, D. J., Sanz, E. J. *et al.* (eds) (1996). *Children, Medicines and Culture*. Pharmaceuticals Products Press (Haworth Press).
61. Trakas, D. J. (1996). Children's accounts of illness: comparisons of children's interviews from the COMAC Childhood and Medicines Project. In: *Disrupted Lives* (D. J. Trakas and E. Sanz, eds), pp. 293–311. University of California Press.
62. Botsis, C. and Trakas, D. J. (1996). Childhood and medicine use in Athens. In: *Disrupted Lives* (D. J. Trakas and E. Sanz, eds), pp. 221–44. University of California Press.
63. Vaskilampi, T., Kalpio, O. and Hallia, O. (1996). From catching a cold to eating junk food: conceptualization of illness among Finnish children. In: *Children, Medicines and Culture* (P. J. Bush, D. J. Trakas, E. J. Sanz *et al.*, eds), pp. 295–318. Pharmaceuticals Products Press (Haworth Press).
64. Aramburuzabala, P., Garcia, M., Polaino, A. and Sanz, E. (1996). Medicine use, behaviour children's perceptions of medicines and health care in Madrid and Tenerife (Spain). In: *Disrupted Lives* (D. J. Trakas and E. Sanz, eds), pp. 245–68. University of California Press.
65. Gerrits, T., Haaijer-Ruskamp, F. and Hardon, A. P. (1996). 'Preferably half a tablet': health-seeking behaviour when Dutch children get ill. In: *Children, Medicines and Culture* (P. J. Bush, D. J. Trakas, E. J. Sanz *et al.*, eds), pp. 209–228. Pharmaceuticals Products Press (Haworth Press).
66. Van der Gest, S. (1996). Grasping the children's point of view? An anthropological reflection. In: *Children, Medicines and Culture* (D. J. Trakas and E. Sanz, eds), pp. 337–46. Pharmaceuticals Products Press (Haworth Press).
67. James, A., Jenks, C. and Prout, A. (1998). *Theorizing Childhood*, pp. 77–9. Polity Press.
68. Hall, E. T. (1984). *The Dance of Life: The Other Dimensions of Time*. Anchor Press.
69. Barrett, T. G. and Booth, I. W. (1994). Sartorial elegance: does it exist in the paediatrician–patient relationship? *Br. Med. J.*, **309**, 1701–1702.
70. Zola, I. K. (1973). Pathways to the doctor: from person to patient. *Soc. Sci. Med.*, **7**, 677–89.
71. Zola, I. K. (1966). Culture and symptoms: an analysis of patients' presenting complaints. *Am. Sociol. Rev.*, **31**, 615–30.
72. Hackett, T. P., Gassem, N. H. and Raker, J. W. (1973). Patient delay in cancer. *N. Engl. J. Med.*, **289**, 14–20.
73. Olin, H. S. and Hackett, T. P. (1964). The denial of chest pain in 32 patients with acute myocardial infarction. *JAMA*, **190**, 977–81.
74. Scott, C. S. (1974). Health and healing practices among five ethnic groups in Miami, Florida. *Public Hlth. Rep.*, **89**, 524–32.
75. Zborowski, M. (1952). Cultural components in responses to pain. *J. Social Issues*, **8**, 16–30.
76. Helman, C. G. (1985). Disease and pseudo-disease: a case history of pseudo angina. In: *Physicians of Western Medicine: Anthropological Approaches to Theory and Practice* (R. A. Hahn and A. D. Gaines, eds), pp. 293–331. Reidel.
77. Mechanic, D. (1972). Social psychologic factors affecting the presentation of bodily complaints. *N. Engl. J. Med.*, **286**, 1132–9.
78. Stimson, G. V. and Webb, B. (1975). *Going to See the Doctor: The Consultation Process in General Practice*. Routledge and Kegan Paul.
79. Balint, M. (1964). *The Doctor, His Patient and the Illness*, pp. 21–5. Pitman.
80. Bell, C. M. (1984). A hundred years of *Lancet* language. *Lancet*, **ii**, 1453.

81. Boyle, C. M. (1970). Difference between patients' and doctors' interpretation of some common medical terms. *Br. Med. J.*, **2**, 286–9.
82. Pearson, D. and Dudley, H. A. F. (1982). Bodily perceptions in surgical patients. *Br. Med. J.*, **284**, 1545–6.
83. Leff, I. P. (1978). Psychiatrists' versus patients' concepts of unpleasant emotions. *Br. J. Psychiatry*, **133**, 306–13.
84. Stimson, G. V. (1974). Obeying doctor's orders: a view from the other side. *Soc. Sci. Med.*, **8**, 97–104.
85. Waters, W. H. R., Gould, N. V. and Lunn, J. E. (1976). Undispensed prescriptions in a mining general practice. *Br. Med. J.*, **1**, 1062–3.
86. Harwood, A. (1971). The hot–cold theory of disease: implications for treatment of Puerto Rican patients. *JAMA*, **216**, 1153–8.
87. Cay, F. L., Philip, A. F., Small, W. P. *et al.* (1975). Patient's assessment of the result of surgery for peptic ulcer. *Lancet*, **1**, 29–31.
88. Hall, E. T. (1977). *Beyond Culture*, pp. 85–103. Anchor Books.
89. Stein, H. F. (1990). Psychoanalytic perspectives. In: *Medical Anthropology* (T. M. Johnson and C. F. Sargent, eds), p. 75. Praeger.

Chapter 6 Gender and Reproduction (pages 108–27)

1. Keesing, R. M. (1981). *Cultural Anthropology*, pp. 27–9. Holt, Rinehart & Winston.
2. MacCormack C. P. and Strathern, M. (eds) (1981). *Nature, Culture and Gender.* Cambridge University Press.
3. Ganong, W. F. (1983). *Review of Medical Physiology*, pp. 342–3. Lange Medical Publications.
4. Keesing, R. M. (1981). *Cultural Anthropology*, pp. 301–10. Holt, Rinehart & Winston.
5. Keesing, R. M. (1981). *Cultural Anthropology*, p. 150. Holt, Rinehart & Winston.
6. Goddard, V. (1987). Honour and shame: the control of women's sexuality and group identity in Naples. In: *The Cultural Construction of Sexuality* (P. Caplan, ed.), pp. 166–92. Tavistock.
7. Dunk, P. (1989). Greek women and broken nerves in Montreal. *Med. Anthropol.*, **11**, 29–45.
8. Shepherd, G. (1982). Rank, gender, and homosexuality: Mombasa as a key to understanding sexual options. In: *The Cultural Construction of Sexuality* (P. Caplan, ed.), pp. 240–70. Tavistock.
9. Ember, C. R. and Ember, M. (1985). *Cultural Anthropology*, pp. 137–56. Prentice Hall.
10. Rosaldo, M. Z. and Lamphere, L. (1974). *Women, Culture, and Society.* Stanford University Press.
11. Parker, R. (1987). Acquired immunodeficiency in urban Brazil. *Med. Anthropol. Q.* (new series), **1**, 155–75.
12. Caplan, P. (1987). Introduction. In: *The Cultural Construction of Sexuality* (P. Caplan, ed.), pp. 1–30. Tavistock.
13. Devisch, R. and Gailly, A. (1985). A therapeutic self-help group among Turkish women: Dertlesmek: 'The sharing of sorrow'. *Psichiatrica e Psicoterapia analitica*, **4**, 133–52.
14. Lewis, I. M (1971). *Ecstatic Religion.* Penguin.
15. McGuire, M. B. (1988). *Ritual Healing in Suburban America.* Rutgers University Press.
16. Stacey, M. (1988). *The Sociology of Health and Healing*, pp. 78–97. Unwin Hyman.
17. Stacey, M. (1988). *The Sociology of Health and Healing*, pp. 177–93. Unwin Hyman.
18. Fry, J., Brooks, D. and McColl, I. (1984). *NHS Data Book.* MTP Press.
19. Royal College of General Practitioners (1999). *Profile of UK General Practitioners.* RCGP Information Sheet No. 1. RCGP.
20. World Bank (1993). *World Development Report 1993*, pp. 208–9. Oxford University Press.
21. Merry, P. (ed.) (1993). *NHS Handbook,,* 8th edn, p. 58. JMH Publishing.
22. Dixon, M. (1996). *Creative Career Paths in the NHS: Report No. 5.* Department of Health.
23. Gamarnikow, E. (1978). Sexual division of labour: the case of nursing. In: *Feminism and Materialism* (A. Kuhn and A. M. Wolpe, eds), pp. 96–123. Routledge and Kegan Paul.
24. Krantzler, N. (1986). Media images of physicians and nurses in the United States. *Soc. Sci. Med.*, **22**, 933–52.
25. Littlewood, J. (1989). A model for nursing using anthropological literature. *Int. J. Nurs. Stud.*, **26**, 221–9.
26. Illich, I. (1976). *Limits to Medicine.* Marion Boyars.
27. Gabe, I. and Calnan, M. (1989). The limits of medicine: women's perception of medical technology. *Soc. Sci. Med.*, **28**, 223–31.
28. Stacey, M. (1988). *The Sociology of Health and Healing*, pp. 253–4. Unwin Hyman.
29. Cooperstock, R. (1976). Psychotropic drug use among women. *Can. Med. Assoc. J.*, **115**, 760–63.
30. Stimson, G. (1975). The message of psychotropic drug ads. *J. Communication*, **25**, 153–60.
31. Titmuss, R. M. (1984). The position of women: some vital statistics. In: *Health and Disease* (N. Black, D. Boswell, A. Gray *et al.*, eds), pp. 71–5. Open University Press.
32. Friseb, R. E. (1985). Fatness, menarche and female fertility. *Perspect. Biol. Med.*, **28**, 611–33.
33. Dalton, K. (1964). *The Premenstrual Syndrome.* Heinemann.
34. Gottlieb, A. (1988). American premenstrual syndrome. *Anthropol. Today*, **4(6)**, 10–13.
35. Johnson, T. M. (1987). Premenstrual syndrome as a Western culture-specific disorder. *Cult. Med. Psychiatry*, **11**, 337–56.
36. Furth, C. and Shu-Yueh, C. (1992). Chinese medicine and the anthropology of menstruation in contemporary Taiwan. *Med. Anthropol. Q.* (new series), **6**, 27–48.

37. Lock, M. M. (1982). Models and practice in medicine: menopause as syndrome or life transition? *Cult. Med. Psychiatry*, **6**, 261–80.
38. Kaufert, P. A. and Gilbert, P. (1986). Women, menopause and medicalisation. *Cult. Med. Psychiatry*, **10**, 7–21.
39. Waldron, I. (1978). Type A behavior pattern and coronary heart disease in men and women. *Soc. Sci. Med.*, **12B**, 167–70.
40. Rintala, M. and Mutajoki, P. (192). Could mannequins menstruate? *Br. Med. J.*, **305**, 1575–6.
41. Low, S. M. (1989). Health, culture, and the nature of nerves. *Med. Anthropol.*, **11**, 91–5.
42. U205 Course Team (1985). *Medical Knowledge: Doubt and Certainty*, pp. 73–81. Open University Press.
43. Hahn, R. A. and Muecke, M. A. (1987). The anthropology of birth in five U.S. ethnic populations: implications for obstetrical practice. *Curr. Probl. Obstet. Gynecal. Fertil.*, **10**, 133–71.
44. Stacey, M. (1988). *The Sociology of Health and Healing*, p. 52. Unwin Hyman.
45. Leavitt, J. W. (1987). The growth of medical authority: technology and morals in turn-of-the-century obstetrics. *Med. Anthropol. Q.* (new series), **1**, 230–55.
46. Davis-Floyd, R. E. (1987). The technological model of birth. *J. Am. Folklore*, **100**, 479–95.
47. Graham, H. and Oakley, A. (1981). Competing ideologies of reproduction: medical and maternal perspectives on pregnancy. In: *Women, Health and Reproduction* (H. Roberts, ed.), pp. 99–118. Routledge and Kegan Paul.
48. Kitzinger, S. (1982). The social context of birth: some comparisons between childbirth in Jamaica and Britain. In: *Ethnography of Fertility and Birth* (C. P. McCormack, ed.), pp. 181–203. Academic Press.
49. Browner, C. H. (1996). The production of authoritative knowledge in American prenatal care. *Med. Anthropol. Q.* (new series), **10(2)**, 141–156.
50. MacCormack, C. P. (1982). Biological, cultural and social adaptation in human fertility and birth: a synthesis. In: *Ethnography of Fertility and Birth* (C. P. McCormack, ed.), pp. 1–23. Academic Press.
51. McGilvray, D. B. (1982). Sexual power and fertility in Sri Lanka: Batticaloa Tamils and Moors. In: *Ethnography of Fertility and Birth* (C. P. McCormack, ed.), pp. 25–73. Academic Press.
52. Pillsbury, B. L. K. (1984). 'Doing the month': confinement and convalescence of Chinese women after childbirth. In: *Health and Disease* (N. Black, D. Boswell, A. Gray *et al.*, eds), pp. 17–24. Open University Press.
53. World Health Organization (1978). *The Promotion and Development of Traditional Medicine.* Technical Report Series 622. WHO.
54. World Health Organization (1979). *Traditional Birth Attendants: An Annotated Bibliography on their Training, Utilization and Evaluation.* WHO.
55. World Health Organization (1990). *Traditional Birth Attendants: A Joint WHO/ UNFPA/UNICEF Statement.* WHO.
56. Rageb, S. (1987). *Daya Training Programme: Trainer's Guide.* Ministry of Health/UNICEF.
57. Sargent, C. and Bascope, G. (1996). Ways of knowing about birth in three cultures. *Med. Anthropol. Q.* (new series), **10(2)**, 213–36.
58. Becker, G. (1997). *Disrupted Lives*, pp. 80–98. University of California Press.
59. Cosminsky, S. (1982). Childbirth and change: a Guatemalan study. In: *Ethnography of Fertility and Birth* (C. P. McCormack, ed.), pp. 205–39. Academic Press.
60. Palgi, P. (1966). Cultural components of immigrants' adjustment. In: *Migration, Mental Health and Community Services* (H. P. David, ed.), pp. 71–82. International Research Institute.
61. Macer, D. R. J. (1994). Perception of risks and benefits of *in vitro* fertilization, genetic engineering and biotechnology. *Soc. Sci. Med.*, **38**, 22–3.
62. Stacey. M. (1991). Social dimensions of assisted reproduction. In: *Changing Human Reproduction* (M. Stacey, ed.), pp. 1–47. Sage Publications.
63. Snowden, R., Mitchell, G. D. and Snowden, F. (1983). *Artificial Reproduction.* George Allen and Unwin.
64. Konrad, M. (1998). Ova donation and symbols of substance: some variations on the theme of sex, gender and the partible body. *J. R. Anthropol. Inst.* (new series), **4**, 643–67.
65. Evans-Pritchard, F. F. (1951). *Kinship and Marriage Among the Nuer*, pp. 98–123. Clarendon Press.
66. Keesing, R. M. (1981). *Cultural Anthropology*, p. 161. Holt, Rinehart & Winston.
67. Miller, B. D. (1987). Female infanticide and child neglect in rural North India. In: *Child Survival* (N. Scheper-Hughes, ed.), pp. 95–112. Reidel.
68. Potter, S. H. (1987). Birth planning in rural China: a cultural account. In: *Child Survival* (N. Scheper-Hughes, ed.), pp. 333–58. Reidel.
69. Heggenhougen, H. K. (1980). Fathers and childbirth: an anthropological perspective. *J. Nurse Midwifery*, **25(6)**, 21–6.
70. Lipkin, M. and Lamb, G. S. (1982). The couvade syndrome: an epidemiological study. *Ann. Intern. Med.*, **96**, 509–11.

Chapter 7 Pain and culture (pages 128–35)

1. Morrell, D. C. (1977). Symptom interpretation in general practice. *J. R. Coll. Gen. Pract.*, **22**, 297–309.
2. Weinman, J. (1981). *An Outline of Psychology as Applied to Medicine*, p. 5. Wright.
3. Engel, G. (1950). 'Psychogenic' pain and the pain-prone patient. *Am. J. Med.*, **26**, 899–909.

4. Fabrega, H. and Tyma, S. (1976). Language and cultural influences in the description of pain. *Br. Med. J. Psychol.*, **49**, 349–71.
5. Hoebel, F. A. (1960), *The Cheyenne. Indians of the Great Plains*, pp. 11–16. Holt, Rinehart & Winston.
6. Zola, I. K. (1966). Culture and symptoms: an analysis of patients' presenting complaints. *Am. Social. Rev.*, **31**, 615–30.
7. Boyle, C. M. (1970). Difference between patients' and doctors' interpretation of some common medical terms. *Br. Med. J.*, **2**, 286–9.
8. Helman, C. G. (1985). Disease and pseudo-disease: a case history of pseudo-angina. In: *Physicians of Western Medicine: Anthropological Perspectives on Theory and Practice* (R. A. Hahn and A. Gaines, eds), pp. 293–331. Reidel.
9. Zborowski, M. (1952) Cultural components in responses to pain. *J. Soc. Issues*, **8**, 16–30.
10. Pugh, J. F. (1991) The semantics of pain in Indian culture and medicine. *Cult. Med. Psychiatry*, **15**, 19–43.
11. Wolff, B. B. and Langley, S. (1977). Cultural factors and the response to pain. In: *Culture, Disease, and Healing: Studies in Medical Anthropology* (D. Landy, ed.), pp. 313–19. Macmillan.
12. Lewis, G. (1981). Cultural influences on illness behaviour: a medical anthropological approach. In: *The Relevance of Social Science for Medicine* (L. Eisenberg and A. Kleinman, eds), pp. 1515–62. Reidel.
13. Levine, J. D., Gordon, N. C. and Fields, H. L. (1978). The mechanism of placebo analgesia. *Lancet*, **2**, 654–7.
14. Landy, D. (1977) In: *Culture, Disease, and Healing: Studies in Medical Anthropology* (D. Landy, ed.), p. 313. Macmillan.
15. Le Barre, W. (1947). The cultural basis of emotions and gestures *J. Personality*, **16**, 49–68.
16. Hawkins, C. F. (1975). The alimentary system. In: *Conybeare's Textbook of Medicine* (W. N. Mann, ed.), p. 326. Churchill Livingstone.
17. Kleinman, A. (1980). *Patients and Healers in the Context of Culture*, pp. 138–45. University of California Press.
18. Skultans, V. (1976). Empathy and healing: aspects of spiritualist ritual. In: *Social Anthropology and Medicine* (J. B. Loudon, ed.), pp. 190–221. Academic Press.
19. Csordas, T. J. (1993). Somatic modes of attention. *Cult. Anthropol.*, **8**, 135–56.
20. McGuire, M. B. (1988). *Ritual Healing in Suburban America*, p. 101. Rutgers University Press.
21. McDougall, J. (1989). *Theatres of the Body*, pp. 140–161. Free Association Press.
22. Brodwin, P. F. (1992). Symptoms and social performances: the case of Diane Reden. In: *Pain as Human Experience: An Anthropological Perspective* (M. D. Good, P. E. Brodwin, B. J. Good and A. Kleinman, eds), pp. 77–99. University of California Press.
23. Kleinman, A., Brodwin, P. B., Good, B. J. and Good, M. J. (1992). Pain as human experience: an introduction. In: *Pain as Human Experience: An Anthropological Perspective* (M. D. Good, P. E. Brodwin, B. J. Good and A. Kleinman, eds), pp. 1–26. University of California Press.

Chapter 8 Culture and pharmacology (pages 136–55)

1. Claridge, G. (1970). *Drugs and Human Behaviour.* Allen Lane.
2. Wolf, S. (1959). The pharmacology of placebos. *Pharmacol. Rev.*, **11**, 689–705.
3. Shapiro, A. K. (1959). The placebo effect in the history of medical treatment: implications for psychiatry. *Am. J. Psychiatry*, **116**, 298–304.
4. Benson, H. and Epstein, M. D. (1975). The placebo effect: a neglected asset in the care of patients. *JAMA*, **232**, 1225–7.
5. Editorial (1972). *Lancet*, **2**, 122–3.
6. Hahn, R. A. (1997). The nocebo phenomenon: concept, evidence, and implications for public health. *Prev. Med.*, **26**, 607–11.
7. Levine, J. D., Gordon, N. C. and Fields, H. L. (1978). The mechanism of placebo analgesia. *Lancet*, **2**, 654–7.
8. Adler, H. M. and Hammett, V. O. (1973). The doctor–patient relationship revisited: an analysis of the placebo effect. *Am. Intern. Med.*, **78**, 595–8.
9. Joyce, C. R. B. (1969). Quantitative estimates of dependence on the symbolic function of drugs. In: *Scientific Basis of Drug Dependence* (H. Steinberg, ed.), pp. 271–80. Churchill.
10. Schapira, K., McClelland, H.A., Griffiths, N.R. and Newell, D.J (1970). Study on the effects of tablet colour in the treatment of anxiety states. *Br. Med. J.*, **2**, 446–9.
11. Branthwaite, A. and Cooper, P. (1981). Analgesic effects of branding in treatment of headaches. *Br. Med. J.*, **282**, 1576–8.
12. Jefferys, M., Brotherston, J. H. F. and Cartwright, A. (1960). Consumption of medicines on a working-class housing estate. *Br. J. Prev. Soc. Med.*, **14**, 64–76.
13. Helman, C. G. (1981). 'Tonic', 'fuel' and 'food': social and symbolic aspects of the long-term use of psychotropic drugs. *Soc. Sci. Med.*, **15B**, 521–33.
14. Claridge, G. (1970). *Drugs and Human Behaviour*, p. 25. Allen Lane.
15. Claridge, G. (1970). *Drugs and Human Behaviour*, p. 126. Allen Lane.
16. Benson, H. and McCallie, D. P. (1979). Angina pectoris and the placebo effect. *N. Engl. J. Med.*, **300**, 1424–9.
17. Lader, M. (1979). Spectres of tolerance and dependence. *MIMS Magazine*, 15 August, 31–5.

18. Parish, P. A. (1971). The prescribing of psychotropic drugs in general practice. *J. R. Coll. Gen. Pract.*, **21**(Suppl. 4).
19. Trethowan, W. H. (1975). Pills for personal problems. *Br. Med. J.*, **3**, 749–51.
20. Hall, R. C. W. and Kirkpatrick, B. (1980). The benzodiazepines. *Am. Fam. Phys.*, **17**, 131–4.
21. Editorial (1973). Benzodiazepines: use, overuse, misuse, abuse? *Lancet*, **1**, 1101–2.
22. Shorter, E. (1997). *A History of Psychiatry*, p. 324. Wiley.
23. Parish, P. A. (1971). The prescribing of psychotropic drugs in general practice. *J. R. Coll. Gen. Pract.*, **21**(Suppl. 4), 29–30.
24. Williams, P. (1981). Areas of concern in the prescription of psychotropic drugs. *MIMS Magazine*, 1 January, 37–43.
25. Smith, M. C. (1980). The relationship between pharmacy and medicine. In: *Prescribing Practice and Drug Usage* (R. Mapes, ed.), pp. 157–200. Croom Helm.
26. Cooperstock, R. and Lennard, H. L. (1979). Some social meanings of tranquillizer use. *Soc. Hlth. Illness*, **1**, 331–45.
27. Pellegrino, E. D. (1976). Prescribing and drug ingestion: symbols and substances. *Drug Intell. Clin. Pharm.*, **10**, 624–30.
28. Warburton, D. M. (1978). Poisoned people: internal pollution. *J. Biosoc. Sci.*, **10**, 309–19.
29. Jones, D. R. (1979). Drugs and prescribing: what the patient thinks. *J. R. Coll. Gen. Pract.*, **29**, 417–19.
30. Tyrer, P. (1978). Drug treatment of psychiatric patients in general practice. *Br. Med. J.*, **2**, 1008–10.
31. Desjarlais, R., Eisenberg, L., Good, B. and Kleinman, A. (1995). *World Mental Health*, pp. 87–115. Oxford University Press.
32. Claridge, G. (1970). *Drugs and Human Behaviour*, p. 231. Allen Lane.
33. Wellcome Institute (1985). *Morbid Cravings: The Emergence of Addiction* (catalogue). Wellcome Institute for the History of Medicine.
34. Wellcome Institute (1985). *Morbid Cravings: The Emergence of Addiction* (catalogue), pp. 27–28. Wellcome Institute for the History of Medicine.
35. Burr, A. (1984). The ideologies of despair: a symbolic interpretation of punks' and skinheads' usage of barbiturates. *Soc. Sci. Med.*, **19**, 929–38.
36. Plummer, K. (1988). Organizing AIDS. In: *Social Aspects of AIDS* (P. Aggleton and H. Homans, eds), pp. 20–51. Falmer Press.
37. Gamella, J. F. (1994). The spread of intravenous drug use and AIDS in a neighborhood in Spain. *Med. Anthrop. Q.* (new series), **8(2)**, 131–160.
38. Robins, L. N., Davis, D. H. and Goodwin, D. W. (1974). Drug use by US army enlisted men in Vietnam: a follow-up on their return home. *Am. J. Epidemiol.*, **99**, 235–49.
39. Jackson, B. (1978). Deviance as success: the double inversion of stigmatised roles. In: *The Reversible World: Symbolic Inversion in Art and Society* (B. A. Babcock, ed.), pp. 258–71. Cornell University Press.
40. Freeland, J. B. and Rosenstiel, C. R. (1974). A socio-cultural barrier to establishing therapeutic rapport: a problem in the treatment of narcotic addicts. *Psychiatry*, **37**, 215–20.
41. Bourgois, P. (1989). Crack in Spanish Harlem. *Anthropol. Today*, **5(4)**, 6–11.
42. Baer, H., Singer, M. and Susser, I. (1997). *Medical Anthropology and the World System*, pp. 125–58. Bergin and Garvey.
43. Razali, M. S. (1995). Psychiatrists and folk healers in Malaysia. *World Health Forum*, **16**, 56–8.
44. Desjarlais, R., Eisenberg, L., Good, B. and Kleinman, A. (1995). *World Mental Health*, pp. 110. Oxford University Press.
45. Desjarlais, R., Eisenberg, L., Good, B., and Kleinman, A. (1995). *World Mental Health*, pp. 91–7. Oxford University Press.
46. Knupfer, G. and Room, R. (1967). Drinking patterns and attitudes of Irish, Jewish and White Protestant American men. *Q. J. Studies Alcohol*, **28**, 676–99.
47. Kunitz, S. J. and Levy, J. F. (1981). Navajos. In: *Ethnicity and Medical Care* (A. Harwood, ed.), pp. 337–96. Harvard University Press.
48. McKeigue, P. M. and Karmi, G. (1993). Alcohol consumption and alcohol-related problems in Afro-Caribbeans and South Asians in the United Kingdom. *Alcohol and Addiction*, **28**, 1–10.
49. O'Connor, I. (1975). Social and cultural factors influencing drinking behaviour. *Irish J. Med. Sci.* (Suppl.), June, 65–71.
50. Greeley, A. M. and McCready, W. C. (1978). A preliminary reconnaissance into the persistence and explanation of ethnic subcultural drinking patterns. *Med. Anthropol.*, **2**, 31–51.
51. Thomas, A. E. (1978). Class and sociability among urban workers. *Med. Anthropol.*, **2**, 9–30.
52. Mars, G. (1987). Longshore drinking, economic security and union politics in Newfoundland. In: *Constructive Drinking* (M. Douglas, ed.), pp. 91–101. Cambridge University Press.
53. Peace, A. (1992). No fishing without drinking. In: *Alcohol, Gender and Culture* (D. Gefou-Madianou, ed.), pp. 167–80. Routledge.
54. Gefou-Madianou, D. (1992). Introduction: alcohol commensality, identity transformations and transcendence. In: *Alcohol, Gender and Culture* (D. Gefou-Madianou, ed.), pp. 1–34. Routledge.
55. Hunt, G. and Satterlee, S. (1986). Cohesion and division: drinking in an English village. *MAN*, **21**, 521–37.
56. Jackson, S. H. D., Bannan, L. T. and Beevers, D. G. (1981). Ethnic differences in respiratory disease. *Postgrad. Med. J.*, **57**, 777–8.

57. United States Department of Health and Human Services (1984). *A Report of the Surgeon General: Chronic Obstructive Lung Disease.* Publication 84-56205. Office of the Assistant Secretary for Health.
58. United States Department of Health, Education, and Welfare (1979). *A Report of the Surgeon General: Smoking and Health.* Publication 79-50066. Office of the Assistant Secretary for Health.
59. Reeder, L. G. (1977). Socio-cultural factors in the etiology of smoking behaviour: an assessment. *Natl. Inst. Drug Abuse Res. Monogr. Set*, **17**, 186–201.
60. Desjarlais, R., Eisenberg, L., Good, B., and Kleinman, A. (1995). *World Mental Health*, pp. 231–33. Oxford University Press.
61. Marsh, A. and Matheson, J. (1983). *Smoking Attitudes and Behaviour: An Enquiry Carried Out on Behalf of the Department of Health and Social Security.* HMSO.
62. Doherty, W.J. and Whitehead, D. (1986). The social dynamics of cigarette smoking: a family systems perspective. *Family Process*, **25**, 453–9.
63. Nichter, M. and Cartwright, F. (1991). Saving the children for the tobacco industry. *Med. Anthropol. Q.*, **5**, 236–56.
64. Health Education Authority (1991). *The Smoking Epidemic: Counting the Cost.* Health Education Authority.
65. Anonymous (1986). Tobacco use and world health: a situation analysis. *Bull. Pan Am. Hlth Org.*, **20**, 409–17.
66. Baer, H., Singer, M. and Susser, I. (1997). *Medical Anthropology and the World System*, pp. 73–124. Bergin and Garvey.
67. Whyse, S. R. and Van Der Geest, S. (1988). Medicines in context: an introduction. In: *The Context of Medicines in Developing Countries* (S. Van Der Geest and S. R. Whyte, eds), pp. 3–11. Kluwer.
68. Ferguson, A. (1988). Commercial pharmaceutical medicine and medicalization: a case study from El Salvador. In: *The Context of Medicines in Developing Countries* (S. Van Der Geest and S. R. Whyte, eds), pp. 19–46. Kluwer.
69. Nakajima, H. (1992). How essential is an essential drugs policy? *World Health*, March/April, 3.
70. Bledsoe, C. H. and Goubaud, M. F. (1988). The reinterpretation and distribution of Western pharmaceuticals: an example from the Mende of Sierra Leone. In: *The Context of Medicines in Developing Countries* (S. Van Der Geest and S. R. Whyte, eds), pp. 253–76. Kluwer.
71. Van Der Geest, 5. (1988). The articulation of formal and informal medicine distribution in South Cameroon. In: *The Context of Medicines in Developing Countries* (S. Van Der Geest and S. R. Whyte, eds), pp. 131–48. Kluwer.
72. World Health Organization (1992). *The Use of Essential Drugs*, WHO Technical Report Series 825. WHO.
73. Antezana, F. S. (1992). Action for equity. *World Health*, March/April, 7–8.
74. Dobkin de Rios, M. (1973). Curing with *ayahuasca* in an urban slum. In: *Hallucinogens and Shamanism* (M. J. Harner, ed.), pp. 67–85. Oxford University Press.
75. Littlewood, R. and Lipsedge, M. (1989). *Aliens and Alienists*, 2nd edn, p. 18. Unwin Hyman.
76. La Barre, W. (1969). *The Peyote Cult.* Schocken Books.
77. Harner, M. J. (1973). Common themes in South American Indian *yagé* experiences. In: *Hallucinogens and Shamanism* (M. J. Harner, ed.), pp. 155–75. Oxford University Press.
78. Schultes, R. F. (1976). *Hallucinogenic Plants*, pp. 142–7. Golden Press.
79. Kennedy, J. G. (1987). *The Flower of Paradise.* Reidel.
80. Rudgley, R. (1993). *The Alchemy of Culture: Intoxicants in Society*, pp. 115–43. British Museum Press.
81. Dobkin de Rios, M. (1999). The *Duboisia* Genus, Australian Aborigines and suggestibility. *J. Psychoactive Drugs*, **31(2)**, 155–161.

Chapter 9 Ritual and the management of misfortune (pages 156–69)

1. Loudon, J. B. (1966). Private stress and public ritual. *J. Psychosom. Res.*, **10**, 101–8.
2. Turner, V. W. (1968). *The Drums of Affliction*, pp. 1–8. Clarendon Press and IAI.
3. Leach, E. (1968). Ritual. In: *International Encyclopaedia of the Social Sciences* (D. L Sills, ed.), pp. 520–26. Free Press/Macmillan.
4. Turner, V. W. (1969). *The Ritual Process*, pp. 48–9. Penguin.
5. McKinstry, B. and Wang, J. (1991). Putting on the style: what patients think of the way their doctor dresses. *Br. J. Gen. Pract.*, **41**, 275–8.
6. Barrett, T. G. and Booth, I. W. (1994). Sartorial elegance: does it exist in the paediatrician–patient relationship? *Br. Med. J.*, **309**, 1710–20.
7. Ngubane, H. (1977). *Body and Mind in Zulu Medicine*, pp. 111–39. Academic Press.
8. Standing, H. (1980). Beliefs about menstruation and pregnancy. *MIMS Magazine*, 1 June, 21–7.
9. Leach, E. (1976). *Culture and Communication*, pp. 33–6, 77–9. Cambridge University Press.
10. Van Gennep, A. (1960). *The Rites of Passage* (trans. M. D. Vizedom and G. L. Caffee). Routledge and Kegan Paul.
11. Ngubane, H. (1977). *Body and Mind in Zulu Medicine*, pp. 78–9. Academic Press.
12. Davis-Floyd, R. E. (1987). The technological model of birth. *J. Am. Folklore*, **100**, 479–95.
13. Kitzinger, S. (1982). The social context of birth: some comparisons between childbirth in Jamaica

and Britain. In: *Ethnography of Fertility and Birth* (C. P. MacCormack, ed.), pp. 181–203. Academic Press.
14. Hertz, R. (1960). *Death and the Right Hand*, pp. 27–86. Cohen and West.
15. Eisenbruch, M. (1984). Cross-cultural aspects of bereavement. II: Ethnic and cultural variations in the development of bereavement practices. *Cult. Med. Psychiatry*, **8**, 315–47.
16. Skultans, V. (1980). A dying ritual. *MIMS Magazine*, 15 June, 43–7.
17. Laungani, P. (1996). Death and bereavement in India and England: a comparative analysis. *Mortality*, **1(2)**, 191–212.
18. Konner, M. (1993). *The Trouble with Medicine*, pp. 138–60. BBC Books.
19. Sayer, C. (ed.) (1990). *Mexico: The Day of the Dead*. Redstone Press.
20. Foster, G. M. and Anderson, B. G. (1978). *Medical Anthropology*, pp. 115–17. Wiley.
21. Beattie, J. (1967). Divination in Bunyoro, Uganda. In: *Magic, Witchcraft and Curing* (J. Middleton, ed.), pp. 211–31. University of Texas Press.
22. Katz, P. (1981). Ritual in the operating room. *Ethnology*, **20**, 335–50.
23. Balint, M. (1974). *The Doctor, His Patient and The Illness*. Pitman.
24. Balint, M. (1974). *The Doctor, His Patient and The Illness*, pp. 24–5. Pitman.
25. Rose, L. (1971). *Faith Healing*, p. 62. Penguin.
26. Davis-Floyd, R. E. (1992). *Birth as an American Rite of Passage*. University of California Press.
27. Eisenbruch, M. (1984). Cross-cultural aspects of bereavement. I: A conceptual framework for comparative analysis. *Cult. Med. Psychiatry*, **8**, 283–309.
28. Parkes, C. M. (1975). *Bereavement*. Penguin.
29. Turner, V. W. (1964). An Ndembu doctor in practice. In: *Magic, Faith and Healing* (A. Kiev, ed.), pp. 230–63. Free Press.
30. Bosk, C. L. (1980). Occupational rituals in patient management. *N. Engl. J. Med.*, **303**, 71–6.
31. Douglas, M. (1973). *Natural Symbols*, pp. 19–39. Penguin.
32. Byrne, P. (1976). Teaching and learning verbal behaviours. In: *Language and Communication in General Practice* (B. Tanner, ed.), pp. 52–70. Hodder and Stoughton.
33. Foster, G. M. and Anderson, B. G. (1978). *Medical Anthropology*, p. 119. Wiley.
34. Simon, C. (1991). Innovative medicine – a case study of a modern healer. *S. Afr. Med. J.*, **79**, 677–8.

Chapter 10 Cross-cultural psychiatry (pages 170–201)

1. Babcock, B. A. (1978). Introduction. In: *The Reversible World: Symbolic Inversion in Art and Society* (B. A. Babcock, ed.), pp. 13–36. Cornell University Press.
2. Abrahams, R. D. and Bauman, R. (1978). Ranges of festival behaviour. In: *The Reversible World: Symbolic Inversion in Art and Society* (B. A. Babcock, ed.), pp. 193–208. Cornell University Press.
3. Lewis, I. M (1971). *Ecstatic Religion*, pp. 178–205. Penguin.
4. Littlewood, R. and Lipsedge, M. (1989). *Aliens and Alienists*, 2nd edn, pp. 174–81. Unwin Hyman.
5. Foster, G. M. and Anderson, B. G. (1978). *Medical Anthropology*, pp. 81–100. Wiley.
6. Kiev, A. (1964). Implications for the future. In: *Magic, Faith and Healing* (A. Kiev, ed.), pp. 454–64. Free Press.
7. Edgerton, R. B. (1977). Conceptions of psychosis in four East African societies. In: *Culture, Disease and Healing: Studies in Medical Anthropology* (D. Landy, ed.), pp. 358–67. Macmillan.
8. Landy, D. (1977). Emotional states and cultural constraints. In: *Culture, Disease and Healing: Studies in Medical Anthropology* (D. Landy, ed.), pp. 333–5. Macmillan.
9. Littlewood, R. and Lipsedge, M. (1989). *Aliens and Alienists*, 2nd edn, p. 207. Unwin Hyman.
10. Kiev, A. (1972). *Transcultural Psychiatry*, pp. 11–25. Penguin.
11. Kiev, A. (1972). *Transcultural Psychiatry*, pp. 78–108. Penguin.
12. Kleinman, A. (1980). *Patients and Healers in the Context of Culture*, pp. 176–7. University of California Press.
13. Kleinman, A. (1987). Anthropology and psychiatry. *Br. J. Psychiatry*, **151**, 447–54.
14. Littlewood, R. (1990). From categories to contexts: a decade of the new cross-cultural psychiatry. *Br. J. Psychiatry*, **156**, 308–27.
15. Waxler, N. (1977). Is mental illness cured in traditional societies? A theoretical analysis. *Cult. Med. Psychiatry*, **1**, 233–53.
16. Rubel, A. J. (1977). The epidemiology of a folk illness: *Susto* in Hispanic America. In: *Culture, Disease and Healing: Studies in Medical Anthropology* (D. Landy, ed.), pp. 119–28. Macmillan.
17. Pichot, P. (1982). The diagnosis and classification of mental disorders in French-speaking countries: background, current views and comparison with other nomenclatures. *Psychol. Med.*, **12**, 475–92.
18. Merskey, H. and Shafran, B. (1986). Political hazards in the diagnosis of 'sluggish schizophrenia'. *Br. J. Psychiatry*, **148**, 247–56.
19. Kendell, R. E. (1975). *The Role of Diagnosis in Psychiatry*, pp. 70–71. Blackwell.
20. Kendell, R. E. (1975). *The Role of Diagnosis in Psychiatry*, pp. 49–59. Blackwell.
21. Temerlin, M. K. (1968). Suggestion effects in psychiatric diagnosis. *J. Nerv. Ment. Dis.*, **147**, 349–53.

22. Kendell, R. E. (1975). *The Role of Diagnosis in Psychiatry*, pp. 9–26. Blackwell.
23. Eisenberg. L. (1977). Disease and illness: distinctions between professional and popular ideas of sickness. *Cult. Med. Psychiatry*, **1**, 9–23.
24. Szasz, T. (1954). Psychiatric justice. *Br. J. Psychiatry*, **154**, 864–9.
25. Wing, J. K. (1978). *Reasoning about Madness*, pp. 167–93. Oxford University Press.
26. Littlewood, R. and Lipsedge, M. (1989). *Aliens and Alienists*, 2nd edn, pp. 249–54. Unwin Hyman.
27. Lewis, G., Croft-Jeffreys, C. and David, A. (1990). Are British psychiatrists racist? *Br. J. Psychiatry*, **157**, 410–15.
28. Thomas, C. S., Stone, K., Osborn, M. *et al.* (1993). Psychiatric morbidity and compulsory admission among UK-born Europeans, Afro-Caribbeans and Asians in Central Manchester. *Br. J. Psychiatry*, **163**, 91–9.
29. Wesseley, S., Castle, D., Der, G. and Murray, R. (1991). Schizophrenia and Afro-Caribbeans: a case–control study. *Br. J. Psychiatry*, **159**, 795–801.
30. Blackburn, R. (1988). On moral judgements and personality disorders: the myth of the psychopathic personality revisited. *Br. J. Psychiatry*, **153**, 505–12.
31. Cooper, I. E., Kendell, R. F., Gurland, B. J. *et al.* (1969). Cross-national study of diagnosis of the mental disorders: some results from the first comparative investigation. *Am. J. Psychiatry*, **125**(Suppl.), 21–9.
32. Katz, M. M., Cole, J. O. and Lowery, H. A. (1969). Studies of the diagnostic process: the influence of symptom perception, past experience, and ethnic background on diagnostic decisions. *Am. J. Psychiatry*, **125**, 109–19.
33. Van Os, J., Galdos, P., Lewis, G. *et al.* (1993). Schizophrenia sans frontiers: concepts of schizophrenia among French and British psychiatrists. *Br. Med. J.*, **307**, 489–92.
34. Copeland, J. R. M., Cooper, J. E., Kendell, R. F. and Gourlay, A. I. (1971). Differences in usage of diagnostic labels among psychiatrists in the British Isles. *Br. J. Psychiatry*, **118**, 629–40.
35. Littlewood, R. and Lipsedge, M. (1989). *Aliens and Alienists*, 2nd edn, p. 117. Unwin Hyman.
36. Scheper-Hughes, N. (1978). Saints, scholars, and schizophrenics: madness and badness in Western Ireland. *Med. Anthropol.*, **2**, 59–93.
37. Littlewood, R. and Lipsedge, M. (1989). *Aliens and Alienists*, 2nd edn, pp. 218–42. Unwin Hyman.
38. Littlewood, R. (1989). Anthropology and psychiatry: an alternative approach. *Br. J. Med. Psychol.*, **53**, 213–25.
39. Swartz, L. (1998). *Culture and Mental Health: A Southern African View*, pp. 121–39. Oxford University Press.
40. Hussain, M. F. and Gomersall, J. D. (1978). Affective disorder in Asian immigrants. *Psychiatric Clin.*, **11**, 87–9.
41. Rack, P. (1990). Psychological and psychiatric disorders. In: *Health Care for Asians* (B. R. McAvoy and L. J. Donaldson, (eds), pp. 290–303. Oxford University Press.
42. Kleinman, A. (1980). *Patients and Healers in the Context of Culture*, pp. 146–78. University of California Press.
43. Kleinman, A. and Kleinman, J. (1985). In: *Culture and Depression* (A. Kleinman and B. Good, eds), pp. 429–90. University of California Press.
44. Krause, I. B. (1989). Sinking heart: a Punjabi communication of distress. *Soc. Sci. Med.*, **29**, 563–75.
45. Helman, C. G. (1985). Psyche, soma, and society: the social construction of psychosomatic disorders. *Cult. Med. Psychiatry*, **9**, 1–26.
46. McDougall, J. (1989). *Theatres of the Body*, p. 139. Free Association Books.
47. Kirmayer, L. J. and Young, A. (1998). Culture and somatization: clinical, epidemiological, and ethnographic perspectives. *Psychosom. Med.*, **60**, 420–30.
48. Lau, B. W. K., Kung, N. Y. T. and Chung, I. T. C. (1983). How depressive illness presents in Hong Kong. *Practitioner*, **227**, 112–14.
49. Ots, T. (1990). The angry liver, the anxious heart and the melancholy spleen. *Cult. Med. Psychiatry*, **14**, 21–58.
50. Payer, L. (1989). *Medicine and Culture*, p. 116–18. Gollancz.
51. Csordas, T. J. (1990). Embodiment as a paradigm for anthropology. *Ethos*, **18**, 5–47.
52. Freud, S. and Breuer, J. (1966). *Studies on Hysteria* (trans. J. Strachey). Avon.
53. Mumford, D. B. (1993). Somatization: a transcultural perspective. *Int. Rev. Psychiatry*, **5**, 231–42.
54. Lipowski, Z. L. (1984). What does the word 'psychosomatic' really mean? A historical and semantic inquiry. *Psychosom. Med.*, **46**, 153–71.
55. Lipowski, Z. L. (1968). Review of consultation psychiatry and psychosomatic medicine. *Psychosom. Med.*, **11**, 273–81.
56. Knapp, P. H. (1975). Psychosomatic aspects of bronchial asthma. In: *American Handbook of Psychiatry* (M. F. Reiser, ed.), 2nd edn, Vol 4, pp. 693–707. Basic Books.
57. McDougall, J. (1989). *Theatres of the Body*, pp. 17, 55. Free Association Books.
58. Engel, G. L. (1977). The need for a new medical model: a challenge for biomedicine. *Science*, **196**, 129–36.
59. Alexander, F., French, T. M. and Pollock, G. H. (eds) (1968). *Psychosomatic Specificity*, Vol 1.University of Chicago Press.
60. Minuchin, S., Rosman, B. L. and Baker, L. (1978). *Psychosomatic Families*. Harvard University Press.
61. Ader, R., Cohen, N. and Felten, D. (1995).

Psychoneuroimmunology: interactions between the nervous system and the immune system. *Lancet*, **345**, 99–103.
62. Simons, R. C. and Hughes, C. C. (eds). (1985). *The Culture-Bound Syndromes.* Reidel.
63. Littlewood, L. and Lipsedge, M. (1987). The butterfly and the serpent: culture, psychopathology and biomedicine. *Cult. Med. Psychiatry*, **11**, 289–335.
64. Acocella, J. (1998). The politics of hysteria. *The New Yorker*, April 6, 64–79.
65. Bose, R. (1997). Psychiatry and the popular conception of possession among the Bangladeshis in London. *Int. J. Soc. Psychiatry*, **43(1)**, 1–15.
66. De La Cancela, V., Guarnaccia, P. J. and Carillo, E. (1986). Psychosocial distress among Latinos: a critical analysis of Ataques de Nervios. *Hum. Soc.*, **10**, 431–47.
67. Swartz, L. (1998). *Culture and Mental Health: A Southern African View*, pp. 162–6. Oxford University Press.
68. Ngubane, H. (1977). *Body and Mind in Zulu Medicine.* Academic Press, pp. 144–50.
69. Kleinman, A. (1980). *Patients and Healers in the Context of Culture*, pp. 82, 360. University of California Press.
70. Lewis, I. M. (1971). *Ecstatic Religion*, pp. 37–65. Penguin.
71. Murphy, J. M. (1964). Psychotherapeutic aspects of Shamanism on St Lawrence Island, Alaska. In: *Magic, Faith and Healing* (A. Kiev, ed.), pp. 53–83. Free Press.
72. Dow, J. (1986). Universal aspects of symbolic healing: a theoretical synthesis. *Am. Anthropol.*, **88**, 56–69.
73. Kleinman, A. (1988). *Rethinking Psychiatry*, pp. 108–41. Free Press.
74. Csordas, T. J. (1983). The rhetoric of transformation in ritual healing. *Cult. Med. Psychiatry*, **7**, 333–75.
75. Moerman, D. E. (1979). Anthropology of symbolic healing. *Curr. Anthropol.*, **20(1)**, 59–66.
76. McGuire, M. (1988). *Ritual Healing in Suburban America.* Rutgers University Press
77. Finkler, K. (1985). *Spiritual Healers in Mexico* p. 8. Bergin and Garvey.
78. Stein, H. (1992). Medical anthropology and the depths of human experience: contributions from psychoanalytic anthropology. *Med. Anthropol.*, **14**, 53–75.
79. McDougall, J. (1989). *Theatres of the Body*, p. 7. Free Association Books.
80. Kleinman, A. (1988). *Rethinking Psychiatry*, pp. 122. Free Press.
81. Kleinman, A. (1988). *Rethinking Psychiatry*, pp. 117. Free Press.
82. McDougall, J. (1989). *Theatres of the Body*, p. 51. Free Association Books.
83 El-Islam, M. F. (1982). Arabic cultural psychiatry. *Transcultural Psychiatry Res. Rev.*, **19**, 5–24.
84. Brown, D. D. (1994). *Umbanda*, pp. 72 92. Columbia University Press.
85. Finkler, K (1981). Non-medical treatments and their outcomes. Part Two: Focus on the adherents of spiritualism. *Cult. Med. Psychiatry*, **5**, 65–103.
86. Kleinman, A. (1988). *Rethinking Psychiatry*, pp. 319–52. Free Press.
87. Campion, J. and Bhugra, D. (1997). Experiences of religious healing in psychiatric patients in south India. *Social Psychiatry Psychiatric Epidem.*, **32(4)**, 215–21.
88. Csordas, T. J. (1987). Health and the holy in African and Afro-Brazilian spirit possession. *Soc. Sci. Med.*, **24**, 1–11.
89. Csordas, T. J. (1983). The rhetoric of healing in ritual healing. *Cult. Med. Psychiatry*, **7**, 333–75.
90. Katz, P. (1981). Ritual in the operating room. *Ethnology*, **20**, 335–50.
91. Etsuko, M. (1991). The interpretations of fox possession: illness as metaphor. *Cult. Med. Psychiatry*, **15**, 453–77.
92. Bilu, Y., Witzum, F. and Van Der Hart, O. (1990). Paradise regained: 'miraculous healing' in an Israeli psychiatric clinic. *Cult. Med. Psychiatric*, **14**, 105–27.
93. Greenfield, S. M. (1992). Spirits and spiritist therapy in southern Brazil: a case study of an innovative, syncretic healing group. *Cult. Med. Psychiatry*, **16**, 23–51.
94. Ember, C. R. and Ember, M. (1985). *Cultural Anthropology*, 4th edn, pp. 171–7. Prentice Hall.
95. Sayer, C. (ed.) (1990). *Mexico: The Day of the Dead.* Redstone Press.
96. Helman, C. G. (1991). The family culture: a useful concept for family practice. *Fam. Med.*, **23**, 376–81.
97. Christie-Seely, J. (1981). Teaching the family system concept in family medicine. *J. Fam. Pract.*, **13**, 391–401.
98. Byng-Hall, J. (1988). Scripts and legends in families and family therapy. *Fam. Proc.*, **27**, 167–79.
99. Prince-Embury, S. (1984). The family health tree: a form of identifying physical symptom patterns within the family. *J. Fam. Pract.*, **18**, 75–81.
100. McGoldrick, M., Pearce, J. K. and Giordano, J. (eds) (1982). *Ethnicity and Family Therapy.* Guildford Press.
101. Maranhao, T. (1984). Family therapy and anthropology. *Cult. Med. Psychiatry*, **8**, 255–79.
102. DiNicola, V. F. (1986). Beyond Babel: family therapy as cultural transition. *Int. J. Fam. Ther.*, **7**, 179–91.
103. Lao, A. (1984). Transcultural issues in family therapy. *J. Fam. Ther.*, **6**, 91–112.
104. Barot, R. (1988). Social anthropology, ethnicity and family therapy. *J. Fam.Ther.*, **10**, 271–82.
105. Tamura, T. and Lau, A. (1992). Connectedness versus separateness: applicability of family therapy to Japanese families. *Fam. Proc.*, **31**, 319–40.

106. Shankar, R. and Menon, M. S. (1993). Development of a framework of interventions with families in the management of schizophrenia. *Psychosoc. Rehabil. J.*, **16**, 75–91.
107. Krupinski, J. (1967). Sociological aspects of mental health in migrants. *Soc. Sci. Med.*, **1**, 267–81.
108. Cox, I. L. (1977). Aspects of transcultural psychiatry. *Br. J. Psychiatry*, **130**, 211–21.
109. Schaechter, F. (1965). Previous history of mental illness in female migrant patients admitted to the psychiatric hospital, Royal Park. *Med. J. Aust.*, **2**, 277–9.
110. Littlewood, R. and Lipsedge, M. (1989). *Aliens and Alienists*, 2nd edn, pp. 83–103. Unwin Hyman.
111. Wright, C. M. (1981). Pakistani family life in Newcastle. *J. Mat. Child Hlth.*, **6**, 427–30.
112. Gelder, M., Gath, D. and Mayou, R. (eds) (1983). *Oxford Textbook of Psychiatry*, p. 289. Oxford University Press.
113. Burke, A. W. (1984). Racism and psychological disturbance among West Indians in Britain. *Int. J. Soc. Psychiatry*, **30**, 50–68.
114. Lopez, S. and Hernandez, P. (1976). How culture is considered in evaluations of psychotherapy. *J. Nerv. Ment. Dis.*, **176**, 598–606.

Chapter 11 Cultural aspects of stress (pages 202–17)

1. Selye, H. (1936). A syndrome produced by diverse nocuous agents. *Nature*, **138**, 32.
2. Selye, H. (1976). Forty years of stress research: principal remaining problems and misconceptions. *Can. Med. Assoc. J.*, **115**, 53–7.
3. Bridges, P. K. (1982). The physiology and biochemistry of stress: some practical aspects. *Practitioner*, **226**, 1575–9.
4. Weinman, J. (1981). *An Outline of Psychology as Applied to Medicine*, pp. 60–84. Wright.
5. Young, A. (1980). The discourse on stress and the reproduction of conventional knowledge. *Soc. Sci. Med.*, **14B**, 133–46.
6. Pollock, K. (1988). On the nature of social stress: production of a modern mythology. *Soc. Sci. Med.*, **26**, 381–92.
7. McElroy, A. and Townsend, P. K. (1996). *Medical Anthropology in Ecological Perspective*, 3rd edn, pp. 252–6. Westview Press.
8. Parkes, C. M. (1971). Psycho-social transitions: a field for study. *Soc. Sci. Med.*, **5**, 101–15.
9. World Health Organization (1971). Society, stress, and disease. *WHO Chron.*, **25**, 168–78.
10. Helman, C. G. (1985). Psyche, soma, and society: the social construction of psychosomatic disorders. *Cult. Med. Psychiatry*, **9**, 1–26.
11. Tyrell, D. A. J. (1981). Respiratory infection: new agents and new concepts. *J. R. Coll. Phys. Lond.*, **15**, 113–15.
12. Baker, G. H. B. and Brewerton, D. A. (1981). Rheumatoid arthritis: a psychiatric assessment. *Br. Med. J.*, **282**, 2014.
13. Ader, R., Cohen, N. and Felten, D. (1995). Psychoneuroimmunology: interactions between the nervous system and the immune system. *Lancet*, **345**, 99–103.
14. Trimble, M. R. and Wilson-Barnet, J. (1982). Neuropsychiatric aspects of stress. *Practitioner*, **226**, 1580–86.
15. Parkes, C. M., Benjamin, B. and Fitzgerald, R. G. (1969). Broken heart: a statistical study of increased mortality among widowers. *Br. Med. J.*, **1**, 740–43.
16. Murphy, F. and Brown, G. W. (1980). Life events, psychiatric disturbance and physical illness. *Br. J. Psychiatry*, **136**, 326–38.
17. Engel, G. (1968). A life setting conducive to illness: the giving-up–given-up complex. *Ann. Intern. Med.*, **69**, 293–300.
18. Karasek, R. A., Russell, R. S. and Theorell, T. (1982). Physiology of stress and regeneration in job-related cardiovascular illness. *J. Human Stress*, **8**, 29–42.
19. Brown, G. W. and Harris, T. (1979). *Social Origins of Depression*. Tavistock.
20. Kiritz, S. and Moos, R. H. (1974). Physiological effects of social environments. *Psychosom. Med.*, **36**, 96–113.
21. Guthrie, G. M., Verstraete, A., Deines, M. M. and Stern, R. M. (1975). Symptoms of stress in four societies. *J. Soc. Psychol.*, **95**, 165–72.
22. Foster, G. M. and Anderson, B. G. (1978). *Medical Anthropology*, pp. 93–4. Wiley.
23. Hahn, R. A. and Kleinman, A. (1983). Belief as pathogen, belief as medicine: voodoo death and the 'placebo phenomenon' in anthropological perspective. *Med. Anthrop. Q.*, **14**, 3.
24. Landy, D. (ed.) (1977). *Culture, Disease and Healing: Studies in Medical Anthropology*, p. 327. Macmillan.
25. Levi-Strauss, C. (1967). *Structural Anthropology*, pp. 161–2. Anchor Books.
26. Engel, G. L. (1971). Sudden and rapid death during psychological stress: folklore or folk wisdom? *Ann. Intern. Med.*, **74**, 771–82.
27. Cannon, W. (1942). Voodoo death. *Am. Anthropologist*, **44**, 169–81.
28. Engel, G. L. (1978). Psychologic stress, vasopressor (vasovagal). syncope, and sudden death. *Ann. Intern. Med.*, **89**, 403–12.
29. Lex, B. W. (1977). Voodoo death: new thoughts on an old explanation. In: *Culture, Disease and Healing: Studies in Medical Anthropology* (D. Landy, ed.), pp. 327–31. Macmillan.
30. Hertz, R. (1960). *Death and the Right Hand*, pp. 27–86. Cohen and West.
31. Goffman, E. (1961). *Asylums*. Penguin.
32. Cassens, B. J. (1985). Social consequences of the acquired immunodeficiency syndrome. *Ann. Intern. Med.*, **103**, 768–71.

33. Waxler, N. E. (1981). The social labelling perspective on illness and medical practice. In: *The Relevance of Social Science for Medicine* (L. Eisenberg and A. Kleinman, eds), pp. 283–306. Reidel.
34. Haynes, R. B., Sackett, D. L., Taylor, D. W. *et al.* (1978). Increased absenteeism from work after detection and labelling of hypertensive patients. *N. Engl. J. Med.*, **299**, 741–4.
35. Long, J., Gillilan, R., Lee, S. G. and Kim, C. R. (1990). White-coat hypertension: detection and evaluation. *Maryland Med. J.*, **39**, 555–9.
36. Campbell, L. V., Ashwell, S. M., Borkman, M. and Chisolm, D. J. (1992). White coat hyperglycaemia: disparity between diabetes clinic and home blood glucose concentrations. *Br. Med. J.*, **305**, 1194–6.
37. Friedman, M. and Rosenman, R. H. (1959). Association of specific overt behaviour pattern with blood and cardiovascular findings. *JAMA*, **169**, 1286–96.
38. Rosenman, R. H. (1978). Role of Type A behaviour pattern in the pathogenesis of ischaemic heart disease, and modification for prevention. *Adv. Cardiol.*, **25**, 35–46.
39. Appels, A. (1972). Coronary heart disease as a cultural disease. *Psychother. Psychosom.*, **22**, 320–4.
40. Waldron, I. (1978). Type A behaviour pattern and coronary heart disease in men and women. *Soc. Sci. Med.*, **12B**, 167–70.
41. Weber, M. (1948). *The Protestant Ethic and the Spirit of Capitalism.* Allen and Unwin.
42. Helman, C. G. (1987). Heart disease and the cultural construction of time: the Type A behaviour pattern as a Western culture-bound syndrome. *Soc. Sci. Med.*, **25**, 969–79.
43. Eitinger, L. (1960). The symptomatology of mental illness among refugees in Norway. *J. Mental Sci.*, **106**, 947–66.
44. Eisenbruch, M. (1988). The mental health of refugee children and their cultural development. *Int. Migration Rev.*, **22**, 282–300.
45. Dressler, W. W. (1985). Psychosomatic symptoms, stress, and modernization: a model. *Cult. Med. Psychiatry*, **9**, 257–86.
46. Cassell, J. (1975). Studies of hypertension in migrants. In: *Epidemiology and Control of Hypertension* (O. Paul, ed.), pp. 41–61. Stratton.
47. Carpenter, L. and Brockington, I. F. (1980). A study of mental illness in Asians, West Indians and Africans living in Manchester. *Br. J. Psychiatry*, **137**, 201–5.
48. Hitch, P. J. and Rack, P. H. (1980). Mental illness among Polish and Russian refugees in Bradford. *Br. J. Psychiatry*, **137**, 206–11.
49. Burke, A. W. (1976). Attempted suicide among the Irish-born population in Birmingham. *Br. J. Psychiatry*, **128**, 534–7.
50. Burke, A. W. (1976). Attempted suicide among Asian immigrants in Birmingham. *Br. J. Psychiatry*, **128**, 528–33.
51. Burke, A. W. (1976). Socio-cultural determinants of attempted suicide among West Indians in Birmingham: ethnic origin and immigrant status. *Br. J. Psychiatry*, **129**, 261–6.
52. Raleigh, V. S. and Balarajan, S. (1992). Suicide levels and trends among immigrants in England and Wales. *Health Trends*, **24**, 91–4.
53. Desjarlais, R., Eisenberg, L., Good, B. and Kleinman, A. (1995). *World Mental Health*, pp. 47–50, 116–35. Oxford University Press.
54. Swartz, L. (1998). *Culture and Mental Health: A Southern Africa View*, pp. 167–88. Oxford University Press.
55. McCally, M. (1993). Human health and population growth. In: *Critical Condition: Human Health and the Environment* (E. Chivian, M. McCally, H. Hu and A. Haines, eds), p. 182. Massachusetts Institute of Technology Press.
56. Desjarlais, R., Eisenberg, L., Good, B., and Kleinman, A. (1995). *World Mental Health*, pp. 136–154. Oxford University Press.
57. Woloshynowych, M., Valori, R. and Salmon, P. (1998). General practice patients' beliefs about their symptoms. *Br. J. Gen. Pract.*, **48**, 885–89.
58. Osler, W. (1897). *Lectures on Angina Pectoris and Allied States.* Appleton.
59. Levin, J. S. and Coreil, J. (1986). 'New Age' healing in the US. *Soc. Sci. Med.*, **23**, 889–97.
60. McGuire, M. B. (1988). *Ritual Healing in Suburban America*, p. 105. Rutgers University Press.
61. Finkler. K. (1991). *Physicians at Work, People in Pain*, pp. 38–40. Westview Press.
62. Low, S. M. (1981). The meaning of *nervios:* a sociocultural analysis of symptom presentation in San Jose, Costa Rica. *Cult. Med. Psychiatry*, **5**, 25–47.
63. Dunk, P. (1989). Greek women and broken nerves in Montreal. *Med. Anthropol.*, **11**, 29–45.

Chapter 12 Cultural factors in epidemiology (pages 218–29)

1. Hahn, R. A. (1995). *Sickness and Healing: An Anthropological Perspective*, pp. 99–128. Yale University Press.
2. Kendell, R. E. (1975). *The Role of Diagnosis in Psychiatry*, p. 64. Blackwell.
3. Murphy, E. and Brown, G. W. (1980). Life events, psychiatric disturbance and physical illness. *Br. J. Psychiatry*, **136**, 326–38.
4. Townsend, P. and Davidson, N. (eds) (1982). *Inequalities of Health: The Black Report.* Penguin.
5. Zaidi, S. A. (1988). Poverty and disease: need for a structural change. *Soc. Sci. Med.*, **27**, 119–27.
6. Gadjusek, D. C. (1963). Kuru. *Trans. R. Soc. Trop. Med. Hyg.*, **57**, 151–69.

7. Marmot, M. (1981). Culture and illness: epidemiological evidence. In: *Foundations of Psychosomatics* (M. J. Christie and P. G. Mellett, eds), pp. 323–40. Wiley.
8. Kark, S. (1981). *The Practice of Community-Oriented Primary Care.* Appleton-Century-Crofts.
9. Marmot, M. G., Syme, S. L., Kagan, A. *et al.* (1975). Epidemiological studies of coronary heart disease and stroke in Japanese men living in Japan, Hawaii and California: prevalence of coronary and hypertensive heart disease and associated risk factors. *Am. J. Epidemiol.*, **102**, 514–25.
10. Marmot, M. G. and Syme, S. L. (1976). Acculturation and coronary heart disease in Japanese Americans. *Am. J. Epidemiol.*, **104**, 225–47.
11. Fletcher, C. M., Jones, N. L., Burrows, B. and Niden, A. H. (1964). American emphysema and British bronchitis: a standardised comparative study. *Am. Rev. Resp. Dis.*, **90**, 1–13.
12. Van Os, J., Galdos, P., Lewis, G. *et al.* (1993). Schizophrenia sans frontieres: concepts of schizophrenia among French and British psychiatrists. *Br. Med. J.*, **307**, 489–92.
13. O'Brien, B. (1984). *Patterns of European Diagnoses and Prescribing.* Office of Health Economics.
14. Zola, I. K. (1966). Culture and symptoms: an analysis of patients' presenting complaints. *Am. Sociol. Rev.*, **31**, 615–30.
15. Fox, R. (1968). Illness. In: *International Encyclopaedia of the Social Sciences* (D. Sills, ed.), pp. 90–96. Free Press/Macmillan.
16. Rubel, A. J. (1977). The epidemiology of a folk illness: *Susto* in Hispanic America. In: *Culture, Disease and Healing: Studies in Medical Anthropology* (D. Landy, ed.), pp. 119–28. Macmillan.
17. Wagley, C. (1969). Cultural influences on population: a comparison of two Tupi tribes. In: *Environment and Cultural Behavior*, pp. 268–79. Natural History Press.
18. MacCormack, C. P. (1982). Biological, cultural and social adaptation in human fertility and birth: a synthesis. In: *Ethnography of Fertility and Birth* (C. P. MacCormack, ed.), pp. 1–23. Academic Press.
19. Korbin, J. (1980). The cultural context of child abuse and neglect. *Child Abuse and Neglect*, **4**, 3–13.
20. Underwood, P. and Underwood, Z. (1981). New spells for old: expectations and realities of Western medicine in a remote tribal society in Yemen, Arabia. In: *Changing Disease Patterns and Human Behaviour* (N. F. Stanley and R. A. Joshe, eds), pp. 271–97. Academic Press.
21. Qureshi, S. M. (1980). Health problems of Asian immigrants. *Medicos*, **5**, 19–21.
22. Zheng, W., Blot, W. J., Shu, X. O. *et al.* (1992). Diet and other risk factors for laryngeal cancer in Shanghai, China. *Am. J. Epidemiol.*, **136**, 178–91.
23. Peckham, M., Pinedo, H. and Veronesi, U. (eds) (1995). *Oxford Textbook of Oncology*, Vol. 2, pp. 1325–7. Oxford University Press.
24. Skegg, D. C. G., Corwin, P. A., Paul, C. and Doll, R. (1982). Importance of the male factor in cancer of the cervix. *Lancet*, **2**, 581–3.
25. Brabin, L. and Brabin, B. J. (1985). Cultural factors and transmission of hepatitis B virus. *Am. J. Epidemiol.*, **122**, 725–30.
26. Alland, A. (1969). Ecology and adaptation to parasitic diseases. In: *Environment and Cultural Behavior* (A. P. Vayda, ed.), pp. 80–89. Natural History Press.
27. Parker, R. (1987). Acquired immunodeficiency syndrome in urban Brazil. *Med. Anthropol. Q.* (new series), **1**, 155–75.
28. Vayda, E., Mindell, W. R. and Rutkow, I. M. (1982). A decade of surgery in Canada, England and Wales, and the United States. *Arch. Surg.*, **117**, 846–53.

Chapter 13 Medical anthropology and global health (pages 230–64)

1. Mars, G. (1975). A social anthropological approach to health problems in developing countries. In: *Health and Industrial Growth*, pp. 219–35. Ciba Foundation Symposium 32 (new series). Elsevier.
2. World Health Organization. (1995). *The World Health Report 1995 – Bridging the Gaps*. WHO.
3. Smith, R. and Leaning, J. (1993). Medicine and global survival. *Br. Med. J.*, **307**, 693–4.
4. McCally, M. (1993). Human health and population growth. In: *Critical Condition* (E. Chivian, M. McCally, H. Ho and A. Haines, eds), pp. 171–91. Massachusetts Institute of Technology Press.
5. Warwick, D. P. (1988). Culture and the management of family planning programs. *Stud. Fam. Plan.*, **19**, 1–18.
6. Snow, L. F. and Johnson, S. M. (1977). Modern day menstrual folklore. *JAMA*, **237**, 2736–9.
7. Good, B. (1977). The heart of what's the matter: the semantics of illness in Iran. *Cult. Med. Psychiatry*, **1**, 25–58.
8. Scott, C. S. (1975). The relationship between beliefs about the menstrual cycle and choice of fertility regulating methods within five ethnic groups. *Int. J. Gynaecol. Obstet.*, **13**, 105–9.
9. MacCormack, C. P. (1985). Lay concepts affecting utilisation of family planning services in Jamaica. *J. Trop. Med. Hyg.*, **88**, 281–5.
10. Snow, L. F. (1993). *Walkin' over Medicine*, pp. 145–69. Westview Press.
11. Sobo, E. and Russell, A. (1997). Editorial: contraception today: ethnographic lessons. *Anthropol. Med.*, **4(2)**, 125–30.

12. Dyson, T. and Moore, M. (1983). On kinship structure, female autonomy, and demographic behavior in India. *Population Dev. Rev.*, **9**, 35–60.
13. Renne, E. P. (1997). The meaning of contraceptive choice and constraint for Hausa women in a north Nigerian town. *Anthropol. Med.*, **4(2)**, 159–175.
14. Harpham, T., Lusty, T. and Vaughan, P. (eds) (1988). *In the Shadow of the City: Community Health and the Urban Poor*, pp. 1–23. Oxford University Press.
15. Harpham, T., Lusty, T. and Vaughan, P. (eds) (1988). *In the Shadow of the City: Community Health and the Urban Poor*, pp. 40–88. Oxford University Press.
16. Kendall, C., Hudelson, P., Leontsini, E. *et al.* (1991). Urbanization, dengue, and the health transition: anthropological contributions to international health. *Med. Anthropol. Q.* (new series), **5**, 257–68.
17. Kark, S. (1981). *The Practice of Primary Health Care.* Appleton-Century-Crofts.
18. Mann, J. M., Tarantola, D. J. M. and Netter, T. W. (eds) (1992). *AIDS in the World.* Harvard University Press.
19. Sontag, S. (1988). *AIDS and its Metaphors.* Penguin.
20. Frankenberg, R. (1990). Disease, literature and the body in the era of AIDS – a preliminary exploration. *Soc. Hlth. Illness*, **12**, 351–60.
21. Clatts, M. C. and Mutchler, K. M. (1989). AIDS and the dangerous other: metaphors of sex and deviance in the representation of disease. In: *The AIDS Pandemic: A Global Emergency* (R. Bolton, ed.), pp. 13–22. Gordon and Breach.
22. Miller, D., Green, J., Farmer, R. and Carroll, G. (1985). A 'pseudo-AIDS' syndrome following from fear of AIDS. *Br. J. Psychiatry*, **146**, 550–1.
23. Miller, E. (1998). The uses of culture in the making of AIDS neurosis in Japan. *Psychosom. Med.*, **60**, 402–9.
24. Ingstad, B. (1990). The cultural construction of AIDS and its consequences for prevention in Botswana. *Med. Anthropol. Q.* (new series), **4**, 28–40.
25. Flaskerud, J. and Rush, C. (1989). AIDS and traditional health belief and practices of black women. *Nursing Res.*, **38**, 210–15.
26. Farmer, P. (1990). Sending sickness: sorcery, politics, and changing concepts of AIDS in rural Haiti. *Med. Anthropol. Q.* (new series), **4**, 27.
27. Smithson, R. D. (1988). Public health staff knowledge about AIDS. *Comm. Med.*, **10**, 221–7.
28. Temoshok, L., Sweet, D. M. and Zich, J. (1987). A three city comparison of the public's knowledge and attitudes about AIDS. *Psychol. Hlth.*, **1**, 43–60.
29. Snow, L. F. (1993). *Walkin' over Medicine*, pp. 213–15. Westview Press.
30. Webb, D. (1993). Community responses to HIV/AIDS in Owambo, Namibia. Paper presented at the VIIIth International Conference on AIDS in Africa. Marrakech, December.
31. De Souza, R. P., De Almeida, A. B., Wagner, M. B. *et al.* (1993). A study of the sexual behaviour of teenagers in south Brazil. *J. Adolescent Hlth.*, **14**, 336–9.
32. Lyttleton, C. (1994). Knowledge and meaning: the AIDS education campaign in rural northeast Thailand. *Soc. Sci. Med.*, **38**, 135–46.
33. Katz, I., Hass, G., Parisi, N. *et al.* (1987). Lay people's and health care personnel's perceptions of cancer, AIDS, cardiac and diabetic patients. *Psychological. Rep.*, **60**, 615–29.
34. Stanley, L. D. (1999). Transforming AIDS: the moral management of stigmatized identity. *Anthropol. Med.*, **6(1)**, 103–20.
35. Parker, M., Ward, H. and Day, S. (1998). Sexual networks and the transmission of HIV in London. *J. Biosoc. Sci.*, **30**, 63–83.
36. Neaigus, A., Friedman, S. R., Curtis, R. *et al.* (1994). The relevance of drug injectors' social and risk networks for understanding and preventing HIV infection. *Soc. Sci. Med.*, **38**, 67–78.
37. Thomas, P. A., Weisfus, I. B., Greenberg, A. E. *et al.* and the New York City Dept of Health AIDS Surveillance Team (1993). Trends in the first ten years of AIDS in New York City. *Am. J. Epidemiol.*, **137**, 121–33.
38. Parker, R. (1987). Acquired immunodeficiency syndrome in urban Brazil. *Med. Anthropol. Q.* (new series), **1**, 155–75.
39. Skegg, D. C. G., Corwin, P. A., Paul, C. and Doll, R. (1982). Importance of the male factor in cancer of the cervix. *Lancet*, **2**, 581–3.
40. Carrier, J. M. (1989). Sexual behavior and the spread of AIDS in Mexico. In: *The AIDS Pandemic: A Global Emergency* (R. Bolton, ed.), pp. 37–50. Gordon and Breach.
41. Whitehead, T. L. (1997). Urban low-income African-American men, HIV/AIDS, and gender identity. *Med. Anthropol. Q.* (new series), **11(4)**, 411–47.
42. Schoepf, B. G. (1995). Culture, sex research and AIDS prevention in Africa. In: *Culture and Sexual Risk: Anthropological Perspectives on AIDS* (H. ten Brummelhuis and G. Herdt, eds), pp.29–51. Gordon and Breach.
43. Obbo, C. (1995). Gender, age and class: discourses on HIV transmission and control in Uganda. In: *Culture and Sexual Risk: Anthropological Perspectives on AIDS* (H. ten Brummelhuis and G. Herdt, eds), pp. 79–95. Gordon and Breach.
44. Preston-Whyte, E. M. (1995). Half-way there: anthropology and intervention-oriented AIDS research in Kwazulu/Natal, South Africa. In: *Culture and Sexual Risk: Anthropological Perspectives on AIDS* (H. ten Brummelhuis and G. Herdt, eds), pp. 315–37. Gordon and Breach.
45. Waddell, C. (1996). HIV and the social world of female sex workers in Perth, Australia. *Med. Anthropol. Q.* (new series), **10**, 75–82.

46. Leonard, T. L. (1990). Male clients of female street prostitutes: unseen partners in sexual disease transmission. *Med. Anthropol. Q.* (new series), **4**, 41–55.
47. Pickering, H. and Wilkins, A. (1993). Do unmarried women in African towns have to sell sex: or is it a matter of choice? In: *Health Transition Review. Sexual Networking and HIV/AIDS in West Africa* (J. C. Caldwell, G. Santowm, I. O. Oruboloyc *et al.*, eds), 3(Suppl.), 17–27.
48. Carael, M., van der Perre, P., Clumeck, N. and Butzler, J. P. (1987). Urban sexuality changing pattern in Rwanda: Social determinants and relations with HIV infection. International Symposium on African AIDS, Brussels, 22–23 November.
49. Page, B., Chitwood, D. D., Prince, P. C. *et al.* (1990). Intravenous drug use and HIV infection in Miami. *Med. Anthropol. Q.* (new series), **4**, 56–71.
50. Gamella, J. F. (1994). The spread of intravenous drug use and AIDS in a neighborhood in Spain. *Med. Anthrop. Q.* (new series), **8(2)**, 131–160.
51. Newmeyer, J. A., Feldman, H. W., Biernacki, P. and Watters, J. K. (1989). Preventing AIDS contagion among intravenous drug users. In: *The AIDS Pandemic: A Global Emergency* (R. Bolton, ed.), pp. 75–83. Gordon and Breach.
52. Sibthorpe, B. (1992). The social construction of sexual relationships as a determinant of HIV risk perception and condom use among injection drug users. *Med. Anthropol. Q.* (new series), **4**, 255–70.
53. Eisenberg, D., Kessler, R. C., Foster, C. *et al.* (1993). Unconventional medicine in the United States. *N. Engl. J. Med.*, **328**, 246–52.
54. Furin, J. J. (1997). 'You have to be your own doctor': sociocultural influences on alternative therapy use among gay men with AIDS in West Hollywood. *Med. Anthropol. Q.* (new series), **11(4)**, 498–504.
55. O'Connor, B. B. (1995). *Healing Traditions*, pp. 109–60. University of Pennsylvania Press.
56. Ember, C. R. and Ember, M. (1985). *Cultural Anthropology*, pp. 158–78. Prentice Hall.
57. Daly, J. and Horton, M. (1993). Take prevention to the people. *AIDS Action*, **21**, 2–3.
58. Lang, N. G. (1989). AIDS, gays and the ballot box: the politics of disease in Houston, Texas. In: *The AIDS Pandemic: A Global Emergency* (R. Bolton, ed.), pp. 111–17. Gordon and Breach.
59. Tauer, C. A. (1989). AIDS: human rights and public health. In: *The AIDS Pandemic: A Global Emergency* (R. Bolton, ed.), pp. 85–100. Gordon and Breach.
60. Fitzpatrick, R., Dawson, J., Boulton, M. *et al.* (1994). Perceptions of general practice among homosexual men. *Br. J. Gen. Pract.*, **44**, 80–82.
61. World Health Organization (1979). *Formulating Strategies for Health for All by the Year 2000: Guiding Principles and Essential Issues.* WHO.
62. Mull, J. D. (1990). The primary care dialectic: history, rhetoric and reality. In: *Anthropology and Primary Health Care* (J. Coreil and J. D. Mull, eds), pp. 28–47. Westview Press.
63. Rubinstein, R. A. and Lane, S. D. (1990). International health and development. In: *Medical Anthropology* (T. M. Johnson and C. F. Sargent, eds), pp. 367–90. Praeger.
64. Pillsbury, B. L. K. (1991). International health: overview and opportunities. In: *Training Manual in Applied Medical Anthropology* (C. E. Hill, ed.), pp. 54–87. American Anthropological Association.
65. Green, E. C. (1986). Diarrhea and the social marketing of oral rehydration salts in Bangladesh. *Soc. Sci. Med.*, **23**, 357–66.
66. Heggenhougen, H. K. and Clements, C. I. (1990). An anthropological perspective on the acceptability of immunization services. *Scand. J. Infect Dis. Suppl.*, **76**, 20–31.
67. Nichter, M. (1992). Of ticks, kings, spirits, and the promise of vaccines. In: *Paths to Asian Medical Knowledge* (C. Leslie and A. Young, eds), pp. 224–56. University of California Press.
68. Nichter, M. and Nichter, M. (1996). *Anthropology and International Health: Asian Case Studies*, pp. 329–65. Gordon and Breach.
69. Agency for International Development (1983). *Proceedings of the International Conference on Oral Rehydration Therapy (ICORT)*, 7–10 June 1983. Agency for International Development.
70. Weiss, M. G. (1988). Cultural models of diarrheal illness: conceptual framework and review. *Soc. Sci. Med.*, **27**, 5–16.
71. Nichter, M. (1991). Use of social science research to improve epidemiologic studies of and interventions for diarrhea and dysentery. *Rev. Inf. Dis.*, **13**(Suppl. 4), S265–71.
72. Coreil, J. (1988). Innovation among Haitian healers: the adoption of oral rehydration therapy. *Hum. Organization*, **47**, 48–57.
73. Nichter, M. (1993). Social science lessons from diarrhea research and their application to ARI. *Hum. Organization*, **52**, 53–67.
74. World Health Organization (1993). *Focused Ethnographic Study of Acute Respiratory Infections.* World Health Organization, Programme for Control of Acute Respiratory Infections.
75. Kochi, A. (1991). The global tuberculosis situation and the new control strategy of the World Health Organization. *Tubercle*, **72**, 1–6.
76. World Health Organization (1995). The World Health Report 1995 – Bridging the gaps. *World Health Forum*, **16**, 377–85.
77. De Cock, K. M. and Dworkin, M. S. (1998). HIV infection and TB. *World Health*, **6**, 14–15.
78. Rubel, A. J. and Garro, L. C. (1992). Social and cultural factors in the successful control of tuberculosis. *Public Hlth. Rep.*, **107**, 626–36.

79. Vecchiato, N. L. (1997). Sociocultural aspects of tuberculosis control in Ethiopia. *Med. Anthropol. Q.* (new series), **11(2)**, 183–201.
80. Walt, G. (ed.) (1990). *Community Health Workers in National Programmes*. Open University Press.
81. Storey, P. B. (1972). *The Soviet Feldscher as a Physician's Assistant*. DHEW Pub. No. (NIH) 72-58. United States Department of Health, Education, and Welfare.
82. Heggenhougen, H. K. and Magari, F. M. (1992). Community health workers in Tanzania. In: *The Community Health Worker: Effective Programmes for Developing Countries* (S. Frankel, ed.), pp. 156–77. Oxford University Press.
83. World Health Organization (1992). *The Use of Essential Drugs*, pp. 9–10. WHO Technical Report Series 825.
84. Donahue, J. M. (1990). The role of anthropologists in primary health care: reconciling professional and community interests. In: *Anthropology and Primary Health Care* (J. Coreil and J. D. Mull, eds), pp. 79–97. Westview Press.
85. Zaidi, S. A. (1988). Poverty and disease: need for structural change. *Soc. Sci. Med.*, **27**, 119–27.
86. World Bank (1993). *World Development Report 1993*, p. 137. Oxford University Press.
87. Nichter, M. and Cartwright, E. (1991). Saving the children for the tobacco industry. *Med. Anthropol. Q.*, **5**, 236–56.
88. Browne, M. W. (1993). Land mines called a world menace. *New York Times*, 15 November.
89. Foster, G. M. (1982). Applied anthropology and international health: retrospect and prospect. *Hum. Organization*, **41**, 189–97.
90. Coreil, J. (1990). The evolution of anthropology in international health. In: *Anthropology and Primary Health Care* (J. Coreil and J. D. Mull, eds), pp. 3–27. Westview Press.
91. Foster, G. M. (1987). World Health Organization behavioral science research: problems and prospects. *Soc. Sci. Med.*, **24**, 709–17.
92. Trigg, P. and Kondrachine, A. (1998). The Global Malaria Control Strategy. *World Health*, **3**, 4–5.
93. Liese, B. H. (1998). A brake on economic development. *World Health*, **3**, 16–17.
94. Van der Vynckt, S. and Reuganathan, E. (1998). Mobilizing the teachers. *World Health*, **3**, 18–19.
95. Tenner, E. (1997). *Why Things Bite Back*, pp. 106–110. Fourth Estate.
96. Muela, S. H., Ribera, J. M. and Tanner, M. (1998). Fake malaria and hidden parasites – the ambiguity of malaria. *Anthropol. Med.*, **5(1)**, 43–61.
97. Winch, P. J., Makemba, A. M., Kamazima, S. R. *et al.* (1996). Local terminology for febrile illnesses in Bagamoyo district, Tanzania, and its impact on the design of a community-based malaria control programme. *Soc. Sci. Med.*, **42**, 1057–67.
98. Lobo, L. and Kazi, B. (1997). *Ethnography of malaria in Surat*. Surat, Gujurat, India: Centre for Social Studies.
99. Agyepong, I. A (1992). Malaria: ethnomedical perceptions and practice in an Adangbe farming community and implications for control. *Soc. Sci. Med.*, **35**, 131–7.
100. Mwenesi, H., Harpham, T. and Snow, R. W. (1995). Child malaria practices among mothers in Kenya. *Soc. Sci. Med.*, **49**, 1271–7.
101. Baer, H.A., Singer, M., and Susser, I. (1997). *Medical Anthropology and the World System*, pp. 53–5. Bergin and Garvey.
102. Bledsoe, C. H. and Goubaud, M. F. (1988). The reinterpretation and distribution of Western pharmaceuticals: an example from Sierra Leone. In: *The Context of Medicines in Developing Countries* (S. van der Geest and S. R. Whyte, eds.), pp. 253–76. Kluwer.
103. Targett, G. A. T. and Greenwood, B. M. (1998). Impregnated bed nets. *World Health*, **3**, 10–11.
104. Meek, S. and Rowland, M. (1998). Malaria in emergency situations. *World Health*, **3**, 22–3.
105. Slim, H. and Mitchell, J. (1992). The application of RAP and RRA techniques in emergency relief programmes. In: *Rapid Assessment Procedures* (N. S. Scrimshaw and G. R. Gleason, eds), pp. 251–7. International Nutrition Foundation for Developing Countries (INFDC).
106. Piddington, R. (1957). Malinowski's theory of needs. In: *Man and Culture* (R. Firth, ed.), pp. 33–51. Routledge and Kegan Paul.
107. Christiani, D. C. (1993). Urban and transboundary air pollution: human health consequences. In: *Critical Condition: Human Health and the Environment* (E. Chivian, M. McCally, H. Ho and A. Haines, eds), pp. 13–30. Massachusetts Institute of Technology Press.
108. Baer, H. A., Singer, M. and Susser, I. (1997). *Medical Anthropology and the World System*, pp. 55–7. Bergin and Garvey.
109. Bowen, E. L. and Hu, H. (1993). Food contamination due to environmental pollution. In: *Critical Condition: Human Health and the Environment* (E. Chivian, M. McCally, H. Ho and A. Haines, eds), pp. 49–69. Massachusetts Institute of Technology Press.
110. Miller, D. (1994). *Modernity – An Ethnographic Approach*, pp. 236–45. Berg.
111. Chivian, E. (1993). Species extinction and biodiversity loss: the implication for human health. In: *Critical Condition: Human Health and the Environment* (E. Chivian, M. McCally, H. Ho and A. Haines, eds), pp. 193–224. Massachusetts Institute of Technology Press.
112. Keesing, R. M. (1981). *Cultural Anthropology*, pp. 493–7. Holt, Rinehart & Winston.
113. Etkin, N. L. (1988). Cultural constructions of efficacy. In: *The Context of Medicines in Developing Countries* (S. Van der Geest and S. R. Whyte, eds), pp. 299–326. Kluwer.
114. Nichter, N. (1987). Kyasanur Forest Disease: an

ethnography of a disease of development. *Med. Anthropol. Q.* (new series), **1**, 406–23.

115. Cortese, A. D. (1993). Introduction: human health, risk, and the environment. In: *Critical Condition: Human Health and the Environment* (E. Chivian, M. McCally, H. Ho and A. Haines, eds), pp. 1–11. Massachusetts Institute of Technology Press.

Chapter 14 New research methods in medical anthropology (pages 265–71)

1. Helman, C. G. (1991) Research in primary care: the qualitative approach. In: *Primary Care Research* (P. G. Norton, M. Stewart, F. Tudiver *et al.*, eds), pp. 105–1124. Sage Publications.
2. Hudelson, P. M. (1994). *Qualitative Research for Health Programmes.* Division of Mental Health, World Health Organization.
3. Keesing, R. M. (1981) *Cultural Anthropology: A Contemporary Perspective*, pp. 1–8. Holt, Rinehart & Winston.
4. Anderson, R. (1996). *Magic, Science and Health*, p. 120. Harcourt Brace.
5. Helman, C. G. (1991). Limits of biomedical explanation. *Lancet*, **337**, 1080–83.
6. Helman, C. G. (1996). The application of anthropological methods in general practice research. *Fam. Pract.*, **13**(Suppl. 1), S13–S16.
7. Hall, E. T. (1984). *The Dance of Life*, pp. 230–31. Anchor Press.
8. Scrimshaw, N. S. and Gleason, G. R. (eds) (1992). *Rapid Assessment Procedures.* International Nutrition Foundation for Developing Countries (INFDC).
9. Scrimshaw, S. and Hurtado, E. (1987). *Rapid Assessment Procedures for Nutrition and Primary Health Care: Anthropology Approaches for Improving Programme Effectiveness.* University of California Latin American Center, and United Nations University.
10. Pelto, G. H. and Grove, S. (1992). Developing a focused ethnographic study for WHO acute respiratory infection (ARI) control programme. In: *Rapid Assessment Procedures*, pp. 215–25. International Nutrition Foundation for Developing Countries (INFDC).
11. Smith, G. S. (1989). Development of rapid epidemiological assessment methods to evaluate health status and delivery of health services. *Int. J. Epidemiol.*, **18(2)**, S2–14.
12. Chambers, R. (1981). Rapid rural appraisal. *Publ. Admin. Dev.*, **1**, 95–106.
13. Eisenbruch, M. (1990). The cultural bereavement interview: a new clinical research approach to refugees. *Psychiatr. Clin. North Am.*, **13**, 715–35.
14. Griffiths, M. (1992). Understanding infant feeding practices: qualitative research methodologies used in the weaning project. In: *Rapid Assessment Procedures*, pp. 95–103. International Nutrition Foundation for Developing Countries (INFDC).
15. Pelletier, D. I. (1992). The role of qualitative methodologies in nutritional surveillance. In: *Rapid Assessment Procedures*, pp. 51–9. International Nutrition Foundation for Developing Countries (INFDC).
16. Bentley, M.E., Gittelson, J.G., Nag, M. *et al.* (1992). Use of qualitative methodologies for women's reproductive health data in India. In: *Rapid Assessment Procedures*, pp. 241–50. International Nutrition Foundation for Developing Countries (INFDC).
17. Ramos, L. (1992). Rapid assessment procedures and the Latinas and AIDS research project. In: *Rapid Assessment Procedures*, pp. 147–66. International Nutrition Foundation for Developing Countries (INFDC).
18. Gray, R. H. (1992). Interview-based diagnosis of illness and causes of death in children. In: *Rapid Assessment Procedures*, pp. 263–78. International Nutrition Foundation for Developing Countries (INFDC).
19. Long, A., Scrimshaw, S. C. M. and Hernandez, N. (1992). Transcultural epilepsy services. In: *Rapid Assessment Procedures*, pp. 205–14. International Nutrition Foundation for Developing Countries (INFDC).
20. Rifkin, S., Annett, H. and Tabibzadeh, I. (1992). Rapid appraisal to assess community health needs: a focus on the urban poor. In: *Rapid Assessment Procedures*, pp. 357–64. International Nutrition Foundation for Developing Countries (INFDC).
21. Krueger, R. A. (1988). *Focus Groups: A Practical Guide for Applied Research.* Sage.
22. Asbury, J. E. (1995). Overview of focus group research. *Qual. Hlth. Res.*, **5(4)**, 414–20.
23. Hudelson, P. M. (1994). *Qualitative Research for Health Programmes*, pp. 15–20. Division of Mental Health, World Health Organization.
24. Blumhagen, D. (1980). Hyper-tension: a folk illness with a medical name. *Cult. Med. Psychiatry*, **4**, 197–227.
25. Good, B. (1977). The heart of what's the matter: the semantics of illness in Iran. *Cult. Med. Psychiatry*, **1**, 25–58.
26. Christie-Seely, J. (1981). Teaching the family system concept in family medicine. *J. Fam. Pract.*, **13**, 391–401.
27. Helman, C. G. (1991). The family culture: a useful concept for family practice. *Fam. Med.*, **23**, 376–81.
28. Crane, J. G. and Angrosino, M. V. (1974). *Field Projects in Anthropology: A Student Guide*, pp. 74–95. Scott, Foresman & Co.
29. Snow, L. D. (1993). *Walkin' over Medicine.* Westview.
30. Crane, J. G. and Angrosin, M. V. (1974). *Field*

Projects in Anthropology: A Student Guide, pp. 42–50. Scott, Foresman & Co.
31. Prince-Embury, S. (1984). The family health tree: a form of identifying physical symptom patterns within the family. *J. Fam. Pract.*, **18**, 75–81.
32. Scott, J. (1991). *Social Network Analysis: A Handbook*. Sage.
33. Parker, M., Ward, H. and Day, S. (1998). Sexual networks and the transmission of HIV in London. *J. Biosoc. Sci.*, **30**, 63–83.
34. Boyle, C. M. (1970). Difference between patients' and doctors' interpretation of some common medical terms. *Br. Med. J.*, **ii**, 286–9.
35. MacCormack, C. P. (1985). Lay concepts affecting utilization of family planning services in Jamaica. *J. Trop. Med. Hyg.*, **88**, 281–5.
36. Trakas, D. J. and Sanz, E. (eds) (1996). *Childhood and Medicine Use in a Cross-Cultural Perspective: A European Concerted Action*. European Commission.
37. Greenhalgh, T., Helman, C. and Chowdhury, A. M. (1998). Health beliefs and folk models of diabetes in British Bangladeshis: a qualitative study. *Br. Med. J.*, **316**, 978–83.
38. Goffman, E. (1961). *Asylums*. Penguin.
39. Katz, P. (1981). Ritual in the operating room. *Ethnology*, **20**, 335–50.
40. Barrett, R. J. (1996). *The Psychiatric Team and the Social Definition of Schizophrenia*. Cambridge University Press.
41. Kleinman, A. (1980). *Patients and Healers in the Context of Culture*. University of California Press.
42. Finkler, K. (1985). *Spiritualist Healers in Mexico*. Bergin and Garvey.
43. Simon, C. (1991). Innovative medicine – a case study of a modern healer. *S. Afr. Med. J.*, **79**, 677–8.
44. Boone, M. S. and Wood, J. J. (eds) (1992). *Computer Applications for Anthropologists*. Wadsworth.
45. Hudelson, P. M. (1994). *Qualitative Research for Health Programmes*, pp. 99–101. Division of Mental Health, World Health Organization.
46. Carey, J. W. (1993). Practical computing. *Pract. Anthropol.*, **15(3)**, 30–32.
47. Carey, J. W. (1993). Practical computing. *Pract. Anthropol.*, **16**, 34–5.
48. Keesing, R. M. (1981). *Cultural Anthropology: A Contemporary Perspective*, p. 4. Holt, Rinehart & Winston.
49. Pelto, P. J. and Pelto, G. H. (1992). Developing applied medical anthropology in Third World countries: problems and actions. *Soc. Sci. Med.*, **35**, 1389–95.
50. Mumford, D. B. (1993). Somatization: a transcultural perspective. *Int. Rev. Psychiatry*, **5**, 231–42.
51. Kuzel, A. and Like, R. C. (1991). Standards of trustworthiness for qualitative studies in primary care. In: *Primary Care Research: Traditional and Innovative Approaches* (P. G. Norton, M. Stewart, F. Tudiver *et al.*, eds), pp. 138–58. Sage Publications.
52. Pelto, P. J. and Pelto, G. H. (1997). Studying knowledge, culture and behaviour in applied medical anthropology. *Med. Anthropol. Q.* (new series), **11(2)**, 147–63.

Author index

Subject index